Occupational
Lung
Diseases

Occupational Lung Diseases

THIRD EDITION

W. Keith C. Morgan, M.D., F.R.C.P.(Ed.), F.R.C.P.(C), F.A.C.P.
Professor of Medicine
University of Western Ontario
London, Ontario, Canada

Anthony Seaton, M.D., F.R.C.P., F.R.C.P.(Ed.), F.F.O.M.
Professor of Environmental and Occupational Medicine
University of Aberdeen
Honorary Consultant Physician
Aberdeen and Edinburgh, Scotland

W.B. SAUNDERS COMPANY
A Division of Harcourt Brace & Company
Philadelphia   London   Toronto   Montreal   Sydney   Tokyo

W.B. Saunders Company
A Division of
Harcourt Brace & Company

The Curtis Center
Independence Square West
Philadelphia, Pennsylvania 19106

Library of Congress Cataloging-in-Publication Data

Morgan, W. Keith C.

Occupational lung diseases / W. Keith C. Morgan, Anthony Seaton.—3rd ed.

p. cm.

Includes bibliographical references and index.

1. Lungs—Dust diseases. 2. Lungs—Diseases. 3. Occupational diseases. I . Seaton, Anthony. II. Title. [DNLM: 1. Lung Diseases. 2. Pneumoconiosis. 3. Occupational Diseases. WF 600 M8490 1995]

RC773.M67 1995   616.2′4—dc20

ISBN 0–7216–4671–9

DNLM/DLC   94–19777

OCCUPATIONAL LUNG DISEASES   ISBN 0–7216–4671–9

Printed in the United States of America.

Last digit is the print number: 9   8   7   6   5   4   3   2   1

Dedication of the First Edition

To our wives, who have of necessity had to remain
almost completely silent for the past two years,
and who in the end came to share Carlyle's
belief that "Under all speech that is good
for anything there lies a silence that
is better."

Dedication of the Second Edition

To our wives, without whose constant
presence this book would have appeared
two years earlier.

Dedication of the Third Edition

To our wives,
whose conversation, like that of Macaulay,
is punctuated by occasional flashes of silence,
which have given us a rare opportunity to put pen to paper.

Contributors

Brian Boehlecke, M.D., M.S.P.H.
Associate Professor of Medicine,
University of North Carolina School
of Medicine, Chapel Hill,
North Carolina
Respiratory Protection

J. Bernard L. Gee, M.D., F.R.C.P.
Professor of Medicine, Yale
University School of Medicine, New
Haven, Connecticut
*Basic Mechanisms in Occupational
Lung Diseases Including Lung
Cancer and Mesothelioma;
Asbestos-Related Diseases*

Alan Robert Gibbs, M.B., B.S., F.R.C.Path.
Honorary Clinical Teacher,
University of Wales College of
Medicine, Cardiff, Wales; Consultant
Histopathologist, Llandough
Hospital Trust, Penarth, South
Glamorgan, Wales
*Pathological Reactions of the Lung
to Dust*

Brooke T. Mossman, M.S., Ph.D.
Professor of Pathology, University
of Vermont College of Medicine,
Burlington, Vermont
*Basic Mechanisms in Occupational
Lung Diseases Including Lung
Cancer and Mesothelioma*

David M. F. Murphy, M.B., Ch.B., B.A.O.,
M.R.C.P.
Associate Professor of Medicine
(Adjunct Faculty), Hospital of the
University of Pennsylvania,
Philadelphia, Pennsylvania; Chief,
Pulmonary Medicine Department,
Deborah Heart and Lung Center,
Browns Mills, New Jersey
Hypersensitivity Pneumonitis

Robert B. Reger, Ph.D.
Research Professor, Health Sciences,
Alderson-Broaddus College,
Philippi, West Virginia
Occupational Lung Cancer

John A. S. Ross, M.B., Ch.B., Ph.D., F.F.A.R.C.S.
Senior Lecturer, University of
Aberdeen, Aberdeen, Scotland;
Honorary Consultant, Head of
Service for Hyperbaric Medicine,
Aberdeen Royal Hospitals, Aberdeen
Scotland
Toxic Gases and Fumes

Douglas Seaton, M.D., F.R.C.P.
Consultant Physician, Department of
Respiratory Medicine, Ipswich
Hospital, Ipswich, England
*Pulmonary Physiology—Its
Application to the Determination of
Respiratory Impairment and
Disability in Industrial Lung Disease*

James H. Vincent, Ph.D., D.Sc.
Professor of Industrial Hygiene,
Division of Environmental and
Occupational Health, School of
Public Health, University of
Minnesota, Minneapolis, Minnesota
*The Measurement of Workplace
Aerosols*

Stephen J. Watt, B.Sc., M.B., B.S., A.F.O.M.,
F.R.C.P.E.
Senior Lecturer, Department of
Environmental and Occupational
Medicine, University of Aberdeen,
Aberdeen, Scotland; Honorary
Consultant, Aberdeen Royal
Hospital Trust, Aberdeen, Scotland
*Barotrauma and Hazards of High
Pressure*

Preface to the Third Edition

Since the second edition appeared, further interest in occupational lung disease has been generated among the medical profession, those employed in ancillary health services, and lawyers. Many new regulations in the United States, the European Economic Community, Canada, and elsewhere have been introduced for the control of occupationally related lung disease. These have been prompted to some extent by advances in knowledge and better understanding of those conditions which arise from workplace exposures. The third edition has been extensively rewritten, and various new chapters have been added including ones on prevention, barotrauma, and the measurement of aerosols. It is hoped that the new edition will provide a useful and practical reference not only for physicians, but also for industrial hygienists, those concerned with the prevention of disease, and the legal profession.

We are very much indebted to our colleagues who contributed to the text. These include Drs. Brian Boehlecke, Bernard Gee, Alan Gibbs, Brooke Mossman, David Murphy, Robert Reger, John Ross, Douglas Seaton, James Vincent, and Stephen Watt. We would also like to acknowledge the data made available to us relating to the U.S. Federal Black Lung Program. These originated from Mr. Hervey P. Levin. We also acknowledge our many other friends who provided helpful advice. Both of us would like to acknowledge those who have helped with the typing of the text. These include Mrs. Lesley Alexander, Ms. Karen Allen, Mrs. Betty Crolla, and Ms. Kathryn Gillespie. We also thank Drs. Bertha Garcia and Linda Hutton for provision of photomicrographs and radiographs, and Aberdeen University Department of Medical Illustration for photographing many of the figures.

Once again we would like to thank the staff of W.B. Saunders Company, who have been endlessly patient despite the unduly long gestation periods of certain of the chapters. They have been most helpful in the preparation of the manuscript for publication. We hope our readers will find our text helpful, although we realize some defects will be present. As such, we accept the responsibility for them.

W. KEITH C. MORGAN
ANTHONY SEATON

Glossary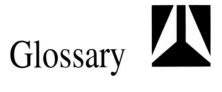

PROPER NAMES

5-HT	5-hydroxytryptamine (serotonin)
AM	Alveolar macrophage
ARDS	Adult respiratory distress syndrome
ATP	Adenosine triphosphate
ATS	American Thoracic Society
BAL	Bronchoalveolar lavage
CWP	Coal workers' pneumoconiosis
DIP	Desquamative interstitial pneumonia
EAA	Exercise allergic alveolitis
GSD	Geometric standard deviation
HDI	Hexamethylene diisocyanate
IgA, IgE, IgG, IgM	Immunoglobulins A, E, G, and M
IL	Interleukin
ILO	International Labor Office
IPF	Idiopathic pulmonary fibrosis
MDI	Diphenylmethane diisocyanate
MMD	Mass median diameter of a particle
MRC	Medical Research Council of Great Britain
NIOSH	National Institute of Occupational Safety and Health
PMF	Progressive massive fibrosis
PMN	Polymorphonuclear leukocyte
SMR	Standard mortality ratio
SRS-A	Slow-reacting substance of anaphylaxis
TDI	Toluene diisocyanate
TMA	Trimellitic anhydride
UICC	Union Internationale Contre le Cancer

PHYSIOLOGICAL MEASUREMENTS

$(A\text{-}a)O_2$	Alveoloarterial oxygen gradient
$(A\text{-}a)CO_2$	Alveoloarterial carbon dioxide gradient
$(a\text{-}v)O_2$	Arteriovenous oxygen difference
ATPS	Ambient temperature and pressure, saturated with water vapor
BTPS	Body temperature and pressure, saturated with water vapor
Cdyn	Dynamic compliance
Cstat	Static compliance
CV	Closing volume
D_L	Diffusing capacity
$D_{L_{CO}}$ or D_LCO	Diffusing capacity for carbon monoxide
D_M	Membrane diffusion coefficient
ERV	Expiratory reserve volume
f	Frequency

$FE(O_2, CO_2,$ etc.)	Fractional concentration of expired gas
$FEF_{25}(\dot{V}max_{25})$	Forced expiratory flow rate at 25 per cent
$FEF_{50}, FEF_{75}, FEF_{90}$	Forced expiratory flow rates at 50, 75, and 90 per cent of forced vital capacity
FEF_{25-75} (MMF)	Forced expiratory flow rate between 25 and 75 per cent of forced vital capacity
$FEV_{0.75}$	Forced expiratory volume exhaled in 0.75 second
FEV_1	Forced expiratory volume exhaled in one second
FEV_3	Forced expiratory volume exhaled in three seconds
FEVM	Forced expiratory volume maneuver
$FI(CO_2, O_2,$ etc.)	Fractional concentration of inspired gas
FRC	Functional residual capacity
FVC	Forced vital capacity
IC	Inspiratory capacity
MEFVC	Maximal expiratory flow volume curve
METS	Multiple of resting metabolic state (if resting O_2 consumption is 250 ml, an O_2 consumption of 1 L is 4 METS)
MV	Minute volume
P	Pressure
Pa_{O_2}, Pa_{CO_2}	Alveolar partial pressure for oxygen, carbon dioxide, etc.
Pa_{O_2}, Pa_{CO_2}	Arterial partial pressure for oxygen, carbon dioxide, etc.
PF or PEF	Peak expiratory flow
Pst	Elastic recoil
Q	Flow in unit time (blood)
Raw	Airways resistance
RQ	Respiratory quotient
TLC	Total lung capacity
μ	Micron
V	Volume flow of gas per unit of time
$\dot{V}A/\dot{Q}$ $(\dot{V}/\dot{Q})$	Ratio between ventilation and perfusion, with each expressed in the same units
V_C	Pulmonary capillary blood volume
V_{D_A}	Anatomical dead space
V_{D_P}	Physiological dead space
V_D/V_T	Ratio of dead space to tidal volume
V_E	Pulmonary ventilation
V_{O_2} (max)	Maximal oxygen uptake
V_T	Tidal volume
Viso $\dot{V}$ (PIF)	Point of identical flow on MEFV curve

Preface to the Second Edition

Since the first edition, there has been increasing interest in occupational lung disease, both within the profession and indeed among laymen. Moreover, many new advances in understanding have occurred. These two facts are our justification for producing an almost entirely rewritten second edition. In doing so, we have tried to take account of a number of comments on the first edition by reviewers and others, in order to satisfy the needs of a wide range of readers within the profession. Several new chapters have been added, and we are indebted to our colleagues Dr. Bernard Gee, Dr. Brian Boehlecke, and Mr. Jim Dodgson for help with these. In addition, Drs. Chris Wagner, Roger Seal, Alan Gibbs, Robert Burrell, and Douglas Seaton have assisted in the rewriting of other chapters. Many other friends have helped with advice, but we should like to mention especially Mr. Bob Boothby and Mrs. Brenda McGovern for photographic and source-tracing help; our long-suffering secretaries, Mrs. Joan Blamires and Mrs. Betty Crolla, without whom the work would not have been possible; and Miss Janet Bronwen Morgan, who compiled the index. We are also indebted to the secretaries of our colleagues, but since so many have been involved, we hope that they will forgive us if we do not name them individually. Once again, Ms. Suzanne Boyd and the staff of W. B. Saunders have proved endlessly patient and helpful in getting our manuscript ready for publication. In spite of all this help, some faults will remain, and for these we must accept responsibility.

W. Keith C. Morgan
Anthony Seaton

Preface to the First Edition

Almost all physicians, pathologists, and radiologists at some time encounter the problem of occupational lung disease, and, not uncommonly, difficulties arise in the course of investigation and diagnosis. Descriptions of the classical features of such diseases are hidden in a multitude of early publications, yet often the disease has been modified by changes in the industrial processes and hygiene. Moreover, new diseases are being described with increasing frequency as modern methods of investigation are brought to bear on new industrial processes and the workers concerned in them. It has become relatively difficult for the practicing clinician to keep in touch with the changes in this expanding field, and this book has been written with the needs of such clinicians primarily in mind. While it is intended especially for those engaged in the practice of internal medicine and the subspecialties of respiratory and occupational medicine, it is hoped that it will be of use also to radiologists and pathologists who may be called upon to assist in the investigation of patients with occupational lung disease.

The preliminary chapters, for two of which we are indebted to our colleagues Drs. Chris Wagner, Roger Seal, and Robert Burrell, are intended more as an outline of current work in the basic subjects of physiology, pathology, immunology, and epidemiology, as applied to occupational lung diseases than as a comprehensive review of those subjects. It is hoped, however, that these chapters illustrate the expanding nature of the subject and the number of different resources that are now being applied to the study of this one increasingly important aspect of the general problem of pollution.

Several other friends and colleagues have contributed to the book. We are particularly grateful to Dr. N. LeRoy Lapp, who contributed the chapter on Industrial Bronchitis, and to Drs. E. P. Pendergrass and C. Dundon for advice, criticism, and help throughout. Drs. D. A. Williams, H. M. Foreman, and J. Lyons also gave help and encouragement. The burden of typing was borne by Mrs. D. Thomas and Miss P. Edwards, to whom we are very much indebted. Many other friends have helped at various stages and to all we extend our thanks.

W. Keith C. Morgan
Anthony Seaton

Contents

A Short History of Occupational Lung Diseases

Anthony Seaton

ANCIENT TIMES

It is only possible to speculate about lung disease in prehistoric times, although the two essential forms of work, agriculture and hunting, would certainly have led to conditions that we would recognize today—allergies to stored grain, and silicosis from the fashioning of flint weapons. It is still possible to visit an excavated prehistoric flint mine in England and see techniques demonstrated of so-called flint knapping which could have caused silicosis. As societies developed from simple tribalism to attain the status of nations, so also developed the concept of the ruling and the working classes, the latter often being slaves, as in the Egyptian civilization. The wealth required to support such dynasties and their conquering armies came ultimately from the earth—food from agriculture, and minerals from mining and quarrying—with their attendant hazards to the health of the exploited classes. The earliest hint of such hazards comes from the 1st century AD, during the Roman Empire, when the historian and writer Pliny the Elder (AD 23–79) recorded in his book *De Rerum Naturum* (Natural History) the dangers to miners from inhalation of fumes and vapors. Ironically, Pliny himself died from suffocation in the eruption of Vesuvius. In his time, mining was regarded as such a dangerous trade as to be suitable only for slaves and for the punishment of criminals.

THE MIDDLE AGES

The bewilderingly exponential advances in technology and science in our lifetime make it difficult to appreciate how slowly these fields developed prior to the present century. From the history of mathematics and astronomy, it is clear that scientific thought was advanced in ancient civilizations and perhaps in prehistoric times; the slow progress in translating theory into its practical consequences of the enrichment and destruction of societies has been due to the disproportionately slow development of technology. Over the first 1700 years of the Christian era, there seems to have been relatively little technological development—cathedrals and houses were built with the same tools and similar methods, agriculture changed little, and mining altered only with the substitution of dynamite for fire as a means of breaking rock. Taken together with this slow change, the development of medicine as a learned profession concerned mainly with the ills of those who could afford to pay appropriate fees ensured that the health of working people attracted little attention from doctors until the 18th century. Of the exceptions, two names stand out, Agricola and Paracelsus.

During the Middle Ages, in Europe, there was a slow change in the status of working people from slaves or serfs to that of tradesmen, often organized into guilds. The status of miners became particularly important as the need for precious metals for coinage and base metals for tools developed in line with the development of trade and commerce. The Erz (or ore) Mountains in Bohemia became an important center for the mining and refining of both precious and useful metals, based round the town of Joachimsthal, now known as Jáchymov. (Indeed, the name of the silver coin, Joachimstaler or taler, from this town is the probable derivation of the word *dollar.*) In 1526, Joachimsthal appointed Georg Bauer (1494–1555), known by his latinized name, Agricola, as town physician. Agricola seems to have been the first doctor to record occupational diseases, having been impressed by the mortality of the miners from lung disease. In his book *De Re Metallica,* published the year after his death,[1] he dealt with all aspects of the technology of mining and refining, including ventilation and drainage. He also discussed the diseases and accidents of miners and their risks of suffocation and lung disease. In his most quoted passage, as translated by Herbert Hoover, later to become President of the United States, he says " . . . some mines are so dry that they are entirely devoid of water and this dryness causeth the workers even greater harm, for the dust, which is stirred and beaten up by digging, penetrates into the windpipe and lungs and produces difficulty in breathing and the disease which the Greeks call asthma. If the dust has corrosive qualities, it eats away the lungs and implants consumption in the body. In the Carpathian mines, women are found who have married seven husbands, all of whom this terrible consumption has carried away.''

The reference to asthma is to the original use of the word as a generic term for shortness of breath. Subsequent studies of miners in this and other regions showed the consumption to be silicosis and tuberculosis. It is also of interest that the first description, in 1879, of occupational lung cancer,[2] later shown to be the consequence of exposure to radon underground, came from the same part of the world.

While Agricola's reputation rests on his contributions in this one book, that of his contemporary Paracelsus is based on a wider yet less secure foundation. Theophrastus Bombastus von Hohenheim (1493–1541) was a Swiss physician who called himself Philippus Aureolus Paracelsus. He studied in Basel and Ferrara and spent much of his life traveling, in the course of which he appears to have become addicted to alcohol before finally dying in a tavern brawl. For part of his life he practiced as town doctor in the mining town of Villach, Austria, also working as a metallurgist. He was a man of independent mind who refused to be constrained by the orthodoxy of the day, which included subscription to the views of Galen, whose works he is said to have burned publicly. He also lectured in German rather than Latin, and it is not difficult to see why he ran into trouble with the medical and academic establishment of his time. Nevertheless, his interests ranged wide, and he was clearly an astute observer and recorder of illness. Some of his ideas were as fanciful as those he repudiated, relating to the concepts of alchemy. However, as a doctor he made important contributions, being the first to describe lung disease in miners in his book *Von der Bergsucht,* published posthumously in 1567,[3] as well as describing the effects of mercury poisoning and recording the relationship between endemic goiter and cretinism. He also made important therapeutic contributions, including the introduction of mercury and laudanum into Western pharmacopoeias and teaching that *vis medicatrix naturae,* the healing power of nature, applied to wounds, stressing simple dressings rather than the use of ointments. From the point of view of occupational medicine, perhaps his fundamental contribution was his recognition that industrial activity brings with it a concomitant risk to health and safety: ''We must have gold and silver, also other metals, iron, tin, copper, lead and mercury. If we wish to have these we must risk both life and body in a struggle with many enemies that oppose us.''

RAMAZZINI AND THE BIRTH OF OCCUPATIONAL MEDICINE

Agricola and Paracelsus were, as far as is known, the first doctors to take an interest in the health of tradesmen, but they confined that interest to miners. The first to take a more general interest in occupational diseases was Bernardino Ramazzini (1633–1714), a doctor who, as the founder of occupational medicine, ranks with Hippocrates, Sydenham, Morgagni, and perhaps even Harvey in the history of medicine. Ramazzini was born in Carpi, near Modena in northern Italy, and studied philosophy and law in Parma before qualifying in medicine in 1659. By 1671 he had been appointed Professor of Medicine in Modena, where he distinguished himself by his epidemiological studies, in the manner of Hippocrates, of local diseases including malaria and lathyrism, a condition of toxic spastic paraplegia caused by excessive consumption of the pea *Lathyrus sativus*. This work, published in a book *De Constitutione Anni* (1690), ensured his international reputation, and he became referred to as the third Hippocrates (his near contemporary Sydenham presumably being the second). However, while making his studies, he also developed a reputation as a humane physician, and it was this aspect of his character that led him to take an interest in the health of tradespeople. While watching a workman furiously cleaning out the cesspit at his house, he became aware of the unhealthy and unpleasant circumstances in which many people worked. His many years of subsequent study of the real and supposed hazards of labor were published in his classic volume *De Morbis Artificum Diatriba* (1700 and 1713),[4] Treatise on the Diseases of Workers, in which he introduced a revolutionary concept into clinical medicine—that doctors should inquire about the work of their patient. Two passages in particular are of importance:

W*hen a doctor visits a working class home he should be content to sit on a three-legged stool, if there isn't a gilded chair, and he should take time for his examination; and to the questions recommended by Hippocrates, he should add one more—what is your occupation?*

Medicine, like jurisprudence, should make a contribution to the well-being of workers, and see to it that, so far as possible, they should exercise their callings without harm. So I for my part have done what I could and have not thought it unbecoming to make my way into the lowliest workshops and study the mysteries of the mechanic arts.

Compared with these original ideas—that doctors should ask about their patients' work and even visit their workplaces—Ramazzini's observations on actual occupational diseases are relatively much less significant, since in the 17th century he lacked the basic technology necessary for investigation, having to rely solely on his powers of observation and inductive logic. Nevertheless, it is possible to find many interesting observations on occupational disease and its management within the pages of the book—descriptions, for example, of dyspnea and metal poisoning in miners, of bronchitis (and probable bronchial hyperreactivity) after inhalation of irritant fumes, of lung fibrosis in potters, of asthma in workers exposed to corn and flour, and of silicosis in stonemasons. Moreover, he drew attention to the general benefits of exercise, good ventilation, and protective clothing and to the harmfulness of prolonged work without adequate rest periods and of awkward postures—matters that are very much the concern of the modern occupational physician.

In the year of publication of *De Morbis Artificum Diatriba,* Ramazzini was invited to the Chair of Medicine in Padua, and occupied this in spite of deteriorating health from cardiac disease and what appears to have been cranial arteritis until his death from stroke at the age of 80.[5] He had started a proud tradition of occupational medicine in Italy which continues to this day.

To place the work of Ramazzini in its historical context, he had been born just 5 years after the publication of *De Motu Cordis* by William Harvey and was a contemporary of Marcello Malpighi, who first described the capillaries that Harvey had postulated, and of Thomas Sydenham, who by his descriptions of the natural history of disease, may be regarded as the founder of modern clinical medicine.

Already, Sanctorius had described a method of measuring the pulse and had adapted Galileo's invention as a clinical thermometer. Thus, the foundations of clinical medicine and physiology were being laid at the same time that Robert Boyle, another contemporary, was translating chemistry from mysticism into a subject of scientific investigation. The early 18th century was a time of great scientific flowering in Europe, and this was reflected in the growth of medical teaching in the universities based on scientific observation of disease, epitomized in the work by Morgagni on morbid anatomy, *De Sedibus et Causis Morborum* (1761). The great advances in science of this era also paved the way for the start of the Industrial Revolution in Europe.

THE INDUSTRIAL REVOLUTION

The early 18th century saw the development of methods for producing steel and for using coke for smelting and the invention of the steam engine. New machinery for more effective production of cotton and woolen materials, for transport, and for pumping water from mines became available, and the concept of application of capital to production led to the rapid spread of factories and to the migration of people from the country to the towns. Populations grew, wealth and life expectancy increased, but, paradoxically, the great changes in prosperity were attended by increasing evidence of ill health and epidemics of disease, especially among the working classes. Tuberculosis and typhoid fever became endemic in the towns and cities of Europe, and regular epidemics of cholera occurred until the second half of the 19th century. The early descriptions of industrial diseases that we would recognize today came from this era. Not surprisingly, the first of these was a consequence of the exploitation of coal—scrotal cancer in apprentice chimney sweeps, described by Percivall Pott in 1775.[6, 7] In 1796, Johnstone described silicosis in people using grindstones to sharpen needles.[8] The previous year had seen the birth of the second most notable figure in the history of occupational disease, Charles Turner Thackrah (1795–1833). Thackrah, in a short book with a long title, *The Effects of the Principal Arts, Trades and Professions, and of Civic States and Habits of Living, on Health and Longevity, with Suggestions for the Removal of Many of the Agents Which Produce Disease and Shorten the Duration of Life* (1831),[9] summarized his observations on health in relation to work in the English city of Leeds. Of particular interest to respiratory physicians are his observations on lung disease in miners and metal grinders and his description of a method of measuring lung volume prior to the invention of the spirometer. Thackrah, as many doctors of his era, was compelled for financial reasons to serve for several years as a town doctor, ministering as best he could to the needs of the poor and indigent. He therefore had firsthand knowledge of the conditions under which the working class labored, and his book is written evidence not just of his powers of clinical observation but also of his desire to do something to ameliorate those conditions. In this he was not alone, as the first half of the 19th century can be looked on as the period during which the conscience of the professional middle class was awakened to the exploitation of the poor on which the prosperity of Britain was based. Doctors played an important role in the campaigns for social change, exemplified by the philosophy of Jeremy Bentham's utilitarianism—that of testing institutions by their ability to promote the greatest happiness of the greatest number. Among these doctors may be numbered many who made important advances: Thomas Percival, whose efforts led to the passage of the first Factories Act; William Farr, who instituted medical statistics of mortality; William Duncan and John Simon, who became Britain's first medical officers of health; Robert Baker, who became the first medical inspector of factories; and Thomas Wakley, the founder and campaigning editor of *The Lancet.*[10, 11]

The efforts of such men were complemented by, and would not have been successful without, the activities of a number of enlightened reformers and legislators. Among these was Sir Robert Peel, who introduced his Health and Morals of Apprentices Act in 1802 in response to discovering the exploitation of child labor in his own factories in Manchester. Most notable, however, was Anthony Ashley Cooper, 7th Earl of Shaftesbury, who, between 1833 and 1875, introduced a series of acts intended to improve the circumstances of those who worked in factories, mines, and chimney sweeping, and thus set in motion a train of legislation that has continued in Britain to this day and has been widely adopted throughout the world.

In becoming the birthplace of the Industrial Revolution, Britain also played a leading role in dealing with the social and health consequences of that endeavor. Occupational medicine may be said to have started with the appointment of doctors to inspect children and to certify their ages for work in factories. However, its real beginnings were with the concern of reforming doctors for the health of workers. An important consequence of this, and a stimulus to industry to improve conditions, came with the institution of Workmen's Compensation Acts. Initially, people injured at work only had recourse to Common Law, which required them to prove their employer negligent in having caused the injury. It can be imagined how rarely in the 19th century such an action might have succeeded, even if a worker could afford the services of a lawyer. In 1897, an act was passed in Britain which gave workers rights to compensation from contributions paid by employers. In the early years of the 20th century, these acts were extended to include certain "scheduled" diseases; the first lung diseases, silicosis and asbestosis, were added to the list in Britain in 1919 and 1931, respectively.

In the early colonial era of the United States, the main industries were agriculture and fishing, and related activities such as shipbuilding. However, toward the end of the 18th century, the cotton industry had begun to establish itself in New England; and in the 19th century, iron, steel, railroads, and exploitation of coal and oil became important sources of employment. The legislation in Britain and other European countries was reflected in the United States with an industrial injury compensation scheme for seamen in 1797 and an 1836 law in Massachusetts requiring schooling for child laborers under the age of 15. The same state introduced factory safeguards against accidents in 1877 and factory inspections in 1879. However, major legislative attempts to prevent occupational lung disease did not take place until the present century.

THE MODERN ERA

The history of North American medicine up until the 20th century is lacking in notable names in occupational medicine, although William Osler, as in so many other areas, made contributions to the understanding of coal miners' diseases. The pre-1900 literature contains a number of individual case reports of pneumoconiosis but no evidence of any systematic investigation of such problems. The first great United States occupational disease specialist was Alice Hamilton (1869–1970), who made outstanding contributions in the field of industrial poisonings and who became, as professor in industrial medicine, the first woman appointed to the faculty of Harvard University. In Britain, her contemporary, Donald Hunter (1898–1978), should be noted as a distinguished London physician whose classic work, *The Diseases of Occupations,* first published in 1955, established the study of occupational diseases firmly in the curriculum of British students and who stimulated a generation of doctors to study occupational medicine. Hunter was one of a continuous line of British physicians interested in the diagnosis and prevention of occupational disease dating back to Thackrah and Robert Baker (1803–1880), the first factory doctor; through J. T. Arlidge (1822–1899), author of *The Hygiene, Diseases and Mortality of Occupations* (1892), in which he gave the classic description of silicosis; T. M. Legge (1863–1932), who did pioneering work on lead poisoning and wrote his book on industrial maladies; E. R. A. Merewether (1892–1970), who established the dangers of asbestos and promoted the first legislation to control it; Ethel Browning (1891–1969), who pioneered the study of solvents; and Andrew Meiklejohn (1899–1970), who fought for the eradication of silicosis and lead poisoning from the pottery industry.

Of the occupational lung diseases, silicosis and coal workers' pneumoconiosis were described early in the industrial revolution. Occupational lung cancer was first described in Germany late in the 19th century in metal miners.[2] At this time, no doubt occupational asthma was occasionally recognized, and anecdotal reports, for example of ipecacuanha asthma in a pharmacist, appeared in medical textbooks in the mid-19th century.[12] One of the earliest American accounts of occupational asthma was of the condition in flour millers described by Duke in 1935.[13] Allergic alveolitis was first described in farmers in Britain and in maple bark strippers in the United States in 1932.[14, 15] Silicosis came to public attention late in the United States, following the notorious episode at Gauley Bridge in West Virginia, where many hundreds of workers died of silicosis during the construction of a hydroelectric tunnel through a sandstone mountain.[16] Berylliosis, in its acute form, was first described in Germany in 1933[17] and in the United States in 1943,[18] and the resemblance of chronic berylliosis to sarcoidosis was described in the United States by Hardy and Tabershaw in 1946, in relation to the manufacture of fluorescent lights.[19] Asbestos was first exploited on an international scale after the discovery of the Canadian and South African deposits in the later decades of the 19th century, and the earliest descriptions of asbestosis date from the turn of the 20th century.[20] A possible association between asbestosis and lung cancer was first commented on in 1934.[21] Occupational lung cancer was also suggested in association with arsenic exposure in sheep dip manufacture in 1934,[22] in relation to exposure to chromates in 1935,[23] and in nickel refining in 1939.[24] Mesothelioma in relation to asbestos exposure was described in South Africa in 1960.[25]

Legislation to control occupational disease in the United States was slow to develop, in spite of the efforts of Alice Hamilton in drawing attention to its need. The Bureau of Mines had been established in 1910, and its studies of silicosis and tuberculosis were probably responsible for attracting the attention of the U.S. Public Health Service, which established an Office of Industrial Hygiene in 1914. This organization, under a number of different names, was responsible for many important studies in occupational health, including those of the granite and anthracite industries and of radiation hazards. Finally, in 1970 under the Occupational Safety and Health Act, it became the National Institute for Occupational Safety and Health (NIOSH). In 1936, the Public Contracts Act was passed, obligating employers receiving federal contracts for more than $10,000 to comply with health and safety standards. It took a major disaster, the coal mine explosion at Farmington, West Virginia, which killed 78 miners in 1968, to stimulate further activity, resulting in the Coal Mine Health and Safety Acts in 1969 and 1972 and the Occupational Safety and Health Act in 1970. Over the same period, interest in occupational lung diseases in the United States was stimulated by public and political concern over asbestos-related disease, following the early studies of Selikoff and his colleagues in the 1960s,[26] although that interest seems to have been related more to litigation and compensation than to prevention. While it is natural for physicians to wish to do all they can on behalf of their patients, including helping them seek legal redress if necessary, it should not be forgotten that the major advances in occupational medicine have come when doctors have taken on a wider role than that of caring for their patients, attempting also to deal with the root causes of the illness. This preventive role is one that should be in the minds of all doctors when faced with a patient with occupational disease, a theme developed further in Chapters 2 and 3.

In contrast, in Britain, there has historically been a much greater legislative effort to prevent occupational disease; indeed, the emphasis has been strongly on prevention rather than on compensation. Starting with the early Factories Acts of 1819 and 1833, which were concerned mostly with the protection of children and women from exploitation, a comprehensive system of legislation to prevent exposure of workers to excessive risk backed by appropriate enforcement agencies has been developed. Much of this legislation was consolidated into a comprehensive Health and Safety at Work, etc. Act of 1974, which put a general duty on employers to ensure, as far as reasonably practicable, the health and safety of employees and others who may be affected by the work of the organization. This act set up the Health and Safety Commission and Executive, which include a medical arm and factory, chemical, nuclear, agricultural, and offshore inspectorates. Regulations under the Act include ones specific to control of asbestos, mining, and radiation hazards, as well as the all-embracing Control of Substances Hazardous to Health Regulations, which put a general duty on employers to assess the risks to their workers from the use of hazardous substances and take steps to reduce that risk. Increasingly, since the Single European Act of the Commission of the European Communities, European legislation has taken an interest in the health and safety of workers. From 1992, it is likely that the main legislation affecting workers' health in Europe will come from the Community, influenced by discussion among representatives of government health and safety organizations of the constituent nations.

In the United States, the role of formulating preventive legislation has traditionally been taken by the individual states, leading to marked differences in the protection of workers in different parts of the nation. In 1970, however, Congress enacted the Occupational Safety and Health Act with objectives that included setting and enforcing preventive exposure standards, encouraging states to improve and enforce their own laws, carrying out research and training in occupational health, and setting up reporting procedures. The workings of the Act are overseen by the Occupational Safety and Health Administration (OSHA) of the Department of Labor.

LESSONS FROM THE PAST

The story of the control of occupational lung diseases is a long and continuing one. Clinicians have traditionally made the major discoveries of associations between occupation and disease, though usually not before their patients have told them of their suspicions. The time lag between description of an association and action to prevent disease has been long, though the pace of this is increasing in developed countries. Even so, the actions of doctors are too often directed at attempts to redress wrong, by means of compensation, than to prevention of disease in others. While action to prevent disease depends primarily on political will, there is much that doctors, having discovered a problem, can do by local action with the company concerned. This is discussed further in Chapter 2.

Ultimately, prevention of occupational disease depends on a partnership between government, industrial management, and workers. It is insufficient to rely on the goodwill of employers—expensive outlay to prevent disease may put an organization at a disadvantage compared to a less scrupulous competitor—so government enforcement of appropriate legislation is essential. So too is research into the efficiency and effectiveness of preventive measures, a neglected area. A pragmatic approach to standard setting is desirable; there is little point in setting a standard to reduce risk to zero (even if that were achievable) if it were so tight as to be unenforceable. Much better information is needed on the quantitative relationships between exposure to hazard and risk of disease, so that an informed judgment on standards can be made. Perhaps the greatest advances of the present century have been the application of epidemiology to the study of occupational lung diseases and the use of techniques of occupational hygiene to quantify exposures in epidemiological populations. The use of these techniques holds hope for the future of formulating standards that can be universally applied to preventing disease in the workplace.

REFERENCES

1. Agricola, G., De Re Metallica, 1556. Hoover, H. C., and Hoover, L. H., trans., The Mining Magazine (London), 1912.
2. Harting, F. H., and Hesse, W., Der Lungenkrebs, die Bergkrankheit in der Schneeberger Gruben. Vjschr. Gerichtl. Med., 31, 102, 1879.
3. Paracelsus, T., On the miners' sickness and other miners' diseases. *In* Sigerist, H. E., ed., Four Treatises of Paracelsus. Baltimore, Johns Hopkins Press, 1941.
4. Ramazzini, B., De Morbis Artificum Diatriba. Geneva, 1713, Wright, W. C., trans., Chicago, University of Chicago Press, 1940.
5. Sakula, A., Ramazzini's De Morbis Artificum and occupational lung disease. Br. J. Dis. Chest, 77, 349, 1983.
6. Pott, P., Chirurgical Observations, Volume 3. London, Hawes, Clark & Collins, 1775, p. 177.
7. Waldron, H. A., A brief history of scrotal cancer. Br. J. Ind. Med., 40, 390, 1983.
8. Johnstone, J., Some account of a species of phthisis pulmonalis, peculiar to persons employed in pointing needles in the needle manufacture. Mem. Med. Soc. London, 5, 89, 1799.
9. Thackrah, C. T., The Effects of the Principal Arts, Trades and Professions, and of Civic States and Habits of Living, on Health and Longevity, with Suggestions for the Removal of Many of the Agents Which Produce Disease and Shorten the Duration of Life. London, Longman, Rees, Orne, Brown and Green, 1831.
10. Lee, W. R., Emergence of occupational medicine in Victorian times. Br. J. Ind. Med., 30, 118, 1973.
11. Rose, M. E., The doctor in the Industrial Revolution. Br. J. Ind. Med., 28, 22, 1971.
12. Seaton, A., Ipecacuanha asthma: an old lesson. Thorax, 45, 974, 1990.
13. Duke, W. W., Wheat hairs and dust as a common cause of asthma among workers in wheat flour mills. J.A.M.A., 105, 957, 1935.
14. Campbell, J. M., Acute symptoms following work with hay. Br. Med. J., 2, 1143, 1932.
15. Tower, J. W., Sweaney, H. C., and Huron, W. H., Severe bronchial asthma apparently due to fungus spores found in Maple bark. J.A.M.A., 99, 453, 1932.
16. Cherniack, M., The Hawk's Nest Incident: America's Worst Industrial Disaster. New Haven, CT, Yale University Press, 1986.
17. Weber, H. H., and Engelhardt, W. E., Uber eine Apparatur zur Erzeugung niedriger Staubkonzentrationen von groser Konstanz und eine Methode zur mikrogravimetrischen Staubbestimung, Andwendung bei der Untersuchung von Stauben aus der Berylliumgewinnung. Zbl. Gew. Hyg., 10, 41, 1933.
18. Van Ordstrand, H. S., Hughes, R. C., De Nardi, J. M., and Carmody, N. G., Beryllium poisoning. J.A.M.A., 129, 1084, 1945.
19. Hardy, H. L., and Tabershaw, I. R., Delayed chemical pneumonitis occurring in workers exposed to beryllium compounds. J. Industr. Hyg., 28, 197, 1946.
20. Murray, M., Departmental Committee for Compensation for Industrial Diseases, Cmd 3495 and 3496. London, Her Majesty's Stationery Office, 1907.
21. Wood, W. B., and Gloyne, S. R., Pulmonary asbestosis: a review of 100 cases. Lancet, 2, 1383, 1934.
22. Legge, T., Industrial Maladies. London, Oxford University Press, 1934, p. 83.
23. Pfeil, E., Lungentumoren als Berufserkrankung in Chromatbetrieben. Dtsch. Med. Wschr., 61, 1197, 1935.
24. Morgan, J. G., Some observations on the incidence of respiratory cancer in nickel workers. Br. J. Ind. Med., 15, 224, 1958.
25. Wagner, J. C., Sleggs, C. A. and Marchand, P., Diffuse pleural mesothelioma and asbestos exposure in the North West Cape Province. Br. J. Ind. Med., 17, 260, 1960.
26. Selikoff, I. J., Churg, J., and Hammond, E. C., Asbestos exposure and neoplasia. J.A.M.A., 188, 22, 1964.

2

Prevention of Occupational Lung Diseases

Anthony Seaton

■

The traditional role of the clinician has been to diagnose and treat disease, with the objectives of cure, amelioration of symptoms, and improvement of prognosis. In the case of occupational lung diseases, cure is rarely possible, leaving the doctor with limited scope for helping the patient. Since occupational lung disease can usually be attributed to a cause in the workplace, and since blame for that risk may be attributed to the patient's employer, it is quite usual for the doctor's efforts on behalf of the patient to be channeled in support of a civil law claim for damages. It may be argued that such claims, if successful, may have a salutary effect on the negligent employer by hitting where it hurts—in the pocket. However, there is little evidence that this is so, in that few industries have reduced workplace risks in response to being found negligent, the costs usually being borne by insurers who pass them on in turn in the form of increased premiums. Thus, it is arguable that, if the toll of industrial illness is to be reduced, clinical doctors should assume a broader role in the management of these conditions and should concern themselves also with preventive aspects. All occupational lung disease represents a failure of preventive measures.

THE SIGNAL CASE

There is something uniquely satisfying to a doctor in identifying the cause of disease in a patient. This seems always to have been the case, even when causes such as possession by demons or imbalance of the humors were more fanciful than most (though not all) of the causes that we recognize today. Understanding of causation may help in planning treatment, usually helps in preventing recurrence or exacerbation, but should always help in preventing disease in others. A patient with occupational lung disease should be looked upon as a signal that all is not well with the workplace, that others may be at risk or already affected, and that something may need to be done about it. This chapter is concerned with what can be done.

The patient's history provides the important clues, and these depend on the disease. Clearly very different actions ensue from seeing patients with, for example, toxic pneumonitis, asthma, or cancer. In the case of cancer and the various pneumoconioses, the exposure may have ceased and certainly started years previously, and current conditions may bear little resemblance to those that caused the disease. In the case of asthma, allergic alveolitis, infections, and toxic pneumonitis, current conditions are always relevant, and sometimes urgent action is necessary. However, this general rule, distinguishing between chronic and acute diseases in the need for prompt action, does not always hold true, as may be seen from two examples.

In 1961, a man aged 34, a lifelong nonsmoker, presented to his doctor with hemoptysis. His chest radiograph showed a tumor which when removed surgically proved to be an oat cell carcinoma. In 1966, a second man, aged 67, who worked in the same factory, which had employed some 500 people, died of anaplastic bronchial carcinoma. He had not smoked for 20 years. In the next 2 years, two more men from the same factory, aged 60 and 62, also died of oat cell carcinoma. In 1970 a 41-year-old nonsmoker, in 1972 two more nonsmokers, aged 40 and 50, and in 1975 a 50-year-old man also died of oat cell carcinoma. In 1971, a 51-year-old man died of cerebral metastasis from an undifferentiated nasal carcinoma. All worked at the same factory. Over the next decade, four men in their 50s died of the same disease. In those two decades, no worker from the factory died from lung cancer of other than undifferentiated type.

This was the sequence of events at a small town in South Wales, site of a factory making ion-exchange resins and using chloromethyl ethers.[1] The possibility of a carcinogenic hazard in the workplace was first raised by a trade union official in 1969, 2 years after the first suspicions were raised in the United States and shortly after the first report in the medical literature of the carcinogenicity of bischloromethyl ether.[2]

This story illustrates a familiar problem—the time taken to suspect a cancer hazard when epidemiological techniques are used, since these require a sufficient number of cases. There is an alternative approach, which in this case would have been dependent on doctors' suspicions being aroused, as they might have been after seeing oat cell carcinoma in relatively young nonsmokers working in a chemical factory. This approach is through clinical investigation, leading to workplace investigation, leading to searches of the literature or toxicological research, leading to the institution of preventive measures. Such action taken early in this case might have saved several relatively young lives.

A 52-year-old man presented to his doctor in 1984 with a 9-month history of dry cough and dyspnea. Crackles were heard over the upper lung zones, and chest radiography showed very fine nodularity in both upper and mid zones with consolidation in the right mid zone. His job was stonemasonry. Silicosis was suspected, though expert opinion was that the x-ray films were not typical, so lung biopsy was carried out. This showed diffuse interstitial fibrosis of mixed usual interstitial pneumonitis (UIP) and desquamative interstitial pneumonitis (DIP) type and little doubly refractile material. The patient deteriorated, dying a year later of respiratory failure.

In 1987 another stonemason working on the same site presented to the same chest physician with similar symptoms and radiographic changes. On this occasion a further occupational history was taken, and an urgent visit to the worksite was arranged. The men were found to be cutting hard sandstone with pneumatic tools; there was no dust extraction, and respiratory protection was wholly inadequate, with quartz levels in the air being over 100 times the threshold limit value. Several other workers at the site had earlier signs of silicosis. Review of the lung tissue of the first man showed it to contain extraordinary amounts of very fine quartz, invisible to polarized light.

This is an episode of accelerated silicosis,[3] which may occur after relatively short periods of very high exposure to quartz—in this case over about 5 years, though exposures of as little as 6 months have been recorded. Clearly, in such cases a visit to the workplace may save many other workers from suffering the same fate.

APPROACH TO THE WORKPLACE

Prior to making any decision or giving advice on preventive measures, a visit to the workplace is necessary. This may be made by the clinician investigating the patient, by a professional in occupational health, or by a representative of a regulatory agency. The objectives of the visit should be to discover the hazard, to estimate the degree of risk to workers, and to advise management on elimination or control of that risk.

The first step should be to seek the patient's agreement. Two matters are of importance here—clinical confidentiality and protection of the patient's interests. Ethical considerations preclude the doctor from divulging any clinical information about the patient without informed consent, while information given to an employer to the effect that an employee has a work-related disease may result in the worker's dismissal. In a large organization it may be possible to conceal the patient's identity, whereas in a small one it may not. For these reasons, it is often better to seek the advice of the appropriate government or state agency responsible for workplace health and safety. Such organizations have powers to order enforcement of relevant legislation and are in a better position to advise the patient of his or her rights under labor and anti-discrimination law. If the workplace is unionized, the patient may also be advised to consult the local representative.

In ideal circumstances, which occur more often than one might be led to believe, having received the patient's agreement to approach management, the doctor should make contact with an appropriate senior manager or with the occupational physician if the company employs one. The problem should be explained, preferably without identifying the patient, and the doctor's wish to help advise on preventing further problems stated. The reasons for requesting a visit, as given above, should be outlined.

In many cases, the doctor will not feel able to make the workplace visit, because of a lack of expertise or understanding of the workings of industry. There are certainly many pitfalls for the unwary, including becoming involved in battles between management and union and becoming identified strongly with one or other party. Moreover, it is easy for the inexperienced to be bewildered by the complexities of many industrial processes. In these circumstances, help may be sought, as mentioned earlier, from government or state agencies (see later), from academic departments of occupational health, or from practicing occupational physicians with appropriate training and expertise.

THE SITE VISIT

In contrast to the occupational physician, who in visiting a workplace is usually looking generally to prevent future risks, the clinical doctor investigating a health problem has more specific objectives, being interested in the particular circumstances that led to the illness. Respiratory disease is almost always caused by inhalation of harmful substances, so interest is focused on possible sources of emission of dusts, fumes, or gases, on ventilation systems, on enclosure of processes, and on personal protective measures employed.

In general, it is sensible when looking at a process to start at the beginning with the raw materials and follow it through to the production and dispatch of the finished product. Particular attention should be paid to areas where emissions might occur, often at points where ingredients are mixed or heat is applied or given off, and where products are bagged. Information on substances used in processes may usually be obtained from data sheets, which in many countries must be made available by law. It is also important to find out what happens when the process breaks down and during maintenance operations—often these are the only times in a well-run factory when workers may be exposed to toxic hazards.

With respect to the specific job being investigated, ideally the patient or a colleague should be watched at work. Are there any airborne hazards given off either by the job or by workers close at hand? What system, if any, is in place to extract such hazardous substances? What is the general ventilation of the workplace? This last question has often been of importance in tracking down mysterious respiratory illnesses, most notably episodes of legionnaires' disease and several outbreaks of asthma in which allergenic chemicals have been drawn into one workplace by ventilation inlets placed close to extraction outlets of another factory.

If a site visit proves impossible, in certain circumstances (the investigation of asthma and allergic alveolitis) it may be possible to arrange for the patient to demonstrate the job, using materials from the workplace, in the hospital laboratory. This is usually done as a challenge test, discussed further in Chapters 17 and 20. At the very least, it is usually possible to get from the patient or from a worker's representative a list of any potentially harmful substances used in the workplace.

Having completed the visit, it is important to explain to the employer the problems that have been identified and means of dealing with them. This will always involve some financial outlay and is therefore likely to meet with some resistance. It is thus important, first, to explain the necessity for change and, second, to be reasonably practical in what is suggested.

PRINCIPLES OF PREVENTION

The principles of preventing occupational lung disease are easily understood, and may be set out in order of efficacy.

1. *Substitution of a harmless or less hazardous substance for a more hazardous one.* The best known examples of the efficacy of such actions came from the pottery industry, when alumina was substituted for powdered silica, and from the widespread substitution of manmade fibers for asbestos. Other examples might be the substitution of *in vitro* tests for animal experiments in preventing animal house asthma, and the introduction of colophony-free solder fluxes in the electronics industry. This simple first principle of prevention is often forgotten—eliminate the hazard.

2. *Enclosure of the process.* When hazardous substances cannot be eliminated, the exposure of workers to them may be prevented by enclosure. This technique is used most notably in the handling of radioactive and carcinogenic substances and has been successfully applied in prevention of asthma in industries using isocyanates and proteolytic enzymes. It is not, of course, as effective as elimination, as no enclosure is 100% efficient. In particular, problems are liable to occur when the process breaks down and during maintenance operations. In such circumstances, maintenance workers and fitters are often more at risk than are the day-to-day process workers.

3. *Exhaust ventilation.* If the process cannot be enclosed, it may still be possible to remove harmful fumes or dusts by appropriate ventilation. A familiar example to many is the use of fume cupboards in chemistry laboratories, where partial enclosure combined with extraction of air allows people to handle chemical reactions in safety. In general, the system for extraction should be sited as close as possible to the source of the fume or dust if partial enclosure is not possible. In some circumstances, such as in coal mines or in painting or welding operations in confined spaces, the system for ventilation relies simply on passing sufficient air through the workplace to dilute the harmful substance to levels that are acceptable in terms of risk. Methods of exhaust ventilation have been used with considerable success in reducing dust levels in, amongst others, the coal and asbestos industries.

4. *Personal protection.* Many doctors and lay people instinctively think first of a mask or respirator when considering ways of protecting individuals from airborne respiratory hazards. Such devices are widely used and of considerable value, as discussed in Chapter 11. However, they have several serious drawbacks:

They depend on the worker's compliance.
They are, often considerably, less than 100% efficient.
They require skilled, regular maintenance.
They impose additional physiological demands on the wearer.
They may interfere with ability to perform the task.

For these reasons, personal respiratory protection should not be relied on to protect workers, unless used in combination with some of the other measures previously outlined. It will be noted that all the other measures put the onus on management to make the workplace safe, whereas use of a respirator moves responsibility to the worker to comply. While it is not bad for responsibility for health and safety to be shared between managers and workers, it is in principle wrong for managers to delegate the responsibility to those who may not be fully aware of the dangers or may take a carefree attitude to risk.

Education and Information

It is no coincidence that the most successful companies take an enlightened attitude to health and safety matters, regarding this as an important part of employer-employee relations. Informing the work force of workplace hazards and educating them on means of reducing risk are part of the policies of such companies. It is also good practice from a legal point of view, should a worker subsequently claim injury due to negligence. It should of course be combined with the practical measures to reduce risk already discussed. Education of workers can take place at induction and up-dating seminars, through trade unions and safety organizations, and especially through notices in the workplace. These should be brief and to the point, announcing hazards and protective measures to be taken.

Screening and Worker Surveillance

There persists in industry, perhaps also among some doctors, a belief that detailed clinical examination of prospective employees will allow a particularly fit and disease-resistant breed of worker to be selected, thus reducing absence due to sickness and increasing resistance to workplace hazard. While there is some substance to this with respect to matching physically or psychologically robust people to particularly stressful jobs and also in ensuring that workers exposed to infective risk (e.g., tuberculosis) have been immunized, there is no evidence of its general worth. Indeed, as can be seen, for example, by the consequences of screening atopic individuals from jobs with an asthma risk, many people may be excluded who would never have developed disease, while the actual incidence of disease is barely if at all affected. Such a screening program may readily run into accusations of being discriminatory, as well as lulling management into a false sense of security with respect to workplace hazards. If pre-employment screening is to take place, it should be with the positive intentions of ensuring that the current health of the worker is suitable for the demands of the job. In these circumstances, it also provides an opportunity for health and safety education, both generally and with respect to the specific workplace.

Regular surveillance of workers may in some countries and in some industries be a legal requirement. Initially introduced in order to detect clinical disease in workers exposed to metals such as lead and phosphorus, it is now used mainly in industry for the biological monitoring of people to detect excessive absorption of toxic substances. In respiratory disease, surveillance is most widely used in workers exposed to asbestos and coal, and usually takes the form of an x-ray and clinical examination. It is also increasingly being used in workers exposed to substances liable to cause asthma. Before embarking on a screening program, it is well to remember a few principles:

That the condition being sought is important.
That, once found, effective management is possible.
That it can be detected at a stage when such management can influence its natural history.
That policy on management of cases is agreed.

These and other matters related to more general population screening are discussed further in Chapter 6.

Surveillance of workers at risk of disease should be instituted only as a back-up to more active preventive measures. It can then be used mainly as a means of ensuring that these measures are working, with a secondary role of intervening in management in the case of those workers who nevertheless develop early signs of disease. This is exemplified by its use in the British coal industry, where primary preventive measures aimed at reducing dust levels in mines have had a dramatic effect in reducing the numbers of new cases of pneumoconiosis, while a program of x-ray examination every four years identifies those miners who have early signs of the disease and leads to action to reduce their subsequent dust exposure, in turn reducing the risks of further progression of their pneumoconiosis. In the case of workers at risk of occupational asthma, an even stronger case for surveillance can be made, since when caught at an early stage, that condition will normally remit if further exposure is prevented, whereas if it is allowed to progress, it may reach a stage when it becomes a chronic condition whether or not exposure ceases.

LEGAL FRAMEWORK FOR PREVENTION

Most countries have decided that, for occupational disease to be prevented, legal rather than voluntary controls are necessary. Such controls are at their most comprehensive and sophisticated in the Scandinavian countries and in the European Community. In order to be effective, laws must also have sanctions available to apply to those who break them and must be supported by an effective regulatory authority. In many developing countries and in the more laissez-faire Western regimes, laws may be better on paper than in application because of the lack of effective enforcement.

United States

The Occupational Safety and Health Act (OSH Act) was enacted in 1970. It puts a general obligation on employers to keep a healthy and safe workplace and makes the Department of Labor, through the Occupational Safety and Health Administration (OSHA), responsible for setting and overseeing compliance with specific workplace standards for hazards. OSHA has paid particular attention to the regulation of carcinogens, most notably asbestos, and its pronouncements have been marked by considerable controversy. The Act does not cover workers who are self-employed or those covered by other acts (such as coal miners) but does make the head of each federal agency responsible for the health and safety of employees within that agency.

OSHA has the right to inspect workplaces and to issue citations when it believes the law is being violated, under either criminal or civil law. However, it emphasizes voluntary efforts to improve health and safety and provides consultative and educational services to industry to this end. In view of the relatively small size of the agency in relation to the vast and complex character of United States industry, enforcement in the face of a financially pressured industrial sector is never going to be more than partially successful, and education of management and the work force seems to be a more promising way forward.

The OSH Act also created a research arm, the National Institute for Occupational Safety and Health (NIOSH), within the Public Health Service of the Department of Health and Human Services. NIOSH has responsibility for gathering information about work-related disease and injury, researching such diseases and their prevention, recommending standards, and training health professionals. Particularly important are its criteria documents, which review the evidence on harmfulness of specific workplace hazards, assessing its scientific merit as a basis for standard setting.

Miners, including coal miners, are covered by a separate act, the Federal Mine Safety and Health Act of 1977, also administered by the Department of Labor. This act prescribes the same general duties in terms of health and safety, mandates regular unannounced inspections of both underground and surface mines, proposes and enforces standards, and provides for safety training of new miners.

In providing help to the practicing doctor wishing to investigate the cause of an occupational lung disease, NIOSH is the most useful nationwide resource. It is able to assist in a practical manner with investigations, provide access to databases for literature searches, and give advice over the telephone about the handling of individual problems.

Britain

The British system is based on a comprehensive Health and Safcty at Work Act 1974, which again puts a general duty on employers and employees to ensure a healthy and safe workplace, qualified by the words "as far as is reasonably practicable." It applies to all workplaces and covers all in those places, including visitors. It is administered by the Health and Safety Commission and Executive (HSC and HSE), the latter containing the various industrial inspectorates (mines, chemicals, radiation, offshore, agricultural, and so on), and the medical arm, the Employment Medical Advisory Service (EMAS). It fulfils similar roles in setting standards, enforcement, education, and advice as does OSHA, the emphasis being strongly on education and information. Under the Act are various regulations, perhaps the most important and pragmatic being the Control of Substances Hazardous to Health Regulations 1989 (COSHH). These put a responsibility on all employers, including the self-employed, to assess all hazardous substances used in the workplace and to keep a written record of an assessment made of the risk to workers from the use of these substances. If risks are perceived to be present, steps are to be taken to reduce them as far as reasonably practicable. If residual risk is present, consideration of further steps including workplace monitoring and worker surveillance is required.

Failure to fulfil the requirements of the COSHH Regulations does not constitute an offense in itself, but is taken into account in legal proceedings if a worker is injured or falls ill. They have proved a reasonably effective means of focusing employers on the need to take care with harmful substances.

The COSHH Regulations do not cover a number of workplace hazards which, because of special perceived danger, have their own regulations. These include radiation, noise, lead, asbestos, underground coal mines, and medicines.

In Britain, the doctor requiring help or advice in the investigation of occupational disease would contact a colleague in EMAS, who has at his or her disposal similar facilities to those of NIOSH.

WORKPLACE STANDARDS

The general principle for setting standards is that a level is set at which exposure of a worker for a normal working lifetime is unlikely to result in disease. Usually it is accepted that for many, if not all, substances, thresholds below which disease will never occur are impossible to define for practical purposes. The aim of standard setting should therefore be to decide on a level which should not be exceeded and which will be likely to prevent most disease, and to encourage industry to adhere to levels as far below that standard as possible.

The process of standard setting is complex. Ideally, for a substance of known hazard to humans, the information linking exposure levels to disease incidence from epidemiological studies should be used to define quantitative relationships between exposure and risk. These scientific data then require comments from management and labor, who will necessarily have divergent views on where, on a continuous curve of risk against dose, an arbitrary line should be drawn. In such debates, with government acting as referee, management is influenced often by the costs of controls, while labor tends to be interested in reducing all risk, no matter what the cost. Resolution of the debate results in a standard which often reflects the general philosophy of the nation's government, be it interventionist or laissez-faire.

In less ideal circumstances, as is the case for many substances, there may be no useful exposure-response data in humans and reliance has to be placed on data on prevalence of disease together with the results of animal and laboratory studies. Sometimes, if a substance has not been in use long enough, or if it has apparently not caused significant disease in people, laboratory studies are all that are available to inform the debate. In such circumstances, it may be useful to argue by analogy— for example, in setting standards for manmade fibers, the knowledge gained from studies of asbestos may be used.

Since the 1940s in the United States, the American Conference of Government Industrial Hygienists (ACGIH) has produced lists of threshold limit values (TLVs) for harmful substances, and these have been adopted widely internationally in the absence of any better alternatives. These values are decided by a committee and are intended to indicate values at which most workers may be exposed for a normal working lifetime without ill effect. They are generally calculated as time-weighted average levels over an 8-hour period; some are designated with a C to indicate that they represent a value that should not be exceeded even for a short period. It is explicit in the ACGIH list that the TLVs are not safe limits and that some workers may be affected at lower levels, for example, as a result of sensitization.

Most countries have an official governmental standard-setting organization, such as OSHA in the United States. OSHA is mandated to promulgate standards at which workers will suffer no ill effects, even if exposed for a lifetime, while taking into account economic feasibility, the need for the products, and the effects of legislation on society as a whole. For practical reasons, it has adopted a number of TLVs as its own standards, though in many cases subsequent revision of the TLV has meant that the two values are now different. To complicate matters further, standards proposed by NIOSH, based on its review of the evidence in the criteria documents, not infrequently differ from both.

In Britain, the Health and Safety Executive publishes what it calls Occupational Exposure Limits (OELs), comprising two types of standards—maximal exposure limits (MELs), which must not be exceeded, and occupational exposure standards (OESs), which are levels at which there is no evidence of harm to workers if exposed over a working lifetime. Thus, MELs refer to substances of known, serious toxicity, while OESs include a much larger list of less harmful (though certainly not innocuous) substances. Exposure of workers must be kept at or below the OES level, and, if the level is exceeded, steps must be taken to reduce it.

Occupational exposure standards assume great importance in litigation. For the practicing doctor, they should be thought of as what they are, an often imperfect guide to industry as to where to aim in controlling workers' exposures, and a reminder that the chemical or dust in question has the potential to do harm. Reference to standards is made in appropriate parts of this book. It should be remembered that they vary considerably from country to country and are subject to periodic revision in the light of new toxicological or epidemiological information.

REFERENCES

1. McCallum, R. I., Woolley, V., and Petrie A., Lung cancer associated with chloromethyl methyl ether manufacture: an investigation at two factories in the United Kingdom. Br. J. Ind. Med., 40, 384, 1985.
2. Van Duren, B. L., Alpha-haloethers: a new type of alkylating carcinogen. Arch. Environ. Health, 16, 472, 1968.
3. Seaton, A., Legge, J. S., Henderson, J., and Kerr, K. M., Accelerated silicosis in Scottish stonemasons. Lancet, 337, 341, 1991.

3

The Clinical Approach

■

Surprisingly little is known of the prevalence or incidence of occupational lung diseases in most countries. Methods of collecting data vary—some countries, such as the United States, have no national system; many have information from sources such as registers of people disabled by industrial disease; and others, such as Sweden, have formal reporting procedures. In the absence of such information, it is difficult to plan appropriate preventive action; and in such circumstances, much responsibility falls on the shoulders of individual physicians to detect occupational disease and to take appropriate action both on behalf of the injured worker and also on behalf of other members of the work force. This latter, preventive role has been discussed in Chapter 2. In this chapter, the doctor's role in diagnosis and management of occupational lung disease is considered.

A glance at the history of development of knowledge about causes of disease will show the primary role that the clinical doctor has played. From the early accounts of the pneumoconioses, to the recognition of asbestosis, asbestos-related lung cancer, mesothelioma, occupational asthma, and farmer's lung, the first clue has come from a clinical doctor who had the curiosity to wonder why particular patients developed particular symptoms and who was also aware that lung disease frequently has external environmental causes.

As industrial processes change and become increasingly complex, we may anticipate a wider range of potentially toxic substances in the air that people breathe in the workplace. At the same time, it is unlikely that the lung will develop many new ways of reacting to inhaled toxic material. Therefore, new occupational lung diseases are likely to be old lung diseases with a new cause—a concept exemplified by the almost daily recognition of a new cause of occupational asthma. An important danger confronting clinicians—and one that is readily apparent to teachers of medicine—is familiarity with a disease, leading to a lack of curiosity about its cause. Thus lung cancer is normally attributed without real thought to cigarette smoking, other possible contributory causes being ignored, and asthma is often regarded more as a consequence of misfortune than of exposure to specific allergens. The good physician will always maintain a curiosity about why patients get the diseases they do, and thus be in a position from time to time to prevent similar occurrences in others.

THE HISTORY

All medical students are taught to take an occupational history, though this process usually becomes, with time and lack of thought, no more than recording the name of the job. A job title is often incomprehensible, varying from district to district and sometimes having been passed down through a trade so that its original meaning and its current meaning are quite distinct. Examples abound—in Scotland's mines a brusher does not operate a brush, but drills into hard rock, while in shipyards caulkers no longer put tar between planks but use electric arc equipment to gouge and fuse metal plates. The real question should not be "What is your job?", but "What do you do at work?". If there is any suspicion that the patient's disease could be work-related (and with lung disease this is an ever-present possibility), further information is necessary. In some cases, particularly where there are medicolegal implications, this may be a time-consuming process.

Is the Illness Work-Related?

In broad terms, work-related lung disease may be considered in two categories, those of short and long induction periods. Into the former category fall asthma, infections, allergic alveolitis, and toxic poisonings, while into the latter fall the pneumoconioses and neoplasms. The key to diagnosis lies in the occupational history, but a different process is required in each of the two situations. The diagnosis of a short-induction disease is suspected from the medical history, and occupational factors are among several that may be responsible for causation. The occupational history should concentrate on details of the current job and workplace and on activities associated with the development of symptoms. Sometimes a very detailed work history is required, and in such circumstances, the patient may be asked to give an account of all activities from going to work at the start of the day (or shift) to leaving at the end. This process should be interspersed with inquiries about any fumes, dusts, chemicals, or other possible causes of the symptoms in question, and about the use of protective measures such as process enclosure or respirators.

CASE HISTORY ■

A 40-year-old man developed his first attack of asthma after cleaning a heat exchanger in a potato chip factory. The work had been very dusty, in that he used a wire brush to scrape incrustations of soot from the machine in a relatively confined space. He had another, severe, attack the next day shortly after doing the same job, and he not unnaturally attributed the disease to the work. He remained off work and claimed industrial injury benefit, which was denied him, as exposure to soot was not recognized as a cause of asthma.

A detailed occupational history revealed that he had in the past worked as a joiner and had been exposed to wood dusts. In his current job, which was as a laborer, he went into work at 7 AM, and his first task was to sweep out the joiners' workshop. Then, after several other tasks, he had been assigned at about 11 AM to cleaning the heat exchanger. On the two days in question, he had swept out a great deal of dust in the joiners' shop, after the tradesmen had been working with Western red cedar. This, rather than soot, proved to be the cause of his asthma, and this knowledge enabled appropriate preventive action to be taken, as well as facilitating his receipt of injury benefit.

Sometimes the cause is only discovered when the patient is asked about other jobs or hobbies, "Do you do any other work?" being an important supplementary question.

CASE HISTORY ■

A young man presenting with asthma gave as his occupation "panel beater." This job involves the repair of damaged cars, and frequently requires the use of paint sprays. He was therefore asked if he did any such painting; he said that he did not, although it was done in the workplace by others in a specially constructed booth. By way of explanation, he was told that some paint sprays could cause the asthmatic symptoms that he had, and at this point he admitted that he had a small second job in his own garage at home. In this he also repaired and spray-painted people's cars, without any appropriate safeguards. This proved to be the cause of his asthma.

In determining whether an illness is work-related, the relationship of the symptoms to the job is crucial. With acute toxic exposures, this is usually obvious even when the symptoms start a few hours after the exposure, as may be the case for example with oxides of nitrogen. Sometimes, however, a delay of several days occurs before the onset of breathlessness, and in these circumstances, if the patient does not volunteer the history of exposure, confusion with infective pneumonia is likely. In occupational asthma, the relationship between work and symptoms often becomes less clear as the condition progresses, and in these circumstances it is advisable to take the patient carefully through the history of development of the symptoms—when did they first start, did they change at weekends or on holidays, did the patient notice anything at work that provoked them, and so on.

With respect to diseases of longer latency, such as lung cancer, mesothelioma, and pneumoconioses, the important point in the history is to establish an adequate likely exposure to a known cause of the condition. Mesothelioma is unique in that it may be caused by relatively brief, if heavy, exposures to asbestos, for as little as 6 months. In this case, it is necessary to ask specifically about exposures to asbestos in such trades as ship repair, insulation, and construction/demolition, over a period some 25 to 50 years previously. With respect to lung cancer and pneumoconioses, relatively prolonged and heavy exposures are usually necessary for causation, and when an occupational cause is found, that occupation is likely to have been the individual's main lifetime activity.

A 65-year-old man presented with cough and shortness of breath over the past month. He had also had a recent episode of hemoptysis. He had smoked 10 cigarettes daily in his early 20s, but none for the past 40 years. His lifelong occupation, until a few months previously, had been as an asphalter, boiling the material and applying it on roofs and floors. Bronchoscopy showed him to have a squamous carcinoma of the right main bronchus, together with dysplastic precancerous changes in his laryngeal epithelium. It seemed likely that his lifetime exposure to asphalt fumes was responsible for this disease.

CASE HISTORY ■

What Has the Patient Been Exposed To?

In coming to a judgment as to whether a patient has occupational disease, the physician needs to find out whether there has been exposure to an agent likely to cause that disease and whether such exposure has been sufficient. Sometimes the patient knows—a farmer will often recognize that the hay is moldy, and a solderer will be aware of the fumes from the flux. Sometimes the exposure will have to be deduced from the history, in that the patient does not know what he or she was exposed to, but can recount what he or she has been doing. In these circumstances, the essential questions relate to the presence of dust, fumes, or gases in the air and to the processes that gave rise to these substances.

In the case of acute illness following exposure to toxic substances, it is rarely possible to obtain from the history an indication of the concentration, other than in very general terms. In differentiating allergic reactions (such as hypersensitivity pneumonitis) from toxic reactions (such as chemical pneumonitis), the effect of the exposure on others is important. Were other people affected to a greater or lesser extent? If so, toxic inhalational injury is more likely. In the case of allergic reactions, both asthma and pneumonitis, it is likewise important to know if prior exposure to the suspected agent has occurred, since it is very rare for such conditions to occur on the first exposure to an antigenic substance.

In the case of diseases of long latency, the total exposure to the toxic agent is likely to be important, and the patient rarely has more than very general knowledge of what the agent was—usually this is confined to memories of working in dusts or fumes, or being exposed to smelly chemicals. Further information may be obtained, if the type of industry is known, from company data sheets, textbooks of occupational hygiene, or the ILO Encyclopaedia of Occupational Health and Safety.[1] If the worker was a member of a trade union, it may be possible to obtain further information on toxic exposures from this source. However, it is reasonable to suspect that someone who has worked many years in a dusty industry will have accumulated some of that dust in his lungs, and that if he has appropriate radiological signs, a connection between the two is likely. In these circumstances, an approximate idea of concentration of dust may be obtained by asking questions about its effect on visibility and on the frequency with which the worker had to wash. An idea of its nature may be obtained by asking about the processes, particularly the raw materials, responsible for the dust. In the case of chemicals, absorption may be important, and questions about retention of smell on the breath or in sweat after coming home from work may be relevant.

Disablement

The clinical history may not only give clues to the causation of lung disease but also contribute to assessment of the patient's disability. The terms *disability* and *dysfunction* are sometimes confused: disability implies an assessment of a person's ability to perform necessary or desirable tasks, and therefore requires qualification by the expected standard, whereas dysfunction is a measurement of impairment of a physiological function compared with the normal expected. Dysfunction is relatively easy to measure—for example, forced expiratory volume in 1 second (FEV_1) expressed as a percentage of that predicted for the individual. However, the same level of functional impairment implies substantial differences in disability in people whose jobs require different levels of physical activity. Disability, moreover, depends not just on a mismatch of physical demands and physical abilities but also on the psychological reaction of the individual to the physical loss. Thus, motivation may allow an individual to overcome considerable dysfunction, and, conversely, there may be exacerbation of disability in a patient who is unmotivated. Negative motivation is commonplace in patients making claims under civil law, in which the greater the disablement, the greater the potential gain.

The clinical history provides an opportunity to assess disability in relation to measurements of dysfunction and to explore factors that might be contributing to a mismatch between them. Apart from the obvious factor, litigation, there are others that are equally important yet frequently missed or ignored by doctors. Depression is common in patients with physical impairment and contributes to worsening of the consequent disablement. A good history will assess for possible symptoms of this complicating disease. Similarly, anxiety may make disability much more severe. Such anxiety is commonly a consequence of ill-considered medical information or advice. It is now commonplace to see people who claim shortness of breath, having been told they have asbestos-caused pleural plaques. The appropriate management of this condition is strong reassurance and encouragement toward exercise rehabilitation, whereas the usual approach is to encourage the person to sue or apply for disability benefits, thus reinforcing the anxiety and the symptoms. Anxiety frequently arises from an incomplete understanding of the disease and its implications, and thus ignorance of whether exercise is likely to be harmful or beneficial; the normal assumption of a breathless patient is that it is likely to be harmful, whereas the reverse is often true.

Shortness of breath is the usual symptom responsible for disability in lung disease, and this should be explored in terms of its development, its severity, and its variability. The pneumoconioses may produce breathlessness, usually of a slowly progressive type. The patient often adapts well to this and is able to perform physical tasks much better than one would expect from the degree of dysfunction. Asthma causes episodic breathlessness, and this is frequently exacerbated by exercise, so that the disability is often greater than would be expected from measurements of function made in the office during remission. A carefully taken history will allow a good assessment to be made of the patient's ability to perform normal tasks at home, such as gardening, repair work, and carrying loads, and at work in relation to the normal demands of the job.

Not infrequently, symptoms may wrongly be attributed to a known radiological abnormality, and the real cause, an unassociated disease, may be missed. In medicolegal work, it is commonplace to find symptoms from cardiac disease or emphysema attributed to simple pneumoconiosis or to pleural plaques, and the physician must always be wary of jumping without proper thought to superficially obvious but incorrect conclusions.

CASE HISTORY ■

A 65-year-old man had worked for 35 years at the coalface and had retired on health grounds 3 years before being referred to the chest clinic. His symptoms were dry cough and increasing shortness of breath, for the past year severe enough to prevent him from leaving the house. The symptoms were worse in the mornings and frequently woke him in the predawn hours. A chest radiograph 3 years previously had shown category 3 simple pneumoconiosis, and he had been told that this was the cause of his symptoms and that nothing could be done.

Knowledge that simple pneumoconiosis is not by itself a cause of breathlessness prompted further investigation. The disability was found to be related to severe airflow obstruction, which was largely relieved by a course of corticosteroids. Subsequent control of his asthma allowed him to return to a fully active life.

Sometimes, concentration on a litigation issue may blind doctors to an alternative diagnosis, with tragic consequences.

CASE HISTORY ■

A 55-year-old man presented with relatively rapid onset of breathlessness. There were no physical signs in his lung, but lung function tests showed a much reduced carbon monoxide transfer factor. Chest radiograph showed no definite abnormality. However, the history revealed that he had worked for several years in rubber tire manufacture and that it was possible that he might have been exposed to talc contaminated with tremolite. A radiologist decided that the radiographs were consistent with asbestosis, and a course of litigation was embarked on. The raised erythrocyte sedimentation rate (ESR) was ignored, as were the rapidly downhill course of the disease over only 3 years, the absence of finger clubbing and crackles, and the lack of a history of adequate asbestos exposure. The patient died of an undiagnosed but potentially treatable pulmonary arteritis, and the litigation was unsuccessful.

PHYSICAL EXAMINATION

The most striking finding in most patients with occupational lung diseases is the relative absence of physical signs. Certain conditions are nonetheless associated with physical signs, and the alert physician will note both their absence when a disease in which they should occur is suspected as well as their presence when the suspected disease is not usually associated with signs. Either finding should give rise to the consideration of an alternative diagnosis.

Clubbing of the digits is a physical sign that is easy to recognize when advanced and equally easy to exclude when the finger ends are completely normal. It should be noted that there are many situations in which it is not possible to be sure. Gross clubbing has always passed through a stage of transformation from normal to abnormal, and many normal nails are in a permanent shape suggestive of this stage of transformation. Repeated injury to the fingers often causes deformity resembling clubbing. It is the author's practice to grade clubbing as present, absent, or ''don't know.'' In these last cases, a tracing of the finger end on the patient's chart or a photograph allows later assessment of any change.

Clubbing occurs in asbestosis and usually appears after other evidence of the disease has become apparent. It does not normally occur in other mineral pneumoconioses or allergic alveolitis, and if it is present when one of these is suspected, it is wise to assume that the diagnosis is wrong or that the patient has an additional disease. The most common nonoccupational causes of clubbing are bronchial carcinoma and cryptogenic pulmonary fibrosis. Other diseases with which it is occasionally associated include hepatic cirrhosis, celiac disease, bronchiectasis, chronic pulmonary tuberculosis complicated by empyema or bronchiectasis, and lung abscess.

Bilateral, repetitive basal crackles (or crepitations) are heard in asbestosis and in acute and chronic allergic alveolitis. They are not heard in silicosis or coal workers' pneumoconiosis. However, the same types of crackles are heard in many nonoccupational diseases, for example, cryptogenic pulmonary fibrosis, bronchiectasis, left ventricular failure, and pneumonia. Similar crackles that clear after a few deep breaths are commonly heard at the lung bases in patients on first waking and in the obese. For this reason, it is important to make the patient take a few deep breaths and cough before listening carefully over the lower parts of the lungs for such crackles. If then they are heard to recur on several breaths, and if cardiac failure has been excluded, organic lung disease is likely to be present.

Distinction must be drawn between the crackles typical of pulmonary fibrosis, allergic alveolitis, and left ventricular failure, which occur in the middle and toward the end of inspiration and are always maximal in the dependent parts of the lung, and those due to bronchiectasis and pneumonia, which occur over the affected site. Moreover, repetitive crackles occurring in early inspiration occur in conditions associated with severe airways obstruction. Mid- and late inspiratory crackles are believed to be generated by delayed opening of small airways, each crackle characteristically occurring at the same transpulmonary pressure in each respiratory cycle.[2, 3] Such crackles are an important finding in suspected asbestosis, their presence in association with an appropriate exposure history considerably increasing the likelihood of the diagnosis. The more advanced the disease, the further up the lung from the bases they are heard. They are also heard when there is extensive asbestos-related pleural fibrosis, when the fibrosis extends into the peripheral parts of the lung. In allergic alveolitis, crackles may be the only physical sign, and, again in the presence of an appropriate exposure history, considerable weight should be attached to this finding.

CASE HISTORY ■

Mrs. W. worked in a pet shop. For the past year she had complained of exertional dyspnea, varying from day to day with no obvious pattern. Bilateral basal crackles were heard at the ends of inspiration. Her chest radiograph and spirometry were within normal limits, and precipitating antibodies to parakeet serum, droppings, and feathers were absent from her serum. In view of the crackles, further investigation was carried out. A slightly reduced lung diffusing capacity was found, and percutaneous lung biopsy showed evidence of extrinsic allergic alveolitis. Finally, a challenge test with parakeet extract produced a rise in temperature and a further fall in transfer factor after 4 hours, confirming the diagnosis. A short course of corticosteroids and avoidance of exposure prevented further symptoms.

Other physical signs are of less importance in occupational lung diseases. Intermittent wheezing may alert the occupational physician to work-related asthma, and the overinflation, quiet breath sounds, and hyper-resonance associated with advanced emphysema may be found in a proportion of patients with either chronic allergic alveolitis or progressive massive fibrosis. The technique of auscultatory percussion[4] may be an aid in the detection of masses in the latter condition, though the general availability of chest radiographs has allowed physicians to manage without this technique.

It should be remembered that physical examination of the chest, though traditionally focusing on anatomical abnormalities, also gives considerable insight into pulmonary function. Measurement of chest expansion gives a good indication of vital capacity; forced expiratory time is the best clinical test of airways obstruction;[5] and noisy breathing at the mouth denotes narrowing of the large airways,[3] while the relative intensity of breath sounds heard over the chest relates to regional ventilation.[6] Moreover, a simple exercise test, such as the 12-minute walking distance, is a useful indication of exercise tolerance. These clinical tests should be among the techniques that a physician can deploy in the assessment of pulmonary disorders.

CLINICAL INVESTIGATION

In most patients in whom an occupational lung disease is suspected, relatively little investigation is required beyond the history and physical examination. A chest radiograph is of course essential and is regarded by most chest physicians as a part of the examination. Some occupational lung diseases (for example, coal workers' pneumoconiosis and silicosis) are in practice diagnosed only on their radiological appearances. In others, such as asbestosis, serious doubts are cast on the diagnosis in the absence of an abnormal radiograph. However, contrary to the belief of some lawyers and even some of their medical witnesses, the chest radiograph is not an infallible guide to diagnosis. A normal radiograph is, of course, to be expected in occupational asthma and byssinosis, but it is not infrequent to find no abnormality in allergic alveolitis, where even quite extensive interstitial pneumonitis can exist in spite of a film regarded as within normal limits. Conversely, small irregular shadows are frequently seen on radiographs of the elderly, especially those with chronic bronchitis, in the absence of dust exposure.[7] Such age-related changes are indistinguishable from the early signs of asbestosis. Moreover, the interpretation of radiographic appearances is subject to wide inter- and intraobserver differences, and the sensible clinician in investigating suspected occupational lung disease will *record* changes seen and only attempt to *interpret* those changes in the light of other evidence from history, lung function testing, and so on. The uncertainties and variability attendant upon radiographic interpretation may be a considerable source of problems in epidemiological studies, and great care has to be taken in designing such studies to overcome this. The use of a standard set of radiographs,[8] several readers, and multiple readings has gone a long way toward solving these problems. However, uncertainty in the interpretation of a radiograph is reduced more by looking elsewhere for evidence than by comparison with standard films.

The role of computer-assisted tomography in the diagnosis of occupational lung diseases is increasing, although it will probably ultimately be judged to make only a marginal contribution to the welfare of patients. It is certainly better able to detect and define the size of pleural plaques and exclude false-positive results on conventional radiographs due to subpleural fat, though this is, of course, of no benefit to the individual's health.[9, 10] It has shown that asbestos-induced diffuse pleural fibrosis may extend into the superficial lung tissue, and it is able to detect pulmonary fibrosis with greater sensitivity than a standard radiograph.[9, 10] Like all new tests, it is very liable to be used uncritically, as though demonstration of a shadow were specific to a particular disease. Before using it, the appropriate question to ask is whether the additional information (and expense) is justified by likely benefit to the patient's health.

The other investigation most likely to be helpful is pulmonary function testing. Here the tests should be determined by the suspected diagnosis. To the non-physiologist, a bewildering array of tests is available; but, fortunately, in clinical practice only a few of these are helpful, and these all are relatively simple. Any organic pulmonary disorder causing disability must be associated with a functional abnormality either of airways caliber or of gas transfer and/or lung volumes. Fixed airways obstruction, as in chronic byssinosis and emphysema, is best demonstrated by simple spirometry, while variable obstruction such as that which occurs in occupational asthma is best diagnosed by asking the patient to record frequent peak flow rates with a portable meter—a process infinitely cheaper and more valuable than body plethysmography. Diseases such as asbestosis and silicosis, which cause pulmonary fibrosis, are best assessed by measurement of vital capacity, lung volumes, and diffusing capacity. Exercise testing is of value in assessing exercise tolerance, and the more complicated exercise tests with arterial gas analysis are useful in excluding the presence of any organic cause for respiratory disability. Measurements of compliance, closing volumes, flow-volume loops, and airways resistance are appealing to the physiologist but are of little additional clinical value, and physicians dealing with occupational lung diseases should think twice, or preferably more often, before putting their patients through the expense of undergoing them.

Blood tests make less contribution to the diagnosis of occupational lung diseases than in many other areas of medicine. Positive diagnostic help may be obtained in allergic alveolitis, in those instances in which precipitating antibody may be found, and in some cases of occupational asthma in which specific IgE antibody may be demonstrated by radioallergosorbent test (RAST). Tests for rheumatoid factors may help in the diagnosis of Caplan's syndrome, and very occasionally measurements of blood or urine levels may help in the diagnosis of acute toxic pneumonitis. In most occupational lung diseases, however, the hazard is known, and the diagnostic problem is to demonstrate whether the disease is present.

The most difficult decisions to make in the investigation of occupational lung disease are whether or not to perform challenge tests or lung biopsy. In general, since both these procedures entail a small hazard, they should not be performed unless there is serious doubt about the diagnosis. Challenge testing needs to be done in occasional cases of allergic alveolitis or asthma in which the diagnosis or the allergen is in doubt. A test approximating most closely the environment of the patient's work (and that may mean a test done at the patient's place of work) is probably the safest, but close medical supervision is always necessary. A proper question for the physician to ask before performing such a test is whether the result, whatever it is, will alter the management of the patient. It is not ethically justifiable to subject one's patient to such procedures for medicolegal reasons alone.

Lung biopsy is potentially more hazardous than challenge testing and rarely needs to be done when an occupational cause is seriously suspected. In the author's practice, biopsies on patients with occupational lung disease have usually been performed when an other than occupational cause was seriously considered and management depended on knowing which condition the patient had. If lung biopsy is considered necessary, the choice should depend on the physician's experience. Probably the most generally used technique since fiberoptic bronchoscopy was introduced has been transbronchial biopsy. This has the disadvantage of producing such small fragments that the pathologist is often unable to narrow the differential diagnosis. It has the advantage of allowing bronchoalveolar lavage, which may occasionally be helpful in the diagnosis of allergic alveolitis and berylliosis. Open lung biopsy provides excellent specimens for the pathologist, though it is much more uncomfortable for the patient; the recent introduction of thoracoscopic lung biopsy has gone some way toward ameliorating this problem. For diffuse disease, which occupational disease usually is, a cutting needle is traumatic and can cause serious hemorrhage. Use of the Steel high-speed drill[11] is less likely to tear the lung and usually produces a good core of lung. If the patient breathes oxygen for a few minutes beforehand, pneumothorax is rarely troublesome, though death from hemorrhage has been reported from this as well as from all other pulmonary and bronchial biopsy procedures. None of these tests should be embarked upon lightly.

MANAGEMENT

An interest in occupational lung disease often extends only to diagnosis of the conditions. The clinician, however, also has the problem of management of the patient once the diagnosis has been made. Management can be divided into assessment of the disability, prognosis, treatment, and advice.

Assessment of disability is essential to making a reasonable prognosis and advising the patient on such matters as future employment prospects. Disability, discussed previously, is a measurement of the patient's inability to perform normal daily tasks, and therefore is more than just a measure of lung function. Its assessment has to take into account lung function, the patient's work requirements, and any psychological reaction to the illness. Prognosis is based on knowledge of the natural history of the patient's illness, information that this book is intended to provide, and of the stage of physiological deterioration that the clinical examination and testing have revealed. Armed with this information, the physician can plan the treatment in order to attempt to alter the course of the disease or palliate its symptoms.

In many cases of occupational lung disease, therapeutics has little part to play, and treatment usually consists of advice on avoiding future exposure to dust or fumes at work. It should not be forgotten, however, that some diseases may be affected by corticosteroids. Berylliosis and, probably, acute toxic pneumonitis respond to these drugs, and allergic alveolitis may require such treatment in addition to avoidance of further exposure. The mineral pneumoconioses in general do not respond to therapy, but they vary considerably in their natural histories; this should be considered when advising the patient. For example, a coal miner developing the early signs of pneumoconiosis 5 years before he is due to retire might well be advised to continue at work, since he is unlikely to progress to massive fibrosis at that stage of his life. Similarly, radiologic shadowing in a welder usually need not cause concern unless it is felt to be due to a nonoccupational cause, as siderosis is a benign condition. However, pneumoconiosis in a 40-year-old coal miner or asbestosis at any age is an indication to cease further dust exposure, since both entail a serious risk of progression to crippling disease.

The most difficult aspect of the management of patients with occupational lung disease is giving sensible advice. The usual explanations of causation, treatment, and prognosis need to be amplified by advice on employment. More harm may be done by well-intentioned but incorrect advice on future employment, based on an imperfect knowledge of the disease, than by the disease itself. Furthermore, the knowledge that the disease was caused by the occupation not infrequently gives rise to resentment in the patient and, with a little help from legal advisers and union officials, to thoughts of compensaition. Society inevitably has to accept some cost in human health for the benefits of industry's productivity, and while in a just society all ill health should attract appropriate compensation whatever its cause, regrettably utopia is not yet with us. Compensation laws and their interpretation differ from country to country and from state to state, and benefits are often inequitable or inadequate. In such a situation, common law claims for injury due to an employer's negligence are an understandable and frequent outcome of the diagnosis of occupational lung disease. The doctor may well be asked by the patient whether to pursue such a claim. In such circumstances, the clinician should advise only on diagnosis, causation, and management and leave legal advice, particularly on matters of liability and negligence, to lawyers. Here, as in other fields, medicolegal considerations can be a dangerous distraction from objectivity in doing one's best for one's patient.

The chest physician is in the unusual position of dealing with an organ of which the diseases are largely caused by outside agents, whether bacteria, allergens, cigarette smoke, or other pollutants. The pollutants to which people are exposed in their occupations are an important source of lung diseases and constitute a challenge to the alert physician. The physician who bears this in mind will not only help his or her patients but will also lead the way in preventing disease in others.

REFERENCES

1. Parmeggiani, L., ed., Encyclopaedia of occupational health and safety, 3rd ed. Geneva, International Labour Office, 1983.
2. Nath, A. R., and Capel, L. H., Inspiratory crackles and mechanical events of breathing. Thorax, 29, 695, 1974.
3. Forgacs, P., Lung Sounds. London, Bailliere Tindall, 1978.
4. Guarino, J. R., Auscultatory percussion of the chest. Lancet, 1, 1332, 1980.
5. Macdonald, J. B., Cole, T. J., and Seaton, A., Forced expiratory time—its reliability as a lung function test. Thorax, 30, 554, 1975.
6. Leblanc, P., Macklem, P. T., and Ross, W. R. D., Breath sounds and the distribution of pulmonary ventilation. Am. Rev. Resp. Dis., 102, 10, 1970.
7. Weiss, W., Cigarette smoking and small irregular opacities. Br. J. Ind. Med., 48, 841, 1991.

8. ILO/UC international classification of radiographs of pneumoconioses. Occupational Safety and Health, Series 22. Geneva, International Labour Office, 1980.

9. Friedman, A. C., Fiel, S. B., Fisher, M. S., et al., Asbestos-related pleural disease and asbestosis: a comparison of CT and chest radiography. Am. J. Roentgenol., 150, 269, 1988.

10. Lozewicz, S., Reznek, R. H., Herdman, M., et al., Role of computed tomography in evaluating asbestos related lung disease. Br. J. Ind. Med., 46, 777, 1989.

11. Steel, S. J., and Winstanley, D. P., Lung biopsy with a high-speed air drill. Thorax, 22, 286, 1967.

4

Legal Aspects of Industrial Disease

W. Keith C. Morgan

■

From the time of Ramazzini (1633–1714), there has been a gradual increase in the awareness of the dangers of certain occupations,[1] but until Victorian times preventive measures were largely voluntary and depended primarily on the conscience of the employer. With the advent of the Industrial Revolution, the problem of industrial injury and disease increased tenfold. It became obvious that the health of the worker had to be safeguarded and, moreover, that this could be effected only by legislation. The hideous conditions in which the British laboring class worked and lived remained largely unknown and ignored until reformers such as Shaftesbury, Owen, Chadwick, and Simon called them to the attention of the government and people. Dickens' graphic descriptions of mill and factory working life disposed the growing middle class to the need for social and industrial reform. Without adequate morbidity and mortality statistics, truly appalling death rates in certain industries were known only to a few persons. In Sheffield, cutlery trade workers were dying of silicosis with as little as 5 years' exposure. The condition became known as "grinders' rot." Because of the horrific conditions which prevailed in many factories in which children were employed, a series of acts concerned with the medical supervision of industrial workers came into existence. The first of these was the Factory Act of 1844, which made provision for the appointment of factory surgeons to certify that children and other young persons employed in the factories were physically capable of working and were not incapacitated by disease. This was followed by the Factory Act of 1891, which introduced special rules and regulations to protect the health of workers in those industries where dangerous materials were in production or being handled. A detailed and excellent account of the various social and industrial reforms which took place in 19th century Britain and slightly later in the United States can be found in Donald Hunter's book *The Diseases of Occupations*.[2]

I was never ruined but twice, once when I lost a lawsuit and once when I won one.

VOLTAIRE

WORKMEN'S (WORKERS') COMPENSATION

In the 19th century, the only recourse open to a workman who was injured while at work was to bring a common law action against the employer. Since the worker had neither the understanding nor the money to finance such litigation, successful actions were rare. To help the workmen, Employer's Liability Statutes came into effect. These made provision for financial compensation in the case of industrial disease or injury, but the employer had three powerful defenses against such actions. Thus, an employer was not held responsible (1) if it could be shown that another worker was wholly or partly responsible for the injury, (2) if the injury occurred as a result of the worker's own negligence, or (3) if the workman knew of or should have known that such injury or illness was an inherent risk in the occupation. With such defenses available to the employer, it was indeed unusual for a worker to win a case.

In 1907, industrial injury was responsible for over 7000 deaths among the U.S. coal miners and railroad workers, yet for the reasons given above, very few if any of the workers' families received compensation. Although recompense was in theory available, the worker's family was usually forced to rely on charity for its existence. Compensation under Common Law for industrially acquired injuries evolved for the most part during a period when most businesses were family concerns with a strictly limited number of employees. When an accident occurred, the employer saw to it that the injured party's medical and financial needs were provided for. Common law suits attracted little attention and still less sympathy, and the courts were for the most part unconcerned about industrial injury.

In the first few years of the 20th century, a series of Workmen's Compensation Acts were put into effect in Britain, and shortly after in the U.S. and Canada. In Britain, the Acts applied to the whole country; in the U.S. and Canada, each state or province enacted its own laws. The prime purpose of the Workmen's Compensation Laws was to provide adequate benefits while limiting the employer's liability to Workmen's Compensation payments. The payments or premiums were to be predetermined so as to avoid uncertainty for the injured man and the employer. Appropriate medical care was to be provided and costly litigation avoided. Most important of all was the establishment of the principle of liability without fault; the cost of the compensation was to be assigned to the employer, not because he was always culpable, but because of the inherent risks of industrial employment. Thus, assent was given to the concept that awards for industrial injury and sickness were part of the cost of production. The introduction of Workmen's Compensation was a tremendous social advance; but even so, in the U.S., obligations for industrial injury and sickness were sometimes inadequate, occasionally evaded, and in addition there were and are large disparities among the various states. From 1932 to 1934, more than 400 workmen were reported to have died from acute silicosis after working on the Gauley Bridge Tunnel in southern West Virginia.[3-5] The bodies were buried in secret so that exhumation was impossible, thereby preventing legal action based on autopsy evidence. Not a single worker received compensation for the illness contracted, and the families were equally unfortunate. The contractor, the state of West Virginia, and Congress itself all were derelict as far as their responsibilities were concerned. This occurred despite the existence of the Workmen's Compensation Laws in the state concerned.

It has become apparent over the years that many other inadequacies exist in the U.S. system, and as a result, a National Commission was appointed by the President to study the effectiveness and operation of Workmen's Compensation Laws in the U.S. The Commission published its report in 1972 and detailed three major deficiencies in the present system.[6] These included the following:

1. *The number of employees covered by Workmen's Compensation.* At that time only 85% of U.S. employees were covered by state and federal programs. In certain areas and in certain states, a little over 50% of the work force was covered. Those excluded from such social programs were usually the lowest paid and the most in need, namely, farm workers, employees of small firms, and casual laborers. Over the past 20 years, only a slight increase in the number of workers covered has occurred. In this regard, some states still permit elective coverage.

2. *The variation in injury and diseases covered.* There is little uniformity from state to state as to which diseases or injuries are regarded as occupationally related. Thus, some states do not recognize byssinosis or farmer's lung, and furthermore, benefits for the same degree of disability differ widely from state to state and in some instances are inadequate. Some states recognize only total disability, while others make provision for partial disability. There is a regrettable but easily understood tendency for industry to move to those states where Workmen's Compensation Laws are less liberal. In addition, certain industries, in particular coal mining,

have their own Federal Coal Mine Health and Safety Acts, which provide infinitely more generous compensation than is available to other workers. Currently, the U.S. taxpayer is paying $1.5 billion a year for black lung benefits.[7] This is approximately 35% to 40% of the total sum being disbursed for all injury and illness.[8]

3. *The provision of medical care and rehabilitation services.* Workmen's Compensation system provides reasonable coverage for medical care; however, only 25% of the beneficiaries receive any form of vocational rehabilitation.

When the National Commission published its report, it made many recommendations, few of which have been put into effect.[6] For the most part, the Commission continued to recommend that each state continue with its own set of laws, failing to realize that the present system guarantees that inequities will persist and that uniformity will not be achieved. In Britain, in contrast to the U.S. and Canada, Workers' Compensation Laws or their equivalent apply to the whole country, benefits are uniform, and there are no regional differences in the administration of compensation.

Separate from State Workers' Compensation regulations and benefits, but nonetheless related to them, is the problem of compensation for coal workers' pneumoconiosis. As a result of the Federal Coal Mine Health and Safety Acts of 1969 and thereafter, a program for compensation for occupationally related respiratory disease of coal miners came into effect. Regulations were established by which miners who had complicated pneumoconiosis were automatically assumed to be totally and permanently disabled. Those with simple coal workers' pneumoconiosis had to have a certain degree of respiratory impairment before they were likewise considered totally and permanently disabled. This created a situation in which a coal miner who happened to be a cigarette smoker and who developed emphysema and significant obstruction and who also had radiographic evidence of coal workers' pneumoconiosis was awarded compensation, while the coal miner with coal workers' pneumoconiosis who happened to be a nonsmoker but who had no significant impairment would fail to be compensated. With the passage of time, the regulations have been amended and now conform to some extent with medical and scientific knowledge.

Initially, the responsibility for compensating disabled coal miners was given to the Social Security Administration (SSA), but the cost became so enormous that it was necessary to introduce what was known as the Black Lung Trust Fund, the administration of which became the responsibility mainly of the Department of Labor. The latter was charged with setting up and administering the Trust Fund with the help of the Department of Health and Human Services and the U.S. Treasury. The Trust Fund came into existence in order to transfer the responsibility of the Black Lung Benefits from the taxpayer, i.e., the federal government, to the coal industry and its insurers. The Black Lung Trust Fund revenues are derived from the coal companies in the form of an excise tax on each ton of coal mined, from the mine owners who owe the Fund money, from refunds for overpayment to claimants, and from repayable advances from the Treasury. At the present time, there is a 4.4% tax on both underground and surface coal. In addition, in 1981 a temporary special tax was added, and this now stands at $1.10 on underground coal and $0.55 on surface-mined coal. The temporary tax will remain in effect until December 2013.

At the end of September 1992, the latest year for which data are available, there were 147,200 primary beneficiaries (miners or their widows) receiving $820 million annually from the Social Security Administration.[7, 8] The average monthly benefit for miners was $593.00 and for widows $414.60. The SSA assumed responsibility for claims up to 1973 and is saddled with the responsibility of processing and paying claims of survivors of this group of miners. The number of beneficiaries who have been receiving benefits from SSA has been slowly declining over the past 15 years. By 1992, the Department of Labor, through the Black Lung Disability Trust Fund, provided benefits for 77,500 beneficiaries each month. At the end of October 1993, the Trust Fund had a balance of $12.4 million, but owed the Treasury $3.9 billion, despite there being a 5-year moratorium on the interest charges due the Treasury on the Trust Fund's accumulated debt.

There are only approximately 95,000 working coal miners in the U.S., as compared to approximately 125 million other workers. It is estimated that approximately 30% to 35% of total disability awards—excluding awards under civil litigation for asbestos and other induced diseases—are going to less than 0.1% of the working population.[9] The precise data are not available, mainly because Workmens' Compensation payments from some states are not available, and because some states award not only total disability but partial disability.[8, 9] In addition, there are offsets for other sources of income. The Black Lung Program also provides for the payment of attorneys' fees and legal costs connected with approved benefit claims. In 1989, there were 1107 fee petitions from lawyers, and more than $3 million was paid to them. In 1992, the fee petitions had fallen to 590, and attorneys' fees from the Trust Fund were $1.8 million. The equivalent expenditure for medical bills for the treatment of coal dust–induced disease in 1989 was $104 million, but this had risen to $112 million by 1992. The total Trust Fund disbursements for 1992 were $973.6 million.

COMPENSATION FOR OCCUPATIONAL LUNG DISEASES IN BRITAIN AND CANADA

Compensation for industrial disease in Britain is administered by the Department of Social Security (DSS). Before a claim is recognized, it must relate to a prescribed disease. As such, any disease may become a prescribed condition if it is shown that it is a risk of specific prescribed employment or occupation and not a risk encountered by the general population. A specific occupational association must be established with reasonable certainty before the disease can be prescribed. The inclusion of new diseases on the prescribed list depends on the deliberations of the Industrial Injuries Advisory Council. This body consists mainly of medical scientists, industrial hygienists, and other experts, but lay representatives are also included. A second requirement must be fulfilled in that the claimant should have been employed as an insured person in an occupation in which the prescribed disease is known to occur.

When a worker believes that he or she has contracted a prescribed disease (e.g., silicosis, asbestosis, hard metal disease), he or she lodges a claim at the nearest DSS Office, where the Social Security Officer checks first that the worker has been employed in a prescribed occupation by ascertaining present or past employment and second that he or she is or has been an insured person. The worker is then referred for medical examination by a panel of doctors known as the Medical Board (Respiratory Diseases) which is responsible for confirming the diagnosis and assessing the level of disablement; however, if the claim is rejected, he or she can appeal to the Pneumoconiosis Medical Board.

If the prescribed disease (e.g., pneumoconiosis) is found to be present in the claimant, then the Medical Board assesses the degree of disablement. This is expressed as a percentage, with the lowest award being 10% and higher awards being multiples of 10%. Disablement is assessed according to (1) the severity of the symptoms; (2) the findings on physical examination; (3) the degree of radiographic abnormality, where appropriate; and (4) the results of biological testing, e.g., lung function. Assessment is based on loss of faculty—that is, the ability to perform physically to that level of a person of the same age and sex, taking into account the demands of that job. The claimant may appeal to a Medical Appeal Tribunal over the Board's decision in regard to the accuracy of the diagnosis and the extent of any disablement that has been awarded.

In Canada, each province has its own Workers' Compensation Board (WCB). A worker or his or her physician lodges a claim with the provincial WCB, which is then considered. If it is felt that the claim may be valid, the worker's occupational history and all relevant medical data are reviewed and a decision is made. In some instances the applicant may be asked by the WCB to return for a further examination and tests. The size of the award is based on the severity of the impairment present. Should the claim be rejected, appeal mechanisms exist, and a worker may request a further hearing. Once the claimant has accepted a WCB award for disability, he or she is precluded from suing the former employer under Common Law. It is stressed that while the general principles of Workers' Compensation laws are similar in all the provinces with the exception of Quebec, individual differences exist as to the diseases and conditions compensated and as to how disability is assessed.

CIVIL LITIGATION

Aside from Workmen's Compensation, workers have the right to bring a lawsuit against a company if they consider that the company or employer has been negligent and has not conformed to the legislated rules and regulations. In Canada such an option is not available in most provinces, and once the worker has been awarded compensation, he or she forfeits the right to sue the employer.

In the U.S. most claims for civil damages under Common Law are tried by jury. Should the claimant reside in one state and the company being sued have a plant or factory in the same state, the action usually takes place in a state court. On the other hand, should the claimant reside in a state where the company has no plant or facility, and its headquarters are located elsewhere, the trial takes place in a Federal court. The rules vary from state to state, and in many the judge who is sitting on the bench is elected by the constituents of his or her county or congressional district. It is not uncommon for claims to be consolidated, and under these circumstances the judge may have 50 to 100 claimants along with their families in attendance at the trial. Many claimants and their families may have voted for the judge in prior elections and intend to keep him or her on the bench provided he or she is suitably compliant. Moreover, the same defense often leads to disparate verdicts according to the state in which the trial takes place, the composition of the jury, whether the trial is held before a state or federal judge, and the extent of leeway permitted counsel by the bench. With every claimant allowed, indeed encouraged, to bring suit and with every case having a different jury, it is impossible to rely on precedent. Thus, while one jury might decide that the first investigation to show conclusively that asbestos was a carcinogen was the 1955 Doll study, at a later date a second jury might decide that the association should have been known as far back as 1934 following the publication of a case report.

In the U.S. many lawyers take cases on a contingency basis, and as such their fee is related to whether they win the suit and on the extent of the damages that the particular claimant is awarded—both of which are strong incentives to enter into litigation. There is little doubt that in the U.S. at the present time an attempt is being made to relate virtually all naturally occurring disease to occupational exposure, and suits for all types of so-called occupational injury and illness are extremely common.[10, 11] The present system has done much to undermine the public's faith in the legal and medical professions, but since vast sums of money are involved, it is likely to persist at least for a time. Under such circumstances, one cannot but sympathize with Jonathan Swift when he defined lawyers as a "breed of men bred up from their youth in the art of proving by words that white is black and black is white, according as they are paid."

Litigation for alleged injury due to exposure to asbestos in the U.S. has become an industry, and fortunes have been and continue to be made. A fair number of claimants' lawyers are making between $1 million and $20 million annually.[12] The firms in which they are partners often own private jets and generally enjoy la dolce vita. All of this has come about through the acceptance of cases on a contingency basis, with the claimant's lawyer taking anything from 30% to over 50% of the award, and the expenses subsequently being deducted from the residue of the award. One humorist defined the contingency fee as follows, "If I lose my lawyer gets nothing, and if I win I get nothing." It has been reliably calculated that the claimant sees approximately 20% to 30% of the total award in the average case in which asbestos-induced injury is alleged. The rest of the award goes for the cost of the trial, many of which last 2 to 3 months or more, to the expert witnesses, and to the other camp followers. As a result, many of the larger U.S. asbestos companies who formerly manufactured products containing asbestos have gone out of business or are operating under Chapter 11, a legal euphemism for modified bankruptcy. In addition, a large number of workers have lost their jobs. In one instance, a company came out of Chapter 11, having set aside a large sum for compensation of workers who it was felt were likely to develop asbestos-related disease over the next 20 years. The welter of claims, and to use one federal judge's term, "the avariciousness of the claimants' lawyers," in 2 years forced the company back into Chapter 11.[13]

In 1985 the Institute for Civil Justice of the Rand Corporation commented on the system of civil justice in the U.S. and its handling of asbestos claims in these terms: "The picture is not a pretty one. Decisions concerning thousands of deaths, millions of injuries, and billions of dollars are entangled in a litigation system and its strengths have been increasingly overshadowed by its weaknesses." While there is a fair bit of hyperbole in this statement, at least in regard to the number of injuries, most authorities felt that otherwise it was an accurate statement. Since then the situation has only worsened, the delays in court have become worse, and many persons who have no significant asbestos-induced disease have been persuaded to seek redress through civil litigation. Nevertheless, although most genuine claims for serious asbestos-induced injury other than mesothelioma have been satisfied, the anticipated decline in litigation has not materialized. The U.S. legal profession, aided and abetted by certain doctors, perhaps realizing that litigation for occupational exposure to asbestos is and will continue to decline, has fostered the notion that the incorporation and use of asbestos in the construction of buildings constitutes a horrendous hazard. As a result, the manufacturers of asbestos-containing building materials are being sued for not placing a warning on the materials used in construction. The notion that asbestos-containing buildings constitute a hazard has been furthered by the Environmental Protection Agency[14] and sundry other U.S. government agencies despite compelling evidence to the contrary.[15] Scientific or rather paratoxicological meetings have been organized for the tendentious purpose of endorsing this view, and in one instance was supported by money from the Claimants' Escrow Fund.[16] Meanwhile, many former manufacturers of asbestos-containing material have gone bankrupt, and the few remaining companies still operating are in a relatively parlous financial state. Jobs have been lost by many, and fortunes made by a cadre of lawyers.

Uncontrolled litigation in the U.S. is stultifying the free market, encouraging dishonesty, and awarding large sums for trivial or nonexistent injuries. According to Evans-Pritchard, "The Protestant ethic of individual responsibility is giving way to the anti-ethic of whingeing fecklessness in which somebody else is always to blame."[17] He describes an incident in which a jury in Long Island ordered an outdoor restaurant to pay $3 million in damages to a customer stung by a bee—a nonresident bee at that! The American Tort Reform Association states that the U.S. has twenty times more lawsuits per person than Japan. It further states that litigation imposes a tax of $117 billion, or 2.6% of the gross national product, on American business, mostly in the form of higher insurance and legal costs. How long such a system can last without bankrupting the country is debatable.

In Canada, should the allegedly injured party seek redress through Workmens' Compensation or its equivalent, then he or she cannot bring suit under the laws of tort. In that country and in Britain, should he or she seek damages under Common Law, the hearing takes place before a judge. In all instances, the judge has been appointed from among the body of practicing advocates and not elected, and is usually experienced and held in esteem by their respective bar associations. Nonetheless, occasional mavericks are found on the bench, and a variety of illogical or wayward verdicts are handed down. In such circumstances, the right to appeal to a higher court is available. Much of the evidence given by expert witnesses involves controversial medical and scientific matters, and as such a judge with broad experience, greater education, and higher intelligence is more likely to render an unbiased and logical verdict than is a jury. Nevertheless, it is easy to underestimate the common sense and fairness of many jurors. Unfortunately, jurors are swayed by sympathy and tend to feel that large companies usually exploit the average worker, and in any case assume that because the company is insured   often an incorrect assumption   the verdict for damages will have little effect on the financial state.

THE PEARSON REPORT

In Britain the issue of tort has been the subject of much discussion, and in 1973 a Royal Commission on civil liability and compensation was set up.[18] The stimulus to the appointment of the Commission was the Report of The Robens Committee on Safety and Health at Work. The charge given to the Commission was to consider to what extent, under what circumstances, and by what means compensation should be payable for death and injuries suffered under the following five circumstances:

1. In the course of employment
2. During the use of a motor vehicle or other means of transportation
3. Through the manufacture, supply, or use of goods and services
4. On property belonging to or occupied by another party
5. Otherwise through an act of omission by another person where compensation is recuperable only on proof of fault or under rules of strict liability

Put more explicitly, the Commission was charged with producing a report which would recommend the first steps to be taken toward the introduction of a unified system that would deal with all injuries and which would apply to the whole country. In time, the system would be extended so that provision would be made to compensate all disabled persons irrespective of cause, that is to say, whether the disability was the result of injury or of acquired or congenital disease.

The recommendations of the Commission were eventually published and have become known as the Pearson Report.[18, 19] Some of the more radical suggestions relate to modifications of the laws of tort, namely those actions arising from private or civil wrongs. While not recommending the complete abolition of tort, the report did seek to limit its role as a means of obtaining redress for injury (e.g., by offsetting Social Security payments against tort damages). They also recommended that compensation awards should be indexed so that the payments did not decrease with inflation. Other suggestions related to the elimination of certain minor claims and changes in the method of assessment of damages. The Pearson Report can be regarded as a landmark and a first step toward achieving a comprehensive and equitable compensation for all forms of disability. It proposes and supports the concept of no-fault and suggests that those who are disabled should be compensated because of their needs rather than because of another's fault.

Inherent in any civilized society is the tenet that such a society should provide its disabled members with sufficient financial support for the necessities of life. Ethically and morally it matters little whether the disability is industrially acquired or not. If this doctrine is accepted, the same impairment and the same disability should receive the same compensation. To continue with the present tort laws suggests that the person who loses a leg in an industrial injury is somehow worthy of greater compensation than the man who through no fault of his own loses a leg in a car accident. In the U.S., it is clear that the only way of realizing a situation in which equal compensation is paid for equal disability is through a Federal Worker's Compensation system administered in the same fashion as Social Security.[20] This would necessitate an actuarial assessment of the frequency of industrial injury and disease throughout the nation. Based on these data, every employer would pay a premium into a centrally administered fund. Also being paid into the same fund would be that portion of each Social Security payment that is put toward premature and permanent disability awards. Such a system would ensure that the employer would be compelled to assume financial responsibility for industrial injury and disease, and premiums could be weighted according to the health and safety record of the company concerned. Impairment would then be determined by a panel of physicians with wide experience in disability assessment rather than being left to the whims of a sympathetic but partial jury and the avarice of a financially involved lawyer.

With the passage of time, more and more industrial hazards are being recognized. Since the 1960s, the etiology of mesothelioma has been recognized, and the role of vinyl chloride monomer in the induction of angiosarcoma of the liver and of many chemicals in the etiology of asthma and pulmonary hemorrhage have been described. Inevitably, there is a delay in the introduction of preventive measures designed to control such diseases, and it is usually even longer before legislative action which gives them official recognition comes into effect. There is little doubt that with advancing technology, new industrial hazards will develop, and as such their initial recognition will depend on somebody asking the time honored question, ''What is your job?''

REFERENCES

1. Ramazzini, B., De Morbis Artificum Diatriba. Geneva, 1713, Wright, W. C., translator, Chicago, University of Chicago Press, 1940.
2. Hunter, D., The Diseases of Occupations, 6th ed. London, English Universities Press, 1978.
3. Skidmore, H., Hawk's Nest. New York, Doubleday, 1941.
4. Subcommittee of the Committee of Labor, House of Representatives. An investigation relating to health conditions of workers employed in construction and maintenance of public utilities, 74th Congress, H.J. Res. 449, 2603, 1936.
5. Cherniack, M., The Hawk's Nest Incident. New Haven, CT, Yale University Press, 1987.
6. Report of the National Commission on State Workmens' Compensation Laws. Washington, D.C., Government Printing Office, 1972.
7. Black Lung Disability Trust Report for Period up to 10/31/93. Washington, D.C., Department of the Treasury, October 1993.
8. Office of Workers' Compensation Programs. Report to Congress 1992. Submitted to Congress, Washington, D.C., May 1993.
9. Nelson, W. J., Workers' Compensation: Coverage, Benefits, and Costs, 1988. Social Security Bulletin, Vol 54, No 3, Washington, D.C., Government Printing Office, March 1991.
10. Morgan, W. K. C., On Disability, Demagoguery, and Dialectic. Forum XIV, 3, 473, 1979. Published by the American Bar Association.
11. Morgan, W. K. C., Compensation for industrial injury and disease. Am. Rev. Respir. Dis., 114, 1047, 1976.
12. Dillon, K., Only 1.5 million a year. The American Lawyer, pp 38–44, October 1989.
13. McAvoy, P. W., The economic consequences of asbestos disease. [Working paper No 27, Series C. Research Program in Government Business Relations.] New Haven, CT, Yale School of Organization and Management, 1982, pp. 85, 86.
14. Nicholson, W., Quoted in: Guidance for Controlling Asbestos Containing Materials in Buildings. EPA 560/5-83-002. U.S. Environmental Protection Agency, Office of Pesticides and Toxic Substances, Washington, D.C., 1983.
15. Mossman, B. T., Bignon, J., Corn, M., et al., Asbestos: scientific developments and implications for public policy. Science 247, 294, 1990.
16. Collegium Ramazzini Conference. Questioned by defendants. Mealey Litigation Reports. Mealey Publications, 5, 49, Oct 19, 1990.
17. Evans-Pritchard, A., Chipping away the USA. Sunday Telegraph, London, June 20, 1993.
18. The Report of the Royal Commission on Civil Liability, Compensation for Personal Injury, Vol 1. London, Her Majesty's Stationery Office, 1978.
19. Collinson, J. M., The Pearson Report. Br. J. Ind. Med. 36, 263, 1979.
20. Morgan, W. K. C., The adversary system: cui bono? Ann. Intern. Med. 97, 919, 1982.

5

Pulmonary Physiology— Its Application to the Determination of Respiratory Impairment and Disability in Industrial Lung Disease*

W. Keith C. Morgan

Douglas Seaton

■

The primary purpose of the lungs is to maintain the oxygen and carbon dioxide content of the arterial blood within a relatively narrow range. This has to be effected despite the fact that both oxygen needs and carbon dioxide production are constantly changing with the degree of activity and metabolic rate of the subject. The lungs achieve this homeostasis by allowing venous blood to come into contact with the alveolar gases, such contact taking place over an enormous surface area, the alveolocapillary bed. Three basic mechanisms are involved in gas exchange, namely, (1) ventilation, or, as it is often known, the bellows function of the lungs, (2) diffusion, or the transfer of gas from the alveolus to the capillary, and (3) perfusion, or pulmonary blood flow.

VENTILATION

The ventilatory capacity of the lungs depends first on the size of the lungs (lung volumes), second, on the resistance to flow present in the airways, and third, on the elastic properties or compliance of the lungs and the chest wall. Movement of air in and out of the lungs can be compared to the action of a pair of bellows and is dependent on the pressure difference between the mouth and the alveoli at various phases of breathing. At times of no flow, alveolar and mouth pressure are equal. During inspiration, the thorax enlarges, the diaphragm descends, and as a result the chest cage increases in volume, as do the lungs. In contrast, expiration is largely passive and depends on the elastic recoil of the chest wall and lungs. The pressure that acts upon the lungs and causes them to expand during inspiration is that which exists in the pleural cavity. Intrapleural pressure is negative as compared to the atmospheric pressure, and during normal breathing varies between -5 and -9 cm H_2O. Much larger pressure changes occur during forced expiratory and inspiratory maneuvers; for example, at total lung capacity, the intrapleural pressure is -35 to -40 cm H_2O, while at residual volume, the pressure may become slightly positive, especially at the lung bases. A detailed description of the mechanical events involved in inspiration is beyond the scope of this chapter but can be found in *The Respiratory Muscles*.[1]

*Portions of this chapter also appear in W. Keith C. Morgan and D. Seaton, Pulmonary ventilation and blood gas exchange. *In* W. A. Sodeman, Jr., and T. M. Sodeman, eds., Sodeman's Pathologic Physiology, 7th ed. Philadelphia, W. B. Saunders Co., 1985.

35

At this stage it is necessary to point out that there is a gradient in pleural pressure from the top to the bottom of the lung. This gradient is largely gravity dependent and is thought to be related to the weight of the lung. Pleural pressure increases from the apex to the base, with a gradient of around 7 to 8 cm H_2O from top to bottom of the lung. This gradient has profound effects on regional ventilation, and perfusion and will be discussed in more detail later in the chapter.

Static Lung Volumes

Certain lung volumes can be measured with a spirometer; however, others require more complicated apparatus. The volume of each breath exhaled during quiet respiration is known as the tidal volume (V_T). The total volume of air that the lungs and bronchial tree contain after maximal inspiration is known as the total lung capacity (TLC). If the subject then exhales as much air as he or she can, the volume of air remaining in the lungs after the expiration is known as the residual volume (RV), while that which has been expelled is known as the vital capacity (VC). It must be stressed that during the measurement of VC, the patient is permitted to take as long as necessary to complete the maneuver. If after maximal inspiration, he or she exhales as rapidly and as forcibly as possible, then the measurement obtained is known as the forced vital capacity (FVC). In normal persons the FVC and the VC are not significantly different; however, in certain types of airways obstruction, e.g., emphysema, the FVC may be considerably less than the VC as a result of collapse of the smaller airways during forced expiration; this is a phenomenon known as air trapping. The volume of air remaining in the lung at the end of a normal tidal expiration is known as the functional residual capacity (FRC), whereas the volume that can be exhaled from FRC is known as the expiratory reserve volume (ERV). Similarly, the volume of air that can be taken in from FRC is known as the inspiratory capacity (IC), and, needless to say, the sum of the ERV and IC equals the VC (Fig. 5–1). The VC, ERV, and IC can be measured with a spirometer; TLC and its derivatives, FRC and RV, require other means, namely, closed-circuit helium equilibration, the nitrogen washout, a radiographic method, or plethysmography. The helium equilibration method depends on the subject rebreathing a known volume of helium in a closed circuit until equilibration is reached. The carbon dioxide produced during the rebreathing is absorbed. If the volume of the helium reservoir is known, and if the initial and final concentrations of the helium in the system are known, it is therefore possible to calculate the FRC. The nitrogen washout depends on giving the subject 100% oxygen and collecting all the expired air in a large spirometer. When the nitrogen has been completely washed out from the lungs and collected along with the expired air in a Tissot spirometer, the volume of the expirate and the nitrogen concentration are measured. Since the concentration of nitrogen in the lungs at the start of the maneuver is known, it is therefore possible to calculate the volume of nitrogen present in the lungs and hence the FRC.

The plethysmographic method is probably the best and most accurate way of determining lung volumes, since it measures all the gas in the thoracic cage. In

Figure 5–1
Lung volumes and spirometric tracing of a slow vital capacity maneuver in a normal subject. (From Sodeman, W. A., Jr., and Sodeman, T. J., eds., Sodeman's Pathologic Physiology, 7th ed. Philadelphia, W. B. Saunders Co., 1985, p. 439.)

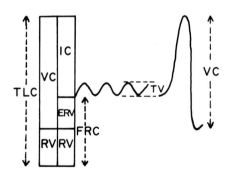

contrast, the helium equilibration and nitrogen washout methods do not include regions of poorly ventilated lung that contain trapped gas, e.g., bullae, and thus falsely low estimates are obtained. A body plethysmograph consists of an air-tight box in which the subject sits. As the subject breathes in and out, the pressure inside the box changes and is recorded by sensitive transducers. If the change in lung volume with each breath is also known, then by simple application of Boyle's law it is possible to calculate the intrathoracic gas volume.

Total lung capacity can also be accurately determined from the chest film. Barnhard and his colleagues have described a method which utilizes anteroposterior and lateral films.[2] The method depends on treating the lungs as a series of elliptical cylindroids and calculating the volume of each. Allowance is made for heart size, pulmonary blood volume, the spine, and domes of the diaphragm. The method has been simplified by Reger and his coworkers,[3] is accurate, and has application to epidemiological surveys. If the VC is determined by spirometry, it then becomes possible to measure the RV and hence the RV/TLC.

In a healthy young adult, the RV is around 20% of the TLC, but as the subject ages, the RV slowly increases so that by the age of 60 it may constitute up to 40% of the TLC. The increase in RV with age is related to the fact that as the subject ages, the lung loses some of its elasticity. This leads to the negative intrapleural pressure exerting a greater "pull" on the lung so that the FRC increases. The RV may be increased in neuromuscular diseases such as amyotrophic lateral sclerosis and myasthenia gravis. This is a consequence of the fact that the affected subject's exhalation is less forceful and is sustained for a shorter period because of neuromuscular weakness. As a result, he or she cannot expel as much of the TLC. The decreased elastic recoil of the lungs of an older person is opposed by an unchanged but relatively greater intrapleural pressure. This maintains the lung at a greater level of inflation than present when the subject was younger. The increased lung volumes and associated radiographic translucency that occur with age used to be known as senile emphysema; however, since there is neither airways obstruction nor disruption of the alveolocapillary surface, this term is a misnomer.

In obstructive airways disease associated with emphysema, the RV/TLC% is increased, and in many instances the RV may be well over 50% of the TLC (Fig. 5–2). An increased RV/TLC% is an almost invariable finding in chronic airflow obstruction, but lesser increases or relatively normal values may be seen in subjects with certain rare diffuse fibroses in which lung volumes are well preserved, e.g., eosinophilic granuloma and lymphangioleiomyomatosis. Similar changes in the RV are also seen in asbestotic subjects who are heavy smokers and who have coincident emphysema. In general, in well established chronic airflow limitation due to either asthma or emphysema, both the TLC and RV are increased; however, the increase in RV is proportionately greater than is the increase in TLC. In subjects with early obstruction, the RV may be increased without detectable changes in the TLC. Under such circumstances, the RV encroaches on the FVC and the VC. When the obstruction becomes more severe, the encroachment becomes more marked, and the VC and FVC may be markedly decreased, but never to the same extent as the

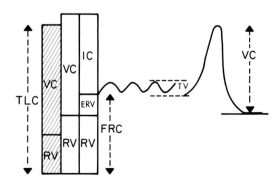

Figure 5–2
Lung volumes and spirometric tracing of a slow vital capacity maneuver in a subject with airways obstruction. The hatched area represents predicted values. (From Sodeman, W. A., Jr., and Sodeman, T. M., eds., Sodeman's Pathologic Physiology, 7th ed. Philadelphia, W. B. Saunders Co., 1985, p. 439.)

forced expiratory volume in 1 second (FEV_1). It is also important to remember that the helium equilibration method usually significantly underestimates static lung volumes in those subjects who have significant airways obstruction that is accompanied by an abnormal distribution of inspired gas. The RV may be increased as a result of air trapping or occasionally muscle weakness, as previously mentioned. The most important factors influencing the TLC are the compliance of the lungs and chest wall.

When the lungs become unduly stiff, in the absence of confounding airways obstruction and emphysema, all lung volumes are decreased, usually to the same extent (Fig. 5–3). When the free movement of the lungs is interfered with by stiffness of the chest wall or pleura or by compromised diaphragmatic function owing to abdominal distention, restrictive impairment results. All of these factors lead to a reduced VC and FVC, and such changes are reflected in a decreased compliance of the chest wall or lungs; however, flow rates are well preserved or occasionally increased owing to the increased elastic recoil of the lungs. In severe abdominal distention, while all lung volumes are reduced, the RV tends to be less affected. Obesity, even only mild to moderate, leads to the reduction of lung volumes, an increase in the alveoloarterial gradient, hypoxemia, and a decreased ERV.[4] In individual subjects, small increases in the RV/TLC% are not necessarily diagnostic of any physiological impairment. In many persons there is a mixed effect, with the effects of the airways obstruction being counteracted to a greater or lesser extent by other areas of the lung which are stiffer and less compliant. In epidemiological studies, a knowledge of the RV/TLC% in large groups of persons is much more useful than it is in the individual. Thus, the demonstration in a particular group of subjects that there is an increased mean RV/TLC% when compared to the RV/TLC% of a comparable reference group indicates a higher prevalence of airways obstruction or of emphysema associated with loss of elastic recoil.

Finally, it must be borne in mind that predicted values for static lung volumes are usually based on a limited number of subjects. This is related to the fact that measurement of static lung volumes takes far longer than it does to measure dynamic lung volumes and that the necessary laboratory equipment is often cumbersome and expensive. By the same token, it is also difficult to find large numbers of nonsmoking subjects over the age of 60 who are not obese and who have neither lung nor cardiac disease. As a result, predicted values for the elderly are based on relatively small numbers of subjects, and as such are likely to be less reliable than the equivalent predictions for younger and middle-aged groups. The reader is referred to an excellent statement from the American Thoracic Society which was published in 1991.[5]

Dynamic Lung Volumes

Ventilatory capacity also depends to a large extent on the resistance to air flow in the bronchial tree. If a normal young subject is asked to take in as big a breath as he or she can, and then to blow it out as rapidly and as forcibly as possible, he

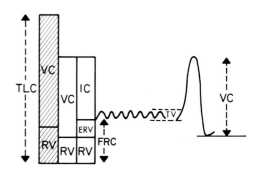

Figure 5–3
Lung volumes and spirometric tracing of a slow vital capacity in a subject with diffuse fibrosis. The hatched area represents predicted values. (From Sodeman, W. A., Jr., and Sodeman, T. A., eds., Sodeman's Pathologic Physiology, 7th ed. Philadelphia, W. B. Saunders Co., 1985, p. 440.)

or she should be able to get out 80% of FVC in 1 second (FEV_1) and 95% in 3 seconds. While this is true for the young subject, there is a fall in the FEV_1/FVC ratio with age, and by the time the subject is 60 or older, the ratio will often be around 67% to 70%. Expiratory flows are most rapid early in the forced expiratory volume maneuver, but as the subject begins to approach RV, there is a marked slowing. This is most evident once the subject gets below the FRC; and when RV is reached, flow ceases entirely (Fig. 5–4). Subjects with airways obstruction, that is to say, those who have an increased resistance to airflow in and out of their lungs, namely, asthmatics, chronic bronchitics, and those with emphysema, all show a flatter curve with decreased flow rates. In some instances, there is also a loss of VC. In asthma, but not in the other two conditions, the use of bronchodilators such as isoproterenol or salbutamol by nebulization will appreciably lessen the obstruction so that the forced expiratory volume curve becomes steeper and more closely resembles that of a normal person. As indices of obstruction, both the 1-second and 3-second timed vital capacity tests (percentage of FVC exhaled in 1 and 3 seconds, respectively) are frequently used. A minority of investigators prefer the actual volume of air exhaled in the first 0.75 second ($FEV_{0.75}$). A less popular but still commonly used measurement is the maximal expiratory flow rate (MEFR), the rate of flow between 200 and 1200 ml on a forced expiratory volume tracing. Another index which has its advocates is the FEF_{25-75} (MMF), or the maximal expiratory flow over the midhalf of a forced expiratory spirogram. The latter is no more sensitive than the FEV_1, is more variable, and is greatly influenced by the duration of the forced expiratory volume maneuver, especially in subjects with chronic airflow limitation. Moreover, although the FEF_{25-75} has been hailed as a means of diagnosing small airways disease, the test has been shown to be nonspecific.[6] Similarly, should flow volumes and, in particular, the FVC change following, for example, the administration of bronchodilators or a challenge test, it is inaccurate and unacceptable to compare the before and after FEF_{25-75} values without carrying out a volume adjustment.[7] Moreover, any minimal increase in sensitivity in the detection of chronic airflow limitation is negated by the lack of specificity of the test.[8] All of the various indices for measuring airways obstruction have their proponents, but there are valid reasons for preferring the FEV_1. These have been fully and well described in a statement from the American Thoracic Society.[5]

An additional method by which the ventilatory capacity can be assessed is the maximal breathing capacity (MBC). This should preferably be known as the maximal voluntary ventilation (MVV) and is the maximal volume of air that can be breathed over 1 minute. As the test is very tiring to subjects with airways obstruction, the volume is usually measured over a period of 15 to 20 seconds and the result multiplied by the necessary factor. This test is effort dependent and has little advantage over the single breath tests. To help those physicians who were trained on this measurement, the simple expedient of multiplying the FEV_1 by 40 yields an excellent approximation to the measured MVV.

The normal respiratory rate (f) of a young adult is around 12 per minute. With increasing age, there is an increase to 14 or 16. Since the tidal volume is normally

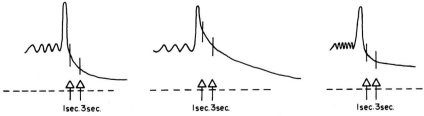

Figure 5–4. Forced expiratory volume maneuvers in a normal subject and in subjects with obstructive and restrictive impairment. (From Sodeman, W. A., Jr., and Sodeman, T. M., eds., Sodeman's Pathologic Physiology, 7th ed. Philadelphia, W. B. Saunders Co., 1985, p. 440.)

around 500 ml, the minute ventilation is 12×500 ml $= 6L$ ($V_T \times f$). Not all of every breath reaches the alveoli, since some air remains in the nose, nasopharynx, and bronchi and therefore does not come into contact with the alveolocapillary surface. The non–gas-exchanging part of the respiratory system is known as the anatomical dead space (V_{D_A}) and is normally around 150 ml. In a normal subject the volume of gas reaching the alveoli with each breath is $500 - 150$ ml $= 350$ ml ($V_T - V_{D_A}$). Alveolar ventilation per minute therefore equals 350 ml $\times 12 = 4.2$ L. The anatomical dead space has to be distinguished from the physiological dead space (V_{D_P}), which consists of the anatomical dead space plus the fraction of each breath which is wasted, either to ventilate underperfused alveolar units or to overventilate alveolar units relative to perfusion. In a normal subject the anatomical and physiological dead spaces are approximately the same, but with mismatching of ventilation and perfusion, the V_{D_P} increases. Lung volumes are generally expressed at the subject's body temperature, saturated with water vapor, and at 760 mm Hg (BTPS). When expressed at BTPS, the various indices represent the actual volume in the lungs.

Air Flow Resistance

During quiet breathing, most of the respiratory effort goes toward overcoming the compliance of the lungs and chest wall. By comparison, the work necessary to overcome air flow resistance is small, but when breathing becomes deeper and more rapid, the work expended overcoming airways resistance increases rapidly. When the airways are narrowed or obstructed by mucus, there may be a huge increase in both the airways resistance and the work of breathing, especially at low lung volumes at which the lumina of the airways are significantly narrowed.

Gas flow in the airways is governed by the same factors that regulate the flow of fluid in tubes or the flow of the electricity in a conductor. Ohm's law ($C = E/R$, where C is the current or flow, E the voltage or pressure gradient, and R the resistance) applies equally well to the flow of gas in the airways. Air flow may be either turbulent or laminar. When flow is turbulent, the pressure gradient necessary to produce a certain flow rate is appreciably higher. With laminar flow, the pressure gradient necessary to produce a certain flow is directly proportional to the viscosity of the gas. In contrast, during turbulent flow, the viscosity of the gas is less important and the density more important. Under normal circumstances, flow in the larger airways tends to be turbulent, and in addition, at the bifurcation of the airways, eddy currents are set up. In contrast, in the smaller airways (from the 12th generation and down), flow is mainly laminar. Thus, flow in the central airways is mainly density dependent, while in the smaller airways it is related more to the viscosity of the gases present. Poiseuille's law ($P = K_1 V$, where P is driving pressure, V is flow, and K_1 is a constant that depends on the viscosity of the gas) applies only to laminar flow in a straight line in a tube whose cross-sectional diameter is not changing. Clearly this situation does not apply in lungs, where the cross-sectional diameter is constantly changing, where the airways are repeatedly dividing, and where, owing to disease, the diameter of the airways may be either narrowed and distorted or occasionally dilated. Nonetheless, despite all these variables, the concept of airways resistance and the basic physical laws can be applied to many clinical situations.

Airways resistance depends not only on the number of patent airways but on the total cross-sectional area of the airways. The intrathoracic resistance of the airways may be partitioned into central and peripheral components. The central component includes the resistance from the trachea to roughly the 11th generation of bronchi. The peripheral component is made up of the resistance from the 12th generation to the alveoli. Central resistance in normal subjects makes up 85% to 90% of the total airways resistance (Raw). Thus, the peripheral resistance constitutes only 10% to 15% of the total resistance and, moreover, at high lung volumes is negligible (Fig. 5–5). It is, therefore, possible for a subject to have diffuse disease

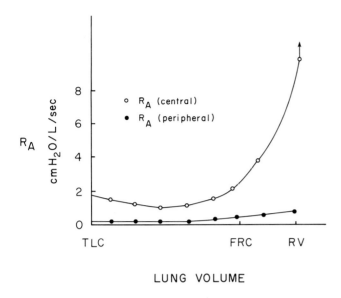

Figure 5–5
Relationship of central and peripheral airways resistance to lung volumes. (From Sodeman, W. A., Jr., and Sodeman, T. M., eds., Sodeman's Pathologic Physiology, 7th ed. Philadelphia, W. B. Saunders Co., 1985, p. 441.)

of the small airways and yet have a normal airways resistance and normal spirometry. When the resistance in the peripheral airways is increased, the lungs become less distensible, although total resistance may still be within normal limits. The peripheral airways are usually not uniformly and diffusely affected; rather, the pathological processes producing small airways disease tend to lead to patchy or regional involvement. Airways resistance is normally expressed at FRC. This is related to the fact that the cross-sectional diameter of the airways varies greatly with lung volume. Thus, at TLC the airways are widely patent, and with expiration there is a fairly minor decrease in a cross-sectional diameter until FRC is approached, at which time the airways start to narrow rapidly. For this reason, Raw remains relatively unchanged until FRC, at which time it starts to rise geometrically. It is also important to remember that in airways obstruction both the Raw and FRC are likely to increase, although not always to the same extent.

Airways resistance can be measured directly in several ways, including the body plethysmograph, the simultaneous recording of alveolar pressure and flow using an esophageal balloon, the interrupter technique, and also the oscillator method. A description of these various techniques is beyond the scope of the present chapter; however, suffice it to say, the plethysmographic method is the preferred, since it is most accurate in the clinical situation. There is little doubt that measurement of Raw in many instances adds little and is not as useful as spirometry in most clinical situations. However, determination of Raw can be most useful in challenge tests and in the assessment of various bronchodilator drugs. Under the latter circumstances, objective measurements of resistance may be preferable to spirometry.

The normal airways resistance is around 1.5 cm H_2O/L/sec. In comparison, the nasal air flow resistance is two to three times as high. In bronchitis and emphysema, the airways are irreversibly obstructed, and Raw may be increased four- to six-fold, under which circumstances most of the increased resistance is located in the respiratory bronchioles and smaller airways. In asthma, even greater increases in Raw occur, but here the obstruction is usually located in both small and large airways.

Compliance of the Lungs

Ventilation also depends on the compliance of the lungs. This is a measurement of the distensibility of the lungs and is expressed as the change in lung volume that occurs when the pressure gradient between the pleura and the alveoli is changed by 1 cm H_2O. It may be measured during breath-holding (static compliance) or during regular breathing (dynamic compliance). If the increase in volume were directly proportional to the pressure change through the range of inflation and deflation, then a single value for static compliance would describe the elastic properties of the lungs. In reality this is not the case; the lungs become less compliant at high lung volumes, and only in the tidal volume range is the relationship approximately linear. Lung compliance also depends on lung size; the larger the lungs, the more compliant they are. Thus, an infant's lung is less compliant than an adult's, and likewise there is disparity in the compliance of the lungs of large and small men. The reason for this can be clearly seen if one considers the hypothetical case of a man whose vital capacity is 5 L and whose static compliance is 0.2 L/cm H_2O. Under such circumstances, increasing his negative intrapleural pressure by 1 cm H_2O increases the volume of his lungs by 200 ml. Were he then to have one lung removed, this would reduce his vital capacity to 2.5 L, and a pressure change of 1 cm H_2O would then increase his lung volume by only 100 ml. In short, his compliance would be halved, although the elastic properties of his lung would be unchanged. This is an oversimplification of the problem, since following pneumonectomy some compensatory overdistention of the remaining lung occurs. The latter phenomenon, nonetheless, is responsible for only a marginal increase in the volume of the remaining lung.

To get around the problem of lung size, a measurement known as specific compliance has been introduced. This relates compliance to lung volume and is obtained by dividing the static compliance by the FRC. If the lungs become stiff and fibrotic, as frequently occurs in asbestosis, sarcoidosis, berylliosis, and certain other diffuse fibroses, the compliance is markedly reduced, and values of 0.04 L/cm H_2O and less may be found. In subjects who have a marked reduction of compliance, the vital capacity is usually concomitantly decreased. In conditions in which the lung has lost elasticity, a small change of pressure may produce a large increase in lung volume (Fig. 5–6). Under such circumstances, the lungs are said to be more compliant than normal. This is the usual state of affairs in emphysema and conditions associated with loss of recoil. Measurement of compliance is usually carried out by relating intrapleural pressure changes as reflected by changes in esophageal pressure to volume change in the lungs. Esophageal pressure is recorded by placing a cylindrical balloon attached to a fine plastic tube in the lower third of the esophagus. The measurement of compliance is objective, but care must be taken to see that the balloon is situated correctly.

Dynamic compliance may be defined as the ratio of tidal volume to the difference between pressure at end inspiration and end expiration at points of no flow during breathing. In normal subjects, measurement of dynamic compliance gives similar values to the static compliance; however, when airways resistance is

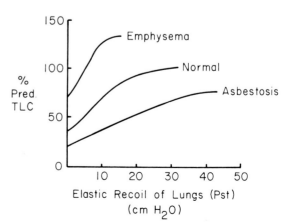

Figure 5–6
Pressure volume curves in a normal subject and in subjects with emphysema and diffuse fibrosis. (From Sodeman, W. A., Jr., and Sodeman, T. M., eds., Sodeman's Pathologic Physiology, 7th ed. Philadelphia, W. B. Saunders Co., 1985, p. 442.)

increased, an appreciable difference is often present. This is best explained by considering a state in which there is partial obstruction of a lobe or lung. In the unobstructed region, flow is maximal and there is an appropriate increase in flow volume for this area. In contrast, the flow of gases into the region with the increased airways resistance takes place more slowly, thereby causing a smaller increase in volume per head of pressure.

Surfactant

The compliance of the lungs is also dependent on the presence of surfactant. This is a substance that lines the alveoli and respiratory bronchioles and tends to prevent their collapse. Radford first demonstrated that the lungs of an animal that had been filled with saline distend more easily than they did with air.[9] This phenomenon suggests that saline either removed or rendered noneffective a substance which regulates the surface tension of the gas-tissue interface. Pattle subsequently showed that pulmonary edema fluid has a much lower surface tension than does plasma, an observation that suggests there is a substance lining the alveoli and influencing surface tension.[10] Subsequently, Clements demonstrated that the surface retractive forces are appreciable during lung expansion, but that during deflation of the lungs and as the surface area contracts, these forces decrease.[11]

In normal subjects, there is a difference between the inspiratory and expiratory limbs of a pressure volume curve, a phenomenon usually referred to as hysteresis. By way of contrast, the saline-filled lung shows only minimal hysteresis, which suggests that the difference in the inspiratory and expiratory limbs in the normal subject is a consequence of a substance which regulates surface tension at the air-liquid interface. This substance has been shown to be surfactant and is a complex of dipalmitoyl-lecithin with protein. It can be extracted from minced lungs or by washing the lungs out with saline. It appears to be secreted by the type II alveolar cells, and it has been shown to be present in decreased amounts in hyaline membrane disease, in conditions in which the blood flow to the lungs is decreased, and in other conditions including the prolonged inhalation of 100% oxygen.

Impairment of the Small Airways Function

The detection of changes in air flow resistance and function in the small airways is a challenge to the ingenuity of the physiologist, but several techniques have been devised which can be used to this end. Moreover, in many subjects such changes have been shown to be reversible, and it has therefore been suggested that if the abnormalities are detected early before there are accompanying spirometric abnormalities and if further exposure to the responsible agent is avoided, irreversible disease may be avoided. Whether such tests will prove useful in prognosticating whether a particular subject is going to develop irreversible airways obstruction remains undecided. Three approaches are presently popular.

1. Flow Volume Loop. The standard method of recording a forced expiratory volume maneuver plots volume against time. In contrast, the flow volume loop, as the name suggests, plots flow against volume. There are several types of flow volume curves and each needs a definition. The maximal expiratory flow volume curve (MEFV) is a plot of maximal expiratory flow ($\dot{V}max$) against volume during a forced expiratory maneuver. The term *flow volume loop* refers to a loop obtained when a maximal forced expiration is followed immediately by forced maximal inspiration, both being presented on the same tracing.

The typical flow volume loop is shown in Figure 5–7. Peak flow is largely effort dependent and is mainly a reflection of the state of the large airways. Flow at 50% of vital capacity (FEF_{50}) reflects both large and small airways function, with the former probably predominating. The latter part of the curve is felt to represent flow in the smaller airways. Also shown in Figure 5–7 is the curve of a subject with airways obstruction.

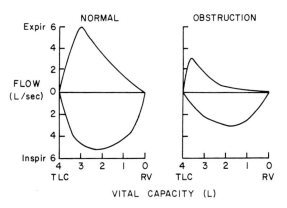

Figure 5–7

Flow volume loops of a normal subject and of a subject with airways obstruction. (From Sodeman, W. A., Jr., and Sodeman, T. M., eds., Sodeman's Pathologic Physiology, 7th ed. Philadelphia, W. B. Saunders Co., 1985, p. 443.)

Figure 5–8 shows a series of curves with different efforts. Although the peak flow varies, it can be seen that eventually the latter part of the curve blends with that of the MEFV; in short, there is a final common pathway. These phenomena stimulated Hyatt to construct isovolume pressure flow curves (IVPF), in which he measured transpulmonary pressure, showing that as driving pressure increased, flow concomitantly increased until a maximal value was attained, after which further increases in pressure produced no further increase in flow (Fig. 5–9).[12] Although flow is usually expressed as a percentage of vital capacity, it is preferable to relate it to TLC for the following reasons. When the MEFV is being used to evaluate bronchodilator drugs or to assess changes in air flow resistance over a relatively short period (e.g., during challenge tests or when subjects may have been exposed to cotton dust or agents likely to produce an acute change in the airways), in some instances, not only do the flow rates decrease, but in addition VC may likewise show a decrease. Thus, it is possible for a "before and after" challenge FEV_{50} when expressed as a percentage of VC to remain relatively unchanged; however, were the FEF_{50} related to TLC, a marked difference would become apparent.

In large airways, because flow is partly turbulent, the pressure necessary to produce a particular flow rate increases with gas density. In contrast, flow in the peripheral airways is for the most part laminar and is therefore independent of gas density. If one measures airways resistance (Raw) when the subject is breathing a helium and oxygen mixture (4:1), it is found that the Raw is substantially decreased. If a subject with peripheral airways obstruction alone breathes a helium oxygen

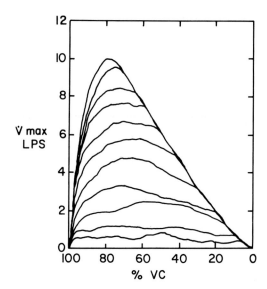

Figure 5–8

Series of flow volume curves showing graded respiratory efforts and different inspiratory volumes. (From Sodeman, W. A., Jr., and Sodeman, T. M., eds., Sodeman's Pathologic Physiology, 7th ed. Philadelphia, W. B. Saunders Co., 1985, p. 444.)

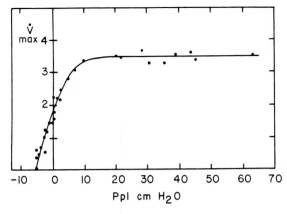

Figure 5–9
Isovolume pressure flow showing
limitation of flow at pressure of 15
cm H$_2$O. (From Sodeman, W. A.,
Jr., and Sodeman, T. M., eds.,
Sodeman's Pathologic Physiology,
7th ed. Philadelphia, W. B.
Saunders Co., 1985, p. 444.)

mixture (HeO$_2$), there is little change in Raw, since flow in small airways is mainly laminar. Since the effective pressure necessary to produce maximal flow is independent of the gas mixture breathed, and since the difference in flow between breathing air and helium oxygen mixture is determined by how much the peripheral airways contribute to the total resistance, the higher the resistance to flow in the peripheral airways, the less will be the helium response (Fig. 5–10).

At a particular lung volume, the flows on HeO$_2$ and air coincide, and this is known as the point of identical flow (PIF, or Viso $\dot{V}$). It is usually expressed as a percentage of vital capacity. In normal subjects it varies from 0% to 6% and is rarely elevated above 10%. In small airways obstruction it may be elevated to around 30% (see Fig. 5–10).

The flow volume curve is also useful in detecting obstructing lesions of the right and left main bronchi, the trachea, and larynx. Figures 5–11, 5–12, and 5–13 show typical examples of the major airways obstruction. Figure 5–11 is a tracing from a subject with a variable extrathoracic obstruction, namely, bilateral vocal cord paralysis. It is obviously apparent that inspiratory flows are more affected than expiratory flows. A variable intrathoracic obstruction, e.g., a tracheal cylindroma,

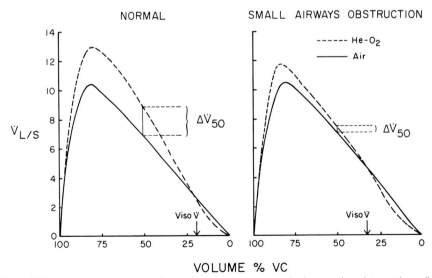

Figure 5–10. Helium oxygen and air flow volume curves in a normal subject and a subject with small airways obstruction. Note the point of identical flow (Viso $\dot{V}$) is farther from RV in the subject with small airways obstruction. (From Sodeman, W. A., Jr., and Sodeman, T. M., eds., Sodeman's Pathologic Physiology, 7th ed. Philadelphia, W. B. Saunders Co., 1985, p. 444.)

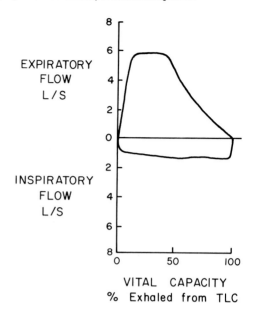

Figure 5–11
Flow volume showing variable extrathoracic obstruction. (From Sodeman, W. A., Jr., and Sodeman, T. M., eds., Sodeman's Pathologic Physiology, 7th ed. Philadelphia, W. B. Saunders Co., 1985, p. 445.)

is represented in the tracing shown in Figure 5–12. Expiratory flows are more affected since the intrathoracic trachea is compressed during exhalation. Figure 5–13 shows a fixed (extrathoracic) obstructive lesion in which inspiration and expiration are both affected, e.g., stenosis of the larynx following surgery or injury.

2. Closing Volume. It has been shown that small airways start to close somewhere between functional residual capacity (FRC) and residual volume (RV). Closure depends on the pressure difference acting on the wall of the airway and on the elastic properties of the small airways. If the lumina of peripheral airways are narrowed by mucus or some pathological process, or if concentration of surfactant is reduced, the surface forces acting on the airways become greater, and a tendency to collapse occurs.

Fowler originally observed that when a person exhaled to residual volume and then took a breath of oxygen and achieved total lung capacity (TLC), during a subsequent slow expiratory maneuver, a tracing of the percentage of nitrogen

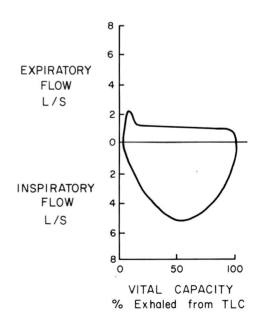

Figure 5–12
Flow volume curve showing variable intrathoracic obstruction. (From Sodeman, W. A., Jr., and Sodeman, T. M., eds., Sodeman's Pathologic Physiology, 7th ed. Philadelphia, W. B. Saunders Co., 1985, p. 445.)

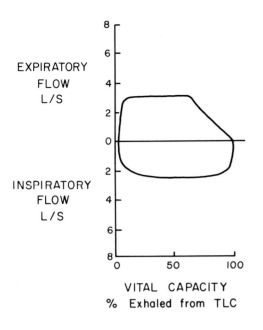

Figure 5-13
Flow volume curve showing fixed extrathoracic obstruction. (From Sodeman, W. A., Jr., and Sodeman, T. M., eds., Sodeman's Pathologic Physiology, 7th ed. Philadelphia, W. B. Saunders Co., 1985, p. 445.)

exhaled showed four distinct phases (Fig. 5–14). In phase 1 there is an absence of nitrogen, owing to the fact that the dead space contains pure oxygen.[13] Phase 2 begins as the subject starts to exhale a mixture of gas from the dead space and alveoli, and is characterized by a sharp increase in the concentration of expired nitrogen. Phase 2 is followed by an alveolar plateau known as phase 3. Finally there is an abrupt increase in the concentration of nitrogen (phase 4). The junction of phases 3 and 4 is thought to be the volume at which the basal airways close, and the volume between the junction of phases 3 and 4 and RV is known as closing volume (CV). CV plus RV is known as closing capacity (CC). The upward inflection at the end of phase 3 is best explained by the effects of gravity on the distribution of inspired gas. In a normal subject there is a gradient of transpulmonary pressure from the top to the bottom of the lung. When a sitting or standing subject takes a breath from RV, the first portion of the breath is distributed to the apices, while the latter portions are distributed to the lower lobes. During a subsequent exhalation the air that is exhaled first comes from the upper and lower zones, but towards the end of the breath small airways in the lower zones close and the

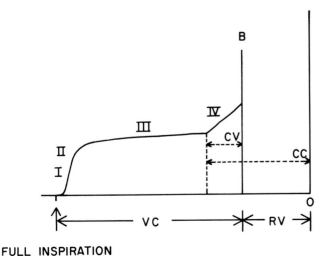

Figure 5-14
Single breath oxygen test showing the four phases, along with closing volume and closing capacity. (From Sodeman, W. A., Jr., and Sodeman, T. M., eds., Sodeman's Pathologic Physiology, 7th ed. Philadelphia, W. B. Saunders Co., 1985, p. 446.)

upper zones make a relatively greater contribution. This principle has been aptly named "first in–last out."[14]

Measurement of closing volume can be carried out in several ways. The most simple is the resident nitrogen method in which the subject takes a breath of 100% oxygen. The nitrogen remaining in the airways forms a bolus of tracer gas. Other methods involve labeling the inspired air with a foreign gas such as argon, xenon, or helium. Differences in measurement of closing volume in the same subject have been noted according to the method used. A normal closing volume implies that the distribution of inspired gases is mainly dependent on gravity and that the lungs empty relatively homogenously. When filling and emptying become discordant, the principle of first in–last out is broken and a closing volume may not be apparent on the tracing. Phase 3 represents gas coming from alveoli, and as such the alveoli must contain different concentrations of nitrogen in order to account for the slope. The steepness of the slope is therefore an indication of abnormal distribution, since the concentration of nitrogen in each alveolus after a breath of oxygen depends on how much oxygen enters each alveolus.

Measurement of CV is influenced by the rate at which the inspired breath is taken, by expiratory flow, and by prolonged breath-holding, which leads to a greater percentage of oxygen being absorbed. Expiratory flow should be regulated to between 0.4 and 0.5 L/sec. CV, CV/VC%, and CC/TLC% all have higher coefficients of variation than do FEV_1 and FVC. In this regard, CV and CV/VC% are the most variable, i.e., 20% to 25%. Moreover, while intelligent subjects have no difficulty in carrying out the CV maneuver, its applicability in field studies is severely limited by the inability of a substantial proportion of the less well-educated population to carry out the respiratory maneuvers in a satisfactory fashion. Abnormalities of CV, in the presence of normal spirometry, have been reported in obesity, cigarette smokers, asthmatics in remission, and coal miners and in skeletal deformities such as kyphosis. As such, an elevated CV is thought to indicate early disease; nonetheless, the prognostic significance of CV remains *sub judice*.

3. Frequency Dependence of Dynamic Compliance. The history of the development of this technique begins with the mechanical time constant theory elaborated by Otis et al. and used to explain the relationship between mechanical factors and the intrapulmonary distribution of inspired gas.[15] Theory suggests that differences in time constants (resistance × compliance) between parallel lung units would be associated with a decrease in dynamic compliance as breathing frequency increased. This would mean that a progressively smaller portion of the lung would be ventilated as breathing frequency increased.

Macklem and Mead reported that the time constants of the distal lung units (airways smaller than about 2 mm) were in the order of 0.01 second.[16] They concluded that a fourfold difference in these time constants would cause dynamic compliance to fall with any increase in respiratory frequency because there would be less time for air to enter and leave the affected regions. Thus, an increased resistance to flow in the smaller airways should lead to a fall in dynamic compliance at faster rates of breathing. This raised the possibility that the frequency dependence of dynamic compliance could be used as a test of obstruction in peripheral airways.

For widespread time constant discrepancies to occur, the obstruction must be unevenly distributed; that is, airways must remain patent while others are narrowed. Other criteria are necessary before it can be assumed that frequency-dependent dynamic compliance is a consequence of peripheral airways narrowing rather than of lesions in large airways or other parts of the lung. If the static pressure/volume (compliance) curve of the lung is normal, then it is not likely that frequency-dependent dynamic compliance is due to abnormal elastic properties of the lung. It has been assumed that regional differences in elastic properties sufficient to cause a detectable fall in dynamic compliance at rapid respiratory rates should result in an abnormal static compliance curve. Thus, if a patient has normal pulmonary resistance, spirometry, and static pressure/volume curve, any fall in dynamic compliance with increased frequency of respiration (frequency-dependent compliance) is assumed to be due to peripheral airways obstruction. The time constants and ventilation of peripheral gas-exchanging units of the lung will be affected by

1. Regional obstruction due to bronchiolar narrowing or obstruction by mucus.
2. Regional increases in elastic recoil produced by interstitial fibrosis; for example, in asbestosis and berylliosis.
3. Regional loss of elastic recoil with airways collapse; for example, in centrilobular emphysema and the focal emphysema of coal workers' pneumoconiosis (CWP).

All three of these pathological processes may lead to unequal time constants in the lung, and hence an uneven distribution of ventilation that is more pronounced at faster rates of ventilation; and all should produce a fall in dynamic compliance at higher respiratory rates.

The detection of frequency-dependent dynamic compliance involves measuring dynamic compliance at various rates of respiration, e.g., 20, 40, 60, and 80 breaths/minute. The dynamic changes in volume are obtained using a pneumotachograph, while the intrapleural pressure changes are measured with an esophageal balloon.

Work of Breathing

A certain amount of energy is expended with each breath we take. Part of the energy expenditure is related to moving air in and out of the lungs, and part to moving the thoracic cage and diaphragm. Normal values for the work of breathing are 0.5 kg/m^2/min at rest and up to 250 kg/m^2/min with a maximal voluntary ventilation maneuver. In asthma and emphysema, the main increase in the work of breathing is related to overcoming the increased air flow resistance; while in pulmonary fibrosis, the additional work is necessary to overcome the stiffness of the lungs. The respiratory muscles under normal circumstances use about 2% to 4% of the energy requirements at rest, but in diseased subjects this may rise to 35% to 40%.

REGIONAL DISTRIBUTION OF VENTILATION AND PERFUSION

Ventilation

Quantitative studies of the regional distribution of gas over large zones of excised lung using radioactive xenon have shown relatively even distribution of inspired gas per unit lung volume. The situation in life, with the lungs suspended within the chest wall, is very different in that the intrapleural pressure is no longer uniform as in the isolated preparation. Instead, in the erect posture there is a vertical gradient of intrapleural pressure, with a progressive reduction in pressure from the base to the apex of the lung.[17] As the static transpleural pressure (i.e., pressure difference between pleural surface and atmosphere, during breath-holding with the glottis open) is more negative at the apex, the upper zone alveoli tend to be more expanded than those in the lower zones. An analogy is a loosely coiled spring which, when suspended by its uppermost coil, becomes progressively more expanded by its own weight from bottom to top (Fig. 5–15). The pleural pressure gradient in the chest always occurs in the direction of gravitational pull; thus, in a supine subject the differences in alveolar expansion occur dorsoventrally.[18] Because of these regional differences in alveolar expansion, the static lung compliance of the more stretched upper zones is less than that of the lower zones in the erect posture; and during tidal breathing at low flow rates, basal ventilation therefore tends to exceed that of the apices.[19] As inspiratory flow rate increases, regional airways resistance is thought to become more influential than compliance in determining regional ventilation, which is then more evenly distributed. It is of note that

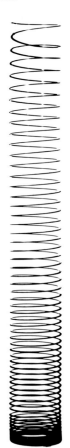

Figure 5–15
A spring suspended from the uppermost coil, showing the relative separation of the coils at the top and bottom. (From Sodeman, W. A., Jr., and Sodeman, T. M., eds., Sodeman's Pathologic Physiology, 7th ed. Philadelphia, W. B. Saunders Co., 1985, p. 447.)

in elderly normal subjects, particularly in the supine posture, regional ventilation may be altered by small airways closure occurring in dependent lung zones during tidal breathing, and this may result in a reduction in arterial oxygen tension.[20]

Perfusion

Studies using a variety of different radioactive tracer techniques have also demonstrated that pulmonary perfusion is not uniformly distributed and that there is a vertical gradient of increasing pulmonary perfusion per unit lung volume from apex to base in the erect posture, apart from some reduction over the most dependent 6 to 10 cm of lung. Hughes et al. and West have explained these regional differences in terms of the interaction of pulmonary arterial, venous, alveolar, and interstitial pressures in the lungs (Fig. 5–16).[20, 21] In zone 1 of the upright lung there is no pulmonary arterial perfusion because pericapillary lung pressure, which under static conditions can be thought of as ''alveolar'' pressure, exceeds pulmonary arterial pressure at this level, and alveolar vessels therefore collapse. The junction of zones 1 and 2, at which pulmonary arterial perfusion commences, is represented by the height of a column of blood in an open manometer tube connected to the pulmonary artery. Below this level, pulmonary arterial pressure exceeds atmospheric pressure and can therefore open the vessels, and perfusion increases down this zone as the hydrostatic pressure of the column of pulmonary arterial blood rises. The amount of perfusion at any level in this zone is determined by the difference between the pulmonary arterial and alveolar pressure which still exceeds pulmonary venous pressure. In the third zone, pulmonary venous pressure now also exceeds alveolar pressure. Here there is a continued slower increase in perfusion probably owing to distention of intra-alveolar vessels as a result of a continued

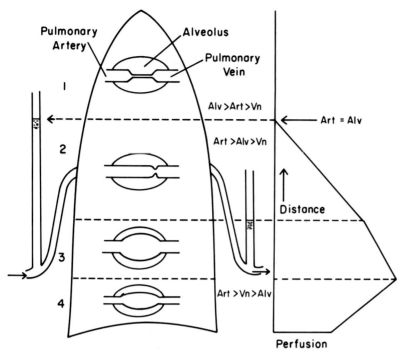

Figure 5–16. Relationship of pulmonary arterial, venous, alveolar, and interstitial pressures in the various zones of the lung (based on West). (From Sodeman, W. A., Jr., and Sodeman, T. M., eds., Sodeman's Pathologic Physiology, 7th ed. Philadelphia, W. B. Saunders Co., 1985, p. 448.)

increase in the hydrostatic pressure in both pulmonary artery and pulmonary vein, whereas alveolar pressure remains atmospheric. A fourth zone was added to this scheme when it was observed that there was some fall-off of basal blood flow, particularly at lung volumes below functional residual capacity. This is attributed to a lung volume–related change in the resistance of extra-alveolar pulmonary vessels, whose caliber is related to changes in surrounding interstitial pressure rather than alveolar pressure.

Regional Variation in the Matching of Ventilation and Perfusion

Although in the normal lung both alveolar ventilation ($\dot{V}A$) and perfusion ($\dot{Q}$) vary regionally in the same direction according to vertical gravity-dependent gradients, the rate of increase of perfusion from apex to base is steeper than that for ventilation. Consequently the regional matching of $\dot{V}A$ to $\dot{Q}$, which may be conveniently expressed as $\dot{V}A/\dot{Q}$ ratios, is not uniform, but decreases down the length of the lung. The total $\dot{V}A/\dot{Q}$ ratio for a normal upright lung with cardiac output of approximately 6 L/min and alveolar ventilation of 5 L/min lies between 0.8 and 0.9; however, regional $\dot{V}A/\dot{Q}$ ratios vary considerably from about 3.3 at the apex to 0.6 at the lung base.[21] The predilection of post-primary pulmonary tuberculosis for the lung apices has been attributed to the high apical $\dot{V}A/\dot{Q}$ ratio, which results in an alveolar oxygen tension and hence tissue tension over 40 mm Hg higher than that at the lung base. This idea is supported by observations of a higher incidence of this disease in patients with pulmonary stenosis whose apical perfusion is still further reduced. Conversely, tuberculosis usually affects the lung *bases* in bats, since they hang upside down. Regional alterations in the normal pattern of $\dot{V}A/\dot{Q}$ matching are important as they determine the overall efficiency of the lung in its principal function as a gas-exchanger. Exercise and the assumption of the supine position even out the regional differences. In disease, most abnormalities of gas exchange result from mismatching of ventilation and perfusion, and these inequalities may be expressed in terms of wasted blood flow or ventilation.

Wasted Perfusion. If an alveolus is totally unventilated but remains perfused ($\dot{V}_A/\dot{Q} = 0$), then the distal end of the capillary supplying it will still contain blood of venous composition, and perfusion will have been useless and is often referred to as a "true shunt." Suppose the supply of fresh air to the alveolus is not completely interrupted, but merely reduced disproportionately to its blood supply. It may be felt intuitively that some of the perfusion is still surplus to the requirements of that alveolus. We can imagine that the reduced amount of inspired gas will be totally accommodated by some fraction of the same volume of perfusing blood, and the rest will remain venous. In both these situations, "venous" blood will mix with arterialized blood, reducing its oxygen content and increasing its carbon dioxide content. This process, which is called "shunting" or "venous admixture," may, if sufficient alveoli are involved, produce measurable changes in the gas tensions of arterial blood. It should be noted that both oxygen and carbon dioxide transfer are impaired in shunting; however, usually the respiratory center responds to hypercarbia by increasing ventilation, which lowers the P_{CO_2} of ventilated alveoli.[22] Since the carbon dioxide dissociation curve is nearly linear (Fig. 5–17), this will be accompanied by an approximately equal fall in CO_2 content for a given fall in P_{CO_2} over the physiological range, and, as a result, in shunts a normal arterial P_{CO_2} can usually be maintained. In the absence of a hyperventilatory response, carbon dioxide retention would occur. Arterial oxygen content is less easily maintained because increasing the P_{O_2} of relatively well-ventilated alveoli on the flat part of the nonlinear oxyhemoglobin dissociation curve (Figs. 5–15 to 5–18) will produce only minimal improvement in the oxygen saturation of the blood perfusing these units, which cannot therefore compensate for unventilated units. The arterial blood gas abnormality most commonly found in significant shunts is a lowered arterial P_{O_2} in the presence of a normal or low arterial P_{CO_2}.

The direct passage of blood from the arterial to the venous side of the pulmonary circulation without any contact with ventilated alveoli is called true shunting, and is physiologically indistinguishable from the small amount of anatomical shunting that occurs in normal individuals through the bronchial circulation and thebesian veins in the heart. Any remaining shunt is due to alveoli with low $\dot{V}_A/\dot{Q}$ ratios and is really a shunt-like effect or physiological shunt. Total shunt in a resting normal individual does not usually exceed 5% of the cardiac output, of which true shunt constitutes about 2%.[23]

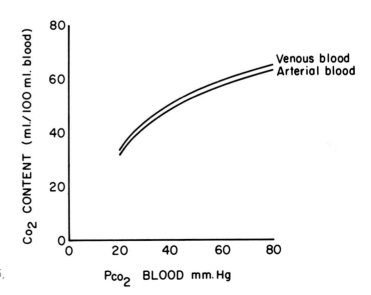

Figure 5–17
Carbon dioxide dissociation curve. (From Sodeman, W. A., Jr., and Sodeman, T. M., eds., Sodeman's Pathologic Physiology, 7th ed. Philadelphia, W. B. Saunders Co., 1985, p. 449.)

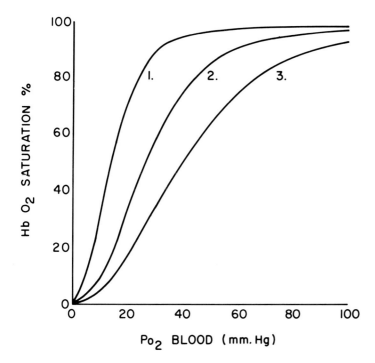

Figure 5–18
Oxygen dissociation curves showing right and left shifts (see text for explanation). (From Sodeman, W. A., Jr., and Sodeman, T. M., eds., Sodeman's Pathologic Physiology, 7th ed. Philadelphia, W. B. Saunders Co., 1985, p. 449.)

Wasted Ventilation. Now consider the opposite situation of a normally ventilated alveolus receiving no perfusion ($\dot{V}A/\dot{Q}$ ratio = infinity). This alveolus will act as an extra space in which air is moved to and fro without participating in gas exchange, and is therefore dead space or wasted ventilation. In terms of function, this dead space produces the same effect as an enlargement of the anatomical dead space, which comprises the whole of the nonalveolated respiratory tract from the mouth and nose to the respiratory bronchioles. If the perfusion of the alveolus is not completely interrupted but only reduced disproportionately to its ventilation, then a fraction of that ventilation will now be sufficient to meet the gas-exchanging potential of the reduced blood flow, and the remaining ventilation is therefore useless. This process will also contribute to alveolar dead space. Alveolar dead space is therefore the volume of inspired gas entering alveoli, but not taking part in gas exchange owing to local $\dot{V}A/\dot{Q}$ imbalance, and is more conceptual and less tangible than anatomical dead space, which, as it is a volume contained within a physical structure, is easier to picture. Alveolar and anatomical dead space together are conventionally referred to as physiological dead space. The measured physiological dead space in healthy individuals is usually not more than 30% of the tidal volume.

If anatomical dead space is increased artificially (e.g., by mouth breathing through a length of tube), and if the rate and depth of breathing are unaltered, then less fresh air will reach the alveoli with each inspiration. It follows that alveolar Po_2 will fall and alveolar Pco_2 will rise, with consequent hypoxemia and hypercapnia. Suppose alveolar dead space is increased by relative underperfusion of a group of normally ventilated alveoli, and that the rate and depth of breathing and overall pulmonary perfusion remain unaltered. Although the oxygen tension of the reduced volume of blood perfusing these alveoli will be increased, it will be insufficient to compensate for a greater reduction of oxygen tension in blood coming from other normally ventilated alveoli, which are now overperfused as they receive additional blood which would normally have been directed to the first group of alveoli. The result will be a reduction in arterial oxygen tension. Even though overall alveolar ventilation may remain normal, wasted regional ventilation will also reduce carbon dioxide exchange, tending to produce a raised arterial carbon dioxide tension.[17] In disease this tendency is often corrected by compensatory hyperventilation, although hypoxemia often persists.

Alveoloarterial Oxygen Gradient [(A-a)O$_2$]

Were the matching of ventilation and perfusion perfect, and assuming gas diffusion occurred across the alveolocapillary membrane to equilibrium, then arterial and alveolar oxygen tensions would be equal. When mismatching occurs, an alveoloarterial oxygen tension difference [(A-a)O$_2$] will develop. The measurement of arterial oxygen tension is easy, but that of average alveolar oxygen tension presents problems. Although end-expiratory samples of alveolar gas may not be contaminated by dead space air in normal subjects, in pulmonary disease some lung units may take much longer to empty than others, so that end-expiratory Po$_2$ measured at the mouth changes continually, and spot sampling introduces error. Consequently, for clinical purposes "ideal" alveolar Po$_2$ is estimated indirectly.[24] This is the alveolar Po$_2$ that would be found in a given subject if, for the same overall rate of consumption of oxygen and production of carbon dioxide, ventilation and perfusion were to become perfectly matched throughout the lung. The calculation requires the analysis of an expired air and arterial blood sample. A simplified version of the ideal alveolar gas equation is

$$\text{ideal } PA_{O_2} = PI_{O_2} - \frac{Pa_{CO_2}}{R}$$

where PI_{O_2} is the inspired oxygen tension, Pa_{CO_2} is the arterial carbon dioxide tension, and R is the respiratory quotient (rate of production of carbon dioxide divided by the rate of uptake of oxygen, which is usually 0.8). The ideal (A-a)O$_2$ underestimates true (A-a)O$_2$ because it fails to account for alveoli with a raised Po$_2$ due to high $\dot{V}A/\dot{Q}$ ratios. It is used as a nonspecific indicator of impaired gas exchange due to diffusion or distribution abnormalities. It remains normal (4 to 15 mm Hg) in patients with overall alveolar hypoventilation, and increases with hyperventilation, whether voluntary or induced by anxiety, and with age (Table 5–1).

Estimation of Shunt

Physiological shunt (anatomical plus alveolar shunt) may be estimated using the following equation:

$$\frac{\dot{Q}s}{\dot{Q}} = \frac{Ci_{O_2} - Ca_{O_2}}{Ci_{O_2} - C\bar{v}_{O_2}}$$

where $\dot{Q}s/\dot{Q}$ is the proportion of total pulmonary flow taking part in the shunt; Ca_{O_2} and $C\bar{v}_{O_2}$ are the arterial and mixed venous oxygen contents, respectively; and Ci_{O_2} is the ideal arterial oxygen content (that which would result from an arterial Po$_2$ equal to the ideal alveolar Po$_2$) which can be obtained from a knowledge of the ideal alveolar Po$_2$ using the oxyhemoglobin dissociation curve. True shunt (anatom-

Table 5–1

■

Changes in Arterial Blood Gases and (A-a)O$_2$ Gradient in Various Physiological Impairments

	Po$_2$	Pco$_2$	(A-a)O$_2$
Regional $\dot{V}/\dot{Q}$ mismatching	↓	↑ or N or ↓	↑
"Pure" diffusion block	↓	N or ↓	↑
Overall alveolar hypoventilation	↓	↑	N
Overall alveolar hyperventilation	N or ↑	↓	↑

From Morgan, W. K. C., and Seaton, D., Pulmonary ventilation and blood gas exchange. *In* Sodeman, W. A., Jr., and Sodeman, T. M., eds., Sodeman's Pathologic Physiology, 7th ed. Philadelphia, W. B. Saunders Co., 1985, p. 450.

ical shunt plus shunt through totally unventilated alveoli) may be separated from shunt-like effects (alveoli with low $\dot{V}_A/\dot{Q}$ ratios) by the administration of 100% oxygen for 20 minutes. This washes out all alveolar nitrogen and fully oxygenates even poorly ventilated alveoli (alveolar P_{O_2} of approximately 670 mm Hg), thereby abolishing shunt-like effects. The only possible cause for persisting hypoxemia in this situation is a true shunt, where venous blood unexposed to ventilated alveoli continues to dilute oxygenated blood. It should be noted that the arterial P_{O_2} will rise to some extent in true shunts owing to the increased alveolar P_{O_2}, and only in large shunts (greater than 25% of the cardiac output) will the blood remain desaturated. A widened $(A-a)O_2$ will persist in true shunts but not in shunt-like effects.

Estimation of Physiological Dead Space and Effective Alveolar Ventilation

Physiological dead space (anatomical dead space plus alveolar dead space) may be estimated using Bohr's equation in terms of alveolar and mixed expired P_{CO_2}:

$$V_{D_P} = V_T \frac{(P_{A_{CO_2}} - P_{\bar{E}_{CO_2}})}{P_{A_{CO_2}}}$$

The difficulties inherent in measuring average alveolar P_{CO_2} are avoided by equating it to arterial P_{CO_2} (equals ideal alveolar P_{CO_2}). The proportion of the tidal volume (V_T) made up by the physiological dead space V_{D_P} may now be given by

$$\frac{V_{D_P}}{V_T} = \frac{P_{a_{CO_2}} - P_{\bar{E}_{CO_2}}}{P_{a_{CO_2}}}$$

Alveolar ventilation has already been defined in terms of anatomical dead space and minute ventilation. If the physiological dead space is known, it is possible to estimate the effective alveolar ventilation, this being the proportion of total ventilation being used effectively in carbon dioxide exchange according to the equation:

$$\dot{V}_A(eff) = \underset{\text{ml/min}}{} \quad \underset{\text{breaths/min}}{f} \quad \times \underset{\text{ml}}{(V_T - \dot{V}_{D_A})}$$

In clinical practice, however, arterial P_{CO_2} alone is generally taken as a reliable and readily available indicator of the level of effective alveolar ventilation. Hypoventilation, by reducing the delivery of fresh air to gas exchanging areas, inevitably reduces arterial P_{O_2} and increases arterial P_{CO_2}. The resultant hypoxemia may be eliminated by the administration of a high concentration of oxygen, but the raised arterial P_{CO_2} cannot be corrected unless the level of alveolar ventilation is increased. Conversely, conditions that result in effective alveolar hyperventilation are associated with a lowered arterial P_{CO_2}. This may be seen in hysterical overbreathing, and occasionally following the hyperventilatory response to hypoxemia due to a diffusion impairment or ventilation-perfusion mismatch in which sufficient normal lung tissue remains to eliminate carbon dioxide.

TRANSPORT OF GASES BY THE BLOOD

In a mixture of different gases, the pressure exerted by each of the constituents, commonly referred to as the partial pressure (P), is the product of its fractional concentration by volume and the total pressure of the mixture. For inspired air, which contains 20.93% oxygen, 0.03% carbon dioxide, 79% nitrogen, and other inert gases, whose total pressure is 760 mm Hg (barometric pressure at sea level) and whose water vapor pressure is 10 mm Hg, the P_{O_2} will be:

$$\frac{20.93}{100} \times (760 - 10) = 157 \text{ mm Hg}$$

Water vapor pressure is subtracted as the volumes of gases are conventionally estimated dry. Similarly the atmospheric P_{CO_2} will be 0.2 mm Hg and the P_{N_2} 592 mm Hg. If a mixture of gases is brought into contact with a fluid, the constituent gases will continue to diffuse into it until their partial pressures in solution are equal to those of the gas phase. At this point, equilibration is said to have occurred. The partial pressure of a gas in fluid is often referred to as its tension.

The content of a gas in a fluid is derived from the product of the gas's solubility coefficient (α) and its partial pressure, and is expressed in milliliters of gas measured at standard temperature and pressure dry (STPD) per 100 ml of liquid or in volume percentage. The solubility coefficient of oxygen is 0.003 ml/dl/mm Hg, and its average partial pressure in the alveoli is approximately 100 mm Hg. This is less than that of atmospheric air because of mixing with oxygen-depleted and carbon dioxide–rich gas already present in the lung, and since it also becomes saturated with water vapor during its passage to the gas exchanging surfaces, with the saturated water vapor pressure at 37°C being 47 mm Hg. The average content of dissolved oxygen in pulmonary capillary plasma at equilibrium with alveolar air will therefore be 0.003 × 100 = 0.3 ml/dl.

A normal resting subject's oxygen requirement is around 300 ml/min, and were all dissolved oxygen in the plasma removed by the tissues on each complete circuit, the minimum cardiac output necessary to support life would be 60 L/min, a level that is impossible to sustain. This difficulty is overcome by the reversible binding of most oxygen to hemoglobin, of which whole blood contains approximately 15 g/dl. Hemoglobin is a tetramer formed by a globulin molecule bound to four heme molecules, each of which may react with a single oxygen molecule. This complex structure is capable of binding 1.34 ml of oxygen/dl, and the hemoglobin capacity is therefore 1.34 × 15 = 20.1 ml/dl. Percentage saturation is the oxygen content, which may be measured by Van Slyke's method, and is expressed as a percentage of the blood oxygen carrying capacity.

Oxyhemoglobin Dissociation Curve

The content of a gas dissolved in fluid, expressed in volume percentage, is related to its partial pressure in a linear fashion (Henry's law). This contrasts markedly with the S-shaped relationship of blood oxygen tension to saturation that results from the presence of hemoglobin (see Fig. 5–18). The curve owes its distinctive shape to the so-called heme-heme reaction, in which the oxygenation of each heme molecule in the tetramer in turn affects the oxygen affinity of the other subunits, so that the molecule as a whole has four successive equilibrium constants.[25] Notice that the upper part of the curve is relatively flat, so that a drop in oxygen tension from 100 to 60 mm Hg is associated with a relatively small fall in oxygen saturation. As a result, persons who live at an altitude of 10,000 feet, at which the alveolar P_{O_2} is about 60 mm Hg, still maintain an oxygen saturation of about 90%, which is clearly to their advantage. Conversely, a rise in the P_{O_2} of arterial blood in this range produces only a minimal increase in oxygen saturation. Consequently hyperventilation of normal lung tissue may be unable to compensate for hypoxemia resulting from areas of impaired gas exchange elsewhere. The lower, steeper part of the curve is also physiologically important, as a small fall in the P_{O_2} of blood is associated with a relatively large change in its oxygen content. Thus, the transfer of oxygen from blood to metabolically active tissues is facilitated.

Factors Affecting the Oxyhemoglobin Dissociation Curve

The relationship of the P_{O_2} of blood to hemoglobin saturation may be altered by a number of factors that are capable of causing a "shift" of the oxyhemoglobin dissociation curve to either the right or the left, so that the flat part of the curve corresponding to high hemoglobin saturations is either expanded or contracted (see Fig. 5–18). The most important of these factors are pH, PCO_2, 2,3-diphosphoglycerate (2,3-DPG) level, and temperature. These shifts may be defined in terms of the PO_2 of blood at which hemoglobin is half saturated (P_{50}). If the oxyhemoglobin dissociation curve shifts to the right, the P_{50} rises, and with a shift to the left, it falls. Although it might at first seem that a raised P_{50} would be disadvantageous, since a smaller amount of oxygen is being transported for the given PO_2, careful examination of the diagram shows that as a result of the shape of curve 3, a raised P_{50} implies that for a given reduction in arterial PO_2 in the physiological range, a greater amount of oxygen becomes available to the tissues. If on passing through the systemic capillaries the PO_2 of arterial blood falls from 90 to 40 mm Hg [arteriovenous O_2 difference, (a-v)O_2], then according to curve 2 the oxygen saturation would fall by only 20%, whereas if curve 3 is applied, the fall would be 40%.

When hemoglobin is oxygenated, hydrogen ions are released from the molecule. If the pH of the red cell, which is linearly related to that of the plasma, is reduced by the addition of hydrogen ions, then by the principle of mass action, this process tends to reverse, hemoglobin reverting to its deoxygenated state with the release of oxygen. In practice, metabolically active tissues constitute a more acid environment for the blood perfusing them as a result of the local production of CO_2 and lactic acid, and this low pH therefore assists the transfer of more oxygen to the tissues for the same arteriovenous fall in PO_2. In other words, a fall in pH results in an increase in P_{50}, or shift of the oxyhemoglobin dissociation curve to the right. This is known as the Bohr effect. It might be thought that the reduced oxygen affinity of venous blood which is more acid would be detrimental to the uptake of oxygen in the lungs; however, at a higher PO_2, the dissociation curves come closer together and oxygen uptake is little affected. P_{50} may be altered by a change of either pH or PCO_2, for the shift to the right will still occur if pH is kept constant and PCO_2 increased, showing that the latter has an effect independent of pH.

The organic phosphate 2,3-DPG is an intermediate in erythrocyte carbohydrate metabolism and constitutes most of the phosphate in red cells. If the concentration of 2,3-DPG is increased, it competes with oxygen for binding sites on deoxygenated hemoglobin, thereby reducing its oxygen affinity, shifting the oxyhemoglobin dissociation curve to the right. The level of 2,3-DPG is regulated by erythrocyte enzyme systems which are pH dependent, so that acidity or alkalinity tends to suppress or stimulate its production, respectively. We have seen that a fall in plasma pH causes an immediate shift of the curve to the right, thereby reducing the affinity of hemoglobin for oxygen. If this fall in pH persists for several hours, 2,3-DPG production is reduced, exerting a counterbalancing effect on the pH-mediated right shift. Consequently, when long-standing acidosis is quickly corrected with bicarbonate, a persisting low 2,3-DPG level may have a deleterious "overshoot effect" by increasing the oxygen affinity of hemoglobin and reducing its supply to the tissues. Deoxygenated hemoglobin, which is a weaker acid and therefore relatively alkaline, stimulates 2,3-DPG production, reducing the affinity of hemoglobin for oxygen and causing the shift to the right that is associated with long-standing hypoxemic conditions such as cyanotic heart disease or chronic bronchitis.[26] Similarly, the rise in plasma alkalinity that occurs at high altitudes causes a shift to the left with increased hemoglobin-oxygen affinity, and also stimulates 2,3-DPG production, which has a counteraction. Other situations in which 2,3-DPG may be depleted with a reduction in blood oxygen–transferring efficiency include the storage of transfusable blood, hypophosphatemia, certain congenital hemoglobinopathies, and the raised blood levels of carboxyhemoglobin associated with cigarette smoking.

A rise in the temperature of blood reduces the oxygen affinity of hemoglobin and facilitates its removal by metabolizing tissues, the temperature of which is slightly higher than that of the lungs.

Carbon Dioxide Transport

The partial pressure gradient between metabolizing tissues and the capillaries perfusing them results in the diffusion of carbon dioxide into the blood in which it is carried in three forms: (1) in solution in plasma, (2) combined with hemoglobin, and (3) as bicarbonate (Fig. 5–19). Plasma alone is an inefficient carrier of carbon dioxide, and only 5% of total carbon dioxide is carried in this way. Although the volume of dissolved carbon dioxide is linearly related to the P_{CO_2} of blood, the slope of this relationship is not steep enough to enable the elimination of sufficient carbon dioxide by the lungs to keep pace with its production by the tissues. A small proportion of dissolved carbon dioxide in the plasma reacts with water to form carbonic acid, which then ionizes according to the equation

$$CO_2 + H_2 \rightleftharpoons H_2CO_3 \rightleftharpoons H^+ + HCO_3^- \qquad \text{(Equation 1)}$$

Carbon dioxide also diffuses into red blood cells, where the above reaction proceeds rapidly as a result of the action of the enzyme carbonic anhydrase. This results in a concentration gradient of bicarbonate between the erythrocyte and the plasma, so that bicarbonate diffuses out of the cell in exchange for chloride, which passes in to maintain electrical neutrality, a process known as the chloride shift. The hydrogen ions are largely buffered by hemoglobin, although venous blood is rendered slightly more acid than arterial blood. Ninety per cent of total blood carbon dioxide is carried as bicarbonate in this way. The remaining 5% combines reversibly with NH_2 on deoxygenated hemoglobin to form hemoglobin carbamate:

$$HbNH_2 + CO_2 \rightleftharpoons HbNHCOOH \rightleftharpoons HbNHCOO^- + H^+$$

When venous blood in the lungs comes into contact with alveolar gas, carbon dioxide in the plasma diffuses into the air spaces, causing the equations illustrated in Figure 5–19 to proceed in the opposite direction. It is clear that the red blood cell is essential for not only oxygen but also for carbon dioxide transport.

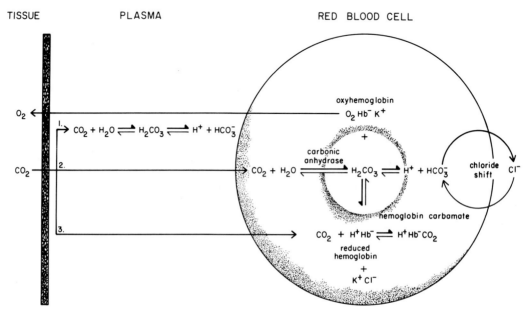

Figure 5–19. Modes of carriage of carbon dioxide in the blood. (From Sodeman, W. A., Jr., and Sodeman, T. M., eds., Sodeman's Pathologic Physiology, 7th ed. Philadelphia, W. B. Saunders Co., 1985, p. 453.)

ACID-BASE BALANCE

The acidity or alkalinity of blood is expressed as pH, which is the negative logarithm of the hydrogen ion concentration [H^+]. If an acid is added to water (pH 7), it dissociates and the hydrogen ion concentration increases, producing a fall in pH.

$$HCl \rightleftharpoons H^+ + Cl^-$$

The addition of a base has the opposite effect, reducing hydrogen ion concentration and therefore increasing pH:

$$NaOH + H^+ \rightleftharpoons Na^+ \ H_2O$$

There is a constant tendency for the body to increase its acidity by the production of both gaseous and nongaseous acid metabolites. This tendency is controlled by the excretion of hydrogen ions indirectly by the lungs and by the kidneys, and involves a number of chemical buffering systems. These mechanisms are normally able to maintain the pH in a narrow range between 7.36 and 7.44; a departure above or below these limits is referred to as alkalosis or acidosis, respectively.

A buffer solution is one whose pH is relatively unchanged following the addition of an acid or alkali. In general, buffers are effective only over a certain range of pH. An example of such a buffer system is a solution containing a weak acid (one that does not completely dissociate in solution) and a salt of that acid. A buffer system substitutes the stronger, more dissociable acid with one that is weaker and less dissociable, therefore reducing the hydrogen ion concentration. In humans there are a number of buffers, the most important of which is the carbonic acid/bicarbonate system, which buffers nongaseous acidic metabolites such as lactic and pyruvic acids. Thus, sodium bicarbonate reacts with lactic acid to produce carbonic acid and sodium lactate:

$$NaHCO_3 + HLac \rightleftharpoons NaLac + H_2CO_3$$

Since carbonic acid is a weaker acid, it is less dissociated than lactic acid and fewer hydrogen ions are released into solution. The buffer system has therefore "mopped up" a number of hydrogen ions that would otherwise have been released were lactic acid alone dissociated in solution.

In addition to nongaseous tissue metabolites, it can be seen from Equation 1 that the continual production of carbon dioxide also has an extremely important influence on pH, in that each molecule of carbon dioxide produced releases one hydrogen ion. We have seen (see Fig. 5–19) how this is buffered by reduced hemoglobin and its neutral salt:

$$H_2CO_3 + KHb \rightleftharpoons HHb + KHCO_3 \xrightarrow{\text{chloride shift}} Cl^-$$

Reduced hemoglobin is an even weaker, less dissociable acid than carbonic acid, and necessarily reduces hydrogen ion concentration, thereby preventing acidemia. Although the role of hemoglobin in buffering tissue carbon dioxide is important, the overall level of carbon dioxide retained in the body depends upon the rate at which it can be eliminated from the blood, and this in turn is dependent upon the level of alveolar ventilation. If alveolar ventilation is reduced disproportionately to the rate of carbon dioxide production, then Equation 1 moves to the right, with a consequent fall in pH.

The ability of these buffer systems to maintain pH within a given range is related to the readiness with which the weak acid dissociates. This may be expressed mathematically:

$$K' = \frac{[H^+] \times [A^-]}{[HA]} \qquad \text{(Equation 2)}$$

where K' is the dissociation constant of HA, which is a weak acid, the brackets denoting concentration. The higher the value of the dissociation constant, the more readily the acid dissociates. Just as hydrogen ion concentration is for convenience expressed as the logarithm of its reciprocal ($-\log_{10}$ [H^+] or pH), so the dissociation constant is conventionally written as $-\log_{10}K'$ or pK'. Equation 2 may therefore be rewritten

$$- \log K' = - \log[H^+] - \log\frac{[A^-]}{[HA]}$$

or:

$$pK' = pH - \log\frac{[A^-]}{[HA]}$$

By adding the last term to both sides of this equation we obtain:

$$pH = pK' + \log\frac{[A^-]}{[HA]} \qquad \text{(Equation 3)}$$

The relationship of the pH of blood to its carbon dioxide content and tension may be derived by substituting carbonic acid from Equation 1 as the weak acid in Equation 3

$$pH = pK' + \log\frac{[HCO_3^-]}{[H_2CO_3]} \qquad \text{(Equation 4)}$$

This is the Henderson-Hasselbalch equation. The dissociation constant of carbonic acid at 37°C is 6.10, and measurement of the remaining two factors will allow the pH to be calculated. In practice, the concentration of carbonic acid in plasma is about 700 times lower than that of dissolved CO_2, as the reaction in Equation 1 is driven to the left by HCO_3^- ions derived from sodium and potassium salts.

$$NaHCO_3 \rightleftharpoons Na^+ + HCO_3 \qquad \text{(Equation 5)}$$

Dissolved CO_2 also bears a constant relationship to carbonic acid concentration, and it can therefore be substituted for it in Equation 4:

$$pH = pK' + \log\frac{[HCO_3^-]}{[CO_2]} \qquad \text{(Equation 6)}$$

The quantity of CO_2 in solution is the product of its solubility coefficient ($\alpha = 0.03$) and partial pressure, and the latter can be measured directly with a CO_2 electrode. Carbonic acid contributes insignificantly to the plasma concentration of HCO_3^- ions which are largely accounted for by the reaction shown in Equation 5. The plasma bicarbonate of arterial blood may be derived by subtracting dissolved from total carbon dioxide content and is normally 24 mM/L. Substituting these values in Equation 6

$$pH = 6.10 + \log\frac{24}{40 \times 0.03}$$
$$= 7.4$$

The practical importance of the Henderson-Hasselbalch equation is that in order for pH to remain constant, any change in bicarbonate (the numerator) has to be matched by a proportional change in CO_2 (the denominator). If this ratio, which is normally 20:1, is altered, a change in pH is inevitable. Disturbances of pH primarily due to alteration in CO_2 are referred to as respiratory, and those primarily due to alteration in HCO_3^- are called metabolic. Any primary change in one component of the HCO_3^-/CO_2 ratio leads to a similar change in the other component in an attempt to maintain normal pH. If for some reason the lungs are unable to remove CO_2 as fast as it is produced, arterial P_{CO_2} will rise and pH will fall. In order to correct this respiratory acidosis, the kidneys act by conserving HCO_3^- and excreting H^+ ions, leading to a compensatory rise in HCO_3^-. In disturbances of acid-base balance, the compensatory change in HCO_3^- or CO_2 is less than the primary change and is also usually insufficient to return the pH to the normal range. The following analyses of arterial blood samples will illustrate this:

Example One: P_{CO_2} = 60 mm Hg, plasma bicarbonate = 26 mM/L

Here the rise in P_{CO_2} is greater than that of bicarbonate and is therefore likely to reflect respiratory acidosis rather than a metabolic alkalosis. The pH of 7.29 confirms this. Normally a rise in P_{CO_2} leads to an increase in output of the medullary respiratory center, resulting in increased ventilation which "blows off" CO_2. A failure of this homeostatic mechanism to compensate can commonly occur with widespread airways obstruction, producing ventilation-perfusion mismatching as seen in chronic bronchitis, or with failure of the bellows function owing to muscle weakness as in myasthenia gravis or depression of the respiratory center by drugs.

Example Two: P_{CO_2} = 50 mm Hg, plasma bicarbonate = 40 mM/L

Here the greatest rise has occurred in bicarbonate with a smaller compensatory rise in P_{CO_2} and is therefore likely to result from a metabolic alkalosis rather than a respiratory acidosis. This is confirmed by the pH of 7.53. This situation might follow the excessive ingestion of alkali or after repeated vomiting, and may also occur in hypokalemia in which depleted intracellular potassium is replaced by hydrogen ions, resulting in extracellular alkalosis.

Example Three: P_{CO_2} = 30 mm Hg, plasma bicarbonate = 12 mM/L

Here the major fall is in bicarbonate, with a smaller compensatory fall in P_{CO_2}. This is therefore likely to be a nonrespiratory or metabolic acidosis rather than a respiratory alkalosis. This is confirmed by the pH of 7.24. This situation is commonly seen in renal failure and in diabetic ketoacidosis, in which the excretion of hydrogen ions fails to keep pace with the production of nongaseous acid metabolites.

Example Four: P_{CO_2} = 25 mm Hg, bicarbonate = 20 mM/L

Here the major change is in P_{CO_2} with only a small fall in bicarbonate, and the fact that this is a respiratory alkalosis is confirmed by the pH of 7.53. This situation may be seen in hysterical hyperventilation or with overbreathing due to other causes such as salicylate poisoning or diffusion defects.

GAS TRANSFER

Diffusing Capacity

The rate of diffusion of a gas in a gaseous medium is inversely proportional to the square root of its density (Graham's law). Thus, in such a medium, CO_2 diffuses less easily than does oxygen; however, diffusion in the lungs involves a gaseous phase and a liquid phase. For this reason, the solubility of the gas in the liquid is an important factor and is governed in this instance by Henry's law. This law states that the volume of the gas that dissolves in a given volume of a liquid is directly proportional to the partial pressure of that gas. CO_2 being 24 times more soluble than oxygen, it has a greater rate of diffusion.

Factors Influencing the Diffusing Capacity of the Lungs[27]
(Table 5–2)

1. The Pressure Gradient Between the Alveoli and the Capillary Blood.
Under normal circumstances, blood remains in the pulmonary capillaries for 0.75

Table 5-2

■

Physiological Factors and Disease Processes Affecting the Diffusing Capacity

	DL_{CO}	Principal Determinants
Loss of lung tissue	$\downarrow$	DM
Emphysema, lung resection		
Diffuse infiltrations	$\downarrow$	DM/VC
Asbestosis, sarcoid, scleroderma		
Altered pulmonary blood volume		
Mitral stenosis	$\uparrow$ or $\downarrow$	DM/VC
Left to right cardiac shunt	$\uparrow$	
Exercise	$\uparrow$	VC
Supine posture	$\uparrow$	
Valsalva maneuver	$\downarrow$	
Altered Hb binding capacity		
Anemia	$\downarrow$	
Polycythemia	$\uparrow$	θ
Reduced Pa_{O_2}	$\uparrow$	
Increased Pa_{O_2}	$\downarrow$	

From Morgan, W. K. C., and Seaton, D., Pulmonary ventilation and blood gas exchange. *In* Sodeman, W. A., Jr., and Sodeman, T. M., eds., Sodeman's Pathologic Physiology, 7th ed. Philadelphia, W. B. Saunders Co., 1985, p. 456.

second. Even this short time is more than enough to allow equilibrium to take place, which is reached in 0.3 second in a normal subject breathing ambient air at sea level. Under these conditions, the alveolar P_{O_2} is around 100 mm Hg. With moderate impairment of diffusion, equilibrium takes longer to occur; but even so, it is still achieved in less than 0.75 second. Only when alveolocapillary block is severe does hypoxemia result. During exercise, however, the time the blood remains in the capillaries is shortened, so although the subject may not be hypoxemic at rest, he or she may become so with exercise. The pressure difference responsible for the diffusion of oxygen is not as might be expected—the initial alveoloarterial gradient (100 − 40 = 60 mm) or the end capillary gradient (100 − 99.9 = 0.01 mm)—but is an integrated mean value that depends on a variety of complex factors including the time oxygen takes to traverse the membrane and combine with hemoglobin.

2. The Length of the Pathway of Diffusion. Before an oxygen molecule can combine with hemoglobin it must traverse the following:

Surfactant lining of alveoli
The alveolar membrane
The capillary endothelium
The plasma in the capillary
The RBC membrane
The intracellular RBC fluid

The distance across the membrane is usually about 0.2 micron. In certain disease states this distance may be increased by edema fluid, fibrous tissue, or the presence of additional alveolar cells.

3. The Surface Area Available for Diffusion. The area available for diffusion depends on the number of functioning alveoli rather than the total number of alveoli present in the lungs. In humans, it is approximately 70 square meters. Thus, loss of diffusing surface occurs in emphysema, following resection, and in a fibrothorax with compression of the adjacent lung. Owing to the fact that in exercise many nonfunctioning alveoli open up, the diffusing capacity increases with exercise.

4. The Number and Character of the Red Blood Cells Available to Accept Diffused Oxygen. Anemia reduces the diffusing capacity since there are fewer red blood cells to take up the diffused gas. In addition, were the red cells affected in some anatomical or physiological way which impaired the acceptance of diffused oxygen, then the diffusing capacity would likewise be reduced. This is mainly a theoretical concept.

Measurement of Diffusing Capacity

To measure the diffusing capacity, it is necessary that the gas used be more soluble in blood than in the alveolocapillary membrane and the tissue fluid. Both oxygen and carbon monoxide fulfill this criterion because they combine with hemoglobin. Other gases such as N_2O are equally soluble in tissues and blood and therefore can be used to measure pulmonary capillary blood flow. They are not, however, suitable for the management of the diffusing capacity.

The equation for measurement of the diffusing capacity for oxygen is expressed thus:

$$D_{O_2} = \frac{ml/O_2 \text{ taken up by capillaries/min}}{\text{alveolar } P_{O_2} - \text{pulmonary capillary } P_{O_2}} = ml\ O_2/min/mm\ Hg$$

Measuring D_{O_2} requires a knowledge of the P_{O_2} of mixed venous blood, since this datum is necessary in order to calculate the alveolocapillary gradient. In addition, since the capillary P_{O_2} rises as the blood traverses the capillary, the gradient and hence rate of diffusion fall. To calculate the D_{O_2} requires that a knowledge of the P_{aO_2} is available at every moment as the blood traverses the capillary. Although these data can be derived mathematically, the calculations are tedious and many assumptions are made. Thus, for the most part, the diffusing capacity of the lungs for oxygen is seldom measured. In this regard, CO is far more convenient and is almost exclusively used now. The advantages of the use of CO are that the P_{CO} in mixed venous blood is zero except in the case of heavy smokers and hence need not be measured. In addition, CO has 210 times the affinity for hemoglobin and consequently only very low concentrations of inhaled CO (0.3%) are necessary to measure the $D_{L_{CO}}$.

There are a number of methods for obtaining $D_{L_{CO}}$, of which the most commonly used is the single breath technique.[28] This requires the subject to make a vital capacity inspiration of a mixture containing 0.3% carbon monoxide, 10% helium, and 21% oxygen, and to breath-hold at total lung capacity for 10 seconds, so that some of the carbon monoxide diffuses into the blood. A forced expiratory volume maneuver is then made, and once dead space gas has been displaced, an "alveolar" sample is taken and is analyzed for the final carbon monoxide concentration ($F_{E_{CO}}$). The carbon monoxide concentration that was present in the alveolar gas before transfer had taken place is estimated from the dilution of inspired helium (He) according to the equation

$$\underset{\text{(initial CO concentration in alveolar gas)}}{F_{I_{CO}}} = \frac{F_{E_{He}} \times F_{I_{CO}}}{F_{I_{He}}}$$

where:
$F_{E_{He}}$ = He concentration in expired alveolar sample
$F_{I_{He}}$ = Inspired He concentration
$F_{I_{CO}}$ = Inspired CO concentration

The change in carbon monoxide concentration during breath-holding is now known, and so $D_{L_{CO}}$ can be calculated according to Krogh's equation:

$$\underset{\text{(ml/min/mm Hg)}}{D_{L_{CO}}} = \frac{\text{alveolar volume (L)} \times 160}{\text{time (secs)}} \times \log 10 \frac{F_{I_{CO}}}{F_{E_{CO}}}$$

Alveolar volume in this equation may be taken as the sum of the inspired volume and the residual volume (measured separately), or the "effective" alveolar volume ($V_{A_{eff}}$) may be calculated from the dilution of helium contained in the mixture according to the equation:

$$\dot{V}A_{eff} = \frac{FI_{He}}{FE_{He}} \times (VI - VD_A) \times 1.05$$

where:

VI = inspired volume

VD_A = anatomical dead space

1.05 = correction for CO_2 absorbed before analysis of expired gas

The "effective" alveolar volume tends to give a lower value for DL_{CO} in obstructive lung disease than does the other method.

DL_{CO} may also be measured by a steady-state technique in which the subject rebreathes a mixture containing a small concentration of carbon monoxide in air, during which the rate of removal of the gas is measured.[29] This method has the advantage that it may be used during exercise; however, errors may occur in the estimation of alveolar PCO, particularly at rest when the tidal volume is small and dead space gas may not be entirely flushed out when sampling is made.

DL is analogous to an electrical conductance, and its reciprocal is therefore comparable to a resistance. Resistances arranged in series may be added to give the overall resistance; and so in the lungs

$$\frac{1}{DL} = \frac{1}{D \text{ alveolar walls}} + \frac{1}{D \text{ capillary walls}} + \frac{1}{D \text{ plasma}} + \frac{1}{D \text{ red cells}}$$

Although it is not possible to estimate each of these smaller values separately, they may be incorporated into two measurable terms to give

$$\frac{1}{DL} = \frac{1}{DM} + \frac{1}{\theta VC}$$

where DM is the diffusing capacity of the alveolocapillary membrane, and θVC is the diffusing capacity of the blood (VC being the volume of alveolocapillary blood to which the gas is exposed in the lungs, and θ being the rate of reaction of the gas with hemoglobin in ml/min).[30] DL_{CO} falls following oxygen breathing because the value of θ, which can be determined *in vitro*, depends on the degree of saturation of hemoglobin, which in turn determines the number of binding sites available for carbon monoxide. If two measurements of DL_{CO} are made after breathing first room air and then oxygen, and θ is known for each level, then simultaneous equations may be solved for the two unknowns DM and VC. The membrane component (DM) falls in diseases in which the surface area available for diffusion is reduced, e.g., emphysema or following lung resection. It is also reduced in conditions causing abnormal thickening of the alveolocapillary membrane such as fibrosing alveolitis or sarcoidosis. The alveolocapillary blood volume (VC) is labile, as the pulmonary circulation has a large reserve capacity, and it may not fall until pulmonary disease is advanced. It tends to increase in normal subjects when they exercise or lie flat. It is also increased in patients with left to right cardiac shunts. In mitral stenosis, DL_{CO} may be initially raised owing to an elevation of VC (see Table 5–2). This may later fall owing to "pruning" of the lungs' vasculature as a result of pulmonary hypertension. The situation may be further complicated by pulmonary edema, which leads to a reduction of DM. The rate of reaction with hemoglobin (θ) is slower in anemia and faster in polycythemia, and DL_{CO} may be corrected for hemoglobin concentration by the equation

$$DL,C = DL,O \, (14.6a + Hb) \div (1 + a)Hb$$

where DL,C and DL,O are corrected and observed DL_{CO}, respectively, Hb is the hemoglobin concentration, and a is the DM/VC ratio, which is assumed to be 0.7.

In bronchial asthma, the DL_{CO} is normal, which is a useful point in distinguishing this condition from irreversible air flow obstruction due to emphysema. The measurement of DM, VC, and θ is laborious, and for clinical purposes, the simpler measurement of DL_{CO} usually suffices. It should be clear that this is influenced by a variety of factors other than thickening of the alveolocapillary membrane as was once thought, and it is therefore sometimes called the gas transfer factor (TL_{CO}).

Carbon Dioxide

Because of its solubility, carbon dioxide diffuses from the pulmonary capillaries to the alveoli about 20 times more rapidly than oxygen. For this reason, diffuse pulmonary fibrotic or granulomatous diseases such as asbestosis or sarcoidosis, which are associated with impaired diffusion of oxygen, do not affect the diffusion of carbon dioxide sufficiently to cause a rise in arterial P_{CO_2}. By the time that this stage is reached, the arterial P_{O_2} is too low to support life. A raised arterial P_{CO_2} usually indicates alveolar hypoventilation.

Control of Respiration

The regulation of ventilation, by which the arterial P_{O_2} and P_{CO_2} are maintained within a fairly narrow range, is complex and incompletely understood. The involuntary rhythmic nature of breathing depends primarily upon the integrity of collections of interrelated, reciprocally acting inspiratory and expiratory neuronal pathways contained in the reticular formation of the medulla oblongata. These are known as the medullary respiratory centers, although they have no distinct anatomical boundaries. Their output to the respiratory neurons in the spinal cord is modified by cortical and pontine activity, by the aortic and carotid body chemoreceptors, and by vagus-mediated signals from the lungs and chest wall. They are extremely sensitive to the arterial P_{CO_2} level, and a 5% increase causes the minute ventilation to double. Carbon dioxide will cross the blood-brain barrier more readily than bicarbonate, and the subsequent dissociation of carbonic acid releases hydrogen ions into the cerebrospinal fluid (CSF), which is less able to buffer them than blood. The medulla possesses receptors on its ventral surface which, when bathed with acid CSF, respond by increasing first tidal volume and later respiratory rate. If the acidity of the CSF is prolonged, as may occur in respiratory acidosis due to chronic obstructive airways disease, a compensatory change occurs in which CSF bicarbonate is increased, raising the pH again. As a result, a patient with an elevated arterial P_{CO_2} due to emphysema may have a diminished hyperventilatory response to carbon dioxide, and depends instead upon hypoxic drive. Uncontrolled oxygen therapy in such a patient may produce apnea by raising arterial P_{O_2} above the normal level, thereby leading to secondary hypoventilation and a further rise in P_{CO_2}, which raises the intracranial pressure and acts as a respiratory depressant. Depression of the respiratory center also occurs physiologically during sleep and may be deepened by hypnotic drugs or anesthetics.

The carotid body and aortic arch chemoreceptors are stimulated mainly by hypoxia and to a lesser extent by hypercarbia. The carotid bodies are also sensitive to a fall in pH. These peripheral chemoreceptors are highly active metabolically, and it has been suggested that they are stimulated by the local accumulation of products of anaerobic metabolism, occurring either as a consequence of a reduction in arterial P_{O_2} or from diminished perfusion in the presence of normoxemia as may occur in hemorrhagic shock. Their afferent signals are carried to the medulla by the glossopharyngeal and vagus nerves. The peripheral chemoreceptor response to hypoxia is not as sensitive as the medullary carbon dioxide response, and the alveolar P_{O_2} is usually reduced to about 50 mm Hg before the chemoreceptors take over. Variation in the intensity of hypoxic drive among normal individuals has been reported, and it is possible that this might explain the differing clinical presentations of chronic obstructive airways disease, in which the ''blue bloater'' with a poor hypoxic response may be found at one end of the scale, and the ''pink puffer'' with a normal response at the other.

A number of vagally mediated afferent stimuli pass to the respiratory centers from the lungs and chest wall. The Hering-Breuer reflex is initiated by receptors in the bronchial and bronchiolar walls and in the diaphragm. Inhibitory signals are generated when these are stretched on inspiration. These do not affect central respiratory drive, but modify tidal volume and breathing rate during exercise and hypoxic or hypercarbic stimulation; and their role during quiet breathing is minimal. In addition to brain stem and cortical controls, the diaphragm and intercostal and abdominal muscles, which drive the "respiratory pump," are also subject to reflex influences at spinal level. Like other voluntary muscles, they contain length-sensitive spindle fibers, which when stretched produce signals that are transmitted to the spinal cord by γ-afferent fibers. Here these synapse with α-motor neurons supplying the corresponding muscle fibers. It is thought that the γ-afferent system may have a coordinative function, providing proprioceptive information about the respiratory muscles, so that motor output may be modified accordingly.

In metabolic acidosis, as occurs in renal failure or diabetic ketosis, nongaseous acid metabolites which do not cross the blood-brain barrier may stimulate respiration by acting on the peripheral carotid body chemoreceptors, leading to Kussmaul breathing. Cheyne-Stokes breathing is characterized by a cyclical waxing and waning of tidal volume and respiratory frequency and is commonly seen in severe cardiac failure associated with hypotension and following cerebrovascular accidents. This instability of the ventilatory control system may result from a variety of causes, such as prolonged circulation time resulting in delayed feedback signals to the respiratory centers, or from increased sensitivity of the CO_2 control system as a consequence of damage to higher centers, or paradoxically from depression of CO_2 responsiveness due to brain stem disease, enabling the less stable O_2 control system to take over.

PHYSIOLOGY OF EXERCISE

Under basal conditions, a normal person requires approximately 250 ml of oxygen and produces approximately 200 ml of carbon dioxide every minute. When he or she starts to exercise or do strenuous work, oxygen requirement and carbon dioxide production increase, and the degree of change is related to the extent of increased activity. Sustained work requires adequate gas exchange. Although the body is capable of working under anaerobic conditions for short periods, this method of metabolism is inefficient and results in the build-up of toxic metabolites such as lactic acid. With an increased workload, delivery of oxygen to the tissues depends on the integrity of the three basic processes of respiration, namely, ventilation, perfusion, and diffusion. Also necessary is an intact and properly functioning respiratory center, so that any increase in workload is accompanied by an appropriate increase in ventilation along with a selective redistribution of the oxygenated blood. The factors limiting working capacity are admirably discussed by Jones and Campbell in their book *Clinical Exercise Testing*.[31]

Work performance is best quantified by measuring oxygen consumption. The latter is influenced by body size, but can be standardized by expressing oxygen consumption as ml/kg of body weight or as a multiple of resting oxygen uptake (Mets). During exercise the oxygen demand of the muscles involved increases. Since the oxygen saturation of arterial blood is almost complete, the additional oxygen requirements of the muscles can be met by increasing blood flow or by increasing the arteriovenous oxygen difference [(a-v)O_2], or both. Increased blood flow to the muscles is effected partly as an increase in cardiac output and partly as a consequence of a redistribution of peripheral blood so that the muscles receive a significantly greater proportion of the cardiac output. Cardiac output may be increased as a result of either an increase in heart rate or an increased stroke volume. In practice, increasing the load usually results in both of these responses.

The increased (a-v)O_2 in turn necessitates greater ventilation, with the result that the minute volume increases. The expected increases in heart rate and ventilation that occur in healthy subjects in response to maximal exercise have been well studied, and there are numerous prediction formulae available in the literature. In contrast, during submaximal exercise, the increase in both heart rate and ventilation is variable, may be greatly influenced by anxiety and other factors, and hence cannot be predicted accurately.

In healthy subjects, maximal exercise is limited by the cardiac output and not by limitations of the respiratory reserve. During maximal exercise, minute ventilation does not approach maximal voluntary ventilation (MVV) and is usually only 65% to 75% of the latter. By the same token, arterial oxygen saturation does not fall, at least under normal circumstances, although there is some evidence that in an exceptionally well-trained distance runner with extreme exertion, there may be slight reduction. Certainly there is no fall in the arterial oxygen saturation in a normal person even with maximal exercise. During maximal exercise when the cardiac output can increase no further, anaerobic metabolism takes over, and lactic acid and other metabolites are produced. The lactic acid has to be buffered by bicarbonate, so that ventilation has to increase still further to eliminate the excess CO_2 produced. The additional ventilation is "inappropriate," and the breathlessness which the subject experiences becomes intolerable. Maximal oxygen consumption reaches a peak in the late teens, remains relatively constant to around 25 to 30 years of age, and then slowly decreases. The decrease in maximal oxygen consumption occurs mainly as a consequence of the age-related decrease in heart rate (Fig. 5–20). Maximal oxygen consumption can be predicted fairly accurately from the heart rate response to submaximal exercise, provided the subject has reached a steady state.

As already mentioned, the relationship of heart rate and ventilation to exercise varies appreciably in the healthy individual. Such differences depend on many factors, including body size, hemoglobin content, physical fitness, and the level of training. It is for these reasons that work done is best quantified by oxygen consumption rather than by external workload. Obese subjects use more energy for the same workload than do lean persons in good physical shape. Although some variations occur in the response to the same level of exercise in the same individual, such variations are relatively limited. Finally, the type of exercise performed may affect heart rate and oxygen consumption.

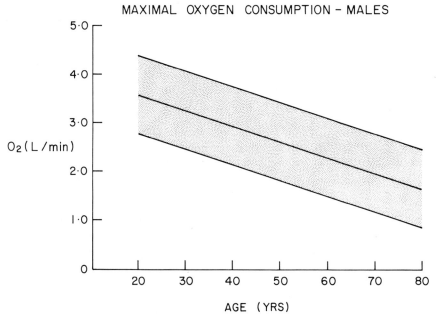

Figure 5–20. Relationship between maximal oxygen consumption and age.

Thus, the performance of the same amount of work on a bicycle and on a treadmill may lead to differing work outputs and oxygen consumptions. This is a consequence of the fact that certain people use one group of muscles more than another, and as a result, one particular muscle group becomes more efficient. With the decline in use of the bicycle in the United States, very few Americans are used to cycling and as a result their thigh muscles are inefficient. Hence, treadmill exercise is better tolerated by most Americans. Lack of training and physical fitness influences the body's ability to adapt to exercise. Thus, inactivity leads to reduced levels of mitochondrial enzymes and energy stores, and should oxygen delivery be inadequate, greater use is made of anaerobic metabolism. Rarely, an enzyme defect in the muscles themselves affects the ability to exercise, the classic example of which is McArdle's syndrome.

In the healthy person, the $(a-v)O_2$ becomes greater with increasing oxygen uptake. The resting value is around 50 ml/L and increases to about 130 to 150 ml/L with maximal work. Thus, the saturation of venous blood during maximal work is around 30%. In a fully trained athlete, venous oxygen saturation may be appreciably lower, indicating that virtually all the oxygen that is carried to the muscles has been used by muscles. In subjects with heart disease, it is even more essential that the removal of oxygen from blood-perfusing muscles is as great as possible. For a more detailed review of exercise physiology, the reader is referred to the paper by Wasserman and Whipp.[32]

RELATIONSHIP BETWEEN PULMONARY IMPAIRMENT AND DISABILITY

When the problem of industrial lung disease is viewed as a whole, it is evident that it matters little whether the physiological defect is obstructive or restrictive in nature; the presenting symptom is virtually always shortness of breath. Moreover, it is this symptom which is almost always the cause of respiratory disability and is therefore of paramount importance. Some elaboration is, therefore, necessary concerning the relationship between dyspnea and respiratory impairment.

Shortness of breath, like pain, is a subjective sensation, and its intensity depends on both the attitude and the personality of the patient. The sensation of shortness of breath does not always correlate well with tests of pulmonary function, sometimes because the person who is affected is relatively stoical, in other instances because he or she has ulterior motives, but most often because no single test or even battery of tests has been devised that can quantify dyspnea. Not uncommonly, the severity of the symptoms is exaggerated in order to obtain financial gain, usually in the form of compensation.

In obstructive airways disease, it can be shown that there is a fairly good relationship between those tests that measure, directly or indirectly, an increased airways resistance (MVV and FEV_1) and the presence of dyspnea. This is especially true of patients who are referred to hospital for nonoccupationally related disease. In restrictive impairment this relationship is sometimes not as clear-cut. It has been suggested that the presence of dyspnea is related to the work of breathing, and indeed there is appreciable evidence in favor of this contention. Nonetheless, there are certain facts which are not easily explained by this hypothesis, in particular the dyspnea experienced by a subject on a ventilator where the work of breathing is nonexistent. Campbell and Howell have suggested that length tension inappropriateness provides a better explanation for the sensation of dyspnea.[33] This theory postulates that dyspnea is experienced when there is an imbalance between the demand of the respiratory center for ventilation and the actual ventilation that takes place; in short, the ventilatory response is inappropriate and inadequate for the stimuli received. At the present time, this hypothesis provides the best explanation for the sensation of shortness of breath. Even so, much needs to be learned about this problem. It must be stressed that with moderate or severe exercise some shortness of breath is normal, and it is the degree of shortness of breath relative to the workload that needs to be assessed. Provided that the above facts are borne in mind, it becomes useful to characterize the types of respiratory impairment that are found in the pneumoconioses and other occupational lung diseases.

Nowhere is there more confusion than in the field of disability determination, and no professional group has done more to foster this confusion than lawyers. Physicians find themselves more and more frequently asked to assess disability, and with few exceptions their level of understanding and experience in this field is often an embarrassment to both themselves and the party for whom they are appearing. In no discipline in medicine is it more important to have a clear understanding of terms and nomenclature, and for this reason, a few definitions are in order.

The loose and imprecise use of the terms *impairment* and *disability* is often a seminal source of confusion. *Impairment* when used correctly in connection with respiratory disease refers to a physiological abnormality of function which persists after treatment. It is therefore best defined as ''an inability of the human respiratory apparatus to perform satisfactorily one or more of the three components of respiration—ventilation, diffusion, and perfusion.'' Anatomical deficiencies, for example, the loss of lung, also constitute an impairment, but in the case of lung disease it is more appropriate to think in terms of physiological function. For the accurate quantification of impairment, the level of either function or performance prior to the injury or illness must be known or an accurate prediction for such dysfunction in health must be available. In contrast, *disability* is best defined as ''an inability to carry out a specific task or job'' or, alternatively, ''the development of undue distress during the performance of the job or task.'' The latter more accurately describes what is generally referred to as handicap. What constitutes distress is, however, a subject of contention, since many perfectly normal persons may suffer some shortness of breath while performing heavy work. In this context it is vital to bear in mind that the same impairment does not necessarily lead to the same disability. Thus, were a ballet dancer to lose a leg, he or she would be completely disabled for the vocation. In contrast, the loss of a leg in a civil servant or governmental bureaucrat would interfere little with the ability to work. By the same token, because the lungs have a tremendous reserve, minimal and even moderate respiratory impairment seldom interferes with the capacity to work unless the subject earns a living as a professional athlete or in an extraordinarily physically demanding job.

While quantification of impairment is the physician's responsibility, the assessment or adjudication of disability should not be left entirely to physicians, since it requires the assessment of the role of additional factors such as educational status, job requirements, propensity for vocational training, and availability of suitable alternative work. With these provisos in mind, it is now pertinent to consider in more detail some of the factors that determine whether a particular impairment is likely to lead to disability.[34]

Educational State and Motivation

The development of shortness of breath sufficient to put a worker at a disadvantage for a particular job need not always be disabling, since in some instances the person can be moved to a less demanding job. An elderly steel worker with obstruction of the airways might be quite capable of carrying out the duties of a storekeeper or janitor, but such a simple solution is not always attainable. Thus, the coal miner who is unable to continue working in the mines might have sufficient respiratory reserve to work as a bank teller or as a salesman, but may have neither the education nor the intellectual attainment for such alternative employment even should such a position be available. Should suitable alternative employment not be possible, the miner must be regarded as disabled despite his having sufficient respiratory reserve to enable him to perform a less demanding job.

In a similar context, it has been clearly established that the likelihood of a worker with a particular impairment continuing to work depends on educational and social background. The better educated the subject, the less likely he or she is to stop working. LeRoy-Ladurie and colleagues have shown that following a pneumonectomy about 20% of laborers return to work, while 70% to 80% of those with a profession return to their job.[35] In the case of children undergoing pneumonectomy, virtually all go on to obtain a job. While the loss of earnings is usually greater in the disabled professional, and this obviously provides some stimulus to return to work, it is not the only factor, and there is little doubt that if a worker finds his job interesting and stimulating, he or she has less desire to remain off work and claim compensation. With increasing age there is decreasing adaptability, and older persons may find it more difficult to acquire new skills. In addition, pulmonary function and reserve decline with age. These changes have an effect on working capacity and will be alluded to again.

Energy Requirements

Clearly the energy or work necessary to perform a specific task is important, since in some instances a subject's respiratory reserve may be insufficient for a particular job. As mentioned earlier, the resting requirements for oxygen in a normal person are around 250 to 300 ml/min. A coal miner operating a continuous miner during maximal effort has an O_2 consumption of around 1.2 L/min, while farming is somewhat more arduous and demanding, and the requirement for oxygen is around 1.5 L/min and under certain circumstances appreciably higher. Heavy labor in many iron and steel foundries necessitates an oxygen consumption of around 2.1 L/min. Athletic activities require a far greater oxygen consumption, and the most arduous of all, such as cross-country skiing and running, require up to 5.0 L/min. Sustained moderate effort is tolerated less well in the subject with respiratory impairment than are short bursts of high-energy output followed by prolonged low expenditure of energy. In deciding whether a worker is capable of carrying out a task, it is therefore essential to know the physical demands of the job as well as his or her exercise tolerance. Many jobs which were formerly regarded as arduous, e.g., coal and metal mining and construction, have become much less so with the advent of mechanization.

Pulmonary Impairment

The assessment of functional deficits in relation to disability is most often required in occupational pulmonary disease. In subjects being examined for occupationally related disability, it is necessary to bear in mind that naturally occurring diseases such as asthma and emphysema may complicate the issue, since they occur concomitantly in a fair number of subjects. It thus becomes important to separate the effects of occupation from those of naturally acquired disease. To achieve this requires a knowledge of the type and site of the impairment produced by the hazard. It is necessary therefore to know whether the particular hazard induces a response in the airways or in the lung parenchyma. Tests that enable one to diagnose and quantify the degree of impairment in a subject who is exposed to toluene diisocyanate are inappropriate for characterizing the respiratory defects in subjects with asbestosis or silicosis.

The most useful tests in the assessment of respiratory disability are those which are objective and not influenced by the behavior of the subject. This aspect of pulmonary function testing has been dealt with in detail in Chapter 6, and the reader is referred to the appropriate section. Although it is often maintained that there is a poor relationship between pulmonary impairment and dyspnea, such a pronouncement is a quarter truth. Granted that there are some individuals in whom this is true, provided one makes allowance for personality, educational status, and whether or not the subject is claiming compensation, an acceptable correlation exists in the majority of subjects. *Faute de mieux*, in the determination of disability, we have to rely on the degree of impairment to indicate how short of breath a person is likely to be. The comprehensive review in which Gaensler and Wright relate symptoms to various grades and types of pulmonary impairment is still the most useful reference, despite the advent of a plethora of so-called sensitive tests for the detection of minor and insignificant degrees of pulmonary insufficiency.[36] Another useful review is that of Hansen and Wasserman.[37]

Turning to the grading of the severity of impairment, in general the patient's or claimant's measured value is expressed as a percentage of the predicted value for a person of the same age, height, sex, and race. That this is less than ideal and discriminates against the older worker is not apparent at first sight. Since pulmonary function declines with age, for a given percentage of the decrement to represent the same disability in an elderly man as it does in a young man would require that the ventilatory cost of performing a certain job declines with age. The reverse is true, and in reality, the young man who has an MVV which is 30% of his predicted figure utilizes less of this respiratory reserve to carry out a certain task than does a 60-year-old man with the same percentage loss of MVV. The regulations devised by the United States Bureau of Disability of the Social Security Administration take this into account and award disability on the basis of a certain absolute reduction of pulmonary function, with the reduction being related only to the subject's height and sex. This appears to be a scientific approach when it is realized that considering age alone might lead to a situation in which the subject is judged disabled or prevented from doing a particular task despite the presence of normal pulmonary function.

Assessment of Shortness of Breath. Since shortness of breath is a cardinal symptom in subjects with pulmonary impairment, some attempt should be made to quantify it. Many factors render this task difficult, in particular the fact that dyspnea is a subjective sensation analogous to pain and, as previously mentioned, this symptom is often exaggerated. The criteria shown in Table 5–3 are helpful in quantifying or grading the severity of impairment.

There is a fairly good relationship between the FEV_1 and dyspnea, especially in chronic air flow obstruction, but it is remaining function rather than loss of function which governs the ability of the subject to work. Our studies in male patients who were not claiming compensation showed that the FEV_1 is closely related to exercise tolerance (Table 5–4). Other symptoms such as cough and wheeziness can seldom be regarded as disabling except under unusual circumstances.

In disability claimants, the reliability of the relationship between pulmonary function and shortness of breath breaks down. This is especially true when the financial rewards exceed what the subject earns at work. Our experience with black lung claimants is shown in Figure 5–21. It is quite clear that disability claimants

Table 5–3

■

Assessing Shortness of Breath

Grade	Criteria
0	No shortness of breath with normal activity. Shortness of breath with exertion, comparable to a well person of the same age, height, and sex.
1	More shortness of breath than a person of the same age while walking quietly on the level or on climbing an incline or two flights of stairs.
2	More shortness of breath than, and unable to keep up with, persons of the same age and sex while walking on the level.
3	Shortness of breath while walking on the level and while performing everyday tasks at work.
4	Shortness of breath while carrying out personal activities, e.g., dressing, talking, walking from one room to another.

Table 5–4

■

Relationship Between Grade of Dyspnea and FEV_1 in Subjects Not Seeking Disability Awards

Grade of Dyspnea	Mean FEV_1
0	3.2 L
1	2.4 L
2	1.8 L
3	1.2 L
4	0.75 L

markedly exaggerate their symptoms, and as such, the symptom of shortness of breath can no longer be relied upon as an index of impairment.[38]

Physical Examination. The physical examination provides limited help in the assessment of impairment and disability. Obvious wasting and shortness of breath at rest or with minor exertion are helpful pointers. The respiratory rate is often useful in the assessment of restrictive impairment when the latter is due to pulmonary fibrosis. In many instances, the subject will apparently be comfortable at rest despite the fact that he or she is breathing with a respiratory rate of 30 to 35 per minute. Minor exercise will often render him or her markedly short of breath. The presence of hyperinflation and increased resonance, the use of the accessory muscles of respiration, and certain physical findings such as the decreased distance between the cricothyroid membrane and the suprasternal notch all are helpful indications of the severity of chronic irreversible airways obstruction. In contrast, cyanosis is an unreliable sign. Decreased breath sounds, especially at the bases, often indicate emphysema and may be helpful. Diaphragmatic excursion is difficult

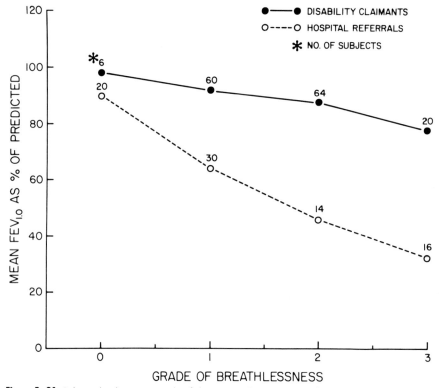

Figure 5–21. Relationship between grade of dyspnea and FEV_1 expressed as a percentage of predicted FEV_1 in black lung claimants and hospital patients. (From Morgan, W. K. C., Disability or disinclination? Impairment or importuning? Chest, 75, 712, 1979. Used by permission.)

to assess and inaccurate.[39] The presence of wheezes indicates turbulent flow and correlates poorly with ventilatory capacity. Persistent crackles, especially medium or coarse in character, which are audible throughout mid- and late inspiration are important and suggest the presence of fibrosis. Early and persistent inspiratory crackles at the bases indicate severe airways obstruction with overdistention.

Chest Radiograph. This is an unreliable method of diagnosing impairment and disability, and nowhere is this more true than in the field of occupationally related disease. While overdistention can be detected in the standard posteroanterior and lateral film, these changes are late and tend to be nonspecific. In the simple pneumoconioses, with the exception of asbestosis, there is little or no relationship between radiographic changes and pulmonary impairment.[40] In asbestosis there is some relationship between the severity of the radiographic changes and both symptoms and pulmonary function, at least in categories 2 and 3. The relationship becomes more tenuous in the lower categories—1/0, 1/1, and 1/2.[41, 42] In conglomerate silicosis and progressive massive fibrosis of coal miners, there is a relationship between shortness of breath and the size of the conglomerate opacities, and in most subjects with stages B and C there is obvious pulmonary impairment.[40]

Pulmonary Function in Determination of Impairment and Disability

Pulmonary function tests can be used in two ways to help in disability determination. First, residual function may be compared to the demands of a specified activity or a given job. Second, pulmonary function values may be related to independent indices of disability such as respiratory symptoms. Thus, the results of pulmonary function tests are often related to the degree of shortness of breath that is present when the subject is performing a certain activity. In this regard, it must be remembered that a significant loss of function may be present before shortness of breath is experienced. Pulmonary function tests tend to be most useful in assessing disability in chronic conditions such as emphysema, in which the airways obstruction is irreversible. They have less application in conditions in which the functional impairment tends to wax and wane or undergo exacerbations, such as occurs in asthma.

Spirometry. The derivation of certain indices of ventilatory capacity is the most commonly used method of assessing lung function. The various indices and the method of measurement have been described elsewhere in this chapter. Suffice it to say, the FVC, the FEV_1 and the FEV_1/FVC ratio are the most useful indices in the assessment of disabling pulmonary impairment. The tests are easily performed, simple, reproducible, sensitive, and fairly specific. Lack of effort is easily detected, and even a neophyte should have some idea that cooperation is lacking when there are disparate values. The tracings should always be inspected for reproducibility, and in every instance there should be three tracings which are reproducible and within 5% of the highest. The curve should be flat when the subject ceases to exhale, indicating the maneuver has been completed. ''Bumps'' along the course of the curve indicate changes in flow rates and are usually caused by attempts by the subject to produce falsely low values. A straight line over the first 75% of the forced vital capacity indicates malingering and can be produced if the subject deliberate limits flow by pursing the lips. If reversible airways obstruction is suspected, the forced expiratory volume maneuver should be repeated following administration of a bronchodilator. Numerous prediction formulae exist. Those based on nonsmoking subjects are recommended. Nonetheless, when a claimant's value is compared to a particular predicted value, only if the claimant's value is markedly reduced is disability likely to be present, and in the context of disability determination, the choice of a particular prediction formula is not of great moment.

The MVV, although often used in disability evaluation, has certain drawbacks. First, the test requires considerable effort from the patient and is tiring and distressing; and second, it is much more difficult to assess whether the subject is making a maximal effort. Even with maximal cooperation, many nonpulmonary factors influence the MVV, including muscle coordination, heart disease, neurological function, and chest wall compliance. If the FEV_1 is multiplied by 40, this gives an accurate prediction of the MVV and enables one to see whether the subject has exerted a maximal effort during the performance of the maneuver. Because of these problems, the MVV is now used less often than previously; however, it does help in assessing the validity of the other measurements. When there is a disparity between the FEV_1 and the MVV, the latter measurement is nearly always found to be depressed, usually because of a submaximal effort.

Diffusing Capacity. This test is most useful in the determination of impairment and disability in subjects with restrictive impairment resulting from fibrotic changes in the lung. It is an overall index of gas transfer and does not measure the diffusing capacity per se but rather the ability of the lungs to transfer gas from the alveolus to the pulmonary capillary. Though fairly reproducible, technically it is not so easily performed and is also somewhat lacking in specificity.[42] Even so, it is an essential part of the investigation of subjects with restrictive impairment in conditions such as asbestosis.[41, 42]

Arterial Blood Gases. Despite the insistence of some United States governmental agencies, blood gas analysis is not recommended, since it is nonspecific, lacking in sensitivity, invasive, and influenced by hyperventilation and the position in which the blood sample is drawn. There is, moreover, an extremely wide variation in the values obtained by different laboratories.[43] Subjects with normal lungs may have a decrease in their Pa_{O_2} tension, and falls of between 10 and 30 mm in the Pa_{O_2} are common when an obese subject assumes the supine position.[44] In addition, correction factors for altitude should be applied to predicted Pa_{O_2} values, since normal values in high-altitude cities such as Denver or Johannesburg differ markedly from the values obtained at sea level. Age likewise has a profound effect on Pa_{O_2}. While the expected Pa_{O_2} of a 25-year-old at sea level is 95 mm, that of a 60-year-old is 76 mm, with the lower limit of normality being 70 mm (Fig. 5–22).

Alveoloarterial Oxygen Gradient [$(A-a)O_2$]. Although the $(A-a)O_2$ is a sensitive method for detecting abnormalities of gas exchange, it has little use in the assessment of disability. It is, moreover, nonspecific and affected by nonpulmonary diseases, such as left ventricular failure and cirrhosis of the liver, and obesity. The size of the gradient is affected by venous admixture, ventilation-perfusion mis-

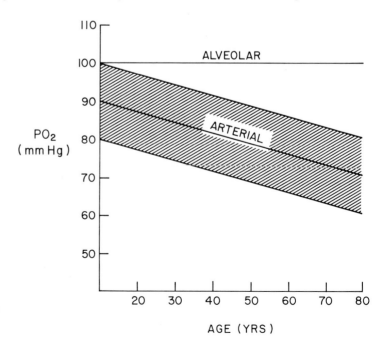

Figure 5–22
Relationship of arterial PO_2 and age. Although the standard deviation is shown as the same for young and older subjects, in practice it is greater in the older subject.

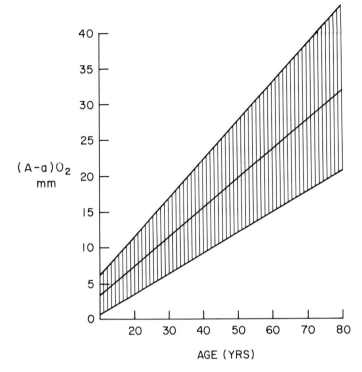

Figure 5–23
Relationship of age to the alveoloarterial gradient for oxygen (A-a)O_2. The predictions are based on observations made in a selected group of older hospital patients with normal spirometry and no chest disease. Some subjects, however, were overweight, and some may have had coronary artery disease in the absence of overt failure. The figure indicates that the standard deviation of the test increases with age.

matching, and a reduction of the diffusing capacity, with each of these factors exerting a different effect varying with the Pa_{O_2} and FI_{O_2}. Measurement of the resting (A-a)O_2 is unreliable as an index of impairment and may uncommonly improve with exercise.[41] The average (A-a)O_2 at the age of 20 is around 8 mm ± 5, but by the age of 60, the mean value is 20 mm ± 8. The normal value in a 60-year-old man ranges between 15 and 28 mm (Fig. 5–23).

The (A-a)O_2 is affected by changes in cardiac output. As the latter changes, different fractions of the cardiac output perfuse the anatomical and physiological shunts which may be present. The coefficient of variation for the (A-a)O_2 is around 19%, in contrast to that of the Pa_{O_2}, which is about 3.5%.[45] The (A-a)O_2 is most useful as a means of detecting disabling impairment during exercise. Even here it is essential to ascertain that the subject has reached a steady state, and only when the (A-a)O_2 is over 50 mm is there any assurance that the impairment is likely to be disabling.[41]

Lung Volumes. These show a poor correlation with shortness of breath and with respiratory disability. They are not recommended as suitable tests to be used in disability assessment.

Tests of Small Airways Function. These have no place in the assessment of disability. The tests may be abnormal despite the complete absence of symptoms.

Ventilatory Equivalent ($\dot{V}E_{O_2}$). In order to extract 100 ml of oxygen, a normal person has to breathe about 2.5 L of air. The number of liters of air breathed per 100 ml of oxygen uptake is usually referred to as the ventilatory equivalent ($\dot{V}E_{O_2}$). This index can be measured by simple spirometry. Hyperventilation in the face of normal $\dot{V}E_{O_2}$ is a normal response to exercise and is said to be metabolically justified. In contrast, when the $\dot{V}E_{O_2}$ is increased, the hyperventilation is said to be metabolically unjustified and is a consequence of either cardiopulmonary disease or anxiety. The measurement of $\dot{V}E_{O_2}$ at rest or at low levels of exercise is notoriously prone to inaccuracies and is of little value, but is more useful with high and sustained levels of exercise.[36] It is necessary to bear in mind that virtually every subject hyperventilates to a greater or lesser extent when first starting to breathe on a spirometer, and it is only after some time when the subject has achieved a steady state that the inappropriate hyperventilation disappears.

Dyspnea Index. A formerly popular method of trying to quantify impairment and shortness of breath was known as the dyspnea index. This is the percentage of the MVV required for a stated activity. The dyspnea index for walking on the flat at 2 mph is around 12% ± 4. Elevation of the index can occur as a result of a reduction in the MVV or because of a pathologically increased ventilatory requirement. Any value below 35% suggests that dyspnea is unlikely to be excessive, values between 35% and 50% are in an intermediate zone, and all subjects with a value above 50% can be assumed to be short of breath at abnormally low levels of exercise.

Exercise Testing. Although exercise testing is important physiologically, its usefulness in the determination of occupationally related disability is strictly limited for a variety of reasons. These include the fact that some individuals deliberately misrepresent the severity of their symptoms and stop exercising even though they are capable of further effort. Moreover, results obtained in the exercise laboratory must be related to the individual's job, since performance in the laboratory often bears no relationship to performance in the workplace. Furthermore, although exercise testing may quantify cardiopulmonary impairment, it does not determine the cause of that impairment, e.g., distinguishing asbestosis from fibrosing alveolitis. Subjects are often reluctant to undergo exercise testing. In addition, many subjects have coincident heart disease, and the risk of exercise testing in such subjects limits its usefulness. Moreover, it is unnecessary in subjects who have severe pulmonary impairment which has been brought to light by simple tests such as spirometry, blood gas levels, and measurement of the diffusing capacity.

Indications for Exercise Testing. Exercise testing is best reserved for a small group of individuals in whom the history, physical examination, and standard tests of pulmonary function are equivocal; when the individual's symptoms are inconsistent or out of proportion to the results of standard pulmonary function tests; or if an individual has both cardiac and respiratory disease, and it is necessary to assess the relative contributions of each.[37, 46]

Simple tests such as a Master Two Step test or climbing a flight of stairs have their advocates; they are easily performed and are inexpensive. However, they lack precision, and in addition, it is impossible to quantify the work done. Although the individual's response may be determined by measuring the heart rate and respiratory rate, more sophisticated tests of oxygen uptake and carbon dioxide production cannot be carried out. More useful are incremental three-stage exercise tests as described by Jones and Campbell.[31] By progressively increasing the workload, indices of cardiac and lung function may be related to the work carried out. Thus, the steady-state tests, although safer, are not as helpful in that they are less reliable than incremental three-stage testing, at least as far as the prediction of maximal oxygen consumption is concerned.

End Points Indicating Satisfactory Performance. When an individual is to undergo an exercise test, it is necessary to have in mind appropriate criteria that must be used in order to decide whether the subject has reached an exercise level that is appropriate and is a reflection of what that individual can tolerate. Relatively well-defined cardiac end points are available, with the possible exception of chest pain that occurs without electrocardiographic changes. As far as the lungs are concerned, respiratory end points are less precise. However, if ventilation is 80% or more of the subject's predicted maximal value, it can be assumed with some confidence that the maximal or near maximal load has been obtained. If considerable arterial hypoxemia develops during exercise testing, it can be assumed that the subject is either at or near maximal output. If, on the other hand, the subject complains of shortness of breath and stops because of this symptom, it is difficult if not impossible to know whether he or she has reached the limit of endurance, is unduly anxious, or is resorting to hyperbole in order to obtain a pecuniary reward. Anxiety often causes hyperventilation and lightheadedness, and these may make it difficult for the subject to continue exercising, but as such this is usually reflected as a low CO_2 in the mixed expired air, in an end tidal sample, or in the arterial blood. There is also usually an inappropriately high ventilation for the workload. Exercise testing should aim to achieve 85% or more of the predicted maximal heart rate or 85% or more of the predicted maximal ventilation.

Measurement of Workload.[46] The use of an ergometer enables the work carried out to be quantified directly. Where this is not possible with treadmill exercise in different laboratories, it is necessary to express the work done in terms of either $\dot{V}O_2$ or $\dot{V}CO_2$ to compare results. Ventilatory and cardiac measurements can then be plotted against work done and compared to predicted values. When a cardiac end point is reached, it can be assumed that the cardiovascular system is the limiting factor; however, if the $\dot{V}O_2$ for a particular workload is appropriate to the heart rate or close to the predicted maximal $\dot{V}O_2$, then the subject is normal. If, in contrast, the $\dot{V}O_2$ is low compared to the heart rate, then the circulation is inadequate, and either myocardial disease or, less frequently, peripheral vascular disease is suggested. It needs to be remembered when there is exercise limitation due to cardiac disease that the associated respiratory indices should be at or below those appropriate to the level of oxygen consumption. If ventilation is greater than expected, then the subject is probably limited by respiratory impairment, and this is particularly true if the minute ventilation is approaching 80% of the predicted MVV, always assuming that the heart rate remains within the predicted normal levels for that particular level of exercise. The presence of an elevated VD/VT% and $(A-a)O_2$ provides the necessary confirmation.

Should neither respiratory nor cardiac end points be attained, this places the examiner in a quandary. The subject may have stopped because of symptoms or because of feigned exhaustion. Progressive hyperventilation may be the cause of the symptoms, but some individuals can be persuaded to continue with the exercise and complete the test. Unfortunately, in many instances in subjects being tested for occupational disability, there is no way of knowing whether the individual is malingering or has genuine symptoms that impair the performance.

Measurement of Functional Capacity. The easiest way of estimating functional capacity is to measure oxygen consumption during maximal exercise. This can theoretically be related to the demands of a particular job. This approach, however, takes no account of the fact that an overweight individual requires more energy to carry out a particular job than does a subject of normal weight. Thus, the $\dot{V}O_2$ may be expressed as a percentage of the predicted maximal value for that subject. However, to take obesity into account, it is probably better to express the $\dot{V}O_2$ in terms of Mets. This assumes a linear relationship between increasing body weight and an increase in oxygen requirements. Such an assumption is not entirely justified since the distribution of the extra adipose tissue and the relative fitness of the person also influence oxygen requirements.

The demands of various occupations expressed as Mets have been established.[31] Nevertheless, most of the measurements have been based on relatively few workers, mainly because of the practical problems encountered in measuring O_2 uptake while working. This is particularly true in heavy jobs, such as those of the steel industry. Moreover, the energy requirements of many jobs are not known, and the energy expended in a given job is influenced by the skill of the worker, his or her training, and the worker's ability to adapt. Many jobs may entail a range of activities throughout the working day, and it is necessary to know not only the average demands but also the peak demand of the job. For the most part, peak energy requirements are needed only for brief periods. This problem of quantifying such requirements has been approached in an elegant fashion by Harber, who used a Holter monitor to record the heart rate continuously in underground coal miners during a full work shift.[47] The data related the heart rate to the levels of oxygen uptake when the subject was exercising, and it was shown that the average requirement during the day was 3.3 Mets, but for 10% of the work shift the requirement rose to 6.3 Mets. The study also showed that there was a wide variation between individuals, and indicated that twofold differences existed between two workers who held similar jobs with similar work requirements. It can only be added that making a decision as to whether a particular subject is disabled or not depends as much on the interpretation of the job requirements as it does on any data that are obtained from a reliable exercise study. It is clear that a substantial proportion of well motivated individuals who, according to their pulmonary function and exercise tests, should not be able to manage their job, continue to do so, while others who are physiologically capable of coping claim to be disabled.

When pulmonary impairment causes a limitation of work capacity, exercise tolerance is most often determined by the maximal voluntary ventilation. An increased demand for ventilation may result from impaired gas exchange. The relationship of ventilatory capacity in gas exchange to maximal oxygen consumption was studied by Wright, who was able to derive an equation which predicted maximal O_2 consumption.[48] Armstrong and his colleagues extended Wright's study and were able to predict maximal oxygen consumption from the MVV and the ventilatory equivalent measured during submaximal exercise.[49] The predicted value corresponded closely with the measured value in both healthy and impaired subjects. This approach has been further simplified by Wehr and Johnson and can avoid the problems of maximal exercise.[50] But some doubts have been expressed as to the validity of using submaximal exercise as a means of predicting maximal O_2 consumption.

The use of submaximal exercise to predict maximal oxygen consumption has certain limitations in that heart disease may lead to a lower than normal maximal O_2 consumption. In addition, the ventilatory equivalent depends on the level of exercise, and if the measurements are made while the subject is exercising at too low a level of Mets, then anxiety-induced or voluntary hyperventilation can artifactually elevate the O_2 uptake. At high workloads and nearer to the anaerobic threshold, ventilation increases disproportionately to oxygen uptake, thereby increasing the ventilatory equivalent. In patients with a reduced diffusing capacity, a sudden fall in oxygen saturation often occurs at a particular oxygen consumption, and the level cannot necessarily be predicted by the ventilatory equivalent at lower workloads.

Grading of Impairment

Numerous criteria have been published for grading pulmonary impairment. These differ appreciably, and nowhere more than in the regulations promulgated by various United States governmental agencies. The criteria are listed and discussed by Epler and coworkers.[41] A rough guide to the severity of the various types of pulmonary impairment is shown in Table 5–5. These values are partly based on the work of Gaensler and Wright and partly on our own experience with coal miners applying for black lung benefits. For full details and a lucid discussion of the application of function tests to disability determination, the reader should consult the classic paper of Gaensler and Wright.[36] Elsewhere, Richman gives an excellent description of the legal aspects and definitions of disability and discusses many of the divergent points of view that seem inevitable when physicians and lawyers are involved in lawsuits.[51]

Respiratory disability has been defined by the World Health Organization as a reduction in exercise capacity due to impaired lung function.[52] Any reduction that is found can be rated in the manner proposed by the American Thoracic Society (ATS) for the various indices of lung function.[53] When the ATS criteria are used, zero disability is present when the exercise capacity exceeds the lower limit of normal, while 100% disability is present when there is an inability to increase the oxygen uptake above twice the basal level. This enables a direct rating scale to be devised. Nonetheless, such a system requires exercise testing with all of its vagaries and drawbacks.

In conclusion, the detection of impairment should be done in as noninvasive a

Table 5–5

■

Criteria for Grading Impairment of Pulmonary Function

Test	Mild	Moderate	Severe
Obstructive Impairment			
MVV (% predicted)	65–80	45–60	Less than 45
VC (% predicted)	Normal	Usually normal	Slight to moderate reduction
FEV$_1$ (% predicted)	65–80	45–60	Less than 45
FEV$_1$/FVC%*	55–75	45–55	Less than 45
Blood gases† (% sat)	Normal	Usually normal	Hypoxemia
DL$_{CO}$ (% predicted)	Normal	Normal or slight reduction	Slight to moderate reduction
Restrictive Impairment			
MVV (% predicted)	Normal	Normal	50–80
VC (% predicted)	60–80	50–60	Less than 50
FEV$_1$ (% predicted)	60–80	50–60	Less than 50
FEV$_1$/FVC%*	Normal	Normal	Normal
Blood gases (% sat)	Normal	Normal	Usually normal
DL$_{CO}$ (% predicted)	Normal	50–75	Less than 50
Interstitial Lung Disease			
MVV (% predicted)	Normal	Normal	60 or above
VC (% predicted)	70 or greater	50–70	Less than 50
FEV$_1$ (% predicted)	70 or greater	50–70	Less than 50
FEV$_1$/FVC%*	Normal	Normal	Normal
Blood gases (% sat)	94–96	90–94	90 or less
(A-a)O$_2$ (mm)*	15–30	30–40	Above 40
DL$_{CO}$ (% predicted)	Normal	40–75	Less than 40

*Age related.
†Unreliable in obstructive impairment.

fashion as possible, using simple and objective tests. The use of a battery of tests without regard to the likely cause of the impairment—including blood gas analysis, body plethysmography, and the determination of compliance and lung volumes such as is used in Germany—although objective, is time-consuming and puts the patient or claimant through considerable and for the most part unnecessary discomfort. Moreover, many of the more complex tests correlate poorly with symptoms. This is especially true of the use of blood gas analysis, which has been recommended by the United States Department of Labor for use in coal miners with normal or near normal ventilatory capacity.[43]

Finally, in deciding who is disabled, what is important is not the percentage loss of function but the residual capacity or function, since this determines work capacity.

REFERENCES

1. Campbell, E. J. M., The Respiratory Muscles. Philadelphia, W. B. Saunders Co., 1970.
2. Barnhard, H. J., Pierce, J. A., Joyce, J. W., and Bates, J. H., Roentgenographic determination of total lung capacity. Am. J. Med., 28, 51, 1966.
3. Reger, R. B., Young, A., and Morgan, W. K. C., An accurate and rapid radiographic method of determining total lung capacity. Thorax, 27, 163, 1972.
4. Jenkins, S. C., and Moxham, J., The effects of mild obesity on lung function. Respir. Med., 85, 309, 1991.
5. American Thoracic Society, Statement on lung function testing: selection of reference values and interpretative strategies. Am. Rev. Respir. Dis., 144, 1202, 1991.
6. Handley, D. C., Chronic obstructive pulmonary disease. Disease of the Month, 84, 537, 1988.
7. Olsen, C. R., and Hale, F. C., A method for interpreting the acute response to bronchodilators from the spirogram. Am. Rev. Respir. Dis., 98, 301, 1968.
8. Burger, R., and Smith, D., Acute postbronchodilator changes in pulmonary function parameters in patients with chronic airways obstruction. Chest, 94, 541, 1988.
9. Radford, E. P., Recent studies of the mechanical properties of mammalian lungs. *In* Remington, J. W., ed., Tissue Elasticity. Washington, D. C., American Physiological Society, 1957.
10. Pattle, R. E., Lining layer of the lung. Br. Med. Bull., 19, 41, 1963.

11. Clements, J. A., Surface phenomena in relation to pulmonary function. Physiologist, 5, 11, 1962.
12. Hyatt, R. E., Schilder, D. P., and Fry, D. L., Relationship between maximum expiratory flow and degree of lung inflation. J. Appl. Physiol., 13, 331, 1960.
13. Fowler, W. S., Lung function studies, III. Uneven pulmonary ventilation in normal subjects and in subjects with pulmonary disease. J. Appl. Physiol., 2, 283, 1949.
14. First in-last out in the lung [Editorial]. Br. Med. J., 3, 119, 1973.
15. Otis, A. B., McKerrow, C. B., Bartlett, R. A., et al., Mechanical factors in the distribution of pulmonary ventilation. J. Appl. Physiol., 26, 732, 1969.
16. Mackem, I. T., and Mead, J., Resistance of central and peripheral airways measured by retrograde catheter. J. Appl. Physiol., 22, 395, 1967.
17. Milic-Emili, J., Henderson, J. E. M., Dolovich, M. B., et al., Regional distribution of inspired gas in the lung. J. Appl. Physiol., 21, 749, 1966.
18. Glazier, J. B., Hughes, J. M. B., Maloney, J. E., and West, J. B. Vertical gradient of alveolar size in lungs of dogs frozen intact. J. Appl. Physiol., 23, 694, 1967.
19. Bake, B., Wood, L., Murphy, B., et al., The effect of inspiratory flow rate on the regional distribution of inspired gas. J. Appl. Physiol., 37, 8, 1974.
20. Hughes, J. M. B., Glazier, J. B., Maloney, J. E., and West, J. B., Effect of lung volume on the distribution of pulmonary blood flow in man. Respir. Physiol., 4, 58, 1968.
21. West, J. B., Regional differences in gas exchange in the lung of erect man. J. Appl. Physiol., 17, 893, 1962.
22. Evans, J. W., Wagner, P. D., and West, J. B., Conditions for reduction of pulmonary gas transfer by ventilation-perfusion inequality. J. Appl. Physiol., 36, 533, 1974.
23. Fahri, L. E., and Rahn, H., A theoretical analysis of the alveolar oxygen difference with special reference to the distribution effects. J. Appl. Physiol., 7, 699, 1955.
24. Riley, R. L., and Cournand, A., Ideal alveolar air and the analysis of ventilation-perfusion relationships in the lungs. J. Appl. Physiol., 1, 825, 1949.
25. Perutz, M. F., Stereochemistry of cooperative effects of haemoglobin. Nature, 228, 726, 1970.
26. Lenfant, C., Wayes, P., Aucutt, C., and Couz, J., Effect of chronic hypoxic hypoxia on the O_2-Hb dissociation curve and respiratory gas transport in man. Resp. Physiol., 7, 7, 1969.
27. Comroe, J. H., Diffusion. In Forster, R. E., ed., The Lung, 3rd ed. Chicago, Year Book Medical Publishers, 1986.
28. Ogilvie, C. M., Forster, R. E., Blakemore, W. S., and Morton, J. W., A standardized breath-holding technique for the clinical measurement of the diffusing capacity of the lungs for carbon monoxide. J. Clin. Invest., 36, 1, 1957.
29. Filley, G. F., MacIntosh, D. J., and Wright, G., Carbon monoxide uptake and pulmonary diffusing capacity in normal subjects at rest and during exercise. J. Clin. Invest., 33, 530, 1954.
30. Roughton, F. J. W., and Forster, R. E., Relative importance of diffusion and chemical reaction rates in determining rate of exchange of gases in the human lung, with special reference to true diffusing capacity of pulmonary membrane and volume of blood in the lung capillaries. J. Appl. Physiol., 11, 277, 1957.
31. Jones, N. L., Clinical Exercise Testing, 3rd ed. Philadelphia, W. B. Saunders Co., 1988.
32. Wasserman, K., and Whipp, B. J., Exercise physiology in health and disease. Am. Rev. Respir. Dis., 112, 219, 1975.
33. Campbell, E. J. M., and Howell, J. B. L., Sensation of breathlessness. Br. Med. Bull., 19, 36, 1963.
34. Morgan, W. K. C., Disability or disinclination: impairment or importuning. Chest, 75, 712, 1979.
35. LeRoy-Ladurie, M., Silbert, D., and Ranson-Bitker, B., Factors d'invalidité après pneumonectomie. Bull. Physiopathol. Respir., 11, 182, 1975.
36. Gaensler, E., and Wright, G. W., Evaluation of respiratory impairment. Arch. Environ. Health, 12, 146, 1966.
37. Hansen, J. E., and Wasserman, K., Disability evaluation. In Murray, J. F., and Wade, I. J., eds., Textbook of Respiratory Medicine. W. B. Saunders Co., Philadelphia, 1988, pp. 699–718.
38. Morgan, W. K. C., Lapp, N. L., and Seaton, D., Respiratory disability in coal miners. J. A. M. A., 243, 410, 1980.
39. Williams, T., Ahmad, D., and Morgan, W. K. C., A clinical and roentgenographic correlation of diaphragmatic movement. Arch. Intern. Med., 134, 878, 1981.
40. Morgan, W. K. C., Handelsman, L., Kibelstis, J. A., et al., Ventilatory capacity and lung volumes in U. S. coal miners. Arch. Environ. Health, 28, 182, 1974.
41. Epler, G. R., Saber, F. A., and Gaensler, E. A., Determination of severe impairment (disability) in interstitial lung disease. Am. Rev. Respir. Dis., 121, 647, 1980.
42. Epidemiology Standardization Project. Am. Rev. Respir. Dis., (Suppl.) (Part 2), 118, 7, 1978.
43. Morgan, W. K. C., and Zaldivar, G. L., Blood gas analysis as a determinant of occupationally related disability. J. Occup Med., 32, 440, 1990.
44. Said, S. I., Abnormalities in pulmonary gas exchange in obesity. Ann. Intern. Med., 53, 1121, 1960.
45. Kafer, E. R., and Donnelly, P., Reproducibility of data on spread of steady state gas exchange in indices of maldistribution of ventilation and blood flow. Chest, 71, 758, 1977.
46. Morgan, W. K. C., and Pearson, M. G., Pulmonary function tests in determining disability. In Fishman, A. P. ed., Pulmonary Diseases and Disorders; Vol III. New York, McGraw Hill Co., 1988, p. 2533.
47. Harber, P., Tamimie, J., and Emory, J., Estimation of the exercise requirements of coal mining work. A non-invasive way of determining energy output. Chest, 85, 226, 1984.

48. Wright, G. W., Maximum achievable oxygen uptake during physical exercise of six minutes correlated with other measurements of respiratory function in normal and pathological subjects. Fed. Proc., 12, 160, 1953.
49. Armstrong, B. W., Workman, J. M., Hurt, H. H., and Roemich, W. R., Clinicophysiologic evaluation of physical working capacity in persons with pulmonary disease. Parts I and II. Am. Rev. Respir. Dis., 93, 90 and 223, 1966.
50. Wehr, K. L., and Johnson, R. L., Maximal oxygen consumption in patients with lung disease. J. Clin. Invest., 58, 880, 1976.
51. Richman, S. I., Meanings of impairment and disability. The conflicting social objectives underlying the confusion. Chest (Suppl.), 78, 367, 1980.
52. World Health Organization, International classification of impairment, disability, and handicap. Geneva, WHO, 1980.
53. American Thoracic Society, Evaluation of impairment/disability secondary to respiratory disease. Am. Rev. Respir. Dis., 133, 1205, 1986.

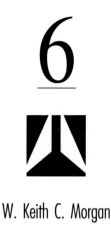

6

Epidemiology and Occupational Lung Disease

W. Keith C. Morgan

■

The identification, characterization, and assessment of the magnitude of both acute and chronic occupational hazards depend for the most part on the intelligent application of epidemiological methods. MacMahon has defined epidemiology as "the study of the distribution and determinants of disease in man." This definition is, however, somewhat restrictive, and much epidemiological research now takes place in normal populations, since only by delineating the range of normality can abnormality or disease be recognized. Epidemiology in more simple terms then becomes the study of normal and diseased states through the acquisition and analysis of pertinent data collected from the community.

Three methods of studying disease are commonly used:

1. Clinical observation of subjects with the disease
2. Controlled laboratory experiments using either humans or animals
3. Epidemiological studies

The use of epidemiology overlaps with the first two methods, and epidemiological observations are clearly important in both controlled laboratory experiments and the clinical observation of subjects with disease. In considering the epidemiological method in the study of disease, Morris[1] described seven standard approaches:

1. *The characterization of historical patterns of disease in populations by determining the relative and absolute frequency of disease in different groups, in different areas, and at different times.* This approach is most useful when there is a single or pre-eminent factor involved in the etiology of the disease, e.g., lung cancer that develops after exposure to bischloromethyl ether or radon daughters. In the case of diseases of multifactorial origin, the problem becomes far more complex and this approach may be inadequate.
2. *The measurement of current differences in the prevalence, incidence, morbidity, and mortality of disease.* By these means it is possible to define the magnitude and effects of the problem or disease.
3. *Study of the efficacy and operation of health services.* This approach involves an assessment of the health services which are used in the prevention and control of disease.
4. *The estimation of risk of disease in individuals and selected groups.* Theoretically attractive, this method is often less than ideal, since at present identification of susceptible subjects is possible only in a few instances.
5. *The identification of disease syndromes from different patterns of disease in the population exposed.* An example of this approach would be the separation of coal workers' pneumoconiosis and industrial bronchitis in coal miners.
6. *The characterization of the range of disease from the subclinical and possibly reversible stage to the irreversible and fatal form.* This implies a full under-

standing of the natural history of disease and is essential when considering prevention and control of the disease.

7. *Establishment of an understanding of the causes of the disease through knowledge of the determinants of disease frequency in different populations.* This approach allows separation of several risk factors, e.g., the role of industrial exposure, air pollution, and cigarette smoking in the etiology of bronchitis.

Morris's methods, while neatly defining the seven approaches which can be used in the epidemiological investigation of disease, are not as precise and well defined as at first appears. Considerable overlap is present in his various defined approaches; nonetheless, they provide a logical and helpful guide to both epidemiologists and clinicians who are concerned with the investigation and prevention of occupational disease.

Before describing the various types of studies that can be carried out on exposed populations, a few definitions of the more commonly used epidemiological terms would be in order. Prevalence means the number of subjects in a population who have a particular condition at a stated time. In occupational lung disease, the prevalence of a condition may be a reflection of recent exposure or of exposure many years previously. Thus, a survey of the prevalence of coal workers' pneumoconiosis (CWP) in 1971–1972 showed that about 12% of working miners had radiographic evidence of the condition.[2] Most of those with CWP had developed it following prolonged exposure. The insult that was mainly responsible for the development of the condition occurred 20 to 30 years previously, when dust levels were much higher than now. A repeat survey, carried out 3 years later in 1974–1975, showed the prevalence rate of CWP to have fallen to 6%. Although this might conceivably be a consequence of improved dust control, this explanation appears most unlikely. The real explanations for the lower prevalence are that many of those who were originally diagnosed as having CWP in the first survey retired and claimed compensation, while those who joined the work force and replaced them were free from disease; in addition, the reading habits of those interpreting the radiographs changed.[2]

The incidence of a condition refers to the number of persons in a particular population—in occupational lung disease it refers to exposed workers—who develop the condition over a designated time. The attack rate is somewhat similar and designates the number of subjects in a defined population who were originally normal but subsequently developed an abnormality over a specific period of observation. Thus, to define the attack rate for silicosis would require a knowledge of the number of men who initially started work with normal chest radiographs and no prior exposure and who then went on to develop radiographic evidence of the disease over a specified time.

From data of this type, attack rates may be calculated, but, here again, it is necessary to remember that the incidence or attack rate of a particular disease may be influenced by conditions prevailing much earlier. Thus, were 5 out of 25 asbestos miners to develop radiographic evidence of asbestosis, one explanation would be that all 25 had approximately the same work history (i.e., cumulative exposure) but that only those who were susceptible developed asbestosis. A more likely explanation would be that the five who contracted asbestosis had been exposed to higher concentrations than the rest, perhaps in a job in which exposure was greater and possibly at a time when dust concentrations were higher. Bearing in mind these caveats, it is useful to consider the different types of epidemiological studies or surveys which may be carried out.

TYPES OF EPIDEMIOLOGICAL STUDIES

Longitudinal Studies

A longitudinal study involves observing or measuring certain biological and medical indices over a period of time. This permits systematic observation of change with time. Such a study allows the incidence or the attack rate for a particular condition to be determined. Longitudinal studies have several drawbacks, the most important of which is the loss of participating subjects from the study. Such a loss may be due to migration, death, disability from the disease being studied, or a slackening of interest in the participants. Because of these losses, the remaining subjects may not necessarily be representative of the original population. Other problems include the high cost of longitudinal studies, the maintenance of standardization in measurements and tests, and the low incidence and prolonged incubation period of certain diseases. Using standard criteria is particularly important. Changing personnel may be a source of bias and may lead to different values for pulmonary function tests. Sometimes a new interviewer will cause subjects to respond differently to the administration of the same questionnaire. Technical lapses and changed equipment, e.g., the type of spirometer, can invalidate several years' work by introducing substantial bias.

In any epidemiological study there must always be an initial hypothesis, and the purpose and design of the study should be to determine as simply as possible whether or not the particular hypothesis is correct. The design of the longitudinal study must take into account the end point sought. Thus, some studies may be concerned with a continuing decline in pulmonary function (a continuous variable) following exposure to a certain hazard, while others seek a definite occurrence or development of a defined event such as the onset of asthma, lung cancer, or, most final of all, death. Yet other studies are concerned with the development of repeated episodes in an exposed population, for example, recurrent attacks of asthma, metal fume fever, or farmer's lung.

Historical Prospective Studies

Although these are longitudinal studies, they are carried out after the event. Thus, a particular cohort identified some time previously is traced to the present, and the attack rate or incidence of a particular disease or condition is then calculated. An example of such an approach would be tracing a group of asbestos miners known to have had a defined dust exposure and consequently ascertaining how many have developed lung cancer. Problems exist, in that the working population tends to be fitter than the population as a whole, since certain conditions which are prevalent in the general population automatically exclude or render a person unable to work. This effect is known as a ''healthy worker effect,'' and much is made of it as a source of potential bias. While the healthy worker effect is important in certain industries, e.g., those involving hard physical work, it is unlikely to influence to any great extent those subjects whose work is relatively sedentary and whose physical demands are far less. Thus, a survey of furnace workers in a steel plant is unlikely to turn up a large number of subjects with emphysema or asthma, since only the mildly affected could continue working. In contrast, such a survey carried out in waiters or taxi drivers would be likely to reveal that both of these occupations have a high prevalence of air flow obstruction.

A popular form of a prospective historical investigation is the case control study. This is designed in such a way as to select two groups of subjects, one with a particular affliction or characteristic and another without it. The frequency of exposure to a particular hazard or predisposing factor is sought, and its incidence or, more commonly, prevalence in both groups is ascertained. Thus, the smoking habits of two groups of middle-aged men, one with lung cancer and the other without, may be compared. Similarly, the prevalence of hypertension can be sought in subjects of normal weight and in those who are obese.

Great care must be taken in defining the population that is to be studied and in the selection of the designated cohort and the reference population. Data must be gathered in the same fashion in both the target population and the referents. For example, it is not acceptable to conduct further investigations as to the cause of death in the target cohort and not to do the same in the referents. Such a biased approach has been used to determine the frequency of respiratory malignancy in a large group of insulators in New York (see Chapter 14).

One modification of the case control approach is the study of matched pairs, triads, or quadrads (see later under Multifactorial Effects). The purpose of a study of matched pairs is to control for several confounding factors such as age, exposure, height, and weight.

Cross-sectional Studies

Cross-sectional studies, as the name implies, look at a cross section of the population on one occasion only. In the case of occupationally related lung disease, the normal practice is to examine those exposed to a particular hazard and to compare them to a nonexposed control group.

The main purpose of such studies is to estimate the prevalence of a particular condition and to characterize the type of impairment in those affected by it. In addition, the effects of various nonoccupational factors, such as cigarette smoking, air pollution, ethnic background, lifestyle, and diet, may be assessed. Occasionally, it is possible to reconstruct past exposures from work histories and to derive a dose-response relationship. Usually, however, the dust exposure data depend on so many intangibles and assumptions that accurate inferences cannot be drawn.

A cross-sectional study has many advantages, including the fact that the study is usually finite in both time and expenditure. The main drawback involves the investigation of a survivor population in which those who have been most affected may have already retired. Missing observations on retired and impaired workers may conceal the most important part of the story, and every effort should be made to trace them so that they may be included. In cross-sectional studies, the prevalence of a particular condition may reflect environmental conditions two or three decades previously, a situation which is particularly true of the pneumoconioses. Although many statistical ploys have been devised to cope with missing or incomplete observations, they are based on a series of assumptions, the accuracy or likelihood of which cannot be vouchsafed.

Meta-analyses

Meta-analyses gather together all published studies dealing with a particular treatment, risk, or disease and analyze the pooled data in an attempt to provide a definitive answer to the question posed, e.g., whether a certain treatment is effective or whether a particular agent is a carcinogen. Such analyses are frequently used, but suffer from several defects. These relate partly to differing subjects and methods chosen or used in the various studies, but more to the fact that negative studies are less likely to be published. Hence, the pooled data are biased by the inclusion of an excess of positive findings.

Multifactorial Effects

When a condition or disease results from multiple exposures or multiple factors, some sort of statistical approach may be necessary to sort out the contribution of these various exposures or factors. Thus, the development of coronary artery disease has been shown to be related to a number of risk factors, including smoking habits, obesity, lack of exercise, diet, and elevated levels serum cholesterol and serum triglycerides. Apportioning the relative contribution of each factor is difficult, but can be effected more or less satisfactorily using certain well-accepted statistical techniques. These include the use of matched pairs, triads, quadrads, and so on. For example, if a large population containing both exposed and nonexposed workers has been studied, it is possible to identify a series of pairs from the exposed and unexposed groups who have certain matching characteristics, e.g., age, height, sex, race, and smoking habits. Thus, when studying the prevalence of airways obstruction in textile workers exposed to cotton fibers, one could compare cardroom workers or spinners exposed to cotton with a comparable group of subjects from the same mill who worked with polyesters. If each exposed subject can be matched with a nonexposed subject of the same age, height, sex, race, and smoking habits, then tests of ventilatory capacity such as the FVC and FEV_1 should be very similar. Provided enough pairs are available and provided the results show a consistent and statistically significant difference between the exposed and nonexposed groups, it is possible to incriminate the particular agent concerned. Some authors have decried the use of matched pairs and claim the method is overused; nevertheless, with proper matching, it can be an effective way of controlling and quantifying the confounding factors.

Other methods of controlling confounding factors include multiple regression analyses and an analysis of covariance. The former may be unduly influenced by a few outlying points, while the latter is also subject to certain inherent influences which may introduce bias. Stratification analysis, in which all the variables are characterized so that strata are formed, thereby permitting comparisons within stratum, has recently become popular. This approach is useful when dealing with retrospective studies, but frequently the number of subjects is insufficient to allow adequate comparisons.

No matter the type of study, the design should be simple and acceptable to the subjects who are being asked to participate. When reliable data have been collected, they should then be subjected to the best form of statistical analysis, i.e., that which will extract the maximal amount of information. Frequently the best analysis is relatively simple, and if an effect is evident only after carrying out multiple different methods of analysis, many of which are obscure, complex, and involve mathematical legerdemain, the likelihood is that the relationship is nonexistent or at best tenuous. Thus, if for example one wishes to sort out the effects on the FEV_1 of exposure to a fibrogenic dust, cigarette smoking, and age, this can be done by using multiple regression analysis. However, when several variables, e.g., cumulative dust exposure, age, and pack-years, are closely interrelated, they will demonstrate collinearity—that is to say, all increase at roughly the same rate—and multiple regression analyses may not be able to separate their various effects.[3] Under such circumstances, if there are enough smokers and nonsmokers and if their dust exposure is likewise known, a more simple comparative analysis will often suffice.

Having carried out an epidemiological investigation of a particular agent and having demonstrated that a particular disease or condition occurs more commonly in certain groups of exposed subjects, the investigators must then go on to confirm their suspicions as to the agent's toxicity. An association between two variables does not mean a cause and effect relationship. Before designating an agent as toxic, it is essential to ascertain whether it meets the equivalent of Koch's postulates for toxicity. These include

1. The disease or effects induced are specific and can be recognized and diagnosed with a reasonable degree of certainty.
2. Although the clinical presentation of the specific disease induced by the toxin may vary to some extent, there are certain symptoms, physical signs, and laboratory tests that are common to the condition. A majority of these symptoms, signs, and laboratory tests need to be present or positive prior to making a diagnosis.
3. In the case of an environmentally induced disease, there needs to be an adequate history of exposure, and such exposure must be to a known and recognized hazard.
4. The agent responsible preferably can be identified in the body tissues or fluids, e.g., blood, urine, and so on.
5. The toxin of concern, when absorbed into the body, should produce the same effects in all susceptible subjects and preferably also in experimental animals.
6. The latency period between exposure to the toxin and the development of

physical effects should be reasonable. As a general rule, the longer the latency period, the more onerous and difficult the task of establishing a causal relationship between a chemical in the environment and the effect that is observed.

RISK ASSESSMENT IN INDUSTRY

The term *risk* implies uncertainty, while *assessment* implies quantification or measurement—ergo, risk assessment becomes the measurement of uncertainty. To measure risk assessment requires the application of statistical probability theory to numerical data.

Risk may be estimated or described in a number of ways.

1. Absolute risks. These are measured as decimal fractions ranging from 9 to unity on a probability scale. While zero characterizes the impossible, unity characterizes certainty. As applied to occupational disease (e.g., asbestosis), a knowledge of the number of workers with and without the disease in conjunction with a calculation of the appropriate fraction or percentage affected can provide direct estimates of the absolute health risks associated with and attributed to the various occupations in which asbestosis occurs.
2. Relative risks. When a particular disease also occurs commonly in the general population, e.g., lung cancer, then a comparison of the absolute risk in an exposed population as compared to the risk experienced by those not exposed permits the calculation of the relative risk.
3. Attributable risk. An alternative method of measuring the excess risk in an occupation is to consider the difference in incidence of the same condition in those exposed and unexposed, e.g., an incidence rate in the exposed group of 6% and in the unexposed of 2%. The fraction of the total risk for this particular condition, therefore, becomes $(6 - 2) = 4$ divided by $6 = 0.667$.
4. Acceptable risks. Many problems exist in the collection of epidemiological data, but in some instances, absolute, relative, and attributable risks can be measured with a fair degree of precision. In other instances, data are less reliable. In practice, useful estimates are often obtained within certain confidence limits, and hence it may be possible to attribute a particular effect to occupational factors when the data are carefully analyzed, and it becomes evident that they are statistically significant. The question of an acceptable risk, however, depends on numerous factors, both social and economic, and, for the most part, what constitutes or is seen as an acceptable risk depends much on the philosophy of the beholder. Agreement on these other social, political, economic, and psychological factors will never be forthcoming, although, in many instances, a reasonable consensus is available. What is necessary, however, in making a reasoned judgment as to what constitutes an acceptable risk depends on having the risk quantified fairly accurately, thereby providing society with the necessary data to separate the unreasonable from the reasonable.

As a rule, epidemiologists compare the risk in those exposed and of the same sex in the whole community rather than in a selected control group.

Data Available to Permit Measurement of Risk

There are three general categories of published statistics that can be used for risk measurement.

Federal and provincial government departments and industry usually collect data on the occurrence of morbidity and mortality in various occupational groups. The example par excellence is the Registrar General Decennial Supplement on Occupational Mortality which used to be published by Her Majesty's Stationery Office in Britain. Unfortunately, this is no longer so. Comparable, but less complete publications are available in Canada and the United States.

Data gathered for purposes other than that related to occupational risk can be useful. Such information is commonly collected by hospital medical record departments, cancer registries, Workers' Compensation Boards, and industry, both as far as industrial hygiene and morbidity and mortality data. In many instances, much useful information is available if it has been properly collected and analyzed.

There are also data gathered for assessment of occupational hazards. These usually result from specific studies and tend to have the drawback that they are observational rather than experimental. Nonetheless, specific occupational risks can come to light through well-performed, controlled epidemiological studies.

EPIDEMIOLOGICAL SURVEYS FOR OCCUPATIONAL LUNG DISEASE

When designing an epidemiological survey, it is essential first to pose the question or questions to be asked; second, to select the appropriate study and control population samples so as to exclude bias; and third, to use those methods which answer the questions posed as simply and as unambiguously as possible. Without a hypothesis, a "fishing expedition" results, and data collection becomes an end in itself. An epidemiological study may be carried out for clinical investigative purposes, for example, to ascertain whether a new industrial process constitutes a hazard, and if so, to identify the factors responsible, while in other instances the main purpose of the study may be to detect or screen for a particular condition or disease so that it can be treated. Here the term *screening* is defined as "the presumptive identification of unrecognized disease by the application of tests, examinations, or other procedures which can be applied rapidly."[4] The purpose of screening is to detect disease in those who are apparently well and who are unaware that they have any disease or impairment. No matter what the purpose of the screening survey, certain methodological principles are inviolate. Before starting a screening study, those concerned need to apply the criteria shown in Table 6–1 to the condition for which they are screening. This is seldom done, and nowhere is this more true than in screening for occupational lung disease.[5] Some of these principles, e.g., the avoidance of bias in sample selection, have been touched upon already, but to date nothing has been said concerning the choice of tests and examinations which should be used. In the practice of clinical epidemiology, it needs to be borne in mind that large numbers of persons are studied and that errors

Table 6–1

■

Principles for Deciding if a Screening Test is Justified

1. The condition being sought should be an important health problem for the individual and the community.
2. There should be an acceptable form of treatment for patients with recognizable disease.
3. The natural history of the condition, including its development from latent to declared disease, should be adequately understood.
4. There should be a recognizable latent or early symptomatic stage.
5. There should be a suitable screening test or examination for detecting the disease at the latent or early symptomatic stage, and this test should be acceptable to the population.
6. The facilities required for diagnosis and treatment of patients revealed by the screening program should be available.
7. There should be an agreed policy on whom to treat as patients.
8. Treatment at the presymptomatic, borderline stage of a disease should favorably influence its course and prognosis.
9. The cost of case-finding (which would include the cost of diagnosis and treatment) needs to be economically balanced in relation to possible expenditure on medical care as a whole.
10. Case-finding should be a continuing process, not a "once and for all" project.
11. The benefits accruing to the true positive should outweigh the harm done as a result of false-positive diagnosis.

Modified from Wilson, M.M.G., and Jungner, G., Principles of Screening for Disease. Geneva, World Health Organization, 1968.

in the collection of physiological or other data and in the answering of specific questions occur at random. Such errors, or perhaps variations would be a more apt description, are acceptable in epidemiology, but not in clinical practice.

All tests that are used in epidemiological surveys or, if it comes to that, in clinical practice, should be judged by the criteria shown in Table 6–2. Thus, the test must be acceptable to the patient, and in this regard should neither cause pain nor be associated with risk. Invasive tests such as arterial puncture are particularly unsuited for community studies. The tests should likewise be simple, so that the patient can carry out the instructions. Closing volume can be measured reproducibly and without difficulty in a fixed laboratory using volunteer medical students and laboratory technicians; however, in a field situation in which the subjects being tested are coal miners or textile workers, reproducibility and cooperation become much more difficult to obtain. Given a well-trained and dedicated technician, fewer than 3% of participants should fail to meet the American Thoracic Society (ATS) criteria. Studies purporting to show higher failure rates[6,7] found in impaired subjects have been vastly exaggerated.[8] The presence of impairment may have a slight effect on reproducibility, but even this is not certain. In a study of over 2000 kaolin workers, failure rates for the FVC and FEV_1 were below 2.5%.[9] Similarly, Enright and coworkers in a large study of over 5887 cigarette smokers with definite impairment, aged 35 to 60 years, who were repeatedly tested in a series of sessions found a very low test failure rate for measurement of the ventilatory capacity.[10] During only 2.1% of the test sessions were participants unable to meet the ATS criteria for reproducibility, i.e., the largest two tests having to be within 100 ml or 5%. The recommended tests should likewise be objective and uninfluenced by patient cooperation or observer bias.

Blood gas analysis and electrocardiography are uninfluenced by patient cooperation, provided that the patient consents to undergo these examinations. However, the interpretation of the electrocardiogram, in contrast to that of blood gas analysis, is greatly influenced by the interpreter. A test should be reproducible, meaning that when measured several times under the same conditions it should yield the same result. Lack of reproducibility may be a consequence of the equipment used or the person making the measurements. When an experienced pulmonary physiologist or technician measures closing volume (CV) tracings on several occasions over a period of a week, there may be considerable intraobserver variation. Such variation may affect those indices which are often assumed to be objective, e.g., CV, CC, and the other tests mentioned above. True biological variability also exists. Thus, the FEV_1 is relatively reproducible and, when the test is repeated 5 to 10 times in an hour in the same subject, will vary only by about 5%. In contrast, the FEF_{50}, the FEF_{75}, and the FEF_{25-75} may yield values that vary from 10% to 25% when repeated under the same conditions.[11] Accuracy is even more important and must not be confused with precision or reproducibility (Fig. 6–1). Accuracy means the ability of a particular test to measure what the investigator requires to know. Accuracy and validity are really one and the same and should be assessed by considering three indices—sensitivity, specificity, and predictive value—all of which contribute to the concept of validity. The appropriate formulae for these indices are shown in Table 6–3.

Table 6–2
■
Criteria for Tests

1. Acceptance by subjects: Test should not cause discomfort.
2. Simplicity: Equipment and procedure should be simple.
3. Objectivity: Results should not be influenced by whether subject cooperates fully or not.
4. Precision (reproducibility): Repetition yields the same value.
5. Accuracy: The test quantifies accurately what one needs to know.
6. Validity: Sensitivity, specificity, and predictive value.

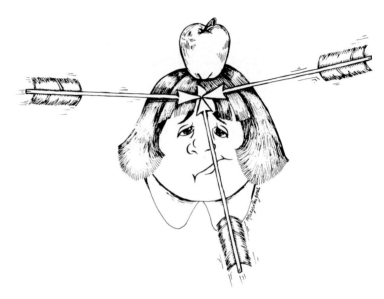

Figure 6–1
Distinction between precision
(reproducibility) and accuracy.

Sensitivity is an index of the number of false-negatives, in short, the ability of the test to give a positive result when the person being tested has the disease. Specificity is an index of the number of false-positives and may be defined as the ability of the test to give a negative result in those who are truly negative. Sensitivity and specificity are competing influences, and the ratio of one to the other is usually referred to by engineers as the signal-to-noise ratio. The predictive value of the test (ability to predict disease) is related to both specificity and sensitivity and is more useful than either of these indices alone. Furthermore, it has special application in screening studies. The predictive value of the test is largely determined by the prevalence of a particular disease in the sample being studied. Even highly specific and sensitive tests lose their predictive value when the prevalence of the condition in the population examined is low (Table 6–4).

The importance of standardization in epidemiological studies has recently received much attention from the Medical Research Council of Great Britain and from the Heart, Lung and Blood Institute of the National Institutes of Health, the American Thoracic Society, and the American College of Chest Physicians. Without adequate standardization, comparisons between different studies are impossible and bias inevitably creeps in. Nowhere is this more of a problem than in longitudinal studies, where personnel and often methods change. Measurement and hence

Table 6–3
■
Formulae for Sensitivity, Specificity, and Predictive Value

$$\text{Sensitivity} = \frac{\text{True-Positives}}{\text{True-Positives} + \text{False-Negatives}}$$

$$\text{Specificity} = \frac{\text{True-Negatives}}{\text{True-Negatives} + \text{False-Positives}}$$

$$\text{Predictive value of a positive test} = 1 + \cfrac{1}{\left(\dfrac{1 - y}{x}\right)\left(\dfrac{1}{z} - 1\right)}$$

Where
Sensitivity = x
Specificity = y
Prevalence = z

Table 6-4
■
Predictive Value of a Positive Test

Sensitivity (%)	Specificity (%)	Prevalence	Predictive Value (%)*
95	95	50/100	95
95	95	5/100	50
95	95	1/100	16
95	95	1/1000	2
60	98	1/1000	3

*Percentage of tests positive.

quantification become impossible unless the methodology has been standardized and is consistently applied. In 1978, the American Thoracic Society (ATS) issued a monograph entitled *The Epidemiology Standardization Project.*[12] This monograph has as its goal the standardization of the most frequently used procedures that are applied in epidemiological surveys of lung disease. Three methods are used for the collection of medical and biological data: first, a standardized questionnaire to elicit the prevalence of respiratory symptoms, smoking habits, and other pertinent information; second, performance of certain pulmonary function tests; and third, radiographic examination of the chest. The Epidemiology Standardization Project has been followed by a number of additional statements.[13, 14] These bring up to date the original recommendations and will be referred to again later.

The Questionnaire

An excellent questionnaire has been devised by the Medical Research Council (MCR) of Great Britain.[15] The questionnaire records the prevalence of certain symptoms including cough, sputum, wheeze, and shortness of breath. The latter is quantified as far as possible. A smoking history is obtained, and here it is important to estimate lifelong smoking habits rather than those which are current. Additional questions concerning past illnesses can be added to the questionnaire. In surveys of occupational lung disease, the standard questions should be supplemented by further questions which record the worker's complete occupational history from the time he or she started work to the present. In addition, if there are doubts as to what each job entailed, supplementary questions asking for details should be put to the worker. The MRC questionnaire has been tested in a variety of different conditions and has been shown to be a reproducible and accurate way of collecting such information. However, the questions have to be asked as written, and the subject being interviewed must not be intimidated or bullied by the tone of the interviewer. In this context, it has been found that subjects who smoke will, when interviewed by a physician who is against the habit, confess more often to cough and sputum than they would have done had they been interviewed by a nurse or disinterested interviewer. For these reasons, the MRC has published a set of instructions describing how these questionnaires should be administered.[16] In addition, some form of training in the administration of the questionnaire is advisable for all interviewers prior to its use. To be an effective instrument in the accumulation of reliable data, the questionnaire should not be too long. When a questionnaire takes 30 to 60 minutes to complete, the patient becomes bored and resentful. As a result, it is often left incomplete and much of the data are useless. Self-administered questionnaires are in general less satisfactory, and their reliability is inversely proportional to their length. It must, however, be conceded that if the questionnaire is short and explicit, it can be self-administered and the data may indeed be useful and accurate.[12]

As previously mentioned, the ATS published a series of recommendations concerning the administration of standardized respiratory questionnaires. In doing so, they devised their own questionnaire, which is a modification of the original

MRC version. This is known as the ATS/DLD/78 Questionnaire and has been shown to be reliable and reproducible in selected groups whether self-administered or administered by an interviewer. Additional questions can be added concerning asthma, family history, and the evaluation of pediatric disease. The ATS/DLD/78 Questionnaire has two components, an initial part designed as a bare minimum to be used in all surveys and a secondary part involving a group of supplementary questions that can be selected as appropriate by the interviewer or study designer. The questionnaire tends to be overly long, and when it is self-administered, the attention of the subject often lapses. Copies of the questionnaire can be found in a supplement to the American Review of Respiratory Disease.[12]

As with the MRC version, instructions for the use of the ATS/DLD/78 Questionnaire have been published. The instructions emphasize the need to ask the questions in an impartial fashion. It is recommended that interviewers be trained for a week or 10 days prior to using the questionnaire in any survey. The ATS/DLD/78 Questionnaire is recommended for use in the United States, but because of nuances in phraseology due to cultural differences and difficulties in translation, the questionnaire is somewhat less useful in Britain and other English-speaking nations, not to mention those countries where English is not the native language.

Tests of Pulmonary Function

The following are the uses of pulmonary function tests in occupational lung disease.

1. The detection of respiratory impairment and disease.
   a. Pre-employment examination.
      In many instances such tests are included as part of the pre-employment or pre-placement examination. The main aim of the tests is to detect impairment and thereby avoid employing those with compromised lung function and those who are at a greater risk of developing pulmonary impairment.
   b. Detection of occupationally related or naturally occurring disease by means of serial examinations.
      This approach represents a form of screening, and the basic purpose of such examinations is to detect disease early and thereby to modify its course and prognosis. Detection in the absence of an ability to change the course of the disease is futile other than to quantify the prevalence and risk in a particular population. The World Health Organization has elaborated certain criteria which should be applied to each and every screening program (see Table 6–1).
2. For epidemiological purposes.
   a. Hazard evaluation.
      If there is a suggestion that a particular job appears to be associated with the development of respiratory symptoms, then by carrying out a limited number of appropriate tests in the exposed population and in a suitable group of nonexposed controls it should be possible to determine whether such a hazard exists. The choice of the test to be used should be decided according to the type of impairment likely to be associated with the hazard. Thus, if several of the subjects are complaining of wheezing and shortness of breath, those tests measuring ventilatory capacity should be selected.
   b. The derivation of standards for specific hazards.
      An environmental standard has as its purpose the elimination or control of a particular hazard. In the promulgation of standards, the risk of exposure has to be weighed against the demand for and the importance of the product that is being manufactured. If it is decided that a particular product is essential, then it becomes necessary to accept a certain risk. In the process of deriving a standard, it is essential to relate biological to environmental measurements; for example, to estimate the concentration of a particular agent that produces a certain decrement in pulmonary function.

3. Disability determination.

Those pulmonary function tests that are most useful in this discipline are those which are both objective and simple. The purpose of such tests should be to determine whether significant impairment is present. Those tests that detect abnormalities not associated with symptoms, e.g., closing volume and frequency dependency of compliance, have no place in the determination of disability.

No matter what the purpose of the particular tests, the criteria already alluded to should be used to assess whether the particular choice of test is appropriate. Simplicity, accuracy, reproducibility, and reliability are the prerequisites for tests that have most use in epidemiological studies of pulmonary disease. To attain these features, some form of standardization of each test in investigation is necessary. The National Institute for Occupational Safety and Health (NIOSH) and the Division of Lung Diseases of the Heart, Lung and Blood Institute have sponsored several workshops and conferences in the hope of achieving this end. That they have been largely successful has depended on the support of a considerable number of persons and organizations, including the Environmental Health and Physiology Committees of the American College of Chest Physicians (which first published the Statement on the Assessment of Ventilatory Capacity),[17] the Division of Lung Diseases of the Heart, Lung and Blood Institute, and the American Thoracic Society.

For several years it has been apparent that not only do the techniques of performing pulmonary function tests require standardization but, in addition, many of the numerous spirometers which are on the market provide unreliable and inaccurate measurements.[18] Because of these technical problems, an effort was made by the ATS to define the appropriate specifications for spirometer performance. A workshop was held on the standardization of spirometry at Snowbird, Utah, and the proceedings were subsequently published.[19] This has been brought up to date.[13, 14] Specifications for pulmonary function tests were subsequently published in the Federal Register, and an excellent paper by Gardner and Hankinson subsequently described the performance characteristics of a number of commonly used spirometers.[20]

As a result of much research and effort, there is now a large measure of agreement as to what tests should be done, how such tests should be done, and what equipment should be used to obtain valid results (Table 6–5).

The Epidemiology Standardization Project of the ATS divided pulmonary function tests into essential tests and optional tests.

Essential Tests for Pulmonary Epidemiological Studies (FEV$_1$, FVC, FEV$_1$/FVC%)

As a minimum, all epidemiological studies involving pulmonary function should include the FVC and FEV$_1$. The equipment used to measure these indices

Table 6–5

■

Rating of Various Respiratory Function Tests

Criteria	FVC	FEV$_1$	FEF$_{25-75}$	Peak Flow	FEF$_{50}$	FEF$_{75}$	Lung Volumes TLC and RV	CV	DL$_{CO_b}$	Blood Gases	(A-a)O$_2$
Acceptability	+ + +	+ + +	+ + +	+ + +	+ + +	+ + +	+ +	+ +	+ +	− −	− −
Simplicity	+ + +	+ + +	+ + +	+ +	−	−	−	±	−	−	− −
Objectivity	+ +	+ +	+ +	−	+ +	+ +	+ + +	+	+ +	+ + +	−
Reproducibility	+ + +	+ + +	− −	+ +	−	− −	+	±	+ +	+ +	±
Accuracy	+ +	+ + +	±	+	±	±	±	−	+ +	−	±
Sensitivity	+	+ +	+ +	+	±	+	− −	+ +	+ +	−	+
Specificity	+ +	+ + +	−	+	−	−	−	− −	±	− − −	−

of ventilatory capacity should provide a permanent record. The system used should graphically record either time versus volume or flow versus volume, preferably both. Time display should be at least 2 cm/sec, volume display 1 cm/L, and flow 4 mm/L/sec. All spirometers should have a thermometer or temperature probe. In adults the tests can be performed either sitting or standing, but children should preferably be seated during the tests. A nose clip is optional but recommended, although there is little evidence to suggest that failure to use nose clips has any significant effect in normal subjects. If tidal volume is being recorded over a period of 30 seconds or more, nose clips are desirable.

At least three acceptable maneuvers should be performed. If a subject shows great variability between the various forced expiratory volume maneuvers (FEVMs), up to eight maneuvers may be necessary before three acceptable FEVMs are obtained.[12, 13] The maneuver should be sustained for at least 10 seconds, and up to 15 seconds if severe obstruction is present. An obvious plateau indicating the advent of residual volume should be sustained for at least 2 seconds. A volume decrease can likewise be regarded as the termination of the FEVM. In subjects with a slow start to the FEVM, the steepest portion of the curve should be extrapolated back to zero.[12, 13] The extrapolated portion should be less than 0.1 L or 5% of the FVC. If it is greater, the FEVM is not acceptable.

Spirometry should be performed only when the ambient temperature is between 17°C and 40°C, since very cold air may induce bronchoconstriction in some susceptible subjects. Subjects may be studied either sitting or standing, but standing volumes are usually slightly larger.[21]

The largest FEV_1 and FVC should be accepted as the subject's value, even if they do not originate from the same curve. Other indices (e.g., the FEF_{25-75}) should be taken from the single best test.

As criteria for acceptability, the largest FVC and second largest FVC should be within 0.1 L or 5% of each other when expressed as a percentage of the larger FVC. The same criteria should be applied to assess the validity of the FEV_1. All curves should be inspected for lack of a smooth contour, coughing, or other artifacts. Despite these rigid criteria, more than 97% of subjects can comply with the ATS criteria.[9, 10] All volumes should be corrected to BTPS. Calibration of the spirometer must be done regularly for both the FVC and the FEV_1.

The rationale for the number of maneuvers to be carried out is discussed elsewhere, and various combinations have been tried.[22, 23] The first FVC maneuver often yields the lowest results, and it is apparent that there is a definite learning effect. This is less evident in regard to the FEV_1.

The FEV_1/FVC% should be derived from the largest FEV_1 and FVC. Many microprocessors use a predicted lower limit of normal for this ratio. This is to be avoided, since the FEV_1/FVC% is inversely related to age.[24] The use of a fixed ratio will increase the prevalence of impairment associated with aging, and this will be particularly marked in elderly smokers or those with occupational exposure. Large, athletic, muscular men or women may have a relatively larger FVC than FEV_1. Finally, to express the FEV_1/FVC% as a percentage of the predicted percentage is meaningless and is to be avoided.

Optional Tests for Pulmonary Epidemiological Studies

Forced Expiratory Flow Between 25% and 75% of Vital Capacity (FEF_{25-75}). In certain instances the additional tests can be obtained from the standard spirometric tracing of the time versus volume maneuver or the flow volume loop. Such tests include the FEF_{25-75}, or maximal midexpiratory flow (MMF). It is often suggested that this test is more sensitive than the FEV_1 or the FEV_1/FVC ratio. The test and the method of calculation are described in Chapter 5. Calibration of the spirometer is essential, as in the case of the FEV_1 and FVC. The FEF_{25-75} is less reproducible than the FEV_1 and FVC,[12, 14] and although it has been suggested that it is more sensitive than the FEV_1, there is good evidence that this is not so.

Thus, when the FEV_1/FVC ratio is normal—between 75% and 85%—by definition the complete FEF_{25-75} is measured within the time required to complete the FEV_1 maneuver. Only if the flow rate during the first 25% of the FVC were supernormal would it be possible for an abnormal FEF_{25-75} to occur. The specificity of the FEF_{25-75} is low, and, moreover, the annual decrement in FEV_1 is exponential and not linear; therefore the FEF_{25-75} is less useful in longitudinal studies. Other problems include the fact that the FEF_{25-75} falls concomitantly with the FVC and with restrictive impairment. It has thus been suggested that a correction factor should be applied for lung volume when restrictive impairment is present.[25, 26] By the same token, when the FVC increases after the use of bronchodilators, the FEF_{25-75} is likewise affected, since the lung volumes often also increase. The several defects are discussed in a recent statement on lung function testing.[14]

The Flow Volume Curve (Peak Flow, FEF_{25}, FEF_{50}, FEF_{75}). The apparatus required for measurement of flow volume curves is more complex than the standard water-filled spirometer. A storage oscilloscope is desirable and a permanent record essential. Calibration for both flow and volume needs to be carried out. The various indices, e.g., FEF_{25} and FEF_{50}, should be taken off the curve in which the sum of the FVC and FEV_1 is largest. Since the equal pressure point migrates peripherally at low lung volumes, flow at these volumes (FEF_{75} and FEF_{90}) is determined by the resistance to flow in the small airways and by the elastic recoil of the lungs. In addition, flows such as the FEF_{50} and the FEF_{75} are affected by changes in lung volume.[12, 25, 26] All of these indices are more variable than the FEV_1 and FVC, but the peak flow is, however, less variable than the others.[11]

Static Lung Volumes Other than Vital Capacity. The measurement of lung volumes, in particular total lung capacity (TLC), residual volume (RV), and functional residual capacity (FRC), in occupationally exposed populations may provide useful information under certain circumstances. In a clinical setting, a knowledge of these volumes has limited usefulness except in the performance of challenge studies, and even then dynamic lung volumes provide more useful information. Nevertheless, changes of RV and TLC often occur following exposure to toluene diisocyanate, cotton dust, and other agents, and may invalidate maximal flow measurements when they are expressed as a percentage of vital capacity. The determination of lung volumes enables flow to be expressed at a percentage of TLC or at absolute lung volumes.[27] Similarly, when the body plethysmograph is being used to determine airways resistance (Raw), it is essential to express Raw at a particular lung volume. In addition, a knowledge of lung volumes enables this index of lung function to be converted to the more satisfactory measurement of specific conductance. In regard to TLC and RV, deviations from predicted values in an individual subject, even when marked, are seldom reliable as a means of assessing impairment. First, the percentage change in TLC and RV is usually less than that which occurs in the vital capacity; and second, predicted values for TLC and RV are less well established and have a larger standard error, and the effects of age and other variables are not so well documented. Moreover, many subjects have a combination of both restrictive and obstructive impairment, with the result that changes in TLC and RV are often inapparent or obscured. For these reasons, it is apparent that in a clinical setting a knowledge of TLC and RV does not always help in differential diagnosis, except insofar as restrictive impairment cannot be diagnosed without a reduction of the TLC.

Other problems exist, in that TLC and RV are not easily determined and the apparatus necessary is complicated and subject to technical errors. This is especially true of the body plethysmograph, which, although the most accurate method, is also the most complex and the one in which technical errors are most difficult to detect. Furthermore, the plethysmograph is relatively immobile and cannot be used easily in the field. The helium single breath and rebreathing methods are technically more simple, but both tend to underestimate TLC, FRC, and RV when there are poorly ventilated areas of lung such as bullae present. Finally, a radiographic method of determining total lung capacity is available. This requires both a posteroanterior and lateral chest film. This method treats the lungs as a series of elliptical cylindroids and calculates the volume in this fashion.[28] If radiographs are available for other reasons, the radiographic method has considerable application, especially in epidemiological studies. It is reasonably clear that in interstitial disease, changes in TLC, RV, and FRC are insensitive and lag behind changes in the VC and diffusing capacity. In addition, they have limited prognostic value and are unsuitable for long-term studies. In obstructive disease and diseases in which the elastic recoil of the lung decreases, a knowledge of FRC and RV is more helpful, especially as a means of relating flows to lung volume.

Diffusing Capacity ($DL_{CO_{sb}}$). There is little doubt that the $DL_{CO_{sb}}$ adds appreciably to the characterization of impairment in occupational lung disease, especially in those diseases leading to restrictive impairment and abnormal gas transfer, such as asbestosis, hard metal disease, and berylliosis. The steady-state method is not suitable for epidemiological purposes but can be used in diagnosis and in the assessment of impairment and disability. In surveys and field work, an automated method using a module is probably best, but here again regular calibration is vitally important. The various methods of carrying out the $DL_{CO_{sb}}$ are described in the Epidemiology Standardization Project.[12] Duplicate values are essential and should agree within 5% to 10%. The $DL_{CO_{sb}}$ is influenced by the size of the inspired volume, and if this differs by more than 10% from the FVC, the value will be invalid, owing to an artifactually reduced alveolar volume. The test is also affected by the duration of breath-holding and by an inadvertent Valsalva maneuver. The values obtained are also influenced by the hemoglobin level, and hence women tend to have lower values. Cigarette smoking also affects the measurement. The specificity and sensitivity in conditions such as asbestosis and interstitial lung disease have been studied in detail by Gaensler et al.[12] They found the sensitivity to be high but the specificity relatively low. More recently, a method for standardization of the single breath diffusing capacity has been described.[29]

Blood Gas Analysis. Blood gas analysis at rest and with exercise is often used to help in the diagnosis of certain conditions and in the assessment of pulmonary impairment and disability. While a reduction of arterial PO_2 may be seen in occupational asthma, byssinosis, asbestosis, and several other occupational lung diseases, blood gas analysis seldom adds any additional diagnostic information and still less frequently is helpful in the assessment of occupationally related pulmonary impairment.[30] Thus, the arterial PO_2 is affected by numerous nonpulmonary conditions, including cardiac disease, obesity, hepatic cirrhosis, and various neurological diseases. This lack of specificity is as great a drawback as is its relative lack of sensitivity. Moreover, there is little correlation between the arterial PO_2 and the presence of dyspnea. Thus, asthmatics or byssinotic subjects may have severe ventilatory impairment and yet have a normal or near normal arterial oxygen tension. Much the same is true for a restrictive impairment, and here again the diffusing capacity is affected earlier than are the blood gases, and in addition correlates far better with the presence of dyspnea. Nonetheless, exercise studies may be helpful in assessing how much oxygen is available to the metabolic sites and as a way of separating cardiac from pulmonary impairment.

Other Indices Derived from Blood Gas Analysis. The alveoloarterial oxygen gradient [$(A-a)O_2$], physiological dead space (VD_P), and ratio of dead space to tidal volume (VD/VT) are indices derived from blood gas analysis, and all may be abnormal in occupational lung disease. Nevertheless, for the most part they are nonspecific and relatively insensitive. The $(A-a)O_2$ has been recommended as a sensitive test for early disease, but it is now clear that its usefulness is strictly limited for a variety of reasons. First, as already mentioned, the test is nonspecific; second, the resting value may be profoundly influenced by hyperventilation and anxiety; third, the $(A-a)O_2$ increases with age; and fourth, the test is invasive. The exercise $(A-a)O_2$ is far more useful and helps to eliminate the confounding factor of hyperventilation. Despite these drawbacks, some subjects with categories 2 and 3 simple coal workers' pneumoconiosis who have an absolutely normal ventilatory capacity will show an increase in the $(A-a)O_2$. Even so, this is a late finding and is always preceded by radiographic changes unless other disease is present.

Tests of Small Airways Function. These tests have been hailed as a means of detecting disease early in its course, thereby providing an opportunity to arrest the condition and prevent the onset of disability. Many problems exist with this approach, not the least of which is the fact that the detection of abnormalities by these tests does not necessarily portend who is going to develop disabling impairment. The proportion of cigarette smokers who have an abnormal closing volume or frequency dependence of dynamic compliance is far in excess of the 12% to 15% who go on to develop significant airways obstruction. Thus, it is apparent that not all subjects who have these abnormalities of small airways function develop significant impairment.

Of the tests of small airways function that are available, frequency dependence of dynamic compliance has the least to recommend it. The test is difficult to carry out and involves swallowing an esophageal balloon; the equipment used in its determination is expensive; and technical misadventures are common. In the presence of normal spirometry, a fall in dynamic compliance at high respiratory frequencies may indicate small airways obstruction or, alternatively, localized changes in the elastic recoil of the lung. Thus, while it is possible for the overall flow pressure volume curve to be normal, this would not preclude a situation in which the presence of localized areas of emphysema and fibrosis balance each other out so that the overall mechanical properties of the lung are normal.

Closing volume is less sensitive but is much simpler to carry out. Nonetheless, the test is nonspecific. While noninvasive, it is technically more difficult to perform than simple spirometry, and around 20% of the general population who are tested in the field cannot follow the instructions necessary to complete the test.[31] The determination of closing volume is influenced by inspiratory and expiratory flow rates during the performance of the tests and also by the duration of breath-holding. Compared to the FEV_1, the test is more variable, less specific, more difficult to carry out, and more time-consuming. Pilot studies using the test in byssinosis and in other conditions in which there is an acute change in ventilatory capacity have shown it to be less sensitive and less reliable than the FEV_1.[31]

Flow volume curves with oxygen-helium mixtures have likewise been advocated as the ideal approach to early diagnosis. The initial enthusiasm for the test has not been vindicated, and at least in some occupationally related diseases, in particular those due to coal dust exposure, the test has been shown to be far more variable and less sensitive than the FEV_1.[32] It is doubtful whether it will prove more useful in other occupationally related disease, although controlled trials may be worthwhile.

Normal Values for Pulmonary Function Tests

Numerous prediction formulae exist for the various indices of ventilatory capacity, the FVC and FEV_1, in particular. For a variety of reasons, it is difficult to recommend one particular set. Probably the most reliable values are those of Morris,[33] Knudson,[34] and Peterson,[35] all of which were derived from nonsmoking populations.

The selection of reference predicted values should depend on methodological, epidemiological, and statistical criteria. Thus, reference values should be obtained by skilled technicians using equipment that corresponds to ATS standards. The population studied should be similar to the cohort being studied. Age, height, sex, and ethnic group should be considered as variables. Weight also should be considered, although it is less important. The statistical model chosen for prediction equations should be simple. A series of predicted values is listed in a recent ATS statement.[14] A similar extensive series of recommendations and prediction formulae for assessment of lung function have been published by the in European Economic Community.[36]

For any given subject, age, height, sex, and race influence his or her ventilatory capacity and lung volumes. Weight and other factors make a far lesser contribution. The FVC and FEV_1 reach their maximum at about the age of 25, remain relatively unchanged to age 30 or so, and then slowly decline. The annual decrement for the FEV_1 is around 25 ml, and that for the FVC around 15 to 20 ml. Although the mean annual decrement in subjects with chronic air flow obstruction tends to be linear over a period of 7 to 10 years, and may range from 30 to 200 ml, over periods of a year considerable fluctuations occur, and in some instances definite improvement takes place for no apparent reason (Fig. 6–2). Furthermore, much greater declines in both the FEV_1 and FVC occur in older subjects.[37, 38] In contrast, maximal expiratory flows tend to reach their maximum at an earlier age, that is to say 17 or 18, and then start to decline in the early 20s. Although it is often not realized, the FEV_1/FVC ratio likewise decreases with age, and it is inappropriate to take an arbitrary cut-off, such as 70%, as the lower limit of normal. A ratio of around 65%, which is definitely abnormal in a 25-year-old, may be entirely normal for a 60-year-old. The larger the subject, the greater the FVC, and the greater the tendency for the person to have a somewhat lower FEV_1/FVC ratio. Appropriate prediction formulae for this index have also been published.[36, 39]

In a disease-free individual of any given height, there is a range of values for normality, and when a large number of subjects of the same age, height, and sex are tested, the values for the FVC and FEV_1 have a gaussian distribution. The lower limit of normality is usually defined as the value which is exceeded by 95% of healthy individuals in the population. This is approximately the mean value minus 1.64 SEE (standard error of the estimate). Black subjects have lung volumes and flow rates that are about 12% to 15% less than white subjects of the same age and height.[40] Other racial differences have been reported in Eskimos, Chinese, and East Indians.[41–43]

Many laboratories report abnormal pulmonary function when the subject being tested has a value that is 80% or less than the predicted figure. The use of 80% as a cut-off irrespective of age and other factors is, however, incorrect. Reasons for this were discussed in an editorial by Sobol and Sobol.[44] A level of 80% of predicted value is based on the assumption that all pulmonary function tests have a variance around the predicted which is a fixed percentage of that figure. Coincidence of 80% of the predicted value and two standard deviations is a matter of chance and occurs at a single point only. It is apparent that small persons with normal function will deviate more readily than those who have normal function and are tall. Thus, the regression line for 80% of the predicted value and the line for the 95% confidence limit do not coincide. In older subjects, the 80% of the predicted line converges on the predicted value, whereas the reverse is true for

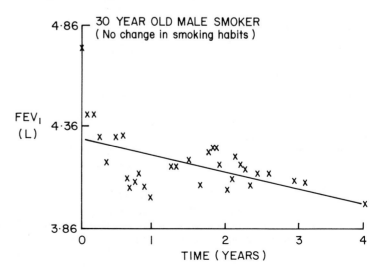

Figure 6–2
Serial measurements of FEV_1 over a period of 4 years in a heavy smoker.

younger subjects. Sobol describes a method that normalizes all subjects to a single value for each function.[44] Thus, for an index whose value is represented by a simple mean and standard deviation (SD), the normalizing process requires determining the value of the mean when the mean minus 2 SD represents 80% of the mean.

Boehlecke and Merchant in an excellent review of the usefulness of pulmonary tests in occupational disease have emphasized certain of the problems that originate from the use of a given percentage predicted in relation to age. Thus, in a group of normal men older than 60 years of age, the prevalence of an abnormal FEV_1 based on an 80% of predicted cut-off will be 12%. The same figure for the FEF_{25-75} would be 28.5%.[45]

Decline in the FEV₁

It has become evident over the years that the FEV_1 is not only an indication of the ability of the lungs to function but also is a reliable predictor of life expectancy in those with respiratory impairment. Its predictive value is based on the observation that in a normal subject the FEV_1 declines with age at a rate of between 25 and 30 ml/year. It is often assumed that there is a steady decline with increasing age, but recently this has been shown to be incorrect. With increasing age the rate of decline increases,[37, 38] moreover, the decline is not smooth, and there are marked systematic differences between the rate of decline from one occasion to another.[46]

A longitudinal study of ventilatory capacity using serial measurements of the FEV_1 can be made by comparing suitable groups of subjects who show a distinctive effect when the subject lives in a particular environment. It must also be assumed that in any subject the effect of living in this environment (i.e., the rate of decline of the FEV_1), is proportional to the number of years he or she is exposed to it. Similarly, it should be possible to show whether there is a diminishing or accelerating effect over the passage of time or with increasing exposure. This is usually determined from the average level of the FEV_1 that corresponds to a specified number of years in a particular environment and is achieved by calculating multiple regressions of FEV_1 on the years lived in these environments, thereby taking into account other variables. It has been pointed out that multiple regression works by discovering how, among persons with the same amount of exposure to all other relevant agents, an index (in this case, the FEV_1) varies as the degree of exposure to a particular agent varies. This it does simultaneously for each relevant agent.[46] The answer depends on the configuration of the set of exposure data. Oldham[46] emphasized that in considering factors related to the decline of FEV_1, it is essential to look for possible hidden links between these various factors and for any fallacies that may arise therefrom.

Obstruction—Reversible or Not?

Some learned societies recommend a certain percentage improvement in the FEV_1 as an indication of reversibility, the usual figures being either 12% or 15%. Defining reversibility on the basis of percentage improvement suffers from the drawback that an 0.5-L increment in a subject who starts off with an FEV_1 of 4 L constitutes a 12.5% increase. In another subject who has an initial FEV_1 of 0.5 L, a 0.5-L increment constitutes a 100% improvement. In assessing the change brought about by bronchodilation, obviously there are occasions when absolute volumes need to be taken into consideration.

One of the major problems in expressing bronchodilator responsiveness is distinguishing a true response to a bronchodilator from the inherent variability in the measurement of airflow.[47] A pattern of change can be determined only by making serial measurements of the FEV_1 in the absence of any drug therapy. Studies of normal subjects, subjects with restrictive impairment, and subjects with obstructive impairment have shown that when such subjects are observed over a period, the variation in the FEV_1 when expressed as a percentage progressively increased as the FEV_1 decreased. Thus, asthmatic subjects are likely to have a higher FEV_1 than are subjects with obstruction due to emphysema, and it becomes evident that it is very difficult to distinguish subjects with asthma from those with chronic airflow limitation due to emphysema solely on the basis of reversibility unless one looks at the changes in FEV_1 when expressed in absolute volumes. What is abundantly clear is the fact that subjects with low lung volumes and chronic airflow limitation due to emphysema (i.e., an FEV_1 less than 1 L), often show a 20% to 35% improvement after bronchodilators. Such a change is usually of no moment and is often best explained by the inherent variability of the subject. In studying each group, it is important first to make serial measurements prior to the introduction of bronchodilator therapy so as to provide a baseline and as an index of the inherent variability, and second, to use a control group who are not on any therapy whatsoever. Even then, it is often impossible to predict whether there is a definite therapeutic response, because the changes may be small and the power extremely limited without the inclusion of a large number of subjects.

Radiographic Examinations

The chest radiograph has for many years been one of the mainstays in the epidemiological investigation of the pneumoconioses. It remains the sole means of detecting pulmonary retention of certain dusts, e.g., silica and coal. For these and other reasons, an abnormal chest film is routinely accepted as the only legal evidence of dust exposure in workmen's compensation cases and in industrial litigation. Seldom, however, is the chest film useful in the assessment of pulmonary function, although there is some correlation between the radiographic category of asbestosis and the degree of pulmonary impairment. It nevertheless provides a measure of the amount of dust retained in the lungs and is especially useful in monitoring coal miners and those exposed to silica.

Before embarking on a respiratory disease survey that relies on chest radiography as one of the means of acquisition of epidemiological data, it is imperative that the techniques for taking and interpreting films be standardized as much as possible.[48] This is especially important in longitudinal studies. The reasons for this are several. The chest radiograph is used as a means of quantifying the amount of dust that is retained in the lungs. The retention of dust leads to the development of certain shadows or opacities in the chest film, and in general, the more opacities, the more retained dust.[49-51] While the radiographic opacities may not always be produced by the dust itself—rather, they may originate as a fibrogenic response to the retained dust—it is reasonable to assume that the more fibrosis present, the more retained dust. Thus, it is evident that there is a continuum from no dust in the lungs to maximal dust, whatever the latter might happen to be. In an attempt to quantify the amount of dust in the lungs, various radiologic classifications of the pneumoconioses have been introduced. Since 1950, the International Labour Office (ILO) has published a series of classifications that have been widely accepted. The latest and most comprehensive is the ILO 1980 classification, which provides the means of classifying not only the pneumoconioses but also pleural thickening and pleural calcification.[48] Classifications rely on the partly arbitrary selection of certain films as being typical of the various stages of the disease. The films used in the 1980 ILO classification have been reproduced and are available from the ILO as standard sets.

The pneumoconioses were originally divided into simple and complicated forms of the disease. The simple form was diagnosed by the presence of either regular or irregular opacities less than 1 cm in diameter, plus a significant exposure history. When one of the opacities was larger than 1 cm in diameter, complicated pneumoconiosis was said to be present. Simple pneumoconiosis was subdivided into categories 1, 2, and 3, according to the extent and profusion of the opacities. Similarly, complicated pneumoconiosis was divided into stages A, B, and C, according to the size of the large opacity or opacities. A group of experts selected a series of chest films that in their opinion could be used as standards for the various stages and categories. It was, moreover, suggested that any unknown, unclassified film that was being categorized should be compared to the standards. While such an exercise is essential when approximating the unknown to the standard, it must be realized that no other radiograph exactly matches any of the standards. The amount of dust retained in the lungs of the subject whose film is being interpreted is bound to be either slightly more or less than that retained in the lungs of the subject from whom the standard film was made. In addition, the volume of the lungs and soft tissue shadows will influence the radiographic appearances.

It subsequently became apparent that a classification that relies on major categories alone (i.e., 1, 2, and 3), lacked sufficient sensitivity for longitudinal epidemiological studies. It also became evident that those studies in which an attempt was made to relate environmental measurements to radiographic progression needed a more sensitive indicator. This led to the introduction, by Liddell and May, of the 12-point scale.[52] This modification subdivides each major category of simple pneumoconiosis into three subcategories (Fig. 6–3). Category 0 is divided into subcategory 0/−, in which the film was absolutely normal and under no conceivable circumstances could anyone consider it otherwise (in British parlance, a "barndoor" normal); 0/0, in which the film was normal; and 0/1, in which the interpreter decided that it was category 0, but considered category 1 as well. Category 1 is made up of subcategories 1/0, 1/1, and 1/2. In the case of subcategory 1/0, it was decided that the film should be placed in category 1, but category 0 was also seriously considered; 1/1 represents a typical category 1, and closely resembles the standard film. In the case of category 1/1, neither category 0 nor category 2 was considered. The classification goes up to category 3/+, in which there are more opacities present in the film than in the midcategory 3/3 standard radiograph. Thus, the numerator represents the category in which the radiograph was placed, while the denominator describes any other category that was considered.

The Liddell classification divides the continuum from no dust to maximal dust into a 12-point scale. Most persons assume that the scale is made up of equal intervals, and that the weight of additional dust retained for each increase in category is the same, i.e., it takes the same amount of dust to change a 0/1 to a 1/0 as it does to change a 2/2 to a 2/3. This assumption may not be valid, but has much to recommend it in practical terms, especially when it comes to the assessment of progression in pneumoconiosis. Moreover, studies have been carried out which have related radiographic subcategories to the coal content of the lungs, and these have shown that for the most part there is a straight line relationship.[49–51]

Extent

The lungs are divided into three zones on each side: upper, mid, and lower. This division is made by projecting horizontal lines drawn at 1/3 and 2/3 of the vertical distance between the lung apices and the domes of the diaphragm. Profusion of small opacities is determined as mentioned earlier by considering all the affected zones of the lungs, and by comparing the unknown film with the standard radiographs. When there is a marked difference in profusion of different zones of

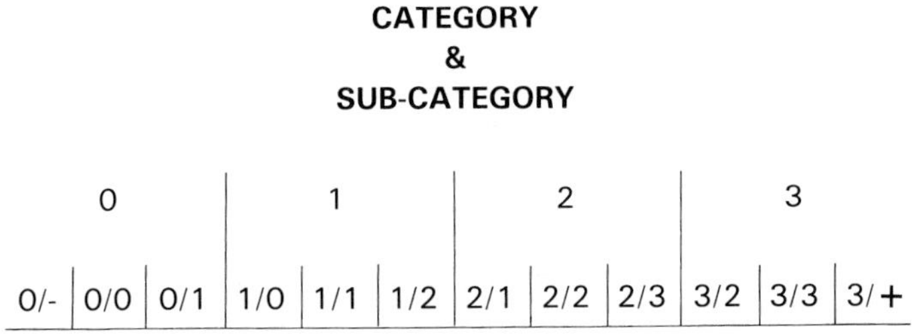

**CATEGORY
&
SUB-CATEGORY**

0			1			2			3		
0/-	0/0	0/1	1/0	1/1	1/2	2/1	2/2	2/3	3/2	3/3	3/+

Figure 6–3
ILO elaboration of the classification of simple pneumoconiosis.

the lungs, the zone or zones showing the lesser involvement or profusion are ignored when classifying the film.

Small Opacities

Those opacities that are present in the lungs and that are found in various pneumoconioses can be classified as either rounded (regular) or irregular.

Small Rounded Opacities. These opacities have a fairly rounded and regular margin, at least when viewed without magnification. They are classified according to their size into p, q, and r; p being up to 1.5 mm, q varying between 1.5 and 3 mm, and r between 3 and 10 mm. While there is usually only one type of opacity present, occasionally mixtures occur. The reading of the film should be based on the predominant type of opacity noted. Provision is made for recording different types of opacity, e.g., p and q or p and r in the same film, and reference to this will be made later. Progression from category 1 to 2 and further up the scale is seldom if ever associated with a change in the type of opacity. When the chest x-ray changes from normal to abnormal and p-type opacities appear, these usually persist should the film progress further to category 2 or 3. While p-type opacities occur for the most part in coal workers' pneumoconiosis (CWP), q-type opacities are seen in both CWP and silicosis, though r-type opacities are more commonly found in silicosis. Progression may occur in silicosis with or without further exposure while in simple CWP the progression and development of more small opacities is seen only with further exposure. Progression rarely occurs in simple silicosis after the subject has been separated for 5 years from exposure to silica. Regression rarely if ever occurs in silicosis, and while regression or clearing is not thought to occur in CWP, the possibility cannot be categorically denied. Regression has been observed in welders' siderosis.

Irregular Opacities. These are classified as s, t, or u and were previously designated without measurements as fine, medium, or coarse opacities; however, in the 1980 ILO classification, dimensions have been given to irregular opacities. Thus, s opacities have a width of up to 1.5 mm, t opacities vary between 1.5 and 3 mm, and u opacities between 3 and 10 mm.

Irregular opacities are characteristically seen in various interstitial fibroses, whether occupationally related or not. They also may be present in cigarette smokers and in subjects with various dust exposures.[53–55] Their presence has been observed in the fibroses induced by asbestos and by hard metal disease, and they are the characteristic type of opacities seen in fibrosing alveolitis, scleroderma-associated pulmonary fibrosis, and lymphangioleiomytosis. Aside from these conditions, the presence of small irregular opacities is associated with increasing age, cigarette smoking, obesity, and nonspecific dust exposure.[55] Thus, there seems little doubt that many dusts, regardless of their fibrogenic properties, may lead to the development of scanty irregular opacities.[55] This is, however, a nonspecific effect that has been observed following exposure to coal, talc, bauxite, silica, polyvinyl chloride, and manmade mineral fibers.[55] In the case of asbestos, sufficient quantities can induce a specific response characterized by the presence of irregular opacities in the lungs, i.e., asbestosis but scanty irregular opacities may be seen in smoking asbestos workers in the absence of interstitial pulmonary fibrosis. In this instance, the presence of irregular opacities appears to be associated with bronchitis. With the exception of asbestosis and hard metal disease, any effects from dust-induced irregular opacities on pulmonary function are slight, and there is little to indicate that the presence of such opacities in a nonsmoking dust-exposed subject ever leads to disabling impairment of lung function. The suggestion that the occurrence of such opacities constitutes a form of pneumoconiosis and that in coal miners their presence should be accepted as a criterion for compensation is based on tenuous evidence. The presence of irregular opacities constitutes a troublesome confounding factor in epidemiological studies of both dust- and non–dust-exposed populations, especially in the older age groups. Nevertheless, it must be borne in mind that in the absence of dust exposure seldom does the radiograph of a smoker rank higher than category 1/1, and more often it is 0/1 or 1/0.

Mixed Opacities. Rounded and irregular opacities may occur in the same film, but one or the other usually predominates. The 1980 ILO classification makes provision for recording both regular and irregular opacities when both are present in the same radiograph. Thus, the designation q/t means that the predominant small opacity is of the q type, but that there are a significant number of small irregular opacities of the t type. In this way, all combinations of opacities may be recorded. Repetition of the same letter (for example p/p, t/t), indicates that the opacities are all predominantly one shape and size. A word of caution should be added in regard to the designation of size of the irregular opacities: it must be remembered that the s, t, and u dimensions are approximations.

Large Pneumoconiotic Opacities

A large opacity is defined as any opacity greater than 1 cm that is present in a film in which there is sufficient evidence to indicate a diagnosis of pneumoconiosis. This definition therefore excludes large opacities due to other causes such as cancer of the lung. Category, or stage, A is defined as a large opacity between 1 and 5 cm in diameter or several opacities each greater than 1 cm in diameter but whose combined diameter is less than 5 cm. Category, or stage, B is present when the combined width of an opacity or opacities is greater than 5 cm and does not exceed the equivalent of the right upper zone. Category, or stage, C is present when there are one or more opacities whose combined area exceeds the equivalent of the right upper zone or a third of one lung field.

Pleural Thickening

The site—the chest wall, diaphragm, or costophrenic angle—and the width and the extent of pleural thickening should be recorded separately.

Chest Wall. Chest wall pleural thickening may be circumscribed (plaques) or diffuse. Both plaques and diffuse thickening can occur in the same subject. Thickening should be recorded separately for the right and left pleural surfaces, and when seen along the lateral chest wall, the maximal width should be recorded. Width is measured from the inner aspect of the chest wall to the inner margin of the shadow cast by the pleural thickening at the border of the lung and pleura. It is subdivided into stages A, B, and C, with A representing a maximal width of 5 mm; B, a maximal width of between 5 and 10 mm; and C, a maximal width of over 10 mm. When pleural thickening is seen *en face*, it should be recorded, although it may also be seen in profile. When viewed *en face* alone, width usually cannot be determined. The extent of pleural thickening is defined in terms of the degree of involvement of the lateral chest wall and is quantified into three grades. Grade 1 indicates involvement of up to a quarter of the lateral projection of the chest wall; grade 2 indicates involvement of between one quarter and one half; and grade 3 more than one half of the lateral projection of the chest wall.

Diaphragm. A plaque involving the diaphragmatic pleura should likewise be recorded as present. Here again, the right or left side should be indicated, and this is as illustrated in the example in the standard radiographs.

Costophrenic Angle. Obliteration of the costophrenic angle should be recorded. If the thickening extends up the chest wall, the findings should be recorded as both costophrenic angle obliteration and pleural thickening, provided the latter is of grade 1 or greater. The site involved should be specified. The scalloping or leafing of the diaphragm that is sometimes seen in severe airways obstruction and that creates a deceptive appearance of costophrenic angle obliteration should not be recorded.

Pleural Calcification. One or both sides may be involved but should be recorded separately. Here again, the site and extent must be documented. In regard to the site, provision is made for recording involvement of the chest wall, diaphragm, and other structures, including the pericardium and mediastinum. The extent of pleural calcification is subdivided into grades 1, 2, and 3, with 1 being an area of calcified pleura with the greatest diameter up to 20 mm, or a number of such areas whose combined diameter does not exceed 20 mm. Grade 2 includes calcification in an area or areas whose greatest diameter exceeds 20 mm but not 100 mm. Grade 3 includes pleural calcification in one or more areas where the greatest diameter exceeds 100 mm.

Equipment and Technique

The ILO classification and guidelines for its use contain a number of recommendations as to the x-ray equipment to be used and the most suitable technique for taking chest radiographs.[48] In regard to certain of the recommendations, unanimity was not forthcoming. The criteria for obtaining a quality film are included in the booklet that accompanies the standard radiographs. Film quality should be assessed and recorded. Four grades are recognized: 1, good quality; 2, acceptable with no technical defect likely to impair the classification of the radiograph for pneumoconiosis; 3, poor with some technical defect, but still acceptable for classification purposes; and 4, unreadable. When a film is unacceptable or of poor quality, some mention should be made as to why it is unsatisfactory, i.e., whether it is overpenetrative or underpenetrative, fogged, or gray.

Classifying Unknown Films

It is recommended that when a reader who is interpreting a series of unknown films sees a film that obviously demonstrates the features of pneumoconiosis, rather than arbitrarily awarding a category to the film, he or she should compare it to the appropriate standard films, trying to match the profusion and type of opacities in the unknown with the appropriate standard. Only in this fashion will the interpretation of films become an objective exercise. Many readers feel that the standard films are so fixed in their minds that they have no need to refer to them when interpreting unknowns. The refusal to use standard films has been shown by Morgan et al. to lead to what they refer to as the "middling" tendency.[56] Thus, when certain readers are faced with interpreting an unknown radiograph that shows pneumoconiosis, instead of comparing it to the standards, they immediately attach a category to it. In doing so, they virtually always use a midcategory (1/1, 2/2, or 3/3). Had they compared it to the standards, an element of uncertainty might have entered their mind. As it is, their mental processes leave them never in doubt but often wrong. Thus, in one study involving several interpreters, all of whom were consultants to the U.S. Public Health Service, all but one showed a pronounced middling tendency.[56] The one exception was the sole reader who regularly used the standards while interpreting unknowns.

Nevertheless, it must be remembered that there is no guarantee that the 12-point scale is made up of equal intervals, and indeed its originators felt that the intervals were probably unequal.[57] If the scale were of equal intervals, the weight of additional dust obtained for each increase in subcategory would be the same. When independent randomized reading is used to determine radiographic progression, should several readers be afflicted with the middling tendency, the bias would tend to eliminate or decrease progression, especially when change is small (1/1 to 1/2). Further references to the problems of reading progression will be found later in the chapter. In the few instances in which progression is marked (i.e., two subcategories), the middling tendency would tend to exaggerate it even further.

Observer Variation

Despite the standardization of techniques for taking and interpreting films, the radiographic interpretation of pneumoconiosis still remains a subjective exercise.

Marked interobserver and intraobserver variations occur,[58-60] as they also do in the interpretation of chest films for tuberculosis, barium enemas for colitis, and electrocardiograms for myocardial infarction. Interobserver variation is usually greater than intraobserver variation, and it is essential in an epidemiological survey to compare and standardize the radiographic interpretations of various readers. Marked differences between British and North American readers have been shown to exist—while the British appear to have been disciplined into conformity with their most experienced reader, the North Americans show too much individuality.[59] Those readers who differ greatly from their colleagues should be excluded. Multiple readings are to be preferred to single readings, but even then the panel of readers should be tested at regular intervals to ensure that their reading habits have not changed. This can be done by having them re-read several series of films at regular intervals. Such a series should range over all categories and should have at least 100 films in it. During the interpretation of the series of unclassified films, all x-rays thought to be positive for pneumoconiosis should be matched with the appropriate standard. When reading an unclassified series of films, the introduction of ''marker films'' at fairly regular intervals, that is to say, good quality x-rays that several readers have read independently and classified in an agreed category, helps keep the readers' ''thermostat'' in line with the consensus. Thus, when a marker film is interpreted, the reader should agree fairly closely with the prior consensus category (within one subcategory). Should the reader deviate by more than one subcategory, the error should be pointed out to him or her. The reader is then aware that his or her readings are out of line with the consensus and can make a conscious effort to adjust the reading scale up or down.

The interpretation of films for pneumoconiosis is greatly influenced by technique, and therefore techniques should be standardized as far as possible prior to starting the survey. Individual radiologists can no more agree on an optimal technique than they can on the degree of pneumoconiosis present in individual films. For these reasons, a uniform technique should be adopted, since were each radiologist allowed to use his or her own preference, the range would be infinite. Such recommendations for standardization of techniques have been published and, while certainly not ideal, can with intelligent application help reduce interobserver variation.[48, 61] Nonetheless, there have been film trials comparing various radiographic techniques using high versus low kilovoltage, and the results have shown that the interpretation is little affected by using high as opposed to low kilovoltage techniques.[62]

The depth of inspiration, the duration of exposure, and the method of developing the film all may influence interpretation. It has been shown that overpenetrative films are likely to decrease the category awarded, whereas if the film is unduly soft or underpenetrative, a higher category is likely to be awarded.[55, 63] The effect of such changes may be profound and may change prevalence and progression rates by as much as 50% (Fig. 6–4).

The Chest Radiograph and Dust Exposure

Serial chest radiographs have been used in numerous epidemiological studies of occupational lung disease as a means of monitoring dust exposure in exposed populations. When conducting studies in which chest radiographs have been made on dust-exposed populations, it is customary to consider several indices, including the prevalence of the condition, the attack rate, and the progression rate. The prevalence rate may not reflect present conditions, and hence is one of the less useful measurements. The attack rate is better as a rule, but in silicosis and CWP, diseases that seldom develop without prolonged exposure, the disease may appear at a time when exposure is decreasing. In certain instances, the main insult may have occurred several years previously, and the onset of abnormalities is related in the main to prior exposure. The best way of relating environmental exposure to the radiographic response is to measure the progression rate, that is to say, the change

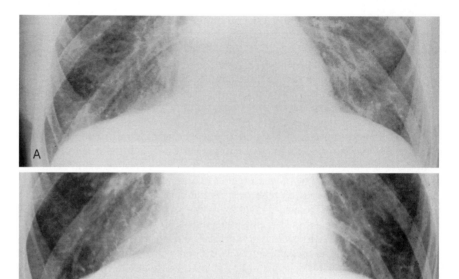

Figure 6–4. Magnified views of the lower zones of a chest radiograph of a non–dust-exposed subject (fruit farmer). A was taken during a submaximal inspiration and was read as category 1/1, t/s opacities. When repeated in full inspiration, (B), the radiograph was read as 0/0. (Reproduced by permission from Dick, J. A., Morgan, W. K. C., Muir, D. C. F., et al., The significance of irregular opacities in the chest roentgenogram. Chest, 102, 251, 1992.)

in category over a period of time during which dust exposure was measured and is known. This is best achieved by comparing diads, triads, or quadrads of films from exposed workers.

Serial films can be used to improve clinical diagnosis and also to determine progression. Thus, when a tentative diagnosis is based on a solitary film which shows only equivocal changes, the diagnosis may subsequently be established when a radiograph is taken at a later date and shows that the characteristic features have appeared. The assessment of radiographic progression and regression needs further description.

Methods of Assessing Progression and Regression

Two kinds of change may be detected through comparison of serial films: first, the appearance of disease or abnormality in previously normal films; and second, progression or regression in a film already interpreted as abnormal.[64] In the first instance, the frequency of abnormalities appearing in a series of previously normal films allows one to calculate an attack rate; while in the second instance, a progression index can be derived. The films may be presented for comparison to the reader in two ways.

Independent Method. This involves presentation to the interpreter of a series of films so that he or she cannot remember when the other radiograph(s) from the same subject was presented. The independent method permits several modes of presentation of the films, namely, immediately, that is to say as soon as the films are available for comparison; serially, with all the first films on one occasion and all the second films on another occasion; and independently randomized, with the films of the first and the second series mixed. Since it is known that the reading habits of an interpreter are subject to change, it is obviously desirable to read all the films of the randomized series within a relatively short time.

Side-by-Side Method. When two or more films of the same subject are available, they may be presented in the correct chronological sequence or the order may be disguised. However, attempts at disguising the order are often unsuccessful, and the technical qualities of the films usually permit recognition of the temporal sequence. When three or more films are available, possible sequences become many and the only useful approach is to completely reverse the order. Two or more films may be interpreted as a simple series (triad, tetrad, pentad) or as separate diads, e.g., as the first and fourth films of a series. The latter involves comparing the first film with the second, then with the third, and so on. The logistics of such complex comparisons become enormous.

The main arguments concerning the reading of progression in pneumoconiosis center around which method is preferred, the side-by-side or the independent. Implicit in the use of the side by side method is the bias introduced by a knowledge of chronological sequence of the films. However, it must not be forgotten that bias exists with the independent method. In any two chest radiographs of the same subject taken at an interval, there are several differences between the films of the diads, for example, the age of the patient examined, weight in certain circumstances, and also technical factors affecting film quality. Experienced readers make allowance for age and technique; but only if these compensatory mechanisms are entirely consistent, which they are obviously not, can it be said that the independent method is without bias. Advocates of the side-by-side method claim it allows readers to compensate for differing techniques, and in addition reduces the variation that is inherent in independent reading.

The problem of bias introduced by knowledge of chronological sequence was investigated by Reger and his colleagues.[65] The results of their studies indicated that the side-by-side method is prone to bias, and the assumed chronological sequence of the diad greatly influenced the progression score. The design of their study was somewhat contrived in that the readers, believing they knew the temporal sequence, were presented with a pair of films showing up to eight steps of regression. This was effected by reversing the order of the films without the interpreter's knowledge. In addition, it was shown that a progression score was often recorded in two copies of the same film when the reader believed that they were taken at different intervals. It is thus apparent that the assumed chronological sequence greatly influences the reading of progression when the side-by-side method is used. Although this trial may be criticized in that it was somewhat foreign to the experience of most readers, a similar investigation utilizing serial radiographs from subjects with tuberculosis and sarcoidosis showed exactly the same findings. In this case it cannot be claimed that regression is unknown, since the interpreters should have known that both tuberculosis and sarcoidosis are prone not only to improve but to regress.[66]

Liddell and Morgan compared side-by-side with independent reading according to standard scientific criteria, and they also reviewed several published series.[64] They did this by comparing the methods in terms of differentiability, consistency, validity, and simplicity. Since there is a continuum from no dust to maximal dust with no exact end point to indicate the presence of disease, the definition of sensitivity has to be modified. The authors concluded that at the present time, side-by-side reading is the method of choice, since independent, randomized reading tends to lack specificity, and the signal-noise ratio is likewise less satisfactory. In general, there is more variability with the independent method of reading, and regression may be recorded in a proportion of the paired films. Comparison of independent and side-by-side reading usually shows that the independent method yields about half as much progression as the side-by-side method.[67] Only when it becomes possible to guarantee exactly the same technique when taking films over a period of several years will it be possible to limit the problem of bias in the independent method.

The few comparative trials that have been carried out in which progression has been read by interpreters from different nations have shown some startling differences. This is especially true of one trial in which British and North American readers were compared. The cause of such variability was not immediately apparent, but clearly much needs to be done in order to obtain more uniform and less variable readings of progression.

It is often assumed that the interpretation of the films for pneumoconiosis requires profound knowledge and perspicacity, and that the ideal interpreter is a god-like blend of Sherlock Holmes, Albrecht Dürer, and Socrates. In reality, the interpretation of a film for pneumoconiosis is a glorified guess or estimate of the number of dots present on it. The more educated the observer, the more likely he or she is to be rigid in interpretation. If the observer happens to have an opinion that coincides with an accepted consensus, this is ideal, but if not, it is most unlikely that he or she will change reading habits. If the latter state of affairs is the case— and this is a frequent occurrence among eminent radiologists and to lesser extent in chest physicians—then that observer must be excluded from epidemiological studies. The distinction between epidemiology and clinical diagnosis is often difficult to explain to radiologists and clinicians, but its importance cannot be overestimated. We have shown that lay readers can be trained to read films for pneumoconiosis.[68] Since they have no preconceived ideas and hence tend to be more open to suggestion, they are more likely to record than to interpret and in many ways are to be preferred.

A report of a workshop sponsored by the National Heart and Lung Institute offers much useful advice for those who are involved in the use of the chest x-ray in epidemiology.[69] The main recommendations are that in epidemiological studies involving radiographic examinations of the chest, at least three readers, whose comparability has been assessed prior to the study, should be used. All readings should be carried out independently, and consensus or collaborative reading sessions should be avoided, since the consensus frequently represents the opinion of the most forceful and biased reader. A mean reading is the best measure of the prevalence of the condition. In addition, standard films should be used in order to achieve comparability, and chest films of unexposed workers should be included in the series for control purposes. A percentage of the films should be recycled to ensure reproducibility.

REFERENCES

1. Morris, J. N., Uses of Epidemiology. New York, Churchill Livingstone, 1975, pp. 318–320.
2. Attfield, M., and Hudak, J., Prevalence of coal workers' pneumoconiosis: comparison of first and second rounds. *In* Rom, W. N., and Archer, V. E., eds., Health Implications of New Energy Technologies. Ann Arbor, MI, Ann Arbor Science, 1980.
3. McGee, D., Reed, D., and Yano, K., The results of logistic analyses when the variables are highly correlated: an empirical example using diet and CHD incidence. J. Chronic Dis., 37, 713, 1984.
4. Whitby, L. G., Screening for disease: definitions and criteria. Lancet, 2, 819, 1974.
5. Morgan, W. K. C., Screening for occupational cancer of the lung. Chest, 74, 239, 1978.
6. Elsen, E. A., Robins, G. A., Greaves, I. A., et al., Selection effects of repeatability criteria applied to lung spirometry. Am. J. Epidemiol., 120, 734, 1984.
7. Eisen, E. A., Oliver, L. C., Christiani, D. C., et al., The effects of spirometry standards on two occupational cohorts. Am. Rev. Respir. Dis., 132, 120, 1985.
8. Morgan, W. K. C., The effect of spirometry standards on two occupational cohorts [correspondence]. Am. Rev. Respir. Dis., 132, 1371, 1985.
9. Morgan, W. K. C., Donner, A., Higgins, I. T. T., et al., The effects of kaolin on the lung. Am. Rev. Respir. Dis., 138, 813, 1988.
10. Enright, P. L., Johnson, L. R., Connett, J. E., et al., Spirometry in the lung health study. Am. Rev. Respir. Dis., 143, 1215, 1991.
11. McCarthy, D. S., Craig, D. B., and Cherniack, R. M., Intraindividual variability in maximal expiratory flow-volume and closing volume in asymptomatic subjects. Am. Rev. Respir. Dis., 112, 407, 1975.
12. Epidemiology Standardization Project. Am. Rev. Respir. Dis, 118(suppl. II), 1–88, 1978.
13. American Thoracic Society. Statement on the standardization of spirometry—1987 update. Am. Rev. Respir. Dis., 136, 1285, 1987.
14. American Thoracic Society. Statement on lung function testing: selection of reference values and interpretative strategies. Am. Rev. Respir. Dis., 144, 1202, 1991.
15. Medical Research Council Committee on the Aetiology of Chronic Bronchitis. Standardized questionnaire on respiratory symptoms. Br. Med. J., 1960, 2, 1965.
16. Medical Research Council Committee on the Aetiology of Chronic Bronchitis. Instructions for the Use of the Questionnaire on Respiratory Symptoms. Dawlish, England, W. J. Holman, Ltd., 1966.
17. Morgan, W. K. C., and Branscomb, B. V., The assessment of ventilatory capacity. Joint statement of the Committees on Environmental Health and Respiratory Physiology. Chest, 67, 95, 1975.

18. Fitzgerald, M. X., Smith, A. A., and Gaensler, E. A., Evaluation of electronic spirometers. N. Engl. J. Med., 289, 1283, 1973.
19. ATS Statement. Snowbird workshop on standardization of spirometry. Am. Rev. Respir. Dis., 119, 831, 1979.
20. Gardner, R. M., Hankinson, J. L., and West, B. J., Evaluating commercially available spirometers. Am. Rev. Respir. Dis., 121, 73, 1980.
21. Townsend, M., Spirometric forced expiratory volume in the standing versus sitting posture. Am. Rev. Respir. Dis., 130, 123, 1984.
22. Tager, I., Speizer, F. E., Rosner, B., and Prang, G., A comparison between the three largest and three last of five forced expiratory maneuvers in a population study. Am. Rev. Respir. Dis., 114, 1201, 1976.
23. Ferris, B. G., Speizer, F. E., Bishop, Y., and Prang, G., Spirometry for an epidemiologic study. Bull. Eur. Physiopath. Respir., 14, 175, 1978.
24. Knudson, R. J., Lebowitz, M. D., Holberg, C., et al., Changes in normal maximal expiratory flow volume curve with growth and aging. Am. Rev. Respir. Dis., 127, 725, 1983.
25. Sherter, C. B., Connolly, J. J., and Schilder, D. P., The significance of volume adjusting the maximal midexpiratory flow in assessing the response to a bronchodilator drug. Chest, 73, 568, 1978.
26. Cockcroft, D. W., and Berscheid, B. A., Volume adjustment of maximal midexpiratory flow. Importance of changes in total lung capacity. Chest, 78, 595, 1980.
27. Hankinson, J. L., Reger, R. B., and Morgan, W. K. C., Maximal expiratory flows in coal miners. Am. Rev. Respir. Dis., 116, 175, 1977.
28. Reger, R. B., Young, A., and Morgan, W. K. C., An accurate and rapid radiographic method of determining total lung capacity. Thorax, 27, 163, 1972.
29. American Thoracic Society. Single breath carbon monoxide diffusing capacity: recommendation for a standard technique. Am. Rev. Respir. Dis., 136, 1299, 1987.
30. Morgan, W. K. C., Lapp, N. L., and Seaton, D., Respiratory disability in coal miners. J.A.M.A., 243, 2401, 1980.
31. Fairman, R. P., Hankinson, J. L., Lapp, N. L., and Morgan, W. K. C., Pilot study of closing volume in byssinosis. Br. J. Ind. Med., 32, 235, 1975.
32. Boehlecke, B., Piccirillo, R. E., and Hankinson, J. L., Use of helium oxygen spirometry in the detection of small airways disease in coal miners. Paper presented at the International Conference on Occupational Lung Disease, sponsored by the American College of Chest Physicians, San Francisco, 1979.
33. Morris, J. F., Koski, A., and Johnson, L. C., Spirometric standards for healthy nonsmoking adults. Am. Rev. Respir. Dis., 103, 57, 1971.
34. Knudson, R. J., Slatin, R. C., and Lebowitz, N. J., et al., The maximal expiratory flow volume curve: normal standards, variability, and effects of age. Am. Rev. Respir. Dis., 113, 587, 1976.
35. Petersen, M. R., Amandus, H., Reger, R. B., et al., Ventilatory capacity in normal coal miners: prediction formulae for the FEV_1 and FVC. J. Occup. Med., 15, 899, 1973.
36. Clinical respiratory physiology. Bull. Eur. Physiopath. Resp., 19(suppl. 5), 7, 1983.
37. Milne, J. S., Longitudinal respiratory studies in older people. Thorax, 33, 547, 1978.
38. Buist, A. S., Evaluation of lung function, concepts of normality. In Simmons, D. H., ed., Current Pulmonology. New York, John Wiley & Sons, 1982, pp. 141–165.
39. Morris, J. F., Temple, W. P., and Koski, A., Normal values for the ratio of one second forced expiratory volume to forced vital capacity. Am. Rev. Respir. Dis., 108, 1000, 1973.
40. Lapp, N. L., Amandus, H., Hall, R., and Morgan, W. K. C., Lung volumes and flow rates in black and white subjects. Thorax, 29, 185, 1974.
41. Rode, A., and Shephard, R. J., Pulmonary function and Canadian eskimos. Scand. J. Respir. Dis., 54, 4, 1973.
42. DaCosta, J. L., Pulmonary function studies in healthy Chinese adults in Singapore. Am. Rev. Respir. Dis., 104, 128, 1971.
43. Corey, P. N., Ashley, M. J., and Chan-Yeung, M., Racial differences in lung function: search for proportional relationship. J. Occup. Med., 21, 395, 1979.
44. Sobol, B. J., and Sobol, P. G., Percent of predicted as the limit of normal in pulmonary function testing: a statistically valid approach. Thorax, 34, 1, 1979.
45. Boehlecke, B. A., and Merchant, J. A., The use of pulmonary function testing and questionnaires as epidemiologic tools in the study of occupational lung disease. Chest, 79(suppl. 4), 114S, 1981.
46. Oldham, P. D., Decline of FEV_1. Thorax, 42, 161, 1987.
47. Editorial. Airflow limitation—Reversible or irreversible? Lancet, 1, 26, 1988.
48. Guidelines for the use of the ILO international classification of radiographs of pneumoconiosis. No 22. (Rev.)., Occupational Safety and Health series. Geneva, International Labour Office, 1980.
49. Rivers, D. E., Wise, M. E., King, E. J., and Nagelschmidt, G., Dust content, radiology, and pathology of simple pneumoconiosis of coal workers. Br. J. Ind. Med., 17, 87, 1960.
50. Rossiter, C. E., Relation of lung dust content to radiological changes in coal workers. Ann. N.Y. Acad. Sci., 200, 465, 1972.
51. Caplan, H., Correlation of radiological category with lung pathology in coal workers' pneumoconiosis. Br. J. Ind. Med., 19, 171, 1962.
52. Liddell, F. D. K., and May, J. D., Assessing the Radiological Progression of Simple Pneumoconiosis. London, National Coal Board (Medical Service), 1966.

53. Carilli, A. D., Kotzen, L. M., and Fischer, M. L., The chest roentgenogram in smoking females. Am. Rev. Respir. Dis., 107, 133, 1973.
54. Amandus, H. E., Lapp, N. L., Jacobsen, G., and Reger, R. B., Significance of irregular small opacities in the radiographs of coal miners in the U.S.A. Br. J. Ind. Med., 33, 13, 1974.
55. Dick, J. A., Morgan, W. K. C., Muir, D. C. F., et al., The significance of irregular opacities in the chest roentgenogram. Chest, 102, 251, 1992.
56. Morgan, W. K. C., Petersen, M. R., and Reger, R. B., The ''middling'' tendency. Arch. Environ. Health, 29, 334, 2974.
57. Liddell, F. D. K., An experiment in film reading. Br. J. Ind. Med., 20, 300, 1963.
58. Reger, R. B., and Morgan, W. K. C., On the factors influencing consistency in the radiologic diagnosis of pneumoconiosis. Am. Rev. Respir. Dis., 102, 905, 1970.
59. Reger, R. B., Amandus, H. E., and Morgan, W. K. C., On the diagnosis of coal workers' pneumoconiosis: Anglo-American disharmony. Am. Rev. Respir. Dis., 108, 1186, 1973.
60. Amandus, H. E., Pendergrass, E. P., Dennis, J. N., and Morgan, W. K. C., Pneumoconiosis: interreader variability in the classification of the type of small opacities in the chest roentgenogram. Am. J. Roentgenol. Radium Ther. Nucl. Med., 122, 740, 1974.
61. Jacobsen, G., Bohlig, H., and Kiviluoto, R., Essentials of chest radiology. Radiology, 95, 445, 1970.
62. Washington, J. S., Dick, J. A., Jacobsen, J., and Prentice, W. M., A comparison of conventional and grid techniques for chest radiography in field surveys. Br. J. Ind. Med., 30, 365, 1973.
63. Reger, R. B., Smith, C. A., Kibelstis, J. A., and Morgan, W. K. C., The effect of film quality and other factors on the roentgenographic categorization of coal workers' pneumoconiosis. Am. J. Roent., 115, 462, 1972.
64. Liddell, F. D. K., and Morgan, W. K. C., Methods of assessing serial films of the pneumoconioses: a review. J. Soc. Occup. Med., 28, 6, 1978.
65. Reger, R. B., Butcher, D. F., and Morgan, W. K. C., Assessing change in the pneumoconioses using serial radiographs. Am. J. Epidemiol., 98, 243, 1973.
66. Reger, R. B., Petersen, M. R., and Morgan, W. K. C., Variation in the interpretation of radiographic change in pulmonary disease. Lancet, 1, 111, 1974.
67. Amandus, H. E., Reger, R. B., Pendergrass, E. P., et al., The pneumoconioses: methods of measuring progression. Chest, 63, 736, 1973.
68. Peters, W. L., Reger, R. B., and Morgan, W. K. C., The radiographic categorization of coal workers' pneumoconiosis by lay readers. Environ. Res., 6, 60, 1973.
69. Weill, H., and Jones, R., The chest roentgenogram as an epidemiologic tool. Arch. Environ. Health, 30, 435, 1975.

The Deposition and Clearance of Dust from the Lungs—Their Role in the Etiology of Occupational Lung Disease

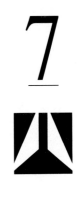

W. Keith C. Morgan

■

An understanding of the pathophysiology of occupational lung disease requires some knowledge of the mechanisms involved in the deposition and disposal of inhaled dust. Over the years, dust physicists have studied pulmonary deposition in much detail, and much is now known concerning the physical processes involved. The subsequent transport of dust from the sites of deposition, in particular the alveoli, to other regions is less well understood.

The basic anatomy of the lung has been known for many years, and by applying this knowledge, certain outstanding workers formulated many of the theoretical concepts of dust deposition and respiratory mechanics long before appropriate fast-response electronic equipment became available to confirm their hypotheses. The advent of sophisticated and sensitive electronic measuring devices has led to a rebirth of the study of the acute and chronic effects of inhaled particles.

DUST DEPOSITION

In 1935, Findeisen[1] constructed a model designed to provide information on how dust particles are deposited in the lungs. The model assumed that deposition depended on Newtonian mechanics and Stokes' law; the latter being the physical law which describes the fall of small particles. It has been known since the days of Lister that, while inhaled air contains numerous bacteria, viruses, and other particles, exhaled air—apart from the early expirate which is composed of the dead space air—is free from bacteria and particles. This was first demonstrated by Tyndall, who, by means of the Tyndalloscope, showed that expired air under normal circumstances contained few, if any, particles and hence was invisible in a strong light. When a person takes a breath, air is drawn through the nares into the nasopharynx and trachea and hence into the conducting system of the lungs. From there it reaches the alveoli by way of the various bronchi, terminal bronchioles, respiratory bronchioles, and atrial ducts. Most of the bronchial surface of the healthy subject is lined by a film of mucus which is continually propelled upward by ciliary action. As the inspired air enters the trachea, its flow rate decreases slightly. A further reduction in velocity takes place in the main segmental bronchi. When the third, fourth, and fifth divisions of the bronchi are reached, there is marked slowing of the air stream, so that, by the time the inspired air reaches the terminal bronchioles, the flow rate is not more than 2 to 3 cm/sec.

The deposition of inhaled particles and the effects of inhaled gases are influenced by the physical and chemical properties of the inhaled agent and also by sundry host factors (Table 7–1). The physical properties of importance include particle size and density, shape and penetrability, surface area, electrostatic charge, and hygroscopicity.[2] Among the more important chemical properties that influence

Table 7–1
■
Factors Influencing the Effects of Inhaled Agents

Physical Properties

1. Physical state—whether particle, mist, vapor, fume, or gas. Sulfur dioxide is adsorbed onto particles of carbon and hence carried into the distal airways.
2. Size and density of particles, mist, or aerosol—determines site of deposition.
3. Shape and penetrability—influences propensity for migration, chrysotile versus crocidolite.
4. Solubility
   a. Particulates—insoluble agents, such as asbestos, produce local action, whereas soluble agents, such as manganese compounds, have systemic effects.
   b. Gases and vapors—relatively insoluble agents, such as oxides of nitrogen, are inhaled into small air passages, while soluble agents, such as ammonia and sulfur dioxide, seldom pass beyond nose and nasopharynx.
5. Hygroscopicity—hygroscopic particles increase in size as they travel down respiratory tract.
6. Electric charge—influences site of deposition.

Chemical Properties

1. Acidity and alkalinity—have a toxic effect on cilia, cells, and enzyme systems.
2. Propensity to combine with substances in lung and tissues—agents, such as carbon monoxide and hydrogen cyanide, have systemic effects, while fluorine compounds may have both local and systemic effects.
3. Fibrogenicity—asbestos and silica are fibrogenic; iron and carbon are nonfibrogenic.
4. Antigenicity—stimulates antibodies.

Host Factors: Genetic, Environmental, and Acquired

1. Lung defenses.
   a. Genetic determinants influence ciliary action, clearance rates, and macrophage function. Slow and rapid clearers exist, and rates of clearance are inherited characteristics.
   b. Acquired determinants, viz., drugs, cigarette smoke, temperature, and alcohol, all influence ciliary and macrophage function.
2. Anatomical and physiological factors—influence of breathing patterns and airways geometry.
3. Immunological state—response to an agent can be influenced by allergic diathesis, atopy, and possibly tissue type.

---

the respiratory tract's response are the acidity or alkalinity of the inhaled agent and its ability to enter into combination with the body's constituents. Various host factors are also of importance and will be referred to later.

When particle deposition is considered, it is useful to divide the respiratory tract into three main regions: (1) the nose and extrathoracic airways that extend to the glottis; (2) the conducting airways, i.e., dead space, or trachea and bronchi to the terminal bronchioles; and (3) the pulmonary parenchyma where gas exchange occurs. The nose is an exceedingly efficient filter, and most large particles are deposited in it, provided the subject is breathing through the nares. Some small particles will, however, reach the intrathoracic dead space, and an even smaller number will reach the parenchyma. Those particles between 0.5 and 6.0 microns are referred to as the respirable fraction, a term which implies their size permits their deposition in the lung parenchyma. While this is true, not all respirable particles are deposited in the gas-exchanging portions of the lung, and many are deposited in the nose and dead space. The particles most likely to be deposited in the alveoli, and of particular concern as a cause of pneumoconiosis, are those between 0.5 and 3.0 microns.

Physical Properties

The respiratory tract's response is influenced by whether the inhaled agent is a particulate, fume, mist, vapor, or gas, and in this connection, a few definitions are in order. An aerosol is a collection of fine particles, either liquid or solid, which is dispersed in a gas. A fume is a fine solid particulate. A mist is a fine liquid particulate. A vapor is the gaseous form of the substance which is normally a liquid; while a gas is a substance whose physical state is without fixed volume. Besides size, on occasion, the shape and penetrability of a particle influence the body's reaction to it. Thus, the sharp and needle-like fibers of crocidolite asbestos are more likely to penetrate and migrate than are the serpentine fibers of chrysotile. Evidence indicates that this may be an important factor in the etiology of mesothelioma and may explain the increased incidence of this tumor following exposure to crocidolite. Solubility is also important, in that, while insoluble particulates such as asbestos and silica produce their effects entirely or nearly entirely owing to a local action, other agents, such as manganese and beryllium, are soluble to a greater or lesser extent and therefore can have systemic effects on the brain, kidneys, and other organs.

The humidity and temperature of the aerosol have important influences on the site of deposition in that hygroscopic aerosols tend to increase their size as they pass down the airways. Hence, the relative humidity of the airways becomes important. In humans, inhaled air in most circumstances becomes fully saturated in the nose, partly because of diffusion and partly because of convective mixing. The large deflecting channels which are present in the anterior nares create turbulence and increase the tendency for deposition from inertial impaction. The turbinates create eddy currents and further turbulence and likewise increase deposition from inertial impaction.

The flow of air through the tracheobronchial tree may be laminar, turbulent, or transitional. In laminar flow the viscosity of the gas or mixture of gases is of prime importance, while in turbulent flow the density of the gases has a greater influence. The Reynolds' number, the ratio of inertial to viscous forces, decides whether flow is turbulent or laminar. In the larger airways, such as the larynx, trachea, and lobar and segmental bronchi, flow is partly turbulent and partly transitional. Increases in air flow that occur during exercise, coughing, or hyperventilation increase turbulence in the large airways. Laminar flow predominates in the small airways, and their flow rates are appreciably less than are those of the larger airways. Respiratory flow rates and the size of the tidal volume affect deposition due to both inertial impaction and diffusion. Diseases which increase turbulent flow, e.g., bronchitis and asthma, increase central deposition of particles. Similarly, obstruction of the airways likewise tends to limit deposition peripherally and to increase central deposition.[3]

Chemical Properties

The chemical properties of the inhaled agents likewise influence the effect of particles, mist, vapors, and gases. Depending on the site of deposition, the acidity or alkalinity of the agent can cause a variety of effects, including paralysis of cilia, delayed particle clearance, and ciliary death, and may in addition interfere with enzyme systems which control cellular metabolism. In a like fashion, certain substances combine with the lung and tissue fluids and exert both systemic and local effects. Thus, carbon monoxide traverses the alveolocapillary membrane to form carboxyhemoglobin. Fluorine and its compounds, while having a local effect, may also be absorbed and exert systemic effects on the skeleton and other organs. The propensity of the deposited particle to induce fibrosis is likewise important, and while some particles, including asbestos, quartz, and cristobalite, are intensely fibrogenic, others, such as stannic oxide, iron, and coal, have little or no fibrogenicity. Other agents, such as *Bacillus subtilis* enzymes, when inhaled, can lead to the development of antibodies and asthma. Fungal spores and other organisms may likewise generate an immunological response.

Host Factors

Host factors may be divided into genetic, environmental, and acquired factors. The lung defenses include ciliary clearance, humoral antibody formation, and other factors which may be compromised by hereditary defects. By the same token, some persons clear particles rapidly from the ciliated airways, while others do so relatively slowly. The rate of clearing is determined to a large extent by genetic factors and is immutable in that slow and fast clearers retain their characteristics throughout life.[4, 5] Lung defenses may also be affected by environmental and occupational insults, including air pollutants, cigarette smoking, drugs, and excessive cold, and by other nonspecific factors. Macrophage function, mucociliary clearance, and smooth muscle sensitivity may all be affected by such extraneous influences. The anatomy and airways geometry of individuals show marked variations. Thus the total cross-sectional area of each generation of the airways varies considerably in persons of the same age and height.[6, 7] Much the same can be said for the angles of bifurcation of the airways. Such anatomical differences affect the degree of turbulence in the airways and also the propensity for particles to settle.

It has been suggested that the likelihood of uranium miners to have lung cancer and of chrysotile asbestos miners to have radiographic evidence of asbestosis varies according to bodily habitus.[8, 9] In both instances those of shorter stature were thought to be at greater risk. It was postulated that the shorter trachea of pyknic asbestos miners put them at greater risk of developing asbestosis. Subsequently a detailed investigation of the relationship between particle deposition and body habitus indicated that deposition was not significantly influenced by the height of the subject when the investigator corrected for ventilated lung volume. No evidence was found to support the hypothesis that shorter workers were more at risk from the inhalation of toxic particles.[10]

Breathing rates and tidal volume likewise vary appreciably and, as such, may have a profound influence on the site and magnitude of particle deposition. Similarly, the immune state of the subject influences the response to inhaled agents. Thus, the presence of atopy or the allergic diathesis may predispose to the development of certain types of occupational asthma, e.g., that due to platinum salts. It has been suggested that tissue type, as determined by histocompatibility antigen testing, is also important to predict the development of certain conditions, such as asbestosis or coal workers' pneumoconiosis. This is now known to be of little or no importance.[11] Smoking, on the other hand, seems to protect against the development of extrinsic allergic alveolitis, perhaps the only beneficial health fact that is known to result from this dangerous habit.[12] Whether this is due to a generalized depression of the immunological responses in smokers or occurs as a result of the fact that particles do not reach the alveoli because of an excess of mucus in the conducting airways remains conjectural.

Mechanisms of Particle Deposition

There are five physical processes involved in particle deposition (Fig. 7–1). These have been ably reviewed by Brain and Valberg[2] and are as follows:

1. Sedimentation or gravitational settling
2. Inertial impaction
3. Diffusion or Brownian movement
4. Electrostatic precipitation
5. Interception

In man, the last two processes are of much less importance in the etiology of occupational lung disease than the others.

Sedimentation. Particles sediment under the influence of gravity, each falling at a constant speed which depends on Stokes' law. The speed at which a particle settles is known as the terminal velocity and is directly dependent on its density and the square of its diameter. Large particles settle more rapidly. Sedimentation is also affected by residence time in the alveoli, particle concentration in the various airways, the incline of the angle with respect to gravity, and the aerodynamic diameter of the particle. It must be borne in mind that under normal conditions monodispersed aerosols do not occur, and particles are not of a single size or shape. The deposition of irregular particles is usually described as a function of their

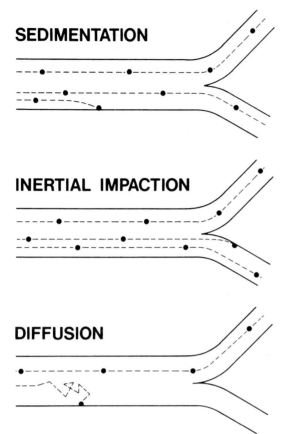

Figure 7–1
Methods of deposition.

aerodynamic diameter, which refers to the diameter of a unit density sphere that has the same terminal velocity as the particle under study. The distribution of aerodynamic diameters of a particular aerosol can be measured experimentally, and the frequency distribution can be determined. Most heterodispersed aerosols fit a log normal distribution in which a plot of particle number density (the number of particles per given size interval, viz., 1 to 2 microns) versus the logarithm of size produces a Gaussian curve. Such an aerosol can effectively be described by two properties, namely, the count median diameter (CMD) and the geometric standard deviation. The mass median diameter (MMD) is larger than the CMD because the larger particles make a greater contribution to the total mass of the aerosol.

Inertial Impaction. When a particle is being carried along in an air current and the latter changes its direction, the momentum of the particle will carry it forward in its initial pathway. As a consequence, some particles are deposited by impaction at those regions of the bronchial tree where a bifurcation or angle is present. Deposition of the particle under such circumstances is mainly determined by its momentum, that is to say, by the product of its weight and speed. Breathing patterns characterized by increased flows tend to lead to greater inertial impaction, especially of larger particles. Turbulent impaction is more important as a cause of deposition in the larger airways and predominantly affects particles greater than 1 micron.

Diffusion or Brownian Motion. Small particles have kinetic energy as a result of being bombarded by molecules of the surrounding air. Their movement is completely random, and if a particle is in close proximity to the alveolar wall, it is likely to be deposited in this fashion. Diffusion is important in the deposition of those particles that measure up to 2 microns, and for particles smaller than 0.5 micron, it is the main physical process involved.

Electrostatic Precipitation. This is a minor process in most instances. The airways are covered by a mucus layer, which is a good conductor and which precludes the development of powerful electric fields, thereby limiting the process of electrostatic precipitation.

Interception. This process involves the noninertial impaction of particles on the airway wall and is related to the physical size and in particular the length of the particle. It is of prime importance in the deposition of certain aerosols that are predominantly composed of fibers, e.g., cotton, hemp, and asbestos.

A number of theoretical models for particle deposition have been developed in which the deposition of inhaled aerosols at a given site in the respiratory tract is expressed as a percentage of the total number of inhaled particles. Most models relate particle size to the anatomical site of deposition, e.g., nose, trachea and bronchi, and lung parenchyma (Fig. 7–2).[13–15] As already mentioned, the site of deposition is influenced by the breathing rate, by tidal volume, by whether breathing is oral or nasal, and by cigarette smoking and the presence of various lung diseases. Exertion tends to increase oral breathing, and the nose no longer acts as the efficient filter it is, with the result that a greater number of larger particles reach and are deposited in the dead space. Since there are regional differences in ventilation between the top and the bottom of the lungs, it is a reasonable assumption that there will also be regional differences in particle deposition. This has been confirmed.[16]

The site of deposition is influenced by the size of the particle, by the flow rates in the varying regions of the lung, by the effect of respiration and other factors on the caliber of the airways, and by the subject's postural position during the time he or she is breathing the particle.[16] It has been shown that the act of drawing air into the lungs from a cigarette selectively redistributes the inhaled particles from the bases to the apices of the lungs.[17] While breathing quietly, larger respirable particles are preferentially deposited in the upper lobes, as compared to particles with a smaller MMD. The penetration of larger particles, e.g., 3.5 microns, is greater to the distal region of the lung and in particular to the apices than it is for smaller particles of around 1 micron.[18] These matters and the vagaries of particle deposition have been discussed at some length.[19] It has also been shown that exercise causes a redistribution of particles to the upper zones, with the resultant increase in deposition in the upper lobes.[20]

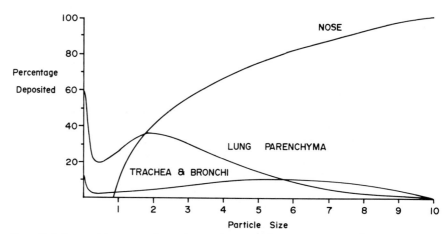

Figure 7–2. Regional deposition of particles as a function of their size in microns. This assumes a respiratory rate of 15 per minute and a tidal volume of 700 to 750 ml. (Based on data from Task Force Group on Lung Dynamics, Committee II IRCP, Deposition and retention models for internal dosimetry of the human respiratory tract. Health Phys., 12, 173, 1966.)

Most of the larger inhaled particles (5 microns or greater) are deposited in the nose or in the dead space long before the respiratory bronchioles are reached. In contrast, many particles smaller than 3 microns tend to reach the gas-exchanging portions of the lung. For the most part, dust settling on the mucous film of the dead space epithelium is conveyed to the pharynx within 2 to 8 hours. Particles that reach the alveoli and gas-exchanging portions are removed by a different mechanism, which will be described later. In a normal adult subject there are 300 to 400 million alveoli, each of which has a diameter of about 250 microns. Not all alveoli are in use at rest, and there is an intrapleural pressure gradient from apex to base which influences alveolar size. A normal person breathes around 5 to 6 L/min. If it is assumed that the tidal volume is 450 ml, then at a respiratory rate of 12, the minute volume will be 5.4 L. Given a dead space of 150 ml, the dead space ventilation in 1 minute will be 1.8 L and the alveolar ventilation, 3.6 L. Considering that the functioning alveoli increase their volume by less than 300 ml with each breath and that the residual volume of most subjects is around 2 L, there is not much of an increase in alveolar volume in inspiration. In practice, the mean increase in the diameter of alveoli during inspiration is probably less than 5% while the subject is breathing quietly. This indicates that, in contrast to the gas in the conducting system and respiratory bronchioles, the gas in the alveoli is turned over at a slower rate and tends to be stagnant. Because of this lower turnover and prolonged residence time, particles that reach the alveoli are likely to be retained sufficiently long to allow sedimentation to occur. Particles between 2 and 5 microns will settle in as little as 2 to 3 seconds. It is for this reason that expired air is almost free from particles of this size. With particles smaller than 0.5 microns, sedimentation is uncommon and deposition from diffusion tends to be the major physical process involved.

Dust Deposition and Occupation

Davies[21] has calculated the likelihood of a particle being deposited in the lungs based on the alveolar volume in different phases of respiration, the rate of breathing, and the tidal volume. He has shown that an atmospheric concentration of 500,000 particles/ml is necessary to ensure that each alveolus will receive at least one particle. This dust concentration far exceeds that found in any industry. Concentrations of particles that are causally related to pneumoconiosis seldom exceed 5000/ml. Thus, under these circumstances, it requires something like 1000 breaths to guarantee that a particle will first reach and second be deposited in an alveolus.

A coal miner working in a mine for 40 hours a week and exposed to an atmosphere containing 800 to 1000 particles/ml, all below 50 microns, for approximately 60% of the time inhales between 100 and 150 g of dust in 1 year. Of the dust inhaled, about 1 to 10 g is deposited in the alveoli, but only about 0.5 g is permanently retained. This is less than one hundredth of the total inhaled.

In some miners exposed to these conditions, radiographic changes would develop in 10 to 15 years. Since the dust levels in the United States and Britain are generally significantly below the hypothetical concentration mentioned earlier, the likelihood of developing category 1 simple pneumoconiosis in less than 30 years is remote. Nevertheless, it must be remembered that factors other than dust concentration influence the development of pneumoconiosis. Individual susceptibility obviously plays a role, and it is apparent that certain subjects are prone to develop the disease more rapidly than others and that such differences may be related to the varying efficiency of the clearing mechanisms and possibly to differing breathing patterns (see previous discussion). It must be remembered too that the chemical properties of the deposited particles and hence their pathological effects are of prime importance. Thus, at death, many coal miners are found to have 20 to 30 g of coal dust in their lungs despite the fact that during life they suffered no respiratory disability or impairment and, moreover, died of an unrelated cause. In contrast, the pulmonary deposition of 5 g of silica would be almost certainly fatal. Although industrial hygienists use the term lifetime dust exposure in such a way as to imply they measure accurately the dust which a worker inhales during life, such quantifications of dust exposure are at best approximations based on a limited number of measurements, often made at a distance from the worker's breathing zone and over a relatively short time. Even were they accurate, the relationship between the dust levels in the air and the weight of dust deposited in the lungs varies greatly from one individual to another, as does the percentage of dust cleared from the lungs.

CLEARANCE OF DUST

The mechanisms by which particulate matter is removed vary according to the site of deposition. If an insoluble particle is deposited in the dead space, it is cleared by the mucociliary escalator; however, should the particle be deposited in the lung parenchyma, it is engulfed by pulmonary macrophages, which in turn migrate either to the ciliated airways and hence to the mucociliary escalator, or to the interstitium of the lungs and from there find their way to the lymphatic vessels.

Mucociliary Clearance

Those particles which are deposited in the anterior third of the nose are removed by blowing, wiping, sneezing, or other mechanical means. Such particles may remain at the site of deposition for 24 to 48 hours. Clearance from the posterior portion of the nose, including the turbinates, depends on the usual mucociliary mechanisms. Soluble particles when deposited in the nose are quickly absorbed.[22] The nasal mucus layer is propelled backward toward the nasopharynx at the rate of 4 to 6 mm/min. There is a 4-minute half-time for particles deposited in the posterior part of the nose.

The remainder of the ciliated airways stretch from the trachea to the terminal bronchioles. The larynx is covered by mucus-secreting squamous epithelium. By way of contrast, the trachea and bronchi are covered by columnar cells, some of which are ciliated, and others of which are not. Respiratory mucus is produced by submucosal mucous glands and by goblet cells. The former are situated predominantly in the large airways, while the latter occur more commonly in the smaller and more distal airways. The relative number of ciliated columnar cells progressively decreases from the trachea to the terminal bronchioles. Each columnar cell has around 200 cilia that emerge from its surface, and each cilium contains longitudinal fibers which are capable of contraction. Two single fibrils form the central core. At the periphery, nine fibrils are arranged in a concentric fashion. The peripheral fibrils converge and unite into a common structure at the top of the core.[22, 23]

It is believed that the respiratory mucus has two layers as follows: (1) a periciliary layer (sol) which surrounds the cilia and (2) a mucus layer which lies on top of the cilia. It was originally thought that the mucus blanket was both continuous and contiguous, but most of the evidence suggests that this is not true and that mucus-free islands are present on the bronchial epithelium. Regeneration of destroyed ciliated epithelium usually takes between 14 and 17 days.

Cilia beat in one plane with a fast propellant stroke and a slow recovery stroke. It is theorized that one of the two subfibers in the nine peripheral filaments is shorter and that bending results from sliding between two subfibers. The gap between subfibers is bridged by dynein arms. The force of the bending filaments is transferred to the ciliary membrane by radial fibers. In the airways, the effective stroke propels the blanket of mucus toward the larynx. Ciliary motion depends on adenosine triphosphate as a source of energy.[23, 24]

A normal person produces around 50 to 150 ml of mucus daily. While secretion of the mucous glands is under parasympathetic control, the goblet cells appear to respond to direct irritation. The clearance rate in humans varies between 5 and

15 mm/min, with a slower rate prevailing in older subjects and a higher rate in the young. Mucus transport rates decrease from the trachea to the peripheral airways, and the same can be said of the frequency of ciliary beating. Mucus clearance rates vary according to age and sex and are also influenced by the viscosity of the sputum and by the site of deposition of the particle. The trachea is usually cleared of particles within 10 minutes; however, the segmental and subsegmental bronchi have half-lives for particle clearance of 20 to 30 minutes. In the smaller airways, from the 10th generation and beyond, the half-life is approximately 100 to 200 minutes.

Factors Influencing Mucociliary Clearance.[24, 25] The more important physicochemical factors that influence ciliary function and clearance are cold and decreased humidity. Cold, dry air greatly depresses ciliary function and clearance and causes many problems in patients with a tracheostomy and in those with reversible bronchospasm or asthma. The upper airways are predominantly affected. Various inorganic salts and radioactivity also depress mucociliary clearance. Acute exposure to cigarette smoke is associated in most studies with decreased mucociliary transport. Occasionally, transient increases in clearance rates have been observed, but these are almost certainly a consequence of the coughing that smoking engenders. Measurements of clearance rates in chronic smokers vary, and such studies tend to yield conflicting results owing to coughing and varying sites of deposition. The deposition pattern in confirmed smokers tends to be abnormal, with significantly more central deposition.[16] Short-term exposure to very high concentrations of air pollutants, such as sulfur dioxide and the oxides of nitrogen and ozone, can be shown to impair ciliary activity transiently, but there is little evidence to suggest that air pollutants in the usual concentrations found in the ambient air of North America or Europe are likely to have a significant effect. High concentrations of oxygen, various inhalation anesthetics, and narcotics likewise depress ciliary activity.

Particle deposition and mucociliary transport are affected in subjects with chronic bronchitis, cystic fibrosis, asthma, and other airways diseases. The removal of foreign particulates by the mucus blanket is slower in these conditions, but the decreases in ciliary activity are often compensated for by increased coughing.

Recently, congenital structural defects in ciliated cells have been reported.[23] Such cells are found in the ependyma of the intracranial ventricles, the fallopian tubes, and the efferent ducts of the testes. Cilia from these different sites have the same ultrastructure as that of the tail of the sperm. Kartagener's syndrome is associated with a defect in the dynein arms on the outer pairs of ciliary microtubules (discussed earlier). Spermatozoa from males with Kartagener's syndrome are immotile. Additional syndromes exist in which the defects affect other parts of the dynein arms.

Alveolar Clearance*

The retention of particles in the lung parenchyma is related not only to deposition but also to clearance. While animals provide a useful model for the study of alveolar clearance, most of the techniques which have been used cannot be applied to humans. Even knowledge about alveolar clearance in animals is fragmentary, and we lack a detailed understanding of the basic mechanisms.

Alveolar transport depends on the alveolar epithelium, the interstitium of the septa, and the fluid and secretory pathways. The alveolar epithelium is composed of two kinds of cells, usually known as type 1 and 2 pneumocytes. The former act as a barrier between the lumen of the alveolus and the interstitium and capillary. It is assumed that their function is the transport of gases through the alveolocapillary membrane. The type 2 cell is a major secretory cell of the primary lobule and is believed by most to be responsible for the synthesis, storage, and secretion of

---

*See also Chapter 11.

surfactant. The latter substance is responsible for the integrity of the alveoli, which is maintained through the low surface tension of surfactant. In its absence, the alveoli collapse, and the lungs become atelectatic. There seems little doubt that surfactant also plays a role in the coating and transport of deposited particles.

The other cell found in the alveoli is the alveolar macrophage. This is a mononuclear cell thought to be derived from the tissue histiocyte and which is responsible for alveolar phagocytosis. It differentiates in a unique fashion in order to adapt to the high oxygen tension that is present in the alveoli. By the same token, its activity and metabolism are seriously affected by hypoxia. After particulate matter has been taken up by the alveolar macrophage, it may be acted upon by the cell's enzyme system or may be retained unchanged prior to being removed from the lung.

The interstitium of the septa is made up of the basement membranes of the epithelium and capillary and the capillary endothelium. It contains connective tissue and stroma and is primarily affected in pulmonary edema. It may act as a pathway whereby the macrophage leaves the alveolus in order to reach the respiratory bronchiole.

As mentioned earlier, particles which may be deposited in the alveoli range from 0.01 to 8 or 9 microns, although deposition of particles larger than 5 microns is uncommon. Once the particle settles in the alveolus or respiratory bronchiole, subsequent clearance takes place by either absorptive or nonabsorptive processes.[26, 27] Absorptive processes involve the selective migration of the particle through the alveolar wall and hence into the bloodstream or lymph channels. Nonabsorptive mechanisms involve phagocytosis of the particle by the alveolar macrophage. Should the dust burden become excessive, clearance rates appear to reach a peak and then plateau, in which case some particles will be seen to lie free in the alveoli. It has been suggested that three phases of clearance exist, all of which have different time courses. The first involves surface transport from the proximal areas of the lobule along the respiratory surface to the respiratory bronchiole. It has been estimated that 50% of the material removed by this process is cleared in 24 hours. A second and slower process has a 50% clearance time of closer to 100 hours. It is suggested that the second process involves septal transport of material that has been phagocytized within the septa. The third mechanism, with a 50% clearance time of around 50 to 100 days, involves foreign particles that have reached dead end pathways in the perivascular and peribronchial spaces. What is becoming increasingly evident is that these generalizations cannot be applied across the board and that the clearance rate is related not only to the size of the particle but also to its density, chemical composition, and toxicity.

Deposited particles may be carried either in a free state or, in some instances, intracellularly. The mode of transport appears to depend on the physical properties and the number of particles deposited. After large challenges with particulate matter, cellular transport, as mentioned previously, is overwhelmed, and many particles will be seen to be lying free on the alveolar surface and interstitial region of the septa.

The means whereby the particle is transported from its site of deposition to the nearest macrophage is unknown, and while it is possible that the macrophage itself chases particles, it has also been suggested that perhaps the particles themselves move as a result of respiratory movements and hence come into contact with the nearest macrophage.

Although it is well recognized that many macrophages migrate from the alveoli by way of the respiratory bronchioles to the terminal bronchiole and hence mount the mucociliary escalator, the exact mechanisms of macrophage migration remain unknown. Macrophage movement entails simple ameboid migration; however, this process is slow, especially when the cells are dust-laden. In addition, the distance from the alveoli to the terminal bronchiole is appreciable. Two pathways of macrophage migration have been suggested, one of which involves passage of the macrophage into the interstitium of the lung and the other of which is a surface route. The former hypothesis assumes that macrophages migrate into the interstitium and wend their way up to the terminal bronchiole in peribronchiolar lymph channels. The subsequent extrusion of the particle-laden macrophage onto the terminal bronchiole has been observed. This process of necessity must involve the migration of free or particle-containing macrophages through the alveolar epithelium by endocytosis. Green[28] has suggested that particles, liquids, and cells all flow through the interstitium in the "liquid" veins of Staub. He suggested that flow results from mechanical tension that acts on alveolar septa as a result of ventilatory movements, in particular, the energy derived from the lung's elastic recoil and from interfacial tension. Gross,[29] on the other hand, favors the surface route. He postulates that a viscosity gradient exists within the surface fluid layer due to evaporation from the fluid surface. Thus, the depth of the alveolar fluid would increase and decrease in phase with the respiratory cycle. The luminal portion of the film, with the macrophages and extracellular particles resting upon it, would tend to move back or retreat less easily during inspiration than the subjacent deeper portion. This would result in the macrophages and entrapped particles being propelled toward the terminal bronchioles.

No matter whether particles are transferred by the interstitial or surface routes or by both routes, the ultimate source of energy must depend on respiratory movements. Similarly, it might be inferred that these processes will be most rapid in those regions of the lung in which, during heavy work, ventilation is most increased; a factor which could explain the predilection of coal workers' pneumoconiosis and silicosis to involve the upper zones of the lungs.[16, 20]

Alveolar clearance seems to proceed in several temporal phases that can usually be described by a series of exponentials, with each presumably corresponding to a different type of clearance mechanism. The earliest lasts from several days or several weeks, while the terminal phase is considerably longer and probably represents sequestration of particulate matter in the interstitial tissues. Mercer[30] has proposed a solubility model that explains long-term clearance by a slow dissolution. This theory applies to relatively insoluble particle burdens that have a log normal distribution. His theoretical results compare well with experimental data for the long-term clearance of particles that are relatively insoluble, such as uranium dioxide, but the process of alveolar clearance seems too complex to be explained by physicochemical factors alone. Part of the terminal phase of alveolar clearance probably relates to the migration of particles into the lymphatic vessels. However, the importance of lymphatic removal for clearing material from the lower respiratory tract has probably been exaggerated. Because particulate matter is slowly cleared from lymphatic channels and lymph nodes, the presence of particulates in these regions may be related to the pathogenesis of certain lung diseases.

In a few studies, humans have been exposed to radiotagged aerosols, with the subsequent retention being followed for several days. Morrow and his colleagues[31] studied clearance of manganese dioxide particles and chromium-labeled ferric oxide and polystyrene particles. The clearance rates for all three particles were slow, ranging from 65 to 35 days, respectively. Camner and Philipson[32] have studied clearance in 10 healthy males using 4-micron Teflon particles tagged with indium. Half the particles were cleared during the first day, but subsequent clearance was slow. Tantalum powder has been instilled into the alveoli of humans. While the trachea and bronchi are cleared within 3 to 4 days and the distal airways within 3 to 4 weeks, alveolar clearing may be incomplete after 3 to 4 years.[26, 27] The author has a patient who still has obvious alveolar retention of tantalum 10 years after a bronchogram. It is thus evident in studies using radioactively tagged particles that there is a fast clearance phase which is usually complete within 24 to 36 hours and a slower phase with a half-time of anything from 3 weeks to 3 months. It is important, however, to realize that other particles, for example, those of tantalum, are cleared far more slowly. Problems also exist with radioactively tagged particles in that it is sometimes difficult to know whether measured clearance is a reflection of alveolobronchiolar transport or is a consequence of dissolution and leakage of the particulate radionucleotide.

Alveolar function and clearance are probably influenced by the same factors and agents, e.g., drugs, that affect tracheobronchial clearance. Cigarette smoke has been shown to delay alveolar clearance in humans.[33]

Detoxification

Aside from the removal of particulates, normal lung defenses are dependent on the detoxification of noxious inhaled particulate matter. This latter process has as its mainstay the alveolar macrophage; however, polymorphonuclear leukocytes and histiocytes can also assume this function should the need arise. Humoral agents, such as specific immunoglobulins, play a dominant role against bacterial invasion, but various surface-active agents, i.e., enzymes such as lysozymes and lipoproteins, probably need to be present for the bactericidal properties of the phagocytes to be fully effective. These mechanisms are pre-eminent in the elimination of inhaled bacteria. The phagocytic properties of the macrophage are inhibited by hypoxia, such as occurs in obstructive airways disease. This may in part explain the predisposition of subjects with chronic bronchitis and emphysema to infection.

The alveolar macrophage is thought to be derived from the bone marrow, although in its adult form it differs significantly in structure, physiology, and metabolism from its parent cell.[34, 35] This differentiation is necessitated by the macrophage's shift to aerobic pathways for metabolic activities. By means of radioactive tagging of inhaled bacteria, it has been shown that 99% of a bacterial challenge is detoxified in the first 24 hours. In contrast, only 50% of the bacteria that are deposited in the lungs are removed.[34] Phagocytosis is adversely affected by the acute and chronic effects of alcohol, by steroids and immunosuppressive agents, by starvation and extreme climatic conditions, and by various air pollutants. Finally, and most deleterious of all, is the effect of cigarette smoking on the function of the alveolar macrophage.

The number of macrophages in the alveoli, as well as the exchange rate from the blood to the interstitium and alveoli, is affected by the presence of inflammation and by the host's immunological response to the inhaled material. Normal macrophages have the capacity to destroy many airborne organisms, including nonpathogenic streptococci and *Escherichia coli*; however, they are unable to kill *Mycobacterium tuberculosis* and *Listeria monocytogenes*. In contrast, when activated by the mechanism of cellular immunity, they acquire the capacity to destroy pathological organisms.

Lymphocyte-mediated activation of macrophages is the chief means of defense against inhaled intracellular parasites that are deposited in the lung parenchyma. This type of acquired immunity is operative in tuberculosis and histoplasmosis and may also play a role in berylliosis. Cellular immunity has the propensity to generate a vigorous and occasionally destructive tissue response in the lung parenchyma, viz., granulomata and sometimes necrosis. The mechanisms that control and affect cell-mediated immunity and its relationship to tissue necrosis need further study.

PATHOPHYSIOLOGICAL RESPONSES TO RESPIRATORY INHALANTS

Given the chemical, physical and host factors described earlier, the ultimate response of the respiratory system still depends to a great extent on the site of deposition of the particle. The range of responses according to the site is listed in Table 7–2.

Table 7–2
■
Pathophysiological Responses of Respiratory Tract to Particles, Mists, and Gases

Site of Deposition	Responses
Nose	Rhinitis, hay fever
	Septal perforation
	Nasal cancer
Trachea and bronchi	Bronchoconstriction
	1. Types I and III immunological reactions
	2. Pharmacologically induced
	3. Reflex; inert particles
	Industrial bronchitis
	Lung cancer
	Acute tracheitis and bronchitis
Parenchyma	Extrinsic allergic alveolitis, types III and IV immunological reactions
	Pneumoconioses
	Acute alveolitis and bronchiolitis: alveolitis, pulmonary edema, and bronchiolitis obliterans
	Pulmonary alveolar proteinosis
	Emphysema

Nose

The deposition of irritants in the nose may lead to rhinitis. Chrome may cause nasal ulcerations and septal perforation, while nasal cancer in furniture workers may result from the inhalation of wood dust.[36] Hay fever results from the deposition of ragweed and other pollens in the nares and is often associated with bronchoconstriction, either reflexly[37] or because some particles bypass the nose during mouth breathing and are deposited in the airways.

Trachea and Bronchi

Several responses may occur and are listed in Table 7–2. The most important and the most frequent is bronchoconstriction. The latter may occur as a result of an immunological reaction or it can be pharmacologically induced, such as probably occurs in byssinosis, in which the deposition of cotton fibers induces the liberation of mediators, for example, leukotrienes and histamine.

When inert particles are deposited in the trachea and bronchi over a prolonged period and if exposure is intense, industrial bronchitis may develop.[38]

In this regard, most particles that are relatively insoluble, e.g., asbestos fibers and silica, and which are deposited in the airways are removed by the mucociliary escalator and hence are inert when deposited in the trachea and bronchi. This would not be the case were they deposited in the alveoli or respiratory bronchioles. When such prolonged and intense exposure occurs, the mucous glands hypertrophy, the goblet cells increase, and excess mucus is produced. This leads to cough and sputum production and, occasionally, some evidence of a minor degree of large airways obstruction.[38] Since the particles are removed by the mucociliary escalator, they leave no radiographic traces.

Radioactive particles, such as radon daughters, may induce lung cancer, as can asbestos, nickel, and other agents. Finally, irritant gases and fumes may induce tracheitis.

Parenchymal Responses

If the particles are organic, they may induce a hypersensitivity pneumonia or what is often referred to as extrinsic allergic alveolitis. The latter is a misnomer in that the condition is characterized not only by alveolitis but also by respiratory bronchiolitis and sometimes a terminal bronchiolitis. Many arguments exist as to the immunological origin and pathogenesis of this condition, but suffice it to say there are features of both type III and IV immunological reactions.

If the particles are inorganic, pneumoconiosis may result. Here the term pneumoconiosis is defined as the deposition of dust in the lungs and the tissue's reaction to its presence. Nonetheless, the response differs according to the chemical and physical properties of the agent which is producing the pneumoconiosis. Four main pathological responses are seen in the pneumoconioses:

1. Interstitial Fibrosis. When this occurs, the particle induces initially an alveolitis and later fibrosis so that the alveolocapillary membrane becomes thickened. In addition, there may be a bronchiolitis. The gas-exchanging part of the lungs and often the respiratory and terminal bronchioles may be affected. The lungs become stiff and inelastic. The causes of this type of reaction are asbestos, beryllium, and cobalt, as found in tungsten carbide (hard metal).

2. Nodular Fibrosis. The classic example of this type of fibrosis is silicosis. In this condition the silica particles are engulfed by the macrophages, which then migrate into the interstitial tissues and the lymphatic channels. There the macrophage dies and liberates toxic enzymes that induce fibrosis. The latter appears as discrete nodules separated from the alveoli but sometimes adjacent to or situated near the respiratory bronchioles and arterioles. Most are at a considerable distance from the gas-exchanging surface. Because the nodules are separated by intervening normal lung tissue, their physiological effects are much less than those from agents which lead to the development of interstitial fibrosis. Most often in the nodular fibroses there are no detectable physiological abnormalities other than a slight increase in the stiffness of the lungs.[39] Even so, simple silicosis is a precursor of the complicated form of the disease, which is associated with both disability and premature death.

3. Interstitial and Nodular Fibrosis. This is a combined response usually only seen in exposure to diatomite, which usually contains a large amount of quartz. When the diatomite is heated and fused, some of the quartz is transformed into cristobalite and tridymite, both of which may induce interstitial fibrosis.

4. Macule Formation and Focal Emphysema. Exposure to coal, carbon, and other air pollutants may lead to the formation of macules around the second division of the respiratory bronchiole. When exposure to relatively nonfibrogenic agents is severe and prolonged, the lungs' defenses are overwhelmed, and there are no longer sufficient macrophages to keep pace with dust removal. The macrophages tend to aggregate around the respiratory bronchiole, especially in the second division, and there they die and liberate their dust burden. Since coal and carbon are only minimally fibrogenic, the fibrogenic response is limited to the production of a few reticulin fibers and occasionally scanty collagen. The pigment that is deposited appears as a mantle around the respiratory bronchiole. The smooth muscle in the latter tends to atrophy, and the respiratory bronchiole subsequently dilates to form a small translucent area in the middle of the macule. This is referred to as focal emphysema and does not extend to the alveoli. Macules, usually smaller than those seen in coal miners, but occasionally with some focal emphysema, may be seen in persons who have grown up in areas with severe urban pollution. Physiologically, the presence of macules and focal emphysema leads only to a slight increase in the alveoloarterial gradient and other minimal evidence of an abnormal distribution of inspired gas.[40] Simple pneumoconiosis does, however, predispose the patient to the development of progressive massive fibrosis.

Irritant gases, such as nitrogen dioxide, chlorine, and other agents, may reach the small airways and alveoli and cause severe damage to the alveolar epithelium and alveolar lining cells. Pulmonary edema may be produced, and subsequently during the recovery phase, bronchiolitis obliterans often supervenes. This is especially common following exposure to relatively insoluble gases, such as the oxides of nitrogen. Massive exposure to silica may induce pulmonary alveolar proteinosis. This condition is fortunately uncommon but in occasional instances is still seen in sandblasters. Finally, the inhalation of cadmium fumes can cause pulmonary edema and tissue destruction and lead to the development of panacinar emphysema.

It should be possible to predict the pathophysiological effects of an inhaled agent that is suspected of being a respiratory hazard by identifying its site of and propensity for deposition, along with its other properties referred to in this chapter. This same knowledge can be used as a means by which the effects of the particular hazard can be either limited or controlled completely.

REFERENCES

00. 1. Findesen, W., Uber das Absetzen kleiner, in der Luft suspendierter Teilchen in der menschlichen Lunge bei der Atmung. Pflugers Arch., 236, 367, 1935.

2. Brain, J. D., and Valberg, P. A., Deposition of aerosol in the respiratory tract. Am. Rev. Respir. Dis., 120, 1325, 1979.

3. Clague, H., Ahmad, D., Chamberlain, M. J., et al., Histamine bronchial challenge: effect on regional ventilation and aerosol deposition. Thorax, 38, 668, 1983.

4. Camner, P., Philipson, K., and Friberg, L., Tracheobronchial clearance in twins. Arch. Environ. Health, 24, 82, 1972.

5. Bohning, A. E., Albert, R. E., Lippman, M., and Forster, W. H., Tracheobronchial deposition and clearance. Arch. Environ. Health, 30, 457, 1975.

6. Lapp, N. L., Hankinson, J. L., Amandus, H., and Palmes, E. D., Variability in size of air spaces in normal human lungs as estimated by aerosols. Thorax, 30, 293, 1975.

7. Matsuba, K., and Thurlbeck, W. M., The number and dimensions of small airways in nonemphysematous lungs. Am. Rev. Respir. Dis., 104, 516, 1971.

8. Archer, V. E., Health concerns in uranium mining and milling. J. Occup. Med., 23, 502, 1981.

9. Becklake, M. R., Toyota, B., Stewart, M., et al., Lung structure as a risk factor in adverse pulmonary response to asbestos exposure. Am. Rev. Respir. Dis., 128, 385, 1983.

10. Graham, D. R., Chamberlain, M. J., and Hutton, L., Inhaled particle deposition and body habitus. Br. J. Ind. Med., 47, 38, 1990.

11. Evans, C. C., Lewinsohn, H. C., and Evans, J. M., Frequency of HLA antigens in asbestos workers with and without pulmonary fibrosis. Br. Med. J. 1, 603, 1976.

12. Morgan, D. C., Smyth, J. J., Lister, R. W., et al., Chest symptoms in farming communities with special reference to farmer's lung. Br. J. Ind. Med., 32, 228, 1975.

13. Landahl, H. D., On the removal of airborne droplets by the human respiratory tract. Bull. Math. Biophysics, 12, 43, 1950.

14. Beeckmans, J. M., The deposition of aerosols in the respiratory tract. Can. J. Appl. Physiol. Pharmacol., 43, 157, 1965.

15. Task Force Group on Lung Dynamics, Committee II IRCP, Deposition and retention models for internal dosimetry of the human respiratory tract. Health Phys., 12, 173, 1966.

16. Chamberlain, M. J., Morgan, W. K. C., and Vinitski, S., Factors influencing the regional deposition of inhaled particles in man. Clin. Sci., 64, 69, 1983.

17. Pearson, M. G., Chamberlain, M. J., Morgan, W. K. C., et al., Distribution and characteristics of particles in the lung during cigarette smoking. J. Appl. Physiol., 59, 1828, 1985.

18. Pityn, P., Chamberlain, M. J., Fraser, T. M., et al., The topography of particle deposition in the lung. Respir. Physiol., 78, 19, 1989.

19. Morgan, W. K. C., Clague, H., and Vinitski, S., On paradigms, paradoxes, and particles. Lung, 161, 195, 1983.

20. Morgan, W. K. C., Ahmad, D., Chamberlain, M. J., et al., The effect of exercise on the deposition of an inhaled aerosol. Respir. Physiol., 56, 327, 1984.

21. Davies, C. N., Deposition of dust in the lungs. In King, E. J., and Fletcher, C. M., eds., Industrial Lung Disease. Boston, Little Brown, 1960. pp. 44–58.

22. Proctor, D. F., The upper airways. Nasal physiology and defense of the lungs. Am. Rev. Respir. Dis., 115, 97, 1977.

23. Afzelius, B. A., and Mossberg, B., Immotile cilia. Thorax, 35, 401, 1980.

24. Wanner, A., Clinical aspects of mucociliary transport. State of the art. Am. Rev. Respir. Dis., 116, 73, 1977.

25. Camner, P., Clearance of particles from the human bronchial tree. Clin. Sci., 59, 79, 1980.

26. Camner, P., Alveolar clearance. Eur. J. Respir. Dis. 107 (Suppl.), 61, 1980.

27. Lippman, M., Yeates, D. B., and Albert, R. E., Deposition retention and clearance of inhaled particles. Br. J. Ind. Med., 37, 337, 1980.

28. Green, G. M., Alveolo-bronchiolar transport mechanisms. Arch. Intern. Med., 131, 109, 1973.

29. Gross, P., The mechanisms of dust clearance from the lung. Am. J. Clin. Pathol., 23, 116, 1953.

30. Mercer, T. T., On the role of particle size in the dissolution of lung burdens. Health Phys., 13, 1211, 1967.

31. Morrow, P. E., Gibb, F. R., and Gazioglu, K. M., A study of particulate clearance from the human lungs. Am. Rev. Respir. Dis., 96, 1209, 1967.

32. Camner, P., and Philipson, K., Human alveolar deposition of 4 μm Teflon particles. Arch. Environ. Health, 33, 181, 1978.
33. Cohen, D., Arai, S. F., and Brain, J. D., Smoking impairs long-term clearance from the lung. Science, 204, 514, 1979.
34. Green, G. M., The J. Burns Amberson lecture—in defense of the lung. Am. Rev. Respir. Dis., 102, 691, 1970.
35. Brain, J. D., The role of pulmonary macrophages. In Brain, J. D., Proctor, D. F., and Reid, L. M., eds., Respiratory Defense Mechanisms, Part II. New York, Marcel Dekker, 1977, pp. 709–967.
36. Acheson, E. D., Hadfield, E. H., and MacBeth, R. G., Nasal cancer in woodworkers in furniture industry. Lancet, 1, 311, 1967.
37. Kaufman, J., and Wright, G. W., The effect of nasal and nasopharyngeal irritation on airway resistance in man. Am. Rev. Respir. Dis., 100, 626, 1969.
38. Morgan, W. K. C., Industrial bronchitis. Br. J. Ind. Med., 35, 285, 1978.
39. Teculescu, D., Stanescu, D. D., and Pilat, L., Pulmonary mechanics in silicosis. Arch. Environ. Health, 14, 461, 1967.
40. Morgan, W. K. C., and Lapp, N. L., State of the art. Respiratory disease in coal miners. Am. Rev. Respir. Dis., 113, 531, 1976.

8

Pathological Reactions of the Lung to Dust

Alan Robert Gibbs

■

Inhalation of foreign materials can cause the lungs to react in a wide variety of ways ranging from a disease such as stannosis, which is asymptomatic but which produces extremely opaque small opacities on chest x-ray, to life-threatening diseases such as silicosis and malignant mesothelioma. Anatomically, the response and damage occur to a varying degree in the large or small conducting airways, the respiratory parenchyma, the pulmonary vascular bed, the pleura, and the reticuloendothelial system. It is not possible in a chapter of this length to describe in detail all the pathological reactions which can occur following exposure to various agents, since the majority of pulmonary pathology would have to be covered. A general overview will have to suffice together with specific examples. However, an occupational exposure should be considered as a possible cause of many pulmonary pathological processes. Sometimes the disease (e.g., asbestosis) may present several years after the patient has left an industry. Table 8–1 gives a list of possible reactions to various inhaled materials.

Table 8–1
■
Types of Pathological Reactions That May Occur with Various Minerals

Compartment	Type of Reaction	Examples
Airways	Asthma	Isocyanates, metals
	Bronchiolitis	Nitrogen dioxide
Airways–parenchyma	Centrilobular dust accumulations	
	Slight fibrosis	Coal, kaolin, talc, mica
	Moderate stellate fibrosis	Silica plus silicates and hematite
	Marked circumscribed fibrosis	Silica
	Diffuse interstitial fibrosis	Asbestos, kaolin, talc
	Extrinsic allergic alveolitis	Farmer's lung
	Sarcoid-like	Beryllium
Parenchyma	Diffuse alveolar damage	Toxic fumes
	DIP	Asbestos, silica, silicates
	GIP	Hard metal
	Pulmonary alveolar proteinosis	Silica
	Emphysema	Coal, cadmium
Diffuse/random	PMF	Coal, kaolin, talc
	Carcinoma	Asbestos, nickel, arsenic
	Infection	Tubercle in silicosis
Pleura	Benign effusion	Asbestos
	Plaques	Asbestos, talc, wollastonite
	Diffuse fibrosis	Asbestos
	Mesothelioma	Asbestos

DIP, desquamative interstitial pneumonitis; GIP, giant cell interstitial pneumonia; PMF, progressive massive fibrosis.

The major factors which influence the lung's reaction to inhaled particulates are the physicochemical properties, the dose of the material, inhalation of other minerals, and host factors. Phylogenetically the mammalian lung has developed efficient defense mechanisms to deal with the majority of inhaled particulates; for example, over 80% of silica particles are eliminated within a short time after exposure, and this process continues for the life of the subject.[1] Overloading of the mechanism, however, leads to retention of particles, with a response that is dependent on the biological activity of the material inhaled. This activity is determined by size and shape of the particles, durability, and surface properties. Inhalation of high doses of finely particulate silica causes an alveolar proteinosis–type of reaction, whereas prolonged exposures to lower doses of coarser silica leads to classical silicosis.[2] Chronic exposure to asbestos fibers, which are durable, can result in pulmonary fibrosis, whereas it appears that glass fibers, which are not durable, do not lead to pulmonary fibrosis.[3] Evidence indicates that the physical dimensions of fibers are important predictors of neoplastic potential, but surface properties may also be important. For example, in experimental systems, inhalation of erionite causes the development of more mesotheliomas fiber for fiber than crocidolite, although they have very similar physical dimensions.[4] The response to a dust may be modified by another—there is both experimental and human evidence to suggest that concomitant inhalation of clay minerals inhibits the effect of silica.[5, 6]

Host factors also form a variable that will modify the consequences of exposure; the intervention of chronic inflammation and ill-understood background states such as the rheumatoid diathesis and atopy are examples. Anatomical variations, for example of the lymphatic drainage, may also alter the site of dust retention in different individuals. Smoking can also alter pulmonary retention of inhaled particles,[7] and this may be a factor in the enhanced risk of lung cancer, which may be either additive or multiplicative, in asbestos workers who smoke.[8]

EXAMINATION AND HANDLING OF PATHOLOGICAL SPECIMENS

The importance of careful macroscopic examination, accurate description, and systematic and representative sampling of surgical or autopsy specimens cannot be overemphasized. Wherever possible specimens should be inflated with formalin via the bronchus, using a simple tube or catheter connected to a container of fixative at a pressure of 25 to 30 cm of water. The specimen should be inflated until the pleura is smooth, unless the latter is grossly diseased, and immersed in formalin for at least 24 hours. Cases of suspected occupational lung disease are often referred to "experts," either in the form of macroscopic or microscopic specimens, and correct assessment is greatly facilitated by adequate preparation of the materials. Table 8–2 provides a schema for the macroscopic assessment and recording of dust lesions, emphysema, and interstitial fibrosis.[9] It can be equally applied to well-inflated lung specimens and to Gough-Wentworth whole lung sections. The final assessment of interstitial fibrosis severity is best conducted on microscopic sections, provided adequate and representative sampling has been performed. Only the more severe degrees are evident macroscopically. The schema adopted here is a modification of the methods proposed by Hinson et al.[10] and the The Pneumoconiosis Committee of the American College of Pathologists and the National Institute for Occupational Safety and Health.[11] The latter recommends that 15 blocks should be taken from the lungs in cases of suspected asbestosis, but this is probably impractical for many nonspecialist laboratories. As a minimum, four routine blocks should be taken, preferably from the lung not involved by tumor or, if not available, well away from any tumor; ideally these should be from the apex of upper lobe, apex of lower lobe, basal segments, and major bronchi (to include nodes), and some should include pleura. Any other pathology present, such as a tumor, should also be carefully described and sampled.

Table 8–2
■
Macroscopic Assessment of Occupational Lung Diseases

Primary Dust Foci
Average size (Grade 0 to 3):
1 = 1–3 mm
2 = 4–5 mm
3 = > 5 mm

Profusion (Grade 0 to 3):
Assessed according to the proportion of lobules involved:
1 = < 33%
2 = 33%–66%
3 – > 66%

Secondary Dust Foci
Number of stellate foci ⎫ To be recorded for each size as follows:
⎪ a = (< 0.5 cm)
⎬ b = (0.5–2 cm)
Number of round foci ⎭ c = (> 2 cm)

Emphysema
Type: centrilobular, panacinar, irregular

Severity (Grade 0 to 3):
1 = 1–3 mm
2 = 4–5 mm
3 = > 5 mm

Profusion (Grade 0 to 3):
Can be graded for upper and lower lobes separately or for the whole lung and is
  similar to that for the primary dust foci.

Interstitial Fibrosis
Severity (Grade 0 to 4):
A histological grading system is used.

Extent (Grade 0 to 3):
1 = up to 10% of the lung involved
2 = between 10% and 25% involvement
3 = > 25% involvement

From Gibbs, A. R., and Seal, R. M. E., Examination of lung specimens. J. Clin. Pathol., 43, 68, 1990.

Role of Mineral Analysis of Lung Tissues

Various techniques can be employed in the evaluation of mineral dusts within the lung tissues, which vary from the simple, such as counting asbestos bodies in lung tissue sections by light microscopy, to the sophisticated and complex, such as the electron microscopic analysis together with energy dispersive x-ray and electron diffraction techniques of tissue digests. All can be useful, but some are more appropriate than others according to the circumstances of the case. Exact identification of a mineral depends upon its physical configuration (fiber, nonfiber, internal crystal structure) and its chemistry. Therefore exact identification may depend on the use of several techniques in conjunction. These techniques have most often been used in relation to the asbestos-related diseases in order to verify or refute claimed exposures, to correlate the mineral content with the pathological changes, and sometimes to determine the source of the exposure. Whenever these techniques are used to determine the mineral content of lung tissues, it is essential that the methods of digestion are performed meticulously, since there are several sources of error.[12–14] Values obtained for individual subjects should be compared to ranges that have been determined for normal subjects and various diseased groups. It is not sufficient to demonstrate the mere presence of a mineral—accurate quantitative data are essential to come to a realistic evaluation of the role of the mineral in causing a particular disease. These investigations should not be performed on a one-off basis, and it should be realized that methods used to examine airborne samples are not suitable for tissue samples. Electron microscopic techniques provide the most comprehensive information, but they are time consuming, expensive, require considerable expertise, and are performed in few laboratories. It is also important when comparing results from one laboratory to another to be aware of the ranges for the various diseases and controls for those laboratories. The results of one laboratory will be different from those of another laboratory, although they will show the same trends, because the preparation, analysis, and expression of results will vary. In the right hands, these analyses can provide extremely useful information. For example, it was mineral analysis of lung tissues of textile workers from Rochdale who were considered initially to be exposed predominantly to chrysotile that revealed considerable quantities of crocidolite, which together with additional information led the plant to be reclassified as a mixed exposure.[15] Generally nonfiber mineral analyses are more difficult than those for fibers and have been performed less often. However, several recent studies have examined the relationship between various minerals such as kaolin, talc, and silica and the pathology of the lungs. Some of these studies will be discussed in the later sections.

PATTERNS OF RESPONSE

Diffuse Alveolar Damage

Diffuse alveolar damage is an acute reaction which follows combinations of variable amounts of injury to the bronchioloalveolar epithelium and endothelium of the lung. A wide variety of agents can cause it, including viruses, radiation, drugs, collagen diseases, oxygen, and industrial materials such as fumes of the oxides of nitrogen, cadmium, beryllium, and ammonia. The pathological appearances are similar, whatever the causative agent.[16] The outcome of the reaction depends on the intensity and duration of the injurious agent. It varies from death during the acute phase to resolution or to interstitial fibrosis with or without obliterative bronchiolitis. Whenever this pathology is encountered, a thorough occupational history should be obtained.

Macroscopic Appearances

The lungs are heavy, edematous, and hemorrhagic, with varying degrees of induration. Similar changes occur in the larynx, trachea, and bronchi. The more soluble the inhaled substance, the more proximal the area of damage.

Microscopic Appearances

The microscopic appearances can be divided into early changes (1 to 7 days after exposure) and late changes (more than 7 days after exposure). These changes may be complicated by secondary bacterial infection.

Early changes:

1. Intra-alveolar and interstitial edema
2. Intra-alveolar hemorrhage and necrosis
3. Hyaline membranes (3 to 7 days)
4. Focal alveolar epithelial hyperplasia (3 to 7 days)
5. Necrosis of bronchiolar epithelium
6. Fibrin thrombi within capillaries or small arteries
7. Interstitial chronic inflammatory infiltrate (after 5 days)

Late changes:

1. Interstitial and intra-alveolar fibrosis
2. Proliferation of smooth muscle fibers

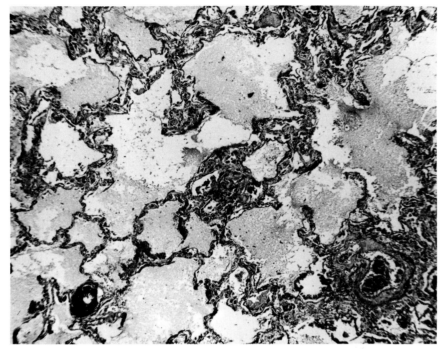

Figure 8–1. Severe, protein-rich edema in the lung of a patient who died after acute exposure to nitrous fumes. (H&E)

3. Vascular changes—subintimal fibrosis of veins and arteries, muscular hypertrophy of pulmonary arterial walls
4. Conspicuous alveolar epithelial hyperplasia

Figure 8–1 illustrates the early changes of diffuse alveolar damage in a subject

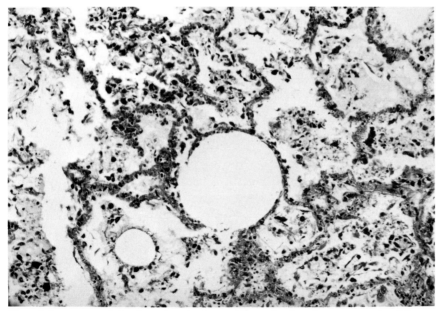

Figure 8–2. Necrosis of alveolar walls with edema and intra-alveolar inflammatory exudate following cadmium fume exposure. (H&E)

who died 2 days after exposure to oxides of nitrogen. Figure 8–2 illustrates a slightly later phase in a patient who died after acute exposure to cadmium fumes while welding. After survival from 6 to 7 days, hyperplasia and metaplasia of the alveolar epithelium become prominent (Fig. 8–3). Although the microscopic changes are similar whether the noxious agent arrived via the airways or bloodstream, the fact that in the least involved lobules the inflammatory changes are more intense in the center and in smaller conducting airways points to an intraluminal route. Some of the late sequelae described may be found in lung biopsies of patients presenting with chronic respiratory disease without a history of a dramatic illness following acute exposure. The clinical picture may not be that of a pure respiratory illness, since many substances affect other organs; for example, cadmium is nephrotoxic, and fluoride has skeletal effects.

Desquamative Interstitial Pneumonia

This term is often used loosely but should be reserved for a relatively rare condition characterized microscopically by uniform filling of alveolar spaces by eosinophilic plump mononuclear cells from field to field with little or no interstitial fibrosis and only minor diffuse alveolar damage.[17] The cells may contain cytoplasmic vacuoles and yellow-brown granules that are periodic acid-Schiff (PAS) positive but negative to iron staining. Electron microscopic studies have demonstrated that the intraluminal cells are mainly macrophages with a smaller proportion of type 2 pneumocytes. Many of these cases are idiopathic, but exposure to a variety of agents, including asbestos, silica, talc, tungsten carbide, aluminum, and a variety of silicates,[18–20] can result in this picture. Whenever this pathological reaction is encountered, it is important to obtain a detailed occupational history and, if possible, to perform a mineral analysis on the tissue to determine the amount and type of minerals present. It is not clear what particular exposure conditions need to occur for this reaction to develop, but high doses appear to be important.

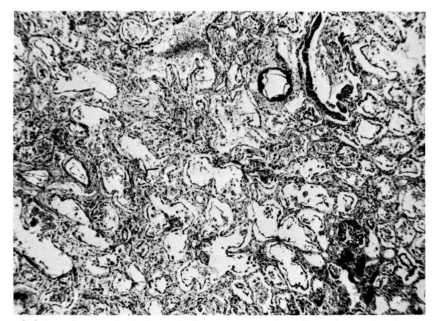

Figure 8–3. Lung of patient who died a week after exposure to cadmium fumes, showing detachment of alveolar epithelial cells and intra-alveolar collections of cells. The alveolar walls are edematous and contain cellular infiltrates. (H&E)

Giant Cell Interstitial Pneumonia

Giant cell interstitial pneumonia is a very rare form of interstitial pneumonia characterized by numerous, bizarre, large, multinucleate giant cells within the alveolar spaces superimposed upon either the desquamative form of interstitial pneumonia or chronic diffuse interstitial fibrosis. A number of these cases have been associated with exposure to hard metal (tungsten carbide).[21, 22]

Pulmonary Alveolar Proteinosis

Pulmonary alveolar proteinosis is an uncommon disease characterized by filling of the alveolar spaces with eosinophilic, amorphous PAS-positive exudate which is rich in lipid. There is a variable amount of interstitial inflammation and fibrosis. The precise roles of the type 2 pneumocytes in excess secretion and the alveolar macrophages in incomplete removal of the intra-alveolar surfactant like material are not understood. There is both experimental and human evidence to show that it can result from exposure to minerals.[23, 24] Finely particulate silica is the best documented, but metal fumes, cement, talc, and aluminum have also been implicated.[24–26] One of the necessary conditions appears to be fine particle size (1 μm or less in diameter).

Occupational Asthma

Occupational asthma is caused by inhalation of a sensitizing agent at work. Agents include platinum salts, isocyanates, chromium, nickel, grain and flour dusts, wood dusts, and anhydrides. There is usually a preliminary period before the onset of symptoms varying from a few days to many years. The symptoms usually come on at work but improve when the individual is not at the workplace. There have been no systematic studies of the pathology of occupational asthma and its relation to severity of the disease, but it is considered to be similar to nonoccupational asthma. Some agents (e.g., isocyanates) can cause both asthma and extrinsic allergic alveolitis (hypersensitivity pneumonitis).

Extrinsic Allergic Alveolitis

This pattern of response is caused by the inhalation of organic antigenic protein of fungal, avian, mammalian, or insect origin. A typical example is farmer's lung. It may be acute or chronic. In the acute form, there is a chronic inflammatory infiltrate which affects the interstitium and the bronchioles and shows a centrilobular accentuation.[27] There are also granulomas which are less compact than those observed in sarcoidosis. The centrilobular accentuation of the disease probably explains the greater dyspnea but minimal radiographic mottling as compared with the greater shadowing and minimal respiratory disability of the sarcoid patient. If the subject is removed from the source of antigen, the condition usually clears, and it has been found that the granulomas disappear within a few months after cessation of exposure. Occasionally a single severe acute episode can lead to the life-threatening chronic form. Usually, however, the chronic form is reached only after repeated acute or prolonged insidious exposures. The chronic form is characterized by diffuse interstitial fibrosis and honeycombing which is most severe in the upper lobes. Granulomas are usually absent in the chronic phase unless there has been recent exposure to the offending antigen.

Some patients following an acute attack appear to proceed to a prominent emphysematous appearance with a fine fibrosis.[28] Such patients have an obstructive profile on lung function testing, and some have been noted to be nonsmokers.

PULMONARY RESPONSES TO SPECIFIC DUSTS

Metals, Metal Salts, Metal Oxides, and Semimetals

Metals are simple minerals containing one element and possess lustre and malleability; under appropriate conditions they react by losing one or more electrons to form cations. They include gold, silver, copper, mercury, lead, platinum, tin, and iron. Semimetals are situated between metals and nonmetals in the periodic table and share properties with both; they can attain stability by either giving up or gaining electrons. They include antimony, arsenic, and bismuth. Most metals and semimetals are chemically combined in compounds and are found most commonly as oxides or sulfides (e.g., beryllium, aluminum, titanium, nickel, cadmium, and chromium).

A number of pathological reactions can follow exposure to these substances in the form of either dusts or fumes.[29, 30] Most of the information comes from case reports or epidemiological studies; there are few systematic studies of the pathology and its relation to mineral burden. Often exposure is to complex mixtures of these and other minerals, which leaves doubt as to the pathogenicity of individual substances. The toxic effects of these substances are due to the strong affinity between the ions of these substances and organic ligands located within the tissue molecules.[29] Respiratory effects are usually due to direct occupational exposure, but occasionally they can occur paraoccupationally; for example, disease has developed in the family contacts of beryllium workers.[31] Table 8–3 is a guide to the reactions that can occur as a result of exposure to some of the substances within this group and indicates the strengths of association in this author's opinion. They can vary from nuisance effects to acute life-threatening disease and prolonged chronic effects and neoplasia. It is not possible to be comprehensive in a chapter of this length, but some of the substances are briefly reviewed, particularly where there are some recent informative studies.

Aluminum

Jederlinic et al.[32] reported a study of nine workers employed in the production of aluminum oxide abrasive grinding wheels and tipped tools who had abnormal chest x-rays. In three who had prolonged heavy dust exposure, there were biopsies

Table 8–3

■

Pathological Responses That Have Been Linked to Exposure to Metals

Agent	\multicolumn{10}{c}{Type of Response}
	1	2	3	4	5	6	7	8	9	10
Aluminum		E		E	Q		Q		E	
Antimony								E		Q
Arsenic										E
Beryllium	E				E		Q		E	Q
Cadmium	E						Q			Q
Chromium						E				E
Hard metal		E	E			E	Q		E	Q
Iron							Q	E		
Mercury	E									
Nickel	E					E			Q	E
Tin								E		
Titanium					Q			E		Q
Uranium	E									E

1 = diffuse alveolar damage; 2 = desquamative interstitial pneumonitis; 3 = giant cell interstitial pneumonia; 4 = pulmonary alveolar proteinosis; 5 = granulomas; 6 = asthma; 7 = airways disease; 8 = dust accumulation with minimal fibrosis; 9 = diffuse interstitial fibrosis; 10 = lung cancer.
E, established; Q, questionable.

which showed interstitial fibrosis and honeycombing, one of which also showed features of desquamative interstitial pneumonitis (DIP). Mineralogical analysis revealed the presence of large amounts of metals, predominantly aluminum oxide and aluminum alloys. The authors considered that the exposure to aluminum oxide was the likely cause of the interstitial fibrosis. Another report found high levels of particulate and fibrous aluminum oxide in a case of DIP.[33] There have also been isolated reports of pulmonary alveolar proteinosis[34] and granulomatous disease[35] occurring in association with aluminum dust exposure.

Beryllium

Exposure to beryllium can result in two types of lung disease: (1) acute exposure to high concentrations causes diffuse alveolar damage, and (2) chronic exposure to low (sometimes extremely low) concentrations causes diffuse interstitial fibrosis and sarcoid-like granulomas.[36] The latter disease is associated with a delayed hypersensitivity (type 4) response evidenced by the elapsed 48- to 72-hour period before the beryllium patch lesions appear, the prominence of granulomas, and the accumulation of beryllium-specific helper/inducer T cells.[37] It may not present for many years after exposure. The *in vitro* beryllium lymphocyte transformation test is positive on blood or lavage samples from subjects with chronic beryllium disease but may also be positive in workers who have been exposed but who have no clinical disease.[38, 39] To date there is no evidence that the latter will definitely progress to overt disease.

The differential diagnosis of chronic berylliosis from sarcoid is difficult, although the extent of the interstitial chronic inflammatory infiltrate is usually less in the latter. Measurement of beryllium within tissues is desirable. The usual microprobe techniques are unsuitable for the detection of beryllium in the tissues because of its low atomic weight and usually low concentration, but the newly developed technique of laser microprobe mass spectrometry can be performed on histological sections.[40] The disadvantage is that it provides only qualitative information.

Cadmium

It is well recognized that inhalation of high concentrations of cadmium fumes can cause diffuse alveolar damage which may lead to death. It is has also been suggested that chronic inhalation may cause emphysema. However, the majority of studies of workers chronically exposed to cadmium have been inconclusive because they have failed to control for smoking. A study of 101 men who had worked for one or more years at a factory making copper-cadmium alloys has controlled for smoking and other factors and has provided convincing evidence that chronic inhalation of cadmium fumes can cause lung function and chest radiograph abnormalities consistent with emphysema.[41]

Chromium

There is a well-recognized association between exposure to hexavalent but not trivalent chromium compounds and increased risks of lung and nasal cancers.[42] The risk appears to increase with increasing exposure and has been observed in chromate production workers[43] and chromium platers.[44] The excess mortality appears about 5 to 9 years after first exposure and rises to its highest level between 35 and 39 years.[43] There is no particular histological type associated with chromium exposure, and there are no published studies of lung tissue levels of chromium in occupationally exposed workers with and without lung cancers. There is a study of pulmonary chromium and nickel levels in autopsy subjects from the Ruhr district and Munster in Germany who were exposed to general air pollution.[45] It was found that there was an increase of chromium and nickel levels with age, and the values were higher in the more polluted area (Ruhr district). Also the six lung cancers in the series were shown to have high levels of these metals in the lungs.

Cobalt–Hard Metal

Hard metal is composed of tungsten carbide set in a cobalt matrix with additional variable quantities of other metals such as nickel, tantalum, titanium, and vanadium. Experimental and human studies of workers exposed to cobalt in the absence of tungsten carbide suggest that cobalt rather than the other metals is the toxic agent.[22] Exposure to cobalt or hard metal can result in asthma, diffuse interstitial fibrosis, desquamative interstitial pneumonia or giant cell interstitial pneumonia.[22] Microprobe techniques have demonstrated in the lung tissues tungsten, titanium, and sometimes the other components of hard metal but not usually cobalt, which is very soluble in biological fluids and is cleared from the lung rapidly.[21, 22]

Nickel

Asthma, diffuse alveolar damage, and lung cancer have been associated with exposure to nickel and its compounds. Large excess risks of lung and nasal cancer have been reported in nickel refinery workers, lesser risks for workers in nickel mining and smelting, but no excess risk for nickel alloy workers.[46] To date, it is unclear which nickel species cause the development of lung cancer. An autopsy study of the Kristiansund, Norway, nickel refinery workers showed elevated levels of nickel within the lung tissues of the exposed workers compared to control subjects but no difference between those with and without lung cancer.[47]

Diseases Associated with Silica and Nonfibrous Silicate Exposure

It is customary to divide these diseases into separate groups such as silicosis, mixed dust fibrosis, and silicatoses; the last category includes talcosis and kaolinosis. However, they can be considered as a spectrum: when the exposure is predominantly to silica, the pathology is usually that of classical silicotic nodules; when predominantly to silicates such as talc, mica, or kaolin, then the lesions consist of interstitial collections of dust-laden macrophages associated with variable amounts of fibrosis. Even in cases of classical silicosis, there is nearly always exposure to substantial quantities of silicates as well as silica. When the effects of silica and silicates are more nearly balanced, the lesions observed are the mixed dust fibrotic nodules. In some exposures, such as in slate workers, the full spectrum of lesions may be encountered (Figs. 8–4 to 8–6).

Silicosis

The physical form of silica is important in determining fibrogenicity;[48, 49] the order of fibrogenicity increasing as follows:

amorphous stishovite < coesite < quartz < cristobalite < tridymite

The most common form encountered is quartz, and this is the major cause of silicosis. The term *silica* will be used in this chapter to mean quartz unless otherwise stated. The development of fibrosis appears to be a two-stage process—phagocytosis of dust particles followed by collagen production by fibroblasts.[50] Particle size is important; particles smaller than 5 μm in diameter will be deposited in the respiratory bronchioles and alveoli, but the most fibrogenic are smaller than 1 μm in diameter,[51] although a more recent study has suggested that the issue is more complex.[52] After deposition the particles are taken up by macrophages whose recruitment is initiated by activation of complement with generation of C5a, a powerful chemoattractant.[53]

This may cause lysosomal rupture and death of the cells, which was previously

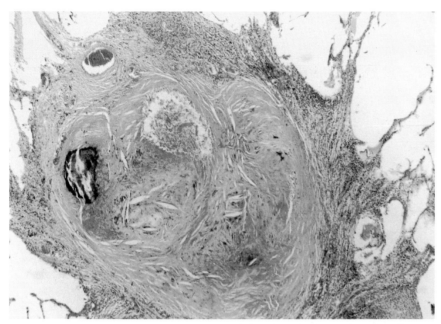

Figure 8–4. Classical silicotic nodule seen in the lung of a North Wales slate worker. The collagen has a whorled arrangement, and there are foci of calcification. There are accumulations of dust-laden macrophages around the periphery of the lesion. (H&E)

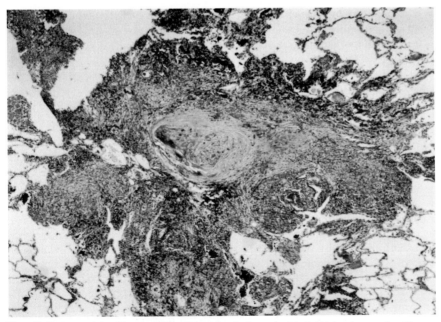

Figure 8–5. A mixed dust fibrotic nodule observed in the lung of a North Wales slate worker. The lesion is stellate, and the center of the lesion does not show as marked whorling as the classical silicotic nodule. There are accumulations of dust-laden macrophages around the periphery. (H&E)

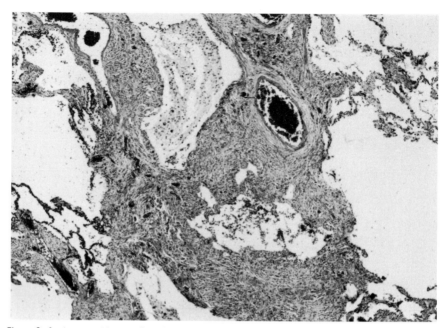

Figure 8–6. The typical lesion of a subject exposed to silicates rather than free silica. There are interstitial collections of dust-laden macrophages with a slight degree of fibrosis. (H&E)

thought to be an important event in the pathogenesis of silicosis.[54] However, recent *in vivo* studies have indicated that the immediate toxicity of silica is reduced by various components of lung fluids and that many of the macrophages survive with particles within them.[55] This will affect macrophage function, which will in turn affect the function of lymphocytes, neutrophils, and epithelial cells with the release of oxidants, fibroblast growth factors, interleukins, and other cytokines, immunoglobulins, and proteolytic enzymes.[1, 55] Precisely how these interact and result in the development of the silicotic nodule is not understood. Many of the macrophages containing silica particles are removed by the mucociliary apparatus or via interstitial planes and lymphatics which begin at the level of the respiratory bronchioles and are then transported to lymph nodes. When there is concomitant damage to type 1 epithelial cells, particles may enter the interstitium, where a proportion may persist for considerable lengths of time. These are probably the most important in stimulating macrophages to produce fibrogenic factors which affect the interstitial fibroblasts.

Silicotic nodules are observed first in the hilar lymph nodes and then in the lung parenchyma. Initially they are discrete and are most common at the apices of the upper and lower lobes, and measure a few millimeters in diameter. As the disease progresses, individual lesions fuse together (conglomerate) to form larger lesions which may, in severe cases, occupy large areas of the lung. Conglomerate silicotic lesions are typically formed by aggregation of smaller nodules, so that if one examines carefully the lesions produced by silica, the individual nodules can be identified.[56] Calcification and necrosis, particularly of the larger lesions, are common. This necrosis can result in ragged cavities which may be due solely to ischemia, although mycobacterial infection may also be responsible.

Microscopically the silicotic nodule consists of a central hyalinized whorled collagenous center, a mid-zone containing circumferentially arranged collagen fibers, and a peripheral zone of randomly arranged collagen fibers admixed with dust-laden macrophages and lymphoid cells (see Fig. 8–4). The cellularity of the nodules tends to decrease with age. Examination of the lesions by polarized light will reveal brightly shining particles toward the periphery of the nodule (silicates) and dull particles at the center (silica).

Mixed Dust Fibrosis

This term has been given to conditions which are characterized by the presence of mixed dust fibrotic nodules and are caused by concomitant exposure to silica and less fibrogenic dusts such as iron, silicates, and carbon. The silica is usually at a lower percentage of the total lung dust than when silicotic nodules occur. In fact, these lesions are frequently seen in association with silicotic lesions. Generally, as the proportion of silica increases, the number of silicotic nodules increase in proportion to the mixed dust nodules. Microscopically the mixed dust fibrotic nodule is characterized by a stellate shape and has a central hyalinized collagenous zone surrounded by linearly and radially arranged collagen fibers admixed with dust-containing macrophages (see Fig. 8–5).

Silicatoses

The typical lesion, observed in subjects exposed to silicates in the absence of or with very low exposures to silica, is an interstitial collection of dust-containing macrophages accompanied by variable amounts of fibrosis (see Fig. 8–6). Often this interstitial fibrosis is mild, but on occasion when there is a heavy dust load within the lung, severe fibrosis with honeycombing can develop. A large number of minerals can be associated with this type of reaction, including kaolin, talc, mica, fuller's earth, bentonite, and feldspar.[2, 57–59]

Other microscopic features that are inconsistently present include ferruginous bodies (which can be mistaken for asbestos) and foreign body giant cells. The precise identification of the minerals present in individual cases cannot generally be determined by morphological techniques and requires sophisticated mineralogical analysis. This is particularly true in secondary industries where the occupational exposures may not be well defined.[60]

Coal Dust Exposure

There are several factors which may influence the number and type of pneumoconiotic lesions in coal workers (Table 8–4). Radiographic studies have shown that cumulative exposure to coal dust is related to the risk and progression of coal workers' pneumoconiosis,[6, 61, 62] but this does not explain all the regional differences in prevalence of pneumoconiosis. Some mines with similar exposures to respirable mine dust produce different rates of pneumoconiosis.[6, 63] This is not surprising, since coals are very complex mineralogically and differ from one mine to another. Coal is customarily classified into ranks according to calorific value. Generally high-rank coals have a greater proportion of carbon and a lower proportion of ash compared to low-rank coals. The ash contains various silicates, such as kaolin and mica, and silica in the form of quartz. It has been found that generally levels of pneumoconiosis are lower in collieries mining low-rank coals than in those mining high-rank coals[6, 61, 64] and that workers exposed to high-rank coals accumulate dust faster than those mining low-rank coals.[65] *In vitro* studies have shown that for a given quartz content the toxicity increases with rank.[66]

Table 8–4
■
Factors Which May Affect the Pulmonary Response to Coal Dust Exposure

1. Cumulative exposure
2. Coal rank
3. Quartz content and surface properties
4. Noncoal content—clays, etc.
5. Individual susceptibility
6. Infection

Attention has also focused on the role of quartz, although there is no consistent direct relationship between the percentage of quartz in the dust and severity and type of pneumoconiosis. In certain coal mines, but not all, where the workers have been exposed to dusts with high quartz contents, there has been a high rate of progressive massive fibrosis (PMF) and an unusually rapid development of pneumoconiosis.[6, 67] Experimental studies have shown increasing pathological effects with increasing quartz contents,[68] but the presence of other minerals such as coal and clay minerals can ameliorate these effects.[5] Among the clay minerals, it has been suggested that illite may have this ameliorating effect. However, there are inconsistencies in the data. Davis et al.[69] conducted an interesting inhalation study on rats which compared the ability of two coal mine dusts to produce pneumoconiotic lesions. One of the dusts was from a Nottinghamshire mine with low levels of pneumoconiosis in the work force but which contained almost 16% quartz and 32% illite. The other dust was from a Scottish mine which was associated with a rapidly progressive pneumoconiosis in the work force and which had a similar quartz content (18.4%) and 17% illite. After 12 and 18 months, there was a higher dust mass in the rats exposed to the Nottinghamshire dust, but although the levels of pathological changes were similar, there was a marked qualitative difference. Fibrotic nodules were present only in the rats exposed to the Scottish dust. Therefore, different coal mine dusts with similar quartz contents caused different biological responses, and this was not reduced by the presence of illite. The reason put forward for this was that the Scottish dust contained quartz which had a greater free surface area than that from Nottinghamshire. Tourman and Kaufmann[70] have demonstrated by single particle analysis of coal mine dusts that toxicity correlates better with the number of ''pure'' quartz particles present than with the gross quartz content (which includes aluminum-contaminated quartz particles). Thus, it is still not completely understood how the various mineralogical components of the coal influence the type and severity of pathology.

Individual susceptibility may also play a part, and this is best examplified by the development of rheumatoid pneumoconiotic lesions (Caplan's syndrome) where dust exposure is often not severe. However, investigative studies for various immunological indices of disease in coal workers have not been helpful.[71] There is a strong association between body build and the development of PMF, it being more frequent in asthenic men.[72]

Mycobacterium tuberculosis has also been implicated in the development of PMF, and several studies in the 1950s reported the finding of these organisms on direct microscopic examination or bacteriological culture of PMF lesions.[73, 74] Experimental studies have demonstrated that the tubercle bacilli result in dust fibrosis indistinguishable from PMF.[75] Nowadays this does not appear to be a significant factor in the pathogenesis of PMF in coal workers from the developed countries. The pathology of coal workers' pneumoconiosis can be conveniently discussed under five headings:

1. Simple pneumoconiosis
2. Complicated pneumoconiosis (PMF)
3. Rheumatoid pneumoconiosis
4. Emphysema
5. Interstitial fibrosis

Simple Pneumoconiosis

The essential lesion of coal workers' pneumoconiosis is the collection of closely packed dust-laden macrophages around the respiratory bronchiole which contains little collagen and is visible macroscopically as a black, stellate, impalpable macule (primary dust focus). These usually measure up to 5 mm in diameter and are profuse but most prevalent in the upper zones of the lungs (Fig. 8–7). They are usually associated with dilatation of respiratory bronchioles—so-called focal

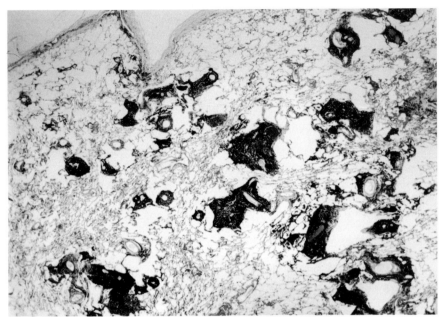

Figure 8–7. Simple coal workers' pneumoconiosis showing the typical black stellate foci with little fibrosis (macules). There is emphysema located at the centers of the acini (lobules). (H&E)

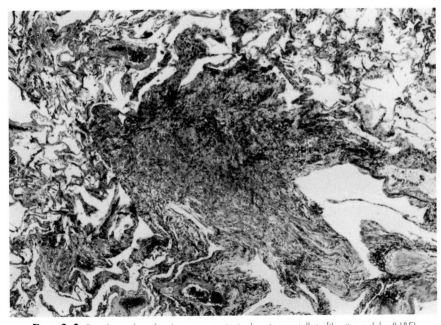

Figure 8–8. Simple coal workers' pneumoconiosis showing a stellate fibrotic nodule. (H&E)

emphysema. Another type of lesion that may be present, but less frequently than the primary dust focus, is the fibrotic nodule (secondary dust focus, micro- and macronodule). These may be rounded or stellate, black and palpable, and scattered more haphazardly than the primary dust foci (Fig. 8–8). Microscopically they contain more collagen, but in some cases they take on a circumferential arrangement similar to silicotic nodules. The lesions are usually evenly pigmented in miners from high-rank collieries, whereas the centers of the lesions from miners of low-rank collieries may lack the central black pigmentation.[76]

Complicated Pneumoconiosis (Progressive Massive Fibrosis)

The transition from simple to complicated pneumoconiosis is arbitrarily determined by the size of the dust foci present. The majority of authorities require a lesion of greater than 1 cm in diameter to be present, although some have set the size at 2 cm.[77] PMF lesions usually occur on a high background of primary dust lesions; if these are not profuse, the lesion should be suspected as an area of pigmented scarring unrelated to coal dust exposure. The PMF lesions tend to occur in the upper zones, can be very large and cavitated, and occupy the majority of a lobe and even cross the fissure into the adjacent lobe (Fig. 8–9). They are usually diffusely black and soft and cut easily with a knife; but if the coal worker has been exposed to low-rank coals, the PMF lesions may appear to have formed by the joining together of individual nodules which are more collagenous.[77] In general, disability occurs only with the complicated type, and then usually with the large lesions. However, it should be kept in mind that the disability attributable to the coal dust lesions appears equal to the severity of emphysema present,[78] although most of the emphysema present in this series was probably due to smoking.

An interesting observation that has been made is that in cases of PMF the central lymph nodes are often heavily dusted and breach their capsules so that their contents extend into the adjacent pulmonary vessels and airways which serve the area where the PMF lesion is located.[79] It has been suggested that this may result in dust-laden activated cells being moved back into the lungs, which might play a part in the development of the PMF by immunological mechanisms.

Rheumatoid Pneumoconiosis

Coal workers with rheumatoid disease may develop nodules rapidly even after relatively low exposures to dust—a condition commonly referred to as Caplan's syndrome.[80] The lesions are typically subpleural, whorled, and large, with a background frequently of relatively sparse dust foci (Figs. 8–10 and 8–11). Microscopically, the lesions show central necrosis with inflammatory debris, circularly arranged bands of coal dust, and a periphery of palisaded fibroblasts and macrophages and collagen. Old lesions can calcify and lose their inflammatory cell activity and mimic silicotic and healed tuberculous lesions.[81]

Emphysema

Focal emphysema is characterized by dilatation of the respiratory bronchioles whose walls are daubed on their internal surfaces by dust, reticulin, and disintegrating cells. This is mild and associated with little destruction, although more modern quantitative techniques would no doubt show loss of the alveolar wall surface area. It is not associated with significant loss of lung function.

Centrilobular emphysema is associated with much more destruction and loss of alveolar wall surface area. This is also observed at the centers of the lobules and therefore acini and is anatomically related to the coal foci. In coal workers, a wide range of combinations may be observed. The dust focus may be insignificant, moderate, or large in size, occupying much of the lobule; and similarly the anatom-

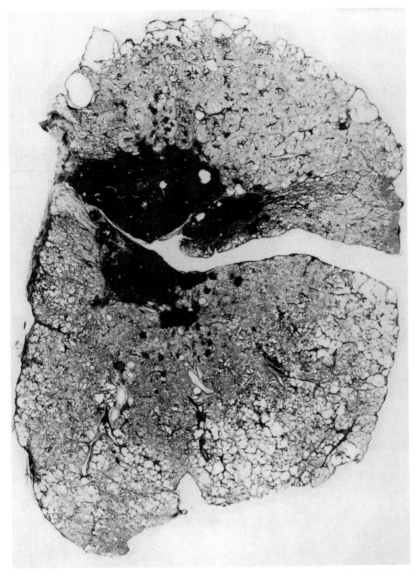

Figure 8–9. Complicated coal workers' pneumoconiosis. The PMF lesion is diffusely black. (Whole lung section)

ically related emphysema may be minimal, moderate, or severe in extent and occupying almost all of the lobule (Figs. 8–12 to 8–18).

There is general agreement that the profusion and size of the dust foci are related to cumulative exposure but have little influence on lung function in the absence of PMF. However, the extent of any concomitant emphysema will influence lung function. There is no disagreement that cigarette smoking is an important factor in its development, but there is argument about whether the coal dust exposure is related. There are now several studies[82, 83] which indicate that coal dust exposure does influence the development of emphysema:

1. There is an increased prevalence of emphysema, including the centrilobular type, among coal workers.
2. Centrilobular emphysema can occur in coal workers who have been lifelong nonsmokers.
3. The severity of emphysema increases with the size and profusion of simple dust lesions, which in turn increase with cumulative respirable dust exposure.

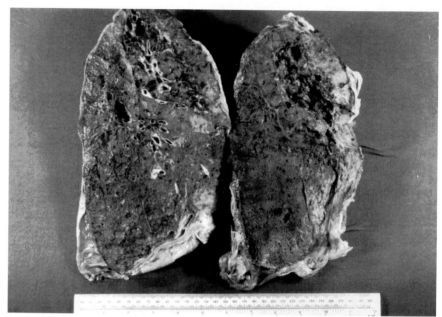

Figure 8–10. Caplan's syndrome. Numerous irregularly distributed whorled nodules, some of which have cavitated. Coal dust macules are sparse.

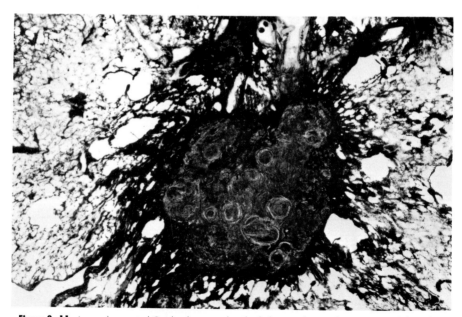

Figure 8–11. A conglomerated Caplan lesion with only slight irregular emphysema around the edge.

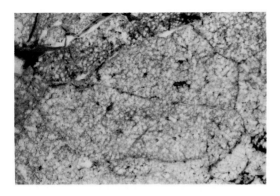

Figure 8–12
Lobules of a normal urban dweller.

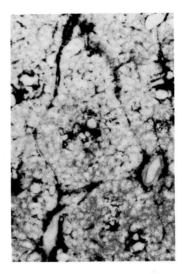

Figure 8–13
A small dust focus with minimal related emphysema barely surpassing that found in a town dweller's lung.

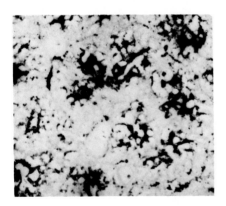

Figure 8–14
Several lobules with moderate central coal dust focus and minimal related emphysema.

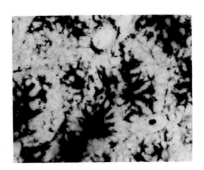

Figure 8–15
Coal dust foci occupying much of the lobule, but without significant related emphysema.

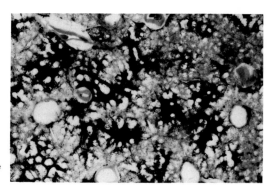

Figure 8–16
Minimal emphysema around a moderate central coal dust focus.

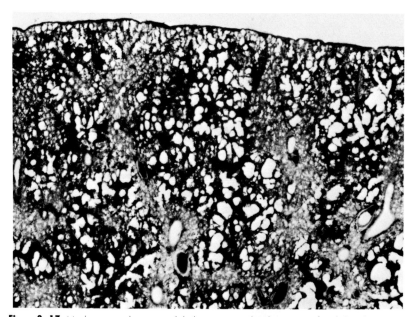

Figure 8–17. Moderate emphysema in lobules associated with extensive focal dust deposition.

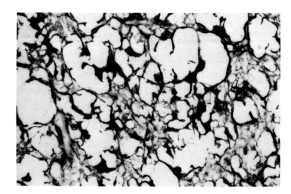

Figure 8–18
Extensive centrilobular emphysema around coal dust foci.

Interstitial Fibrosis

Interstitial fibrosis was found in the lungs at autopsy of approximately 16% of Welsh and West Virginian coal workers.[84] It appears to run a longer clinical course than nonoccupational idiopathic interstitial disease. The reasons for its development in coal workers are not known.

Diseases Associated with Fiber Exposures

There is considerable confusion and controversy concerning the definition of a fiber because there is a different usage of the term between mineralogists and medical practitioners. This has resulted in much argument in the regulatory field, particularly concerning asbestos fibers and their nonasbestosiform counterparts and their potential for causing fibrosis and neoplasia within the lung and pleura. A simple definition of a fiber is an elongated particle which has a length-to-breadth (aspect) ratio equal to or greater than 3:1. Although this definition is simple and easy to apply, it cannot be assumed that anything three times as long as it is wide is biologically harmful. The experimental and human evidence indicates that pleuropulmonary disease is linked with fibers of greater aspect ratio, greater than 8 μm in length and less than 0.25 μm for mesothelioma and greater than 25 μm in length for parenchymal disease.[85] Asbestos fibers are naturally occurring fibers with high tensile strength and flexibility, whereas cleavage fragments are formed by breakage of crystals along planes of fracture following crushing or milling processes. Cleavage fragments may resemble asbestos fibers but are generally of much lower aspect ratio and do not possess the same surface properties and in particular are usually less durable.[86] There is argument as to whether they can cause similar biological effects as natural fibers. Table 8–5 gives a classification of mineral fibers. The asbestos group of minerals is the best studied, and it is this group that is discussed here; it should be realized that other fibers with similar physical and chemical properties might produce similar biological effects. There is particular concern about refractory ceramic fibers which by *in vitro* testing are durable and after inhalation have resulted in lung fibrosis and tumors and mesotheliomas.

Asbestos

Asbestos refers to naturally occurring mineral fibers which have high tensile strength, heat resistance, and durability. There are six major types (see Table 8–5), which occur in two main groups—chrysotile, which has a wavy, coiled configuration, is the only member of the serpentine group; the others are all amphiboles, and

Table 8–5
■
Classification of Mineral Fibers

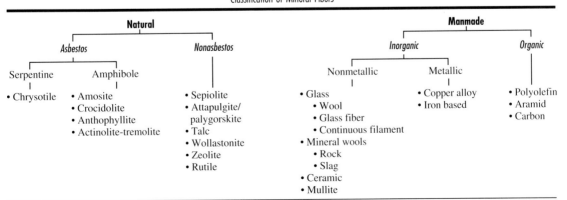

these are long, straight, and rigid. Exposure to asbestos can be associated with the following pulmonary and pleural diseases:

Pulmonary	**Pleural**
Fibrosis (asbestosis)	Effusion
Carcinoma	Plaques
Rounded atelectasis	
	Diffuse fibrosis
	Mesothelioma

ASBESTOSIS

Simply defined, asbestosis is parenchymal (not pleural) fibrosis caused by asbestos exposure. Originally it applied to workers with heavy industrial exposures in whom there was respiratory impairment, irregular opacities on standard chest radiographs, basal crackles on auscultation, and on lung function a restrictive pattern and diffusion defect. It sometimes caused the death of the patient. In these cases, the pathology is that of interstitial fibrosis with fine honeycombing macroscopically, grade 4 microscopic lesions, and numerous clusters of asbestos bodies. Electron microscopic counts of the lung tissues revealed extremely high numbers of asbestos fibers.

Both experimental and human studies demonstrate that the initial lesions of asbestosis commence within the respiratory bronchioles and then spread outward into the adjacent alveoli, eventually to involve all acinar structures. With progression, individual lesions coalesce to form diffuse interstitial fibrosis. Ultimately, dense areas of fibrosis may form, with disorganization of the lung architecture and honeycombing. The established microscopic grading system of asbestosis is based on the severity of fibrosis and not the number of asbestos bodies. It is as follows:[10, 11]

Grade 0—None.
Grade 1—Slight focal fibrosis around respiratory bronchioles.
Grade 2—Lesions confined to respiratory bronchioles of scattered acini, but fibrosis extends into alveolar ducts, atria, and the walls of adjacent airspaces.
Grade 3—Further increase and condensation of the peribronchiolar fibrosis, with early widespread interstitial lesions.
Grade 4—Widespread diffuse fibrosis with few recognizable alveoli, with or without honeycombing.

This understanding of the development of asbestosis has led to the diagnosis of asbestosis being applied to individuals who have no respiratory disability, little or no radiological changes, no macroscopic fibrosis, grade 1 or 2 microscopic lesions, and asbestos bodies found only after prolonged search. Some of these diagnoses are inaccurate, because similar fibrotic lesions can be found in individuals without asbestos exposure and are more common in smokers. This is probably not of clinical importance when there is no lung cancer present, but is of relevance when it comes to linking asbestos exposure to the development of lung cancer. For example, in shipyard workers, there may be grade 1 and 2 fibrotic lesions present which cannot be separated from those observed in the background population unless fiber counts are performed. Even then the evidence suggests that the risk of lung cancer is increased only in those with moderate to severe asbestosis and not in those with minimal or slight asbestosis. Therefore, whenever the term *asbestosis* is used, it should be qualified by the degree. Table 8–6 gives a suggested schema. Ideally when examining tissue for asbestosis or fibrosis due to any other dust, the assessment should be made on the lung which does not contain tumor, since the tumor itself may cause local fibrosis. In surgical specimens this is not possible, but the grading of fibrosis should be made as far away from the tumor as possible.

In general, in cases of asbestosis, the number of asbestos bodies increases with the severity of fibrosis. However, there are certain difficulties which may lead to

Table 8-6

■

Guidelines for the Diagnosis and Grading of Asbestosis

Asbestosis Grade	Clinical and Plain Chest Radiography	Macroscopic Appearance	LM Appearance	Usual LM Count of Fibers*	Usual EM Amphibole Count × 10⁶*
Minimal	None	No fibrosis visible	Grade 1 and 2 lesions. Prolonged search reveals occasional asbestos bodies on average 1 or less per section.	>50,000	>50
Slight	None or mild clinical symptoms, and none or slight radiological changes.	Careful inspection of inflated lung reveals fine interstitial fibrosis occupying less than 25% of the total area. It sometimes appears normal.	Grade 1 to 3 lesions. Asbestos bodies on average 1 to 3 per section.	>100,000	>150
Moderate	None or mild clinical symptoms, and slight radiological changes.	A combination of induration with fine to moderate fibrosis involving 25% to 50% of the total lung area.	Grade 2 to 4 lesions. Asbestos bodies easily found with occasional clumps.	>250,000	>500
Severe	Severely dyspneic. Overt interstitial fibrosis radiologically.	Interstitial fibrosis involving more than 50% of the lung with or without honeycombing.	Grade 3 to 4 lesions. Numerous bodies often in clumps.	>1,000,000	>1,000

LM, light microscopy; EM, transmission electron microscopy.
* Per gram of dried lung tissue.

inaccurate diagnosis. Asbestos bodies are beaded, golden brown, often dumbbell-shaped structures with a straight, thin, transparent core (Fig. 8–19). The golden-brown coat contains glycoprotein and hemosiderin so that a Prussian blue stain, which stains the iron blue, may be helpful in searching for them in tissue sections. These structures may be simulated by other minerals, and then should be called ferruginous rather than asbestos bodies. Examples include erionite, talc, mica, kaolin, carbon, rutile, iron, mullite, and aluminum whiskers.[87] Many of these have cores which differ from those of asbestos—they may be black or yellow or appear round, platy, or irregular. In mixed exposures, such as experienced by arc welders, it may be very difficult to evaluate by light microscopy alone how much asbestos is likely to be present. Electron microscopic mineral fiber analysis is an important and extremely useful tool in these types of cases. I have seen a case where there were ferruginous bodies in the lung tissue which were identical to asbestos bodies by light microscopy but which on mineral analysis were shown to be manmade vitreous fibers—probably glass (Fig. 8–20).

Also, there is a different propensity for developing ferruginous bodies by the different fiber types; they tend to form on longer fibers and amphiboles more easily. Therefore the ratio of asbestos fibers to bodies can be variable. A study by Pooley and Ranson[88] comparing light microscopic to electron microscopic fiber counts of lung tissue digests found that 0.14% of chrysotile, 5% of crocidolite, and 26.5% of amosite fibers formed bodies. They also found that the ratio of ferruginous bodies

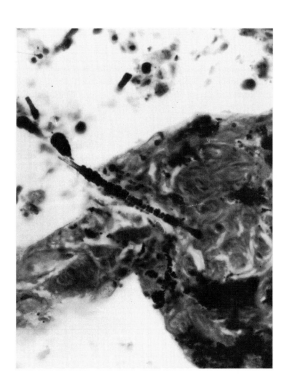

Figure 8–19
A typical beaded asbestos body
with a transparent fibrous core.
(H&E)

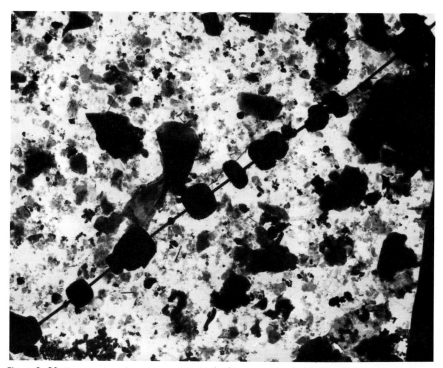

Figure 8–20. Transmission electron micrograph of a ferruginous body which on light microscopy simulated an asbestos body. Energy dispersive x-ray spectrometry showed silica only—probably glass.

to fibers in light microscopic counts was disproportionately high when the fiber counts were low. Therefore, if one finds only an occasional asbestos-type ferruginous body per 5 micron standard histological section, it should be realized that first it is nearly always an amphibole, and that if it is amosite, then the number of fibers actually present will be considerably lower than if it is crocidolite. A study of controls from five British cities of varying industrialization using transmission electron microscopy and energy dispersive x-ray analysis gave the following arithmetic means and ranges (in millions of fibers per gram of dried lung tissue):[89–91]

chrysotile = 7.4 (0–73.9)
amosite = 0.9 (0–137.7)
crocidolitc = 0.5 (0–16.9)
tremolite = 0.1 (0–3.6).

A study of North American controls from the same laboratory found similar results, except that the tremolite value was higher:[92]

chrysotile = 47.5 (0–>1000)
amosite = 1.1 (0–>10)
crocidolite = 0.4 (0–>1)
tremolite = 1.8 (0–>10)

Studies of mineral fiber burdens in lung tissues of workers exposed to asbestos have shown good correlations between the severity of fibrosis and levels of amphiboles, but not with chrysotile.[89, 90, 93]

LUNG CANCER

There is no argument that heavy cumulative exposures to asbestos which lead to asbestosis increase the risk of developing lung cancer. This risk is increased between additive and multiplicative for the two risk factors of smoking and asbestos exposure. What is at issue is whether the risk of lung cancer is increased when asbestosis is not present. I believe that there is now considerable evidence which indicates that the risk of lung cancer only increases when asbestosis is present:

1. In those industries with high rates of lung cancer there is a high prevalence of asbestosis. One such group is the cohort of North American insulators studied by Kipen et al.,[94] who found microscopic evidence of fibrosis in all the cases of lung cancer, although their definition of fibrosis is not that which is commonly accepted. They included pleural fibrosis.
2. In industries where there is a low prevalence of asbestosis, there is no detectable increase in risk of lung cancer. For example, the friction products workers studied by Newhouse and Sullivan showed no excess rates of respiratory disease or lung cancer.[95]
3. In a necropsy study of South African amphibole asbestos miners (crocidolite and amosite), there was no increase of lung cancers in those without asbestosis; but in the group with asbestosis, the rates progressively increased with the severity.[96]
4. A prospective mortality study of men employed in the manufacture of asbestos cement products showed that 20 or more years after hire an excess lung cancer risk occurred only in the group with radiological opacities and not in the group without.[97] This is an important study since it controlled for age, smoking, and exposure to asbestos.
5. There is considerable evidence to indicate that amphiboles are more potent than chrysotile in causing asbestosis and lung cancer.

A hypothesis has been put forward which provides a logical basis for this. It suggests that "asbestosis, lung cancer and mesothelioma result from the single pathological effect of long fibres, which cause release of macrophage mediators after incomplete digestion.[98] The malignant changes do not result from direct genotoxic action.'' It therefore indicates a threshold effect with asbestosis and asbestos-related lung cancer running in parallel as consequences of production of excess growth factors.

A review of the literature by Churg[99] of histological types of lung cancer and asbestos exposure indicated that all the major histological types can occur. One of the problems with this type of analysis and the series in the literature is that those that are genuinely asbestos induced have not been separated from those that are not. Studies are needed that carefully evaluate the location and histological types of the lung tumors in those with and without asbestosis.

ROUNDED ATELECTASIS

These are asymptomatic and usually found radiographically as a sharply defined mass. The pathology is that of an area of pleural fibrosis with infolding of the adjacent lung.

EFFUSION

Exposure to asbestos can cause pleurisy and effusion many years following exposure, but usually within 10 years. The pleura may show florid mesothelial hyperplasia. Many are asymptomatic and often resolve spontaneously. The recurrent ones may lead to diffuse fibrosis.

PLEURAL PLAQUES

These are pearly white, shiny, knobby lesions which are often calcified and situated on the parietal pleura, most commonly in the posterolateral, basal, and diaphragmatic zones. Microscopically they show a basket weave pattern of collagen fibers, beneath which there are focal collections of lymphocytes and plasma cells. They are not uncommon at autopsy and usually not associated with symptoms during life. In my own autopsy practice, I encounter them in approximately 8% postmortem examinations of males. Many but not all are associated with exposure to asbestos. They have occurred in subjects with no history of asbestos exposure and no increase of mineral fibers in their lung tissues.[100] Other suggested causes include exposures to talc, mica, wollastonite, and erionite and inflammation and injury to the pleura.[101–103] In those associated with asbestos exposure, the frequency increases with longer exposure and time since first exposure, but I and others have found no relationship between the presence and degree of asbestosis and the extent and prevalence of pleural plaques.[104] Therefore the presence of pleural plaques is not a predictor of asbestosis. Pleural plaques may also result from environmental exposure to asbestos fibers, particularly tremolite and anthophyllite, located in the soil or through whitewashing of houses. Countries where this has been reported include Austria, Bulgaria, Czechoslovakia, Turkey, Russia and parts of the former U.S.S.R., Corsica, Italy, Greece, and Finland.[105, 106] In some areas such as Finland, Austria, and Bulgaria, there does not appear to be an excess risk of mesothelioma. Also a nested case-control study of a cohort of asbestos-exposed workers found no association between pleural plaques and asbestos-associated malignancies that were independent of other causative factors such as duration of asbestos exposure, age, and cigarette smoking.[107] Therefore, plaques in themselves do not indicate an increased risk of lung cancer development.

DIFFUSE PLEURAL FIBROSIS

Diffuse thickening of the visceral pleura may occur in asbestos-exposed persons without significant parenchymal fibrosis and, if extensive and bilateral, may cause disability and a restrictive defect of lung function. Thickening and adhesions of the parietal pleura may also be present. There is often a history of previous pleurisy and effusion. It usually takes more than 10 years to develop. Microscopically the appearances are similar to a plaque.[108] These appearances are not specific

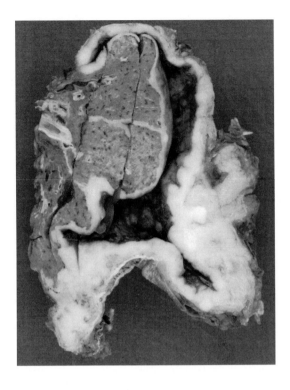

Figure 8–21
Typical macroscopic appearance of a mesothelioma which encompasses the lung and extends along fissures.

and may be caused by previous infections such as tuberculosis and collagen diseases, and there is an idiopathic form. Electron microscopic fiber analysis of the lung tissues usually shows raised levels of amphiboles asbestos, but below the range associated with significant asbestosis.[89, 108]

MALIGNANT MESOTHELIOMA

In North America and the United Kingdom, about 80% to 90% of mesotheliomas can be related to previous asbestos exposure. The latent period from first exposure to death from the tumor averages between 30 and 40 years and is rarely less than 20 years. There is evidence that the risk increases with cumulative exposure, and there is a clear-cut gradient of risk for the different fiber types.[109] Mesothelioma can develop in the absence of asbestosis and at levels of exposure far below those required for the development of asbestosis.

The typical appearance of mesothelioma macroscopically is of a gray, diffuse, often knobby tumor which affects the pleura and encompasses a rather shrunken atelectatic lung (Fig. 8–21). Microscopically the tumor can show many epithelial and connective tissue–like patterns in various combinations.[110, 111]

It should be remembered that other tumors can metastasize to and spread through the pleura to give an appearance exactly like mesothelioma. Also the microscopic patterns of mesothelioma overlap with those of many other tumors. Therefore great care should be exercised and all the clinical and radiological information should be assembled before making a diagnosis of mesothelioma, particularly on biopsy material. Some textbooks state that a history of asbestos exposure is useful in making a diagnosis; this is a misleading statement, and the diagnosis should be made on the pathological appearances of the tumor in combination with the knowledge that there is no other likely site of a primary tumor.

REFERENCES

1. Davis, G. S., The pathogenesis of silicosis. Chest, 89, 166, 1986.
2. Craighead, J. E., and Kleinerman, J., Abraham, J. L., et al., Diseases associated with exposure to silica and nonfibrous silicate minerals. Arch. Pathol. Lab. Med., 112, 673, 1988.

3. Davis, J. M. G., A review of experimental evidence for the carcinogenicity of man-made vitreous fibres. Scand. J. Work Environ. Health, 12(suppl. 1), 12, 1986.

4. Wagner, J. C., Skidmore, J. W., Hill, R. J., and Griffiths, D. M., Erionite exposure and mesothelioma in rats. Br. J. Cancer, 51, 727, 1985.

5. LeBouffant, L., Addison, J., Bolton, R. E., Compared in vitro and in vivo toxicity of coalmine dusts. Relationship with mineralogical composition. Ann. Occup. Hyg., 32, 611, 1988.

6. Hurley, J. F., Copland, L., Dodgson, J., and Jacobsen, M., Simple pneumoconiosis and exposure to dust at 10 British coal mines. Br. J. Ind. Med., 39, 120, 1982.

7. Churg, A., and Wiggs, B., Types, numbers, sizes and distribution of mineral particles in the lungs of urban male cigarette smokers. Environ. Res., 42:121, 1987.

8. McFadden D., Wright, J. L., Wiggs, B., and Churg, A., Smoking inhibits asbestos clearance. Am. Rev. Respir. Dis., 133, 372, 1986.

9. Gibbs, A. R., and Seal, R. M. E., Examination of lung specimens. J. Clin. Pathol., 43, 68, 1990.

10. Hinson, K. F. W., Otto, H., Webster, I., and Rossiter, C. E., Criteria for the diagnosis of and grading of asbestosis. IARC Sci. Publ., 8, 54, 1973.

11. Craighead, J. E., Abraham, J. L., Churg, A., et al., The pathology of asbestos associated diseases of the lungs and pleural cavities: diagnostic criteria and proposed grading scheme. Arch. Pathol. Lab. Med., 106, 542, 1982.

12. Pooley, F. D., and Clark, N. J., Quantitative assessment of inorganic fibrous particulates in dust samples with an analytical electron microscope. Ann. Occup. Hyg., 22, 253, 1979.

13. Gylseth B., Churg, A., Davis, J. M. G., et al., Analysis of asbestos fibres and asbestos bodies in tissue samples from human lung. Scand. J. Work. Environ. Health, 11, 107, 1985.

14. Pooley, F. D., Tissue mineral identification. In Weill, H., and Turner-Warwick, M., eds., Occupational Lung Diseases. Research Approaches and Methods. New York, Marcel Dekker, 1981, pp. 189–235.

15. Wagner, J. C., Berry, G., and Pooley, F. D., Mesotheliomas and asbestos type in asbestos textile workers. B. Med. J., 285, 603, 1982.

16. Katzenstein, A., Bloor, C., and Liebow, A., Diffuse alveolar damage. The role of oxygen, shock and related factors. Am. J. Pathol., 85, 210, 1976.

17. Liebow, A. A., Steer, A., and Billingsley, J. E., Desquamative interstitial pneumonia. Am. J. Med., 39, 369, 1965.

18. Abraham, J. L., and Hertzberg, M. A., Inorganic particles associated with desquamative interstitial pneumonia. Chest, 80, 67S, 1981.

19. Corrin, B., Price, A. B., Electron microscopic studies in desquamative interstitial pneumonia associated with asbestos. Thorax, 27, 324, 1972.

20. Herbert, A., Sterling, E., Abraham, J. L., and Corrin, B., Desquamative interstitial pneumonia in an aluminum welder. Hum. Pathol., 13, 694, 1982.

21. Abraham, J. L., and Spragg, R. G., Documentation of environmental exposure using open biopsy, transbronchial biopsy and bronchopulmonary lavage in giant cell interstitial pneumonia (GIP). Am. Rev. Respir. Dis., 119(suppl.), 196, 1979.

22. Davison, A. G., Haslam, P. L., Corrin, B., et al., Interstitial lung disease and asthma in hard metal workers: bronchoalveolar lavage, ultrastructural and analytical findings and results of bronchial provocation tests. Thorax, 38, 119, 1983.

23. Prakash, U. B., Barham, S. S., Carpenter, H. A., et al., Pulmonary alveolar proteinosis: experience with 34 cases and a review. Mayo. Clin. Proc., 62, 499, 1987.

24. Corrin, B., and King, E., Pathogenesis of experimental pulmonary alveolar proteinosis. Thorax, 25, 230, 1970.

25. McCuen, D. D., Abraham, J. L., Particulate concentrations in pulmonary alveolar proteinosis. Environ. Res., 17, 334, 1978.

26. Miller, R. R., Churg, A. M., Hutcheon, M., and Lam, S., Pulmonary alveolar proteinosis and aluminum dust exposure. Am. Rev. Respir. Dis., 130, 312, 1984.

27. Seal, R. M. E., Hapke, E. J., Thomas, G. O., et al., The pathology of the acute and chronic stages of farmer's lung. Thorax, 23, 469, 1968.

28. Seal, R. M. E., Pathology of extrinsic allergic bronchioloalveolitis. Prog. Respir. Res., 8, 66, 1975.

29. Wright, J. L., and Churg, A., Diseases caused by metals and related compounds, fumes and gases. In Churg, A., and Green, F. H. Y., eds., Pathology of Occupational Lung Disease. New York, Igaku Shoin, 1988, pp. 31–71.

30. Nemery, B., Metal toxicity and the respiratory tract. Eur. Respir. J., 3, 202, 1990.

31. Kniskhowy, B., and Baker, E. L., Transmission of occupational disease to family contacts. Am. J. Ind. Med., 9, 543, 1986.

32. Jederlinic, P. J., Abraham, J. L., Churg, A., et al., Pulmonary fibrosis in aluminum oxide workers. Am. Rev. Respir. Dis., 142, 1179, 1990.

33. Gilks, B., Churg, A., Aluminum induced pulmonary fibrosis: do fibers play a role? Am. Rev. Respir. Dis., 136, 176, 1987.

34. Miller, R. R., Churg, A., Hutcheon, M., et al., Pulmonary alveolar proteinosis and aluminum dust exposure. Am. Rev. Respir. Dis., 130, 312, 1984.

35. DeVuyst, P., Dumortier, P., Schandene, L., et al., Sarcoidlike lung granulomatosis induced by aluminum dusts. Am. Rev. Respir. Dis., 135, 493, 1987.

36. Jones Williams, W., Beryllium disease. In Parkes, W. R., ed., Occupational Lung Disease, 3rd ed. Oxford, Butterworth and Heineman, 1994.

37. Saltini, C., Winestock, K., Kirby, M., et al., Maintenance of alveolitis in patients with chronic beryllium disease by beryllium specific helper T cells. N. Engl. J. Med., 320, 1103, 1989.
38. Jones Williams, W., and Williams, W. R., Value of beryllium lymphocyte transformation tests in chronic beryllium disease and potentially exposed workers. Thorax, 38, 41, 1983.
39. Newman, L. S., Kreiss, K., King, T. E., et al., Pathologic and immunologic alterations in early stages of beryllium disease. Am. Rev. Respir. Dis., 139, 1479, 1989.
40. Williams, W. J., and Wallach, E. R., Laser microprobe mass spectometry (LAMMS) analysis of beryllium, sarcoidosis and other granulomatous diseases. Sarcoidosis, 6, 111, 1989.
41. Davison, A. G., Newman-Taylor, A. J., Darbyshire, J., et al., Cadmium fume inhalation and emphysema. Lancet, 1, 663, 1988.
42. Langard, S., One hundred years of chromium and cancer. Am. J. Ind. Med., 17, 189, 1990.
43. Davies, J. M., Easton, D. F., and Bidstrup, P. L., Mortality from respiratory cancer and other causes in United Kingdom chromate production workers. Br. J. Ind. Med., 48, 299, 1991.
44. Sorahan, T., Burge, D. C., and Waterhouse, J. A., A mortality study of nickel/chromium platers. Br. J. Ind. Med., 44, 250, 1987.
45. Kollmeier, H., Seemann, J. W., Rothe, G., et al., Age, sex, and region adjusted concentrations of chromium and nickel in lung tissue. Br. J. Ind. Med., 47, 682, 1990.
46. Report of the International Committee on Nickel Carcinogenesis in Man. Scand. J. Work Environ. Health, 16, 1–82, 1990.
47. Andersen, I., Svenes, K. B., Determination of nickel in lung specimens of thirty-nine autopsied nickel workers. Int. Arch. Occup. Environ. Health, 61, 289, 1989.
48. King, E. J., Mohanty, G. P., Harrison, C. V., and Nagleschmidt, G., The action of different forms of pure silica on the lungs of rats. Br. J. Ind. Med., 10, 9, 1953.
49. Brieger, H., and Gross, P., On the theory of silicosis. III. Stishovite. Arch. Environ. Health, 15, 751, 1967.
50. Heppleston, A. G., Minerals, fibrosis, and the lung. Environ. Health Perspect., 94, 149, 1991.
51. Kysela, R., Jirakova, D., Holusa, R., and Skoda, V., The influence of the size of quartz dust particles on the reaction of lung tissue. Ann. Occup. Hyg., 16, 103, 1973.
52. Wiessner, J. H., Mandel, N. S., Sohnle, P. G., and Mandel, G. S., Effect of particle size on quartz induced haemolysis and on lung inflammation and fibrosis. Exp. Lung. Res., 15, 801, 1989.
53. Brody, A. R., Roe, M. W., Evans, J. N., and Davis, G. S., Deposition and translocation of inhaled silica in rats. Lab. Invest. 47, 533, 1982.
54. Harrington, J. S., and Allison, A. C., Lysosomal enzymes in relation to the toxicity of silica. Med. Lav., 56, 471, 1965.
55. Bègin, R., Cantin, A., and Masse, S., Recent advances in the pathogenesis and clinical assessment of mineral dust pneumoconioses: asbestosis, silicosis and coal pneumoconiosis. Eur. Respir. J., 2, 988, 1989.
56. Gibbs, A. R., and Wagner, J. C., Diseases due to silica. In Churg A., and Green, F. H. Y., eds., Pathology of Occupational Lung Disease. New York, Igaku Shoin, 1988, pp. 155–175.
57. Wagner, J. C., Pooley, F. D., Gibbs, A. R., et al., Inhalation of china stone and china clay dusts: relationship between the mineralogy of the dust retained in the lungs and pathological changes. Thorax, 41, 190, 1986.
58. Gibbs, A. R., Human pathology of kaolin and mica pneumoconioses. In Bignon, J., ed., Health Related Effects of Phyllosilicates. NATO ASI Series G21. 1990, pp. 217–226.
59. Craighead, J. E., Pathological features of pulmonary disease due to silicate dust inhalation. In Bignon, J., ed., Health Related Effects of Phyllosilicates. NATO ASI Series G21. Berlin, Springer Verlag, 1990, pp. 179–190.
60. Gibbs, A. R., Pooley, F. D., Griffiths, D. M., et al., "Talc pneumoconiosis"—A pathological and mineralogical study. Hum. Pathol, 23, 1344, 1992.
61. Jacobsen, M., Rae, S., Walton, W. H., and Rogan, J. M., The relation between pneumoconiosis and dust exposure in British coalmines. In Walton, W. H., ed., Inhaled Particles III. Old Woking, Surrey, Unwin Bros., 1971, pp. 903–917.
62. Reisner, M. T. R., Results of epidemiological studies of pneumoconiosis in West German coal-miners. In Walton, W. H., ed., Inhaled Particles III. Old Woking, Surrey, Unwin Bros., 1971, pp. 921–931.
63. Reisner, M. T. R., and Robock, K., Results of epidemiological, mineralogical and cytological studies on the pathogenicity of coalmine dusts. In Walton, W. H., ed., Inhaled Particles IV. Oxford, Pergamon Press, 1977, pp. 703–715.
64. Bennett, J. G., Dick, J. A., Kaplan, Y. S., et al., The relationship between coal rank and the prevalence of pneumoconiosis. Br. J. Ind. Med., 36, 206, 1979.
65. Bergman, I., and Casswell, C., Lung dust and iron content in different coalfields in Britain. Br. J. Ind. Med., 29, 160, 1972.
66. Gormley, I. P., Collings, P., Davis, J. M. G., and Ottery, J., An investigation into the cytotoxicity of respirable dusts from British collieries. Br. J. Exp. Pathol. 60, 526, 1979.
67. Jacobsen, M., and Maclaren, W. M., Unusual pulmonary observations and exposure to coal mine dust: a case control study. In Walton, W. H., ed., Inhaled Particles V. Oxford, Pergamon Press, 1982, pp. 735–765.
68. Le Bouffant, L., Daniel, H., and Martin, J. C., The therapeutic action of aluminum compounds on the development of experimental lesions produced by pure quartz or mixed dust. In Walton, W. H., ed., Inhaled Particles IV. Oxford, Pergamon Press, 1977, pp. 389–400.

69. Davis, J. M. G., Addison, J., Brown, G. M., et al., Further studies on the importance of quartz in the development of coalworkers' pneumoconiosis. (IOM Report TM/91/05). Edinburgh, Scotland, Institute of Occupational Medicine, 1991.

70. Tourmann, J. L., and Kaufmann, R., Laser microprobe mass spectrometric (LAMMS) study of quartz and nonquartz related modulating factors of the specific harmfulness of silica and coal mine dusts. Proceedings of the VII Inhaled Particles Meeting, Ann. Occup. Hyg. (in press).

71. Robertson, M. D., Boyd, J. E., Fernie, J. M., and Davis, J. M. G., Some immunological studies on coal workers with and without pneumoconiosis. Am. J. Ind. Med., 4, 467, 1983.

72. Maclaren, W. M., Hurley, J. F., Collins, H. P. R., and Cowie, A. J., Factors associated with the development of progressive massive fibrosis in British coalminers: a case control study. Br. J. Ind. Med., 46, 597, 1989.

73. James, W. R. L., The relationship of tuberculosis to the development of massive pneumoconiosis in coal workers. Br. J. Tuber., 48, 89, 1954.

74. Rivers, D., James, W. R. L., Davies, D. G., and Thomson, S., The prevalence of tuberculosis at necropsy in progressive massive fibrosis of coal workers. Br. J. Ind. Med., 14, 39, 1957.

75. Byers, P. D., and King, E. J., Experimental and infective pneumoconiosis with coal, kaolin and mycobacteria. Lab. Invest., 8, 647, 1959.

76. Davis, J. M. G., Chapman, J., Collings, P., et al., Variations in the histological patterns of the lesions of coal workers' pneumoconiosis in Britain and their relationship to lung dust content. Am. Rev. Respir. Dis., 128, 118, 1983.

77. Kleinerman, J., Green, F., Lacquer, W., et al., Pathology standards for coal workers' pneumoconiosis. Arch. Pathol. Lab. Med., 103, 373, 1979.

78. Ryder, R., Lyons, J. P., Campbell, H., and Gough, J., Emphysema in coal workers' pneumoconiosis. Br. Med. J., 3, 481, 1970.

79. Seal, R. M. E., Cockcroft, A., Kung, I., and Wagner, J. C., Central lymph node changes and progressive massive fibrosis in coalworkers. Thorax, 41, 531, 1986.

80. Caplan, A., Certain unusual radiological appearances in the chest of coal miners suffering from rheumatoid arthritis. Thorax, 8, 29, 1953.

81. Gough, J., Rivers, D., and Seal, R. M. E., Pathological studies of modified pneumoconiosis in coal miners with rheumatoid arthritis (Caplan's syndrome). Thorax, 10, 9, 1955.

82. Cockcroft, A., Seal, R. M. E., Wagner, J. C., et al., Postmortem study of emphysema in coal workers and noncoal workers. Lancet, 2, 600, 1982.

83. Ruckley, V. A., Gauld, S. A., Chapman, J. S., et al., Emphysema and dust exposure in a group of coal workers. Am. Rev. Respir. Dis., 129, 528, 1984.

84. McConnachie K., Green, F. H. Y., Vallyathan, V., et al., Interstitial fibrosis in coal miners—experience in Wales and West Virginia. Ann. Occup. Hyg. 32, 553, 1988.

85. Davies, J. M. G., Mineral fibre carcinogenesis: experimental data relating to the importance of fibre type, size, deposition, dissolution and migration. IARC Sci. Publ., 90, 33, 1989.

86. Wylie, A. G., Relationship between the growth habit of asbestos and the dimensions of asbestos fibres. Society of Mining Engineers Preprint 8885, 1, 1988.

87. Crouch, E., Churg, A., Ferruginous bodies and the histologic evaluation of dust exposure. Am. J. Surg. Pathol., 8, 109, 1984.

88. Pooley, F. D., and Ranson, D. L., Comparison of the results of asbestos fibre counts in lung tissue obtained by analytical electron microscopy and light microscopy. J. Clin. Pathol., 39, 313, 1986.

89. Gibbs, A. R., Stephens, M., Griffiths, D. M., et al., Fibre distribution in the lungs and pleura of subjects with asbestos related diffuse pleural fibrosis. Br. J. Ind. Med., 48, 762, 1991.

90. Wagner, J. C., Pooley, F. D., Berry, G., et al., A pathological and mineralogical study of asbestos-related deaths in the United Kingdom in 1977. Ann. Occup. Hyg., 26, 423, 1982.

91. Wagner, J. C., Newhouse, M. L., Corrin, B., et al., Correlation between lung fibre content and disease in East London asbestos factory workers. Br. J. Ind. Med., 45, 305, 1988.

92. Jones, J. S. P., Roberts, G. H., Pooley, F. D., et al., The pathology and mineral content of lungs in cases of mesothelioma in the United Kingdom in 1976. IARC Sci. Publ., 30, 187, 1980.

93. Gibbs, A. R., Gardner, M. J., Pooley, F. D., et al., Fibre levels and disease in workers from a factory predominantly using amosite. Environ. Health Perspect. (in press).

94. Kipen, H. M., Lilis, R., Suzuki, Y., et al., Pulmonary fibrosis in asbestos insulation workers with lung cancer: a radiological and histopathological evaluation. Br. J. Ind. Med., 44, 96, 1987.

95. Newhouse, M. L., and Sullivan, K. R., A mortality study of workers manufacturing friction materials: 1941–1986. Br. J. Ind. Med., 46, 176, 1989.

96. Sluis-Kremer, G. K., and Bezuidenhout, B. N., Relation between asbestosis and bronchial cancer in amphibole asbestos miners. Br. J. Ind. Med., 46, 537, 1989.

97. Hughes, J. M., and Weill, H., Asbestosis as precursor of asbestos related lung cancer: results of a prospective mortality study. Br. J. Ind. Med., 48, 229, 1991.

98. Browne, K., Asbestos related malignancy and the Cairns hypothesis. Br. J. Ind. Med., 48, 73, 1991.

99. Churg, A., Lung cancer cell type and asbestos exposure. J. A. M. A., 253, 2984, 1985.

100. Warnock, M. L., Orescott, B. T., and Kuwahara, T. J., Numbers and types of asbestos fibres in subjects with pleural plaques. Am. J. Pathol., 109, 37, 1982.

101. Gamble, J., Greife, A., and Hancock, J., An epidemiological-industrial hygiene study of talc workers. Ann. Occup. Hyg., 26, 841, 1982.

102. Huuskonen, M. S., Tossavainen, A., Kosinen, H., et al., Wollastonite exposure and lung fibrosis. Environ. Res., 30, 291, 1983.

103. British Thoracic and Tuberculosis Association and The Medical Research Council Pneumoconiosis Research Unit. A survey of pleural thickening: its relation to asbestos exposure and previous pleural disease. Environ. Res., 5, 142, 1972.

104. Ren, H., Lee, D. R., Hruban, R. H., et al., Pleural plaques do not predict asbestosis: high-resolution computed tomography and pathology study. Mod. Pathol., 4, 201, 1991.

105. Hillerdal, G., Endemic pleural plaques. Eur. J. Respir. Dis., 69, 1, 1986.

106. Boutin, G., Viallat, J. R., Steinbauer, J., et al., Bilateral pleural plaques in Corsica: a marker of non-occupational exposure. IARC Sci. Publi., 90, 406, 1990.

107. Harber, P., Mohsenifar, Z., Oren, A., and Lew, M., Pleural plaques and asbestos associated malignancy. J. Occup. Med., 29, 641, 1987.

108. Stephens, M., Gibbs, A. R., Pooley, F. D., and Wagner, J. C., Asbestos induced pleural fibrosis: pathology and mineralogy. Thorax, 42, 583, 1987.

109. Gibbs, A. R., Role of asbestos and other fibres in the development of diffuse malignant mesothelioma. Thorax, 45, 649, 1991.

110. Gibbs, A. R., and Whimster, W. F., Tumours of the lung and pleura. *In* Fletcher, C. D. M., ed., Histopathology of Tumours. Edinburgh, Churchill Livingstone (in press).

111. Churg, A., Neoplastic asbestos induced diseases. *In* Churg, A., Green, F. H. Y., eds., Pathology of Occupational Lung Disease. pp. 279–326. New York, Igaku-Shoin, 1988.

9

James H. Vincent

The Measurement of Workplace Aerosols

■

Much occupational lung disease is associated with worker exposure to aerosols in the forms of dusts, fumes, mists, and so forth. Measurement of the exposure is central to the assessment of risk and to the establishment and maintenance of standards. For the measurement to be meaningful, however, it must be carried out in a way that properly reflects the nature of the exposure.

In this chapter, attention is focused first on the health-related, particle size–selective criteria that have evolved from knowledge about inhalation and deposition of aerosols in human subjects. We then proceed to summarize the scientific basis of aerosol sampling and the history of the development of technical aerosol sampling devices for use in the occupational environment. This leads in turn to a discussion about how well such instruments conform to the latest criteria and a description of some new instruments that have emerged during recent years, specifically in response to those new recommendations.

The overall approach taken is to deal with general principles and to give a few selected examples of practical applications. Full details of the physics of the sampling process and many practical sampling instruments (for both workplace and ambient aerosol measurement) are described in a more comprehensive text on the subject.[1] For further supplementary information, the latest edition of the handbook on air sampling instrumentation from the American Conference of Governmental Industrial Hygienists (ACGIH) is recommended.[2]

CRITERIA FOR THE MEASUREMENT OF COARSE AEROSOLS

The first part of the process of aerosol exposure is the entry of particles into the respiratory tract. For some types of aerosol, inhaled particles constitute a risk to health irrespective of where they are eventually deposited. So, in the first place, the *inhalable* fraction is frequently an appropriate objective for measurement in itself.

Traditionally, recommendations for the health-related sampling of coarse particles have been based on the concept of the so-called *total aerosol*. In turn, practical sampling instruments for the total aerosol have appeared. Because most such instruments have been developed without particular regard to relevant criteria or indices, however, their performance characteristics have varied greatly. It follows, therefore, that total aerosol has been effectively defined in each particular situation by the instrument chosen to do the job. Eventually, however, in the 1970s, the idea emerged of the human head as an aerosol sampler and, hence, of *inhala-*

*bility** as a quantitative definition of what had previously been known as total aerosol. As will be related later, this now provides the basis for a departure from the inconsistency of the old total aerosol approach and a move toward a more scientific sampling rationale.

Since the concept of inhalability was first suggested, a number of important studies have been conducted in laboratories in Britain and Germany to determine the efficiency with which particles enter the human head during breathing through the nose and/or mouth. All these involved experiments with life-sized human mannequins in large wind tunnels and provided data for a range of wind speeds relevant to workplace exposures and for particles with aerodynamic diameter up to 100 μm.[3-6] It was found that the efficiency of inhalation of a particle can, for practical purposes, be described in terms of a single function of particle aerodynamic diameter (d_{ae}, which embodies not only the geometric size of the particle but also its shape and density). This function starts off at 100% for very small particles and falls to about 50% for particles of around 30 μm and larger.

Data from experiments like these have since been used as the basis of recommendations for replacing the old total aerosol concept with a sampling convention based on human inhalability, at least for the purpose of health-related aerosol sampling. The first was proposed in 1983 by the International Standards Organisation (ISO)[7] in which the inhalation efficiency (or inhalability) of the human head (I) was described as a unique function of d_{ae}. Somewhat later, the more comprehensive data provided by subsequent experimental studies provided the basis of a more representative curve, described in 1985 by the ACGIH,[8] using the empirical expression

$$I = 0.5 \, [1 + \exp(-0.06 \, d_{ae})] \tag{1}$$

for d_{ae} up to and including 100 μm and for wind speeds up to 4 m/sec (Fig. 9–1). It was also recommended that, as a performance band for practical sampling instruments, I may vary by ± 0.1 for each value of d_{ae}.

In both the ISO and ACGIH deliberations, attention appears to have been focused primarily on particle size–selective criteria for aerosol sampling in indoor workplaces where wind speeds even as high as 4 m/sec are uncommon. However, there are some outdoor exposure situations where wind conditions might sometimes lie outside this range.

With this in mind, a modification to Equation 1 has been proposed, based on more recent experimental data which take account of the undersampling that would otherwise occur for wind speeds exceeding 4 m/sec.[6]

---

*The way in which the subject has since evolved has led to some confusion in terminology. Early use of ''inhalable'' in the early 1980s gave way to ''inspirable'' to avoid a clash with other uses of the term (e.g., in the United States in relation to the definition of a finer fraction for the purpose of air pollution measurement). Now, however, there is increasing international consensus on methodology and terminology in this whole area, and there is general agreement on reverting back to the term inhalable.

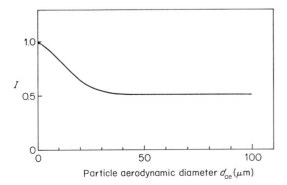

Figure 9–1
Conventional particle size–selection curve for the inhalable fraction (I).[8]

CRITERIA FOR THE MEASUREMENT OF FINER AEROSOL FRACTIONS

Thoracic Aerosol

A *thoracic aerosol* is the fraction of inhaled aerosol which penetrates into the lung. Experimental data are available from the results of inhalation experiments with human volunteer subjects. Figure 9–2 shows the conventional curve proposed by both the ISO and ACGIH (1983 and 1985 versions, respectively) based on these data. It takes the form of a cumulative log-normal function with its median at d_{ae} = 10 μm and has a geometric standard deviation (σ_g) of 1.5. For the ACGIH version, the geometric median value of d_{ae} is allowed to vary by ± 1 μm; σ_g may vary by ± 0.1.

Tracheobronchial and Alveolar Aerosol

For the thoracic aerosol, a further subdivision takes place between what is deposited in the tracheobronchial region and what penetrates down to the alveolar region. The history of particle size–selective criteria for aerosol measurement really began with an identification of the need to make meaningful measurements of fine aerosol fractions in workplaces, which was driven by the high prevalence in some industries (e.g., mining) of *pneumoconioses*. That fine fraction became widely known as the *respirable* fraction, and—in the English language literature at least—is still widely referred to as such. In Figure 9–3, a number of the curves are shown which have been adopted as conventions for the respirable fraction. These include the historically important British Medical Research Council (BMRC) curve, the ACGIH curve, and for completeness, a proposed new version which is expected to appear in the harmonized ISO and ACGIH recommendations when they eventually appear.[9] In regard to tolerance bands, the ACGIH version, for example, allows the geometric median value of d_{ae} to vary by ± 0.3 μm; the σ_g may vary, as before, by ± 0.1.

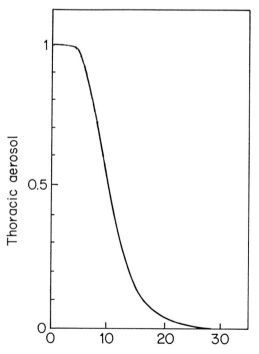

Figure 9–2

Conventional particle size–selection curve for the thoracic fraction.[7, 8]

Particle aerodynamic diameter $d_{ae}(\mu m)$

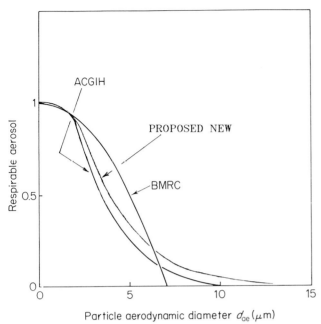

Figure 9–3. Various conventional curves for the respirable fraction: the BMRC curve, the 1985 ACGIH[8] curve, and the proposed new curve.[9]

None of the conventions shown follows exactly all of the trends exhibited by the human deposition data. For example, they do not reflect the downturn associated with the exhalation of some smaller inhaled particles. So they do not reflect true alveolar deposition but, rather, are more representative of the *penetration* of particles to the alveolar region (and hence the *availability* of particles for deposition).

In both the ISO and ACGIH documents, the need to define the tracheobronchial fraction separately is not indicated. However, if desired, a convention for the tracheobronchial fraction may be derived simply by subtracting the alveolar curve from the thoracic curve.

Fibrous Aerosols

Fibrous aerosols can pose extreme risks to health and so are of special interest. Because of their unusual morphological properties and the role of those properties as a cause of lung disease, fibers are specifically excluded from the ISO and ACGIH conventions. Instead, there is a wholly separate rationale for particle size–selective measurement. This is based on an appreciation of both the nature of the particle motion which governs fiber deposition in the deep lung and the biological effects that influence the fate of the particles after deposition. Thus, it has been a widespread convention since the 1960s to assess respirable fibers in terms of the airborne number concentration of particles which, when examined by optical microscopy under phase-contrast conditions, have a length-to-diameter ratio greater than 3, a length greater than 5 μm, and, in some versions, a diameter less than 3 μm.

The practical criteria that have emerged for fibers are based not only on the properties of the particle, which can bear directly on possible health effects, but also on the technical means readily available for assessing them. Optical microscopy is relatively cost effective and straightforward. However, to set an upper limit for fiber diameter smaller than 3 μm (which might be justified in the light of some of the biological evidence) could result in counting problems since a higher proportion would lie beyond the physical limits of detectability by optical means. So the criteria currently in use for routine analysis are based on pragmatic and scientific considerations.

CRITIQUE OF THE VARIOUS SAMPLING CONVENTIONS

As already mentioned, health-related aerosol sampling should include the recognition of the various physical processes by which aerosols come into contact with the human respiratory system. First, it should reflect aerodynamic processes outside the body during inhalation and then the processes inside the body during deposition. That is, inhaled aerosol is a particle size–selected fraction of the total workplace aerosol. In turn, thoracic and respirable aerosols are subfractions of the inhalable fraction. These features which apply to actual human exposure should also be reflected in the performance characteristics of practical instrumentation.

The various criteria have been presented as a set of curves that can be used as "yardsticks" for the performance evaluations of practical aerosol samplers, but the definition of a single curve for defining a particular aerosol fraction raises a difficult question. How do we decide whether or not the performance of a given instrument in relation to the convention is acceptable? In practice, for example, acceptable performance might be defined by requiring that an instrument's efficiency curve falls within a certain range of the ideal (say, within the specified tolerance band). However, this does not represent the full picture, as has been demonstrated numerically for a range of respirable aerosol samplers with performance curves lying within the prescribed ACGIH tolerance bands. For these, the sampled respirable mass of a given aerosol can vary for typical workplace dusts by as much as a factor of five! Such errors can occur for samplers whose performance curves might—on the basis of the sampling efficiency data alone—appear to lie close to a given conventional curve. Therefore, we are alerted to the need, when we test aerosol samplers in relation to specific particle size–selective criteria, to take account not only of the proximity of data points to the target curve but also of possible errors in mass measurement that are dependent on particle size distribution. This is an area in which research is in progress and which clearly needs further work.

STANDARDS FOR AEROSOLS

Standards for airborne contaminants, in the widest sense, are concerned with the whole process of the regulation of exposure and, therefore, should include: (1) criteria for measurement, (2) technical means of measurement, (3) limit values, and (4) sampling strategies. In principle, item 3 cannot be properly prescribed without the others, although much past—and, indeed, some present—practice argues otherwise. Now, however, the emergence of the new health-related aerosol sampling criteria provides a firm basis for a more rational approach to standards.*

Until now, workplace aerosols have usually been thought of in terms of either

---

*Since the preparation of this chapter, there have been significant developments. Recent discussions, involving not only the ISO and ACGIH but also the Comité Européen de Normalisation (CEN), have led to broad international agreement on these conventions. The main elements are as follows:

- The inhalable fraction is described empirically by a single curve relating inhalability, I, and particle aerodynamic diameter (d_{ae}) as given by Equation 1.
- The thoracic fraction takes the form

$$T = I \{1 - F_T\}$$

where F_T is a cumulative log-normal function of d_{ae} with its median at $d_{ae} = 11.64$ μm and having a geometric standard deviation (σ_g) of 1.5.
- Similarly, the respirable fraction takes the form

$$R = I \{1 - F_R\}$$

where $F_R(d_{ae})$ is a cumulative log-normal function of d_{ae} with its median at $d_{ae} = 4.25$ μm and having a geometric standard deviation (σ_g) of 1.5.

Note the important feature in the above is that both the thoracic and respirable fractions are expressed as subfractions of the inhalable fraction.

the old total aerosol or respirable aerosol concepts. The total aerosol approach was applied either where the aerosol in question might be defined as a *nuisance* (that is, posing no specific health risk but recognizing that inhaling high concentrations of any aerosol could present an undesirable challenge to the body's defense mechanisms) or for aerosols that present a risk after they come into contact anywhere in the body. The respirable aerosol approach was applied when the health effect in question produced specific effects in the alveolar region of the lung (e.g., pneumoconiosis).

The recommendations of the ISO and ACGIH have given renewed impetus to the move toward a new set of standards based on the three fractions—*inhalable, thoracic,* and *respirable*—to replace the old total and respirable aerosol combination. To see which aerosol types fall into which categories, we need to reconsider the types of health effects associated with the deposition of particles of various types at the different parts of the respiratory tract. For example, some biologically active particles (e.g., bacteria, fungi, or allergens), if they are deposited in the extrathoracic airways of the head, may lead to inflammation of sensitive membranes in that region, such as symptoms of hay fever (e.g., rhinitis). Other types of particles (e.g., nickel, radioactive material, or wood dust) that are deposited in the same region may lead to more serious local conditions, such as ulceration or nasal cancer. For the health-related measurement of all such aerosols, it is appropriate to sample according to a criterion based on the *inhalable* fraction.

The next class of aerosols includes particles which may provoke local responses in the tracheobronchial region of the lung and lead to such effects as bronchoconstriction, chronic bronchitis, bronchial carcinoma, and so forth. For the health-related measurement of all such aerosols, it is appropriate to sample the *thoracic* fraction.

The third class of aerosols includes particles which deposit in the alveolar region and cause pneumoconiosis, emphysema, alveolitis, pulmonary carcinoma, and so forth. Also, for asbestos fibers, mesothelioma can occur in the nearby pleural cavity. In relation to these, the *respirable* aerosol fraction continues to provide the most appropriate sampling criterion.

Finally, as a general rule, for aerosol substances that are soluble and are known to be associated with systemic effects (in which toxic material can enter the blood after deposition in any part of the respiratory tract and be transported to other organs), standards should be specified in terms of the *inhalable* fraction.

In general, a *limit value* is prescribed in terms of an appropriately time-weighted average airborne concentration of a given fraction of a given aerosol above which "unacceptable" health risks may occur if exposure occurs at that level "day after day." The ACGIH list of threshold limit values (TLVs) is influential not only in the United States but also in other countries throughout the world. In that list, exposure limits are suggested for a wide range of substances which can appear as aerosols. As stated earlier, however, the list currently recommends limits for total and respirable aerosol fractions alone. It is expected that, in the future, such a list will be based on the new particle size–selective sampling criteria. Indeed, in Britain, the old total aerosol concept has already been replaced by the inhalability criterion.

STRATEGIES FOR EXPOSURE ASSESSMENT

Health-related aerosol measurement needs to be carried out with regard not only to such particle size–selective criteria but also to the kinetics of the processes by which the particles can cause harm after inhalation and the variability of exposure. Rappaport has recently addressed these factors in relation to the general problem of occupational exposure.[10] From such considerations, it is clear that, for aerosols, we should be concerned not only with choices about the particle size selectivity of measuring instruments but also about the *duration* and *frequency* of sampling.

In any given sampling exercise, there remains a further question about how best to reflect the true exposures of individual workers (or of groups of workers), either *static* (or *area*) measurement, in which the chosen instrument is located in the workplace atmosphere and provides a measurement of aerosol concentration which is (it is hoped) relevant to the workforce as a whole, or *personal* measurement, in which the chosen instrument is mounted on the body of the exposed subject and moves around with the person at all times. When one or the other of these is chosen, some important considerations need to be taken into account. For a few workplaces (e.g., some working groups in long-wall mining), it has been shown that a reasonably good comparison may be obtained between suitably placed static instruments and personal samplers. More generally, however, static samplers have been found to perform less well and tend to give aerosol concentrations which are consistently low compared with those obtained using personal samplers. One advantage with static samplers is that a relatively small number of instruments may be used to survey a whole work force. If this can be shown to provide valid and representative results, it is a simple and cost-effective exercise. Furthermore, the high flow rates that are acceptable for static samplers mean that, even at very low aerosol concentrations, a relatively large sample mass can be collected in a short sampling period. The use of personal samplers is more labor intensive and requires more instruments and, hence, greater effort in setting them up and in recovering and analyzing the samples afterward. Furthermore, it involves the direct cooperation of the workers themselves. Also, for such samplers, it is inevitable that the capacities of the pumps used will be limited by their portability. So flow rates will usually be low (rarely greater than 4 L/min). However, personal aerosol sampling is the *only* reliable means of assessing the *true* aerosol exposures of individual workers. Therefore, it is by far the most common mode of aerosol measurement in workplaces.

Finally, when personal aerosol sampling is discussed, the *breathing zone* concept is frequently invoked as a practical guide to where the sampler should be placed on the worker's body. However, studies of the physics and aerodynamics of the sampling process have taught us that simple proximity alone does *not* ensure a representative sample.

SCIENTIFIC ASPECTS OF AEROSOL SAMPLING

The technical problems of aerosol measurement may include (1) physical aspiration of particle-laden air into sampling devices, (2) aerodynamic selection and subsequent assessment (e.g., mass determination) of desired fractions, and (3) collection or detection of the selected aerosol.

An important aspect of sampler performance is the efficiency with which particles are aspirated from the air into the sampler through its entry orifice(s). The basic physics of the process of aspiration has been covered extensively elsewhere.[1] It is best illustrated here by referring to the simplest sampling system, a thin-walled sampling probe facing into a moving air stream. This has been the subject of a great deal of research, stimulated primarily by the need to measure true total aerosol concentration in industrial stacks and ducts.

The general nature of the air flow in the vicinity of such a probe is shown simplistically in Figure 9–4 for three contrasting sets of aerodynamic conditions. Figure 9–4A shows what happens when the mean velocity over the plane of the sampler entry (U_s) is less than the free-stream air velocity upwind of the sampler (U). Here, the pattern of the sampled air (the shaded volume) is *divergent*. Approaching particles encounter this distortion, and, as a result of their inertia, some of those from outside the sampled air volume may impact onto the plane of the entry orifice and so pass into the entry orifice. In this way, the net aerosol which

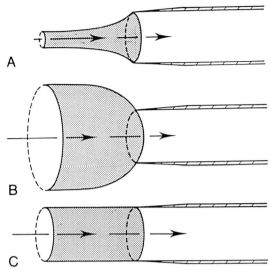

A

B

C

Figure 9–4. Schematic diagram to indicate the nature of the air flow near a simple thin-walled sampling probe facing the wind. *A,* Sampling air velocity less than the wind speed. *B,* Sampling air velocity greater than the wind speed. *C,* Sampling air velocity equal to the wind speed. In this figure, note that the main flow feature is the streamline which divides the sampled flow (the hatched volume) from that which is not sampled. As a result of particle inertial effects, particles approaching the sampler may impact into the sampled flow (in *A*) or out of the sampled flow (in *B*), leading to oversampling and undersampling, respectively. Ideal (or isokinetic) sampling is achieved when the sampling flow is perfectly matched to the wind (as in *C*). (From Vincent, J. H., Aerosol Sampling: Science and Practice, Copyright 1989, London, John Wiley & Sons. Reprinted by permission of John Wiley & Sons, Ltd.)

enters the orifice is *enriched* with particles, especially with larger ones. In Figure 9–4*B*, in which U_s is greater than U, the converse happens. Here, the sampled flow is *convergent* so that particles in the aerosol can impact out of the sampled air volume. The result is a reduction in aerosol concentration in the sampled air, again especially for larger particles. In Figure 9–4*C*, we have U_s = U. The sampled flow is perfectly matched to the wind, and the flow is undistorted. Here, there are no gains or losses caused by impaction, and so, the aerosol concentration in the sampled air will the same as that upstream. The three conditions illustrated in Figure 9–4 may be described as *subisokinetic, superisokinetic,* and *isokinetic,* respectively. The latter is the ideal sampling condition, and thin-walled probes used in this way are referred to as isokinetic samplers.

The nature of the air flow near a sampler that is more typical of those used in occupational hygiene is much more complex than that for the thin-walled probe. From considerations of particle motion in this flow field, it is sufficient for present purposes to state the general functional form for the aspiration efficiency of a blunt sampler thus

$$A = c_s/c_o = f [St, U/U_s, \delta/D, \Theta, B], \qquad (2)$$

where c_s is the sampled aerosol concentration and c_o, the concentration in the undisturbed air outside the sampler. In this expression, St is a dimensionless inertial parameter (a *Stokes' number*) that governs the impaction process and is dependent on the particle's d_{ae}, the wind speed (U), and the width of the sampler body (D). In Equation 2, U_s is the velocity with which air enters the sampler, δ is the width of the sampling orifice, Θ is the orientation of the sampling orifice with respect to the wind, and B is an aerodynamic shape factor (or "bluntness") for the sampler. From qualitative physical reasoning, we can begin to appreciate the factors which influence the performance curves of practical devices. However, it is fair to say that we are still a long way from a full theoretical appreciation of the sampling process. In practice, therefore, design is still a matter of "trial and modification."

After aspiration, the subsequent fate of particles determines which ones reach the filter (or sensing zone) of the sampler. Here, particle size–selective mechanisms may be used in a controlled way to provide classification of the aspirated aerosol into some appropriate health-related subfraction. Some mechanisms which have been employed in this way include the use of gravitational elutriators (based on principles first described by Walton[11]), cyclones, and impactors.

A number of additional factors, not already mentioned, under certain conditions, can have a significant effect on performance. These include instability (or turbulence) in the workplace air, sampler wall effects both outside (''blow-off'' from outer surfaces) and inside (deposition on inside walls), and electrostatic forces associated with particle charge. These are described fully elsewhere.[1]

PRACTICAL SAMPLING FOR COARSE AEROSOL

Static (or Area) Samplers

Over many years, static samplers have been developed for the sampling of coarse aerosols in workplace atmospheres. The simplest are open-filter arrangements mounted on the box which contains the pump (Fig. 9–5), or systems in which the open-filter holder is mounted independently. The sampler shown is widely used in Great Britain. Similar devices have been used elsewhere, both in workplace and in ambient air sampling. The performances of such instruments, originally intended as samplers for total aerosol, should now be assessed in the light of the latest particle size–selective criteria described earlier, in particular in relation to the inhalability curve. Inspection of the available data for these instruments reveals that none comes close to matching the inhalability criterion.

In light of such data, new generations of aerosol samplers are now beginning to emerge, this time designed from the outset to match the inhalability criterion. One designed for use in workplaces is the 3-L/min Institute of Occupational Medicine (IOM) static inhalable aerosol sampler (Fig. 9–6A).[12] It incorporates a number of novel features. First, the sampler contains a single sampling orifice located in a head which, mounted on top of the housing containing the pump, drive, and battery pack, rotates slowly about a vertical axis. The entry orifice forms an integral part of an aerosol collecting capsule which is located mainly inside the head. This capsule also houses the filter.

In the use of the instrument, the whole capsule assembly (tare weight on the

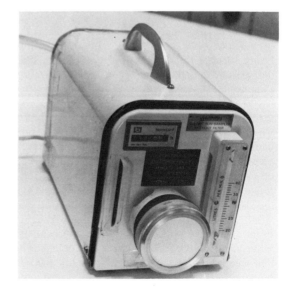

Figure 9–5
Typical open-filter arrangement of the type widely used for the static sampling of coarse aerosol in Great Britain (shown in the pump-mounted version with a recommended flow rate of 60 L/min). (Instrument available in Great Britain from Negretti Automation, Aylesbury, UK). (Reprinted with permission from Mark, D., Vincent, J. H., Stevens, D. C., and Marshall, M., Investigation of the entry characteristics of dust samplers of a type used in the British nuclear industry. Atmos. Environ., 20, 2389, 1986. Reprinted with permission from Pergamon Press PLC.)

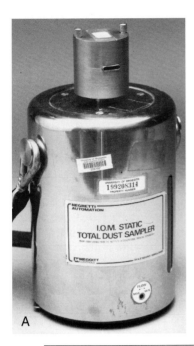

A

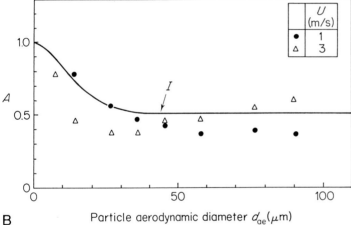

B

Particle aerodynamic diameter $d_{ae}(\mu m)$

Figure 9–6
The IOM 3-L/min static sampler for inhalable aerosol. *A,* The instrument itself. *B,* Performance of the instrument in relation to the inhalability criterion (I), shown in terms of aspiration efficiency (A) as a function of particle aerodynamic diameter (d_{ae}) for various windspeeds (U).[12] (Instrument commercially available in Great Britain from Negretti Automation, Aylesbury, UK). (*A,* Courtesy of Perng-Jy Tsai, from his Ph.D. thesis, University of Minnesota, December 1994. *B,* From Mark, D., Vincent, J. H., Gibson, H., and Lynch, G., A new static sampler for airborne total dust in workplaces. Am. Ind. Hyg. Assoc. J., 46, 127, 1985.)

order of a few grams) is weighed before and after sampling to provide the full mass of aspirated aerosol. This system eliminates the possibility of errors associated with internal wall losses. When the capsule is mounted in the sampling head, the entry itself projects about 2 mm out from the surface of the head, creating a "lip" around the orifice itself. This has the effect of preventing the secondary aspiration of any aerosol particles which strike the outside surface of the head and fail to be retained.

The performance curve of this sampler, shown in Figure 9–6*B,* is in good agreement with the inhalability curve for particles with d_{ae} up to about 100 microns. At present, this is the only static sampler specifically for the inhalable fraction which is commercially available, although prototype higher flow rate versions were built at the IOM during the late 1980s.

Personal Samplers

For the reasons outlined earlier, personal sampling is generally the preferred approach for workplace aerosols. Here, for coarse aerosols, a large number of different devices have been used, again originating—historically—for the purpose of sampling for total aerosol. Again, the simplest is the open-filter arrangement. The one shown in Figure 9–7 is the 25-mm open filter. Other personal samplers for total aerosol that at present are widely used by occupational hygienists in Great Britain are the single (4-mm)-hole sampler recommended by the Health and Safety Executive for lead aerosol and the modified seven-hole version recommended for general coarse aerosol sampling. These too are shown in Figure 9–7. Both of these closed-face samplers also employ 25-mm filters. All three samplers are intended for use at the sampling flow rate of 2 L/min.

Experiments were conducted to compare their performances with the inhalability curve.[13] It is particularly important to note here—and for all the other personal samplers discussed later—that only data obtained with each sampler tested while it is mounted on a life-size torso (e.g., of a mannequin) are considered useful in this context. It should not be assumed that, if such samplers were to be tested independently, they would necessarily provide the same results. The aerodynamic conditions governing the air flow around the sampler would be different. So it follows that devices designed as personal samplers should *not* be used in the static mode. Unfortunately, this common-sense guideline is widely ignored.

Data for the three samplers in Figure 9–7 indicate that all match the inhalability criterion well for particles with d_{ae} up to about 15 μm and for wind speeds of 1 m/sec and less. For conditions outside these ranges, which yet are typical of those found in many workplaces, however, the performance curves are less satisfactory, with strong wind-speed dependence (especially for the single- and seven-hole samplers) and with a tendency toward undersampling. Interestingly, it was found that the performances of these—and, indeed, other personal samplers—are not strongly dependent on *where* the device is mounted on the torso.

The physical and design features of these three samplers are, in one way or another, representative of those exhibited by most of the many others which have been designed and used over the years in many countries. One is the 37-mm plastic cassette which is employed widely—either open or closed faced—by occupational hygienists in the United States (Fig. 9–8). The test results for this sampler are limited in number and range of d_{ae} covered but are sufficient to show that this sampler too provides an inadequate measure of the inhalable fraction (except, again, for fine particles) and tends to undersample with respect to the inhalable fraction.

In the light of the generally poor performance curves of many existing total aerosol samplers with respect to the inhalability criterion, a new personal sampler has been proposed. This is the 2-L/min IOM personal inhalable aerosol sampler (Fig. 9–9*A*).[13] It features a 15-mm diameter circular entry which faces directly

Figure 9–7
Three personal samplers of the type widely used for sampling coarse aerosol in Britain. *A*, Open filter holder. *B*, Single-hole sampler. *C*, Seven-hole sampler. Recommended sampling flow rate for each is 2 L/min. (From Vincent, J. H., Aerosol Sampling: Science and Practice, Copyright 1989, London, John Wiley & Sons. Reprinted by permission of John Wiley & Sons, Ltd.)

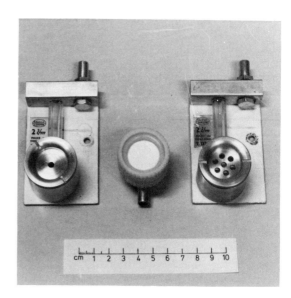

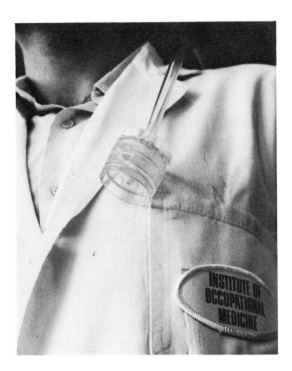

Figure 9–8
The 37-mm cassette of the type widely used in the United States for the personal sampling of coarse aerosol. The recommended sampling flow rate is 2 L/min. (From Vincent, J. H., Aerosol Sampling: Science and Practice, Copyright 1989, London, John Wiley & Sons. Reprinted by permission of John Wiley & Sons, Ltd.)

outward when the sampler is worn on the torso. Like the IOM static inhalable aerosol sampler in Figure 9–6, the entry is incorporated into an aerosol-collecting capsule, which during sampling, is located behind the face plate. The use of this capsule ensures that the overall aspirated aerosol is always assessed. Also, as for the static sampler, the lips of the entry protrude outward slightly from the face plate to prevent the oversampling associated with particle blow-off from the external sampler surfaces. Experimental data for this instrument are shown in Figure 9–9B,

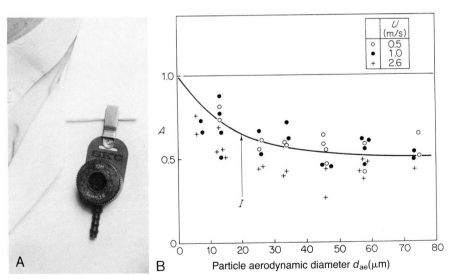

Figure 9–9. The IOM 2-L/min personal sampler for inhalable aerosol. *A,* The instrument itself. *B,* Performance curve of the instrument in relation to the inhalability criterion (I), shown in terms of aspiration efficiency (A) as a function of particle aerodynamic diameter (d_{ae}) for various wind speeds (U).[13] (Instrument commercially available from SKC Inc., Eighty-Four, PA). (*A,* Courtesy of SKC Ltd., England, UK. *B,* From Vincent, J. H., Aerosol Sampling: Science and Practice, Copyright 1989, London, John Wiley & Sons. Reprinted by permission of John Wiley & Sons, Ltd.)

and they show a good match with the inhalability curve. Once again, this instrument is the only one presently available commercially which adequately matches the inhalability criterion.

SAMPLING FOR RESPIRABLE AEROSOL

The history of sampling fine aerosols in workplaces began with the respirable fraction, in particular with the emergence in the 1950s of the BMRC respirable aerosol criterion. A number of types of sampling device have since been developed. Most have in common the fact that they first aspirate a particle fraction which is assumed to be representative of the total workplace aerosol. From this, the desired fine fraction is then aerodynamically separated inside the instrument, using an arrangement (based on one of the physical options mentioned earlier) the particle size–dependent penetration characteristics of which match the desired criterion. It is the fraction which remains uncollected inside the selector and passes through to collect onto a filter (or some other collecting medium) which is the fine fraction of interest.

Static Samplers

A variety of static samplers for the respirable aerosol fraction have been built and successfully used in practical occupational hygiene. Some achieved particle size selection by the mechanism of horizontal gravitational elutriation already mentioned. One example is the British 2.5-L/min MRE type 113A sampler (Casella Ltd., UK) (Fig. 9–10).[14] For such devices, their penetration characteristics can easily be tailored, using elutriator theory, to match the BMRC respirable aerosol curve closely (itself originally derived from elutriator theory).

Other static respirable aerosol samplers have been designed to operate on the principles of cyclone selection. One example is the German 50-L/min TBF50 sampler (Fig. 9–11). Another is the French 50-L/min CPM3. Although such cyclones can be designed that have well-defined penetration characteristics, the prediction of performance from theory is more complicated than that for horizontal elutriators.

Personal Samplers

Horizontal gravitational elutriators are very satisfactory for static respirable aerosol sampling, but they are inevitably rather bulky and not conducive to minia-

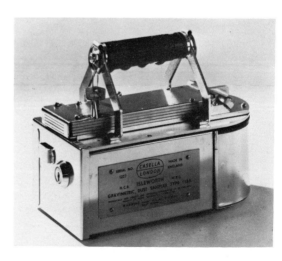

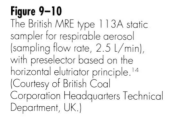

Figure 9–10
The British MRE type 113A static sampler for respirable aerosol (sampling flow rate, 2.5 L/min), with preselector based on the horizontal elutriator principle.[14] (Courtesy of British Coal Corporation Headquarters Technical Department, UK.)

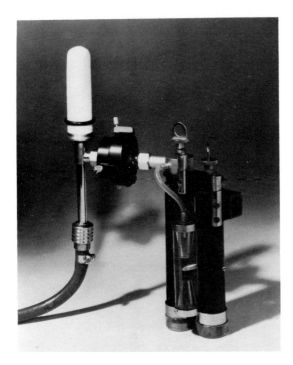

Figure 9–11
The German TBF50 static sampler for respirable aerosol (sampling flow rate, 50 L/min), with preselector based on the cyclone principle (shown in the intrinsically safe version with backing filter and compressed air-ejector air moving system, as commonly used in the mining industry). (Courtesy of British Coal Corporation Headquarters Technical Department, UK.)

turization. Therefore, horizontal gravitational elutriation is not an option for personal respirable aerosol samplers. On the other hand, cyclones are ideally suited for such purposes and have found wide application. Well-known examples are the British 1.9-L/min cyclone (Casella Ltd., UK) (Fig. 9–12) and the American 1.7- to 2.1-L/min cyclone (SKC Inc., USA) (Fig. 9–13), the selection characteristics of which have been shown to be in good agreement with the BMRC curve.

One further device has some interesting and unusual features and so deserves special mention. This is the French CIP10 (Fig. 9–14).[15] Although this instrument is aimed primarily at collecting a finer (respirable) aerosol fraction, it can also provide the concentration of the inhalable fraction. It is particularly interesting because the instrument incorporates its own built-in pumping unit, consisting of a battery-driven, rapidly rotating polyester foam plug. The aerosol is aspirated through a downward anular entry and is collected efficiently by filtration (by a combination of mainly gravitational and inertial forces) in two static, coarse-grade

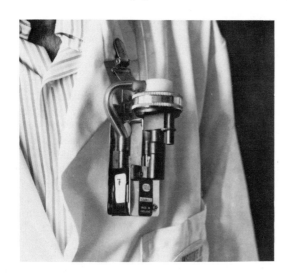

Figure 9–12
The 1.9-L/min cyclone-based personal sampler of the type widely used for respirable aerosol in Britain. (From Vincent, J. H., Aerosol Sampling: Science and Practice, Copyright 1989, London, John Wiley & Sons. Reprinted by permission of John Wiley & Sons, Ltd.)

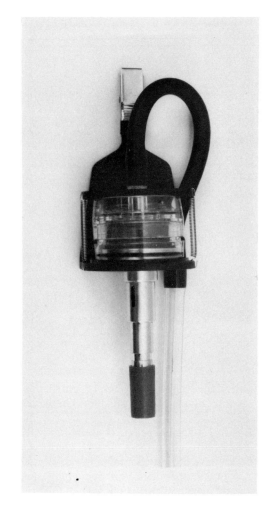

Figure 9–13
A cyclone-based personal sampler for respirable aerosol of the type widely used in the United States. (Courtesy of SKC Ltd.)

foam plugs located inside the entry and on the finer-grade rotating one. As a result of the low-pressure drop characteristics of such foam filtration media, a very high flow rate—by personal sampler standards—can be achieved, up to 10 L/min.

Sampling for Respirable Fibers

As we already indicated, the definition of a respirable fiber is based on purely geometric criteria; therefore, selection is best carried out not aerodynamically but visually under the microscope. This means that, in practical sampling, the main priority is to achieve deposition onto a suitable surface (e.g., a membrane filter) which can then be "cleared" and mounted for subsequent visual analysis. It follows that actual physical sampling can be very simple, usually involving the collection of particles directly onto an open filter (sometimes with the use of a cowl or some other baffle to protect the filter from large airborne material and curious fingers!). Such sampling is carried out routinely in both the static and personal modes.

One important practical aspect is the setting of the sampling flow rate since sufficient flow is required to achieve, over a sampling shift, a sample which is dense enough to provide good counting statistics, yet not so dense as to cause problems with fiber overlap. As far as the effects of sampling flow rate on aspiration efficiency are concerned, it has been demonstrated that, over a very wide range of flow rates, fibrous particles of asbestos are so fine that the aspiration efficiency is nearly always close to unity.[16] Therefore, for practical purposes, sampling bias

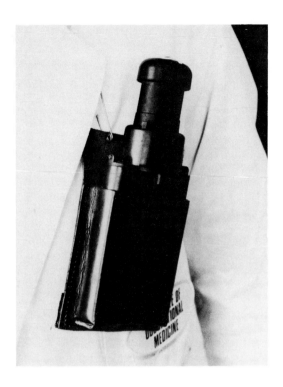

Figure 9–14
The French CIP10 personal sampler for respirable aerosol fraction.[15] It contains its own air-moving apparatus and operates at a sampling flow rate of 10 L/min. (From Vincent, J. H., Aerosol Sampling: Science and Practice, Copyright 1989, London, John Wiley & Sons. Reprinted by permission of John Wiley & Sons, Ltd.)

caused by aspiration effects can be neglected. This provides considerable flexibility in the choice of flow rate in a given situation.

In asbestos measurement, great emphasis is placed on the visual assessment of the sampled fibers. For routine assessment of workplace asbestos, this is usually carried out by using an optical microscope under phase-contrast conditions at a magnification of ×450. An appropriate graticule (e.g., the Walton-Beckett) is used to provide ease of classification of fibers matching the criteria referred to earlier. Sets of "counting rules" have been recommended to aid the microscopist in what—and what not—to count, guiding, for example, the assessment of fibrous aggregates, fibers in the presence of other nonfibrous particles, fibers not fully contained within the microscope field of view, and so forth.[17]

PRACTICAL SAMPLING FOR THORACIC AEROSOL

The methodology for the sampling of the thoracic aerosol fraction in the occupational context was not widely considered before the establishment of the new sampling criteria. For workplaces, the nearest we have come to a thoracic aerosol standard is in the United States cotton industry in which a criterion was established in 1975 by the United States National Institute of Occupational Safety and Health based on a selection curve which falls to 50% at 15 μm (compared with the 10-μm "cut point" in the ISO and ACGIH thoracic fractions). This standard implies recognition of the role of particle deposition in the large airways of the upper respiratory tract in cotton workers' byssinosis. The recommended static sampling method uses the concept of vertical elutriation.[11]

Now, as the ISO and ACGIH recommendations begin to be translated into new standards, more energetic consideration is being given to the development of samplers for the thoracic fraction, and first attempts are being based on a modification of existing respirable aerosol samplers.

SAMPLING FOR MORE THAN ONE FRACTION SIMULTANEOUSLY

The important concept that not only is the thoracic aerosol fraction a subfraction of the inhalable fraction but that the respirable aerosol fraction is a further subfraction of the thoracic subfraction provides a framework by which all three aerosol fractions can be obtained simultaneously. Such aerosol measurements could be important for assessing the aerosol-related risk in certain situations, and appropriate practical sampling devices are just beginning to emerge.

One interesting such personal sampler is the Italian PERSPEC (Lavoro e Ambiente, Bologna, Italy) (Fig. 9–15).[18] The aerosol enters at 2 L/min through a pair of crescent-shaped orifices and, winnowed by a clean air sheath in a strongly divergent flow, is separated by inertial forces into the finer subfractions which are deposited onto different, well-defined parts of the same 47-mm filter. This sampler can provide the inhalable fraction (the whole aspirated catch of aerosol, including that deposited on the internal walls) and the thoracic and respirable subfractions (based on measurements of the mass deposited on different parts of the filter).

A second instrument (Fig. 9–16) is derived directly from the IOM personal inhalable aerosol sampler shown in Figure 9–9.[19] Here, aerosol is again aspirated through a 15-mm circular entry, and as before, the entry forms an integral part of an aerosol-collecting capsule, which acts as a receptacle for the whole inhalable fraction. Now, however, the capsule is extended in length to house two porous polyester foam selectors, each using different grades of foam. The first is chosen (i.e., grade of foam and dimensions) to provide penetration characteristics matching the thoracic fraction. The second selector, placed immediately behind the first, is chosen to provide penetration characteristics matching the respirable aerosol curve. In the practical use of this instrument, the whole capsule is weighed before and after sampling (to provide the inhalable mass fraction). Then the second (fine) foam plug and the backing filter are removed and weighed separately. The sum of the resultant two masses provides the thoracic mass fraction. The mass on the backing filter is the respirable mass sampled.

AEROSOL SPECTROMETERS

In principle, if we know the particle size distribution and the mass of the sampled aerosol, then we can determine the particle size distribution and mass

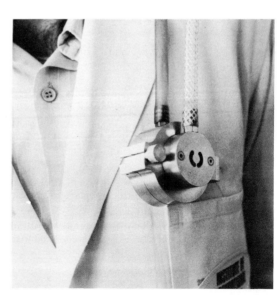

Figure 9–15
The Italian PERSPEC personal sampler,[18] developed primarily as a sampler for the fine thoracic and respirable fractions, but also having the potential for use for inhalable aerosol. Sampling flow rate is 2 L/min. (From Vincent, J. H., Aerosol Sampling: Science and Practice, Copyright 1989, London, John Wiley & Sons. Reprinted by permission of John Wiley & Sons, Ltd.)

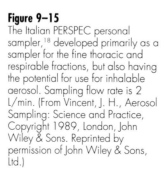

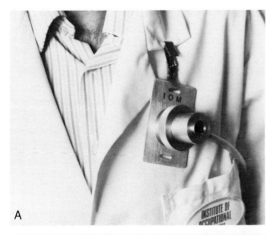

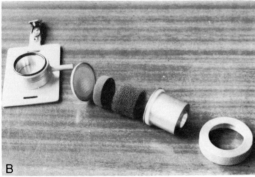

Figure 9–16
The IOM 2-L/min personal sampler developed for the simultaneous sampling of inhalable, thoracic, and respirable aerosol fractions.[19] It incorporates an inhalable entry, like that shown in Figure 9–9, and two porous foam preselectors (located inside the nosepiece of the sampling head) that operate on filtration principles. (From Vincent, J. H., Aerosol Sampling: Science and Practice, Copyright 1989, London, John Wiley & Sons. Reprinted by permission of John Wiley & Sons, Ltd.)

contained in any subfraction. Aerosol spectrometers that can provide such information are more versatile than the dedicated samplers described earlier since they can provide data about any number of subfractions from just *one* sample. This can have important implications, in particular for epidemiological research. For example, in one recent study, the approach outlined before has been used to examine the effects on the dust uptakes in mine workers of changing breathing patterns, and hence different lung deposition characteristics, associated with different work rates.[20]

A wide range of physical possibilities exists on which to base a family of aerosol spectrometer devices. A number of them, including horizontal elutriators, centrifuges, and inertial devices, have been reviewed by Mark et al.[21] More recently, the potential role of such instruments in investigating dust-related health effects in the mining industry has been the subject of a five-nation, six-laboratory study sponsored by the Commission of European Communities.[22]

The class of spectrometer which has achieved the greatest popularity since it first emerged in the 1940s is the cascade impactor. In this device, sampled aerosol passes through a succession of impactor stages, each taking the form of a jet directed onto a solid surface. Particle deposition takes place by impaction onto the surface and is strongly dependent on the particle's aerodynamic size and jet width. Decreasing the jet width at each successive stage ensures that smaller and smaller particles are deposited as the aerosol penetrates from stage to stage. From the masses of aerosol collected at each stage, together with knowledge of the deposition (or "cut") characteristics of the impactor stages, the cumulative—and, in turn, the frequency—size distribution of the sampled aerosol can be obtained. More detailed information of the principles, performances, and types of cascade impactors and on data reduction appears widely elsewhere in the literature.

Here just two specific instruments are mentioned. Since they take the form of personal samplers, they are of particular potential value for applications in the investigation of aerosol-related occupational lung disease and, indeed, are finding increasing use as such.

The first is the sampler proposed by Marple and his colleagues (Fig. 9–17).[23] It is an eight-stage device, with four slot-shaped jets at each stage where aerosol is collected onto polycarbonate membrane films. By weighing the films before and after sampling, the mass of aerosol collected on each is assessed gravimetrically.

The second device is the IOM personal inhalable dust spectrometer (PIDS) (Fig. 9–18).[24] The general configuration is similar to that for the Marple device, except that the slot jets are replaced by circular ones. The aerosol is collected directly onto the back of each disk-shaped aluminum impactor surface, which also incorporates the jets for the next stage. All the collection surfaces are greased before sampling, and the masses of collected aerosol are obtained by weighing each disk itself before and after.

The key feature of the PIDS instrument, which distinguishes it from the previous one, is that it incorporates a 15-mm circular entry like that for the IOM inhalable aerosol sampler; therefore, it begins by aspirating the inhalable fraction. This entry is incorporated into a ''cassette'' which, by also being weighed before and after sampling, provides the mass of aerosol which is collected between the entry and the first impactor stage. Using this mass together with knowledge of the penetration characteristics of the entry stage, the particle size distribution obtained from the cascade impactor part of the instrument may be corrected to allow for deposition (of both coarse and fine particles) in the entry, thus providing the particle size distribution of the inhalable fraction. Thus, the performance of this instrument matches closely the health-related sampling rationale outlined earlier.

SAMPLING SYSTEM COMPONENTS

Pumps

Most samplers require a source of air movement so that particulate-laden air can be aspirated into the instrument. We have discussed both personal and static

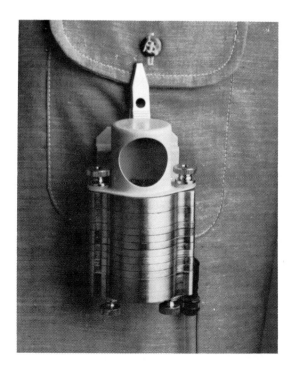

Figure 9–17
The Marple 2-L/min personal cascade impactor.[23] (Courtesy of Andersen Instruments Inc., Atlanta, GA.)

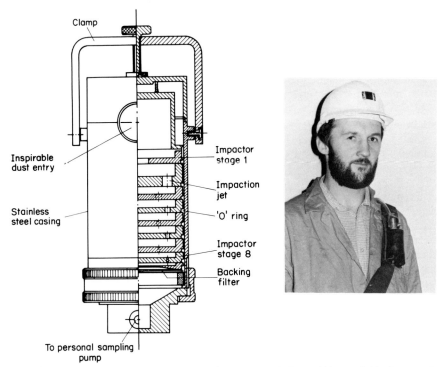

Clamp

Inspirable
dust entry

Stainless
steel casing

Impactor
stage 1

Impaction
jet

'O' ring

Impactor
stage 8

Backing
filter

To personal sampling
pump

Figure 9–18. The IOM 2-L/min PIDS.[24] (From Gibson, H., Mark, D., and Vincent, J. H., A personal inspirable dust spectrometer for applications in occupational hygiene research. Ann. Occup. Hyg. 31, 463, 1987.)

(or area) sampling. The main difference in terms of pump requirements is the flow rate, which tends to be low for personal sampling (usually from 1 to 4 L/min) and larger (up to 100 L/min and even higher) for static sampling. The main limiting factor for a personal sampling pump is its weight; it must be light enough to be worn on the body (usually on a belt) without inconvenience to the wearer.

A wide range of lightweight, battery-powered pumps is available for personal sampling (and also static sampling, if desired). These instruments are based on diaphragm, piston, and rotary pumping principles, and all those in practical use are equipped with damping devices to reduce the effects of flow pulsations. The actual volumetric flow rate depends first on sampling considerations (e.g., entry conditions to provide the desired performance) and then on the amount of material to be collected for accurate assessment, analytical requirements, and so forth. Internal flow meters, usually of the rotameter type or digital counters, are incorporated into most pumps, but these must always be calibrated against a primary flow-rate standard (e.g., a spirometer). It should also be noted that the flow rate may vary with the resistance imposed by the filter and its collected aerosol mass. For this reason, flow rates should be checked periodically during sampling and adjusted if necessary. However, flow-controlled pumps are now available which eliminate the need for such regular attention during sampling. Finally, for sampling in potentially explosive atmospheres (e.g., coal mines and chemical plants), intrinsically safe or flame-proof pumps should be used.

Filters

A filter is the most common means of collecting the aerosol sample in a form suitable for assessment. That assessment might include gravimetric weighing on an analytical balance before and after sampling to obtain the sampled mass. It might also include visual assessment using an optical or electron microscope and a whole range of analytical and chemical techniques. The choice of filter type for a given application depends greatly on how it is proposed to analyze the collected sample. Many different filter materials, with markedly different physical and chemical properties, are now available, including fibrous (e.g., glass), membrane (e.g., cellulose nitrate), and sintered (e.g., silver). Membrane filters have the advantage that they can retain particles effectively on their surface (which is good for microscopy), whereas fibrous filters have the advantage of providing in-depth particle collection and hence a high load-carrying capacity (which is good for gravimetric assessment).

Such filters are available in a range of dimensions (e.g., 25- to 100-mm diameter) and pore sizes (e.g., 0.1 to 10 μm). The mass collection efficiency is usually close to 100% for particles in most size ranges of interest, although sometimes some reduction in efficiency might be traded against the lower pressure drop requirements of a filter with a greater pore size. For some types of filter, an electrostatic charge can present aerosol collection and handling problems. In such cases, the use of a static eliminator is recommended. For other types, weight variations caused by moisture absorption can cause difficulty, especially when the filters are used for the gravimetric assessment of low masses. It is therefore recommended that the stabilization of filters overnight in the laboratory should be carried out before each weighing, together with the use of blank ''control'' filters to establish the level of variability. In certain cases, humidity control in the balance room and desiccation of filters prior to weighing might be recommended.

The chemical requirements of filters depends on the nature of the analysis which is proposed. As we already mentioned, weight stability is important for gravimetric assessment. If particle counting by optical microscopy is required, then the filters used must be capable of being rendered transparent (i.e., cleared). Direct on-filter measurements of mineralogical composition (e.g., by infrared spectrophotometry, x-ray diffraction, scanning electron microscopic and energy-dispersive x-ray analyses, x-ray fluorescence, and so forth) are often required. For these, filters must allow good transmission of the radiation in question, with low background scatter and interference. Collected samples may also be extracted from the filter before analysis, using a range of wet chemical methods, ultrasonication, ashing, and so forth, each of which imposes a range of specific filter requirements.

DIRECT-READING AEROSOL INSTRUMENTATION

In all of the instruments described before, the sampled aerosol is collected on a filter or some other substrate, which may be assessed separately after sampling has been completed. Such instrumentation is suitable when time-averaged measurement can be justified. However, there are occasions in which short-term (or even real-time) measurement is required. Direct-reading instrumentation can be valuable in such cases.

Optical techniques, based on the principles of light extinction and scattering,[25] provide an effective means by which aerosol can be assessed in real time. They provide the great advantage that the measurement can be made without disturbing the aerosol—provided, of course, that the particles can be introduced into the sensing zone of the instrument without distortion. Their disadvantage is that interactions between light and airborne particles are strongly dependent on particle size and type, and so the results are frequently difficult to interpret.

One class of instrument based on such principles is that of *aerosol photometers*, in which the instrument responds to a whole group of particles. The simplest version is based on the principles of light extinction in which the particle concentration is estimated from the attenuation of a beam of light as it passes through the aerosol. In workplaces, however, aerosol concentrations are usually too low to provide significant attenuation. So extinction-based optical instruments have not been widely used in the monitoring of workplace aerosols.

Optical instruments operating on the basis of the detection of the *scattered*, rather than the *transmitted*, light are altogether more sensitive at lower concentrations. There are many possibilities (e.g., optical geometry, scattering angle, and so forth) on which to base an instrument. Therefore, a correspondingly wide range of instruments has appeared on the market. The most successful have been those designed to monitor aerosol fractions within specific particle size ranges, in particular, the respirable fraction.

These include the British Safety in Mines Scattered Light Instrument (SIMSLIN), which is based on the horizontal elutriator system of the MRE type 113A gravimetric respirable dust sampler described earlier but with the elutriated aerosol entering an optical sensing zone in which scattered infrared light from a diode laser is collected within the angles 12° to 20° from the forward direction and focused onto a photodiode. SIMSLIN has been shown to provide a response that is approximately proportional to the instantaneous respirable mass concentration of mine dusts. A more recent version is the Optical Scattering Instantaneous Respirable Dust Indication System (OSIRIS), in which the data can be telemetered to a central monitoring station.

A somewhat different approach is adopted in the German TM-Digital. The aerosol enters the sensing region by direct convection (without the aid of a pump). In the sensing region, scattered infrared light is detected at an angle of 70° to the forward facing. This instrument also has been shown to respond directly to the respirable dust mass concentration in mine environments.

In the American Respirable Aerosol Monitor (RAM), the aspirated aerosol is passed through a cyclone which allows the respirable fraction to penetrate to the sensing zone, where infrared light scattered in the near-forward direction is detected by a photodiode. Like SIMSLIN, OSIRIS, and TM-Digital, the response of the RAM correlates well with the respirable particulate mass for mine dust. An important extension of the RAM is a personal device—the Mini-RAM—which, like the TM-Digital, is an essentially "passive" device without a pump.

The second type of instrument is based on the interaction between a focused light beam and each individual single particle. Such instruments are referred to as *optical particle counters*. From light scattering principles, if an individual particle can be detected and registered electronically, it can be not only counted but also sized (i.e., placed into a given size band or "channel" based on the magnitude of the signal arising from the scattered light). By such means, instruments can be designed that are capable either of counting particles within specified size ranges or of providing an overall particle size distribution. As with aerosol photometers, many practical instruments have evolved within this category and have been widely used in research, both in laboratories and in workplaces. The Fibrous Aerosol Monitor is a version that sets out to provide counts of fibrous particles that conform to the respirable fiber definition (as discussed earlier), even in the presence of nonfibrous particles.

A wide range of other types of direct-reading instruments is available. One is based on the beta-attenuation concept, in which the mass of particulate material deposited on a filter or some other surface is determined by the reduction in intensity of beta-particles passing through the accumulated layer. In such instruments, the change in attenuation reflects the rate at which particles collect on the filter and, hence, on the concentration of the sampled aerosol. One advantage of this approach over optical instruments is that the attenuation of beta-particles is directly dependent on particulate mass and is almost independent of aerosol type or particle size distribution.

Another class of devices is what might be referred to as "vibrational mass balances," the most common of which is the piezo-balance. It is well known that the frequency of mechanical oscillation of a piezoelectric crystal (e.g., quartz) is directly proportional to the mass of the crystal. A change in the effective mass of the crystal, such as that caused by the deposition of particles on its surface, is reflected in the change in its mechanical resonance frequency.

Table 9–1
■
Short Summary of the Various Practical Aerosol Samplers Referred to in This Text and Their Availability

Sampler	Aerosol Fraction	Source
Open filter (static)	Coarse	Negretti Automation
MRE (static)	Coarse/respirable	Casella
TBF50 (static)	Coarse/respirable	Not known
IOM (static)	Inhalable	Negretti Automation
Open filter (personal)	Coarse	Gelman
Single hole (personal)	Coarse	Casella
Seven hole (personal)	Coarse	Casella, Negretti Automation
37 mm (personal)	Coarse	SKC, Millipore
CIP10 (personal)	Coarse/respirable	MSA (France)
PERSPEC (personal)	Inhalable/thoracic/respirable	Lavoro e Ambiente (Italy)
IOM (personal)	Inhalable	SKC
British cyclone (personal)	Respirable	Casella, Negretti Automation, SKC
American cyclone (personal)	Respirable	MSA, Sensidyne, SKC
IOM (personal)	Inhalable/thoracic/respirable	Institute of Occupational Medicine (Edinburgh, UK)
Marple cascade impactor (personal)	All	Andersen Instruments Inc.
IOM inhalable dust spectrometer (personal)	All	Institute of Occupational Medicine (Edinburgh, UK)

For full details about the availability of these samplers, or about others not listed, see the ACGIH handbook on air sampling.[2]

COMMERCIAL AVAILABILITY

The availability of the instruments described earlier, whether commercially or otherwise, is summarized in Table 9–1. For the wider range of instruments not covered by this inevitably concise review, the ACGIH handbook on air sampling instrumentation[2] provides an excellent source of contacts.

REFERENCES

1. Vincent, J. H., Aerosol Sampling: Science and Practice. London, Wiley, 1989.
2. Hering, S. V., ed., Air Sampling Instruments for Evaluation of Atmospheric Contaminants, 7th ed. Cincinnati, American Conference of Governmental Industrial Hygienists, 1989.
3. Ogden, T. L., and Birkett, J. L., The human head as a dust sampler. In Walton, W. H., ed., Inhaled Particles IV. Oxford, Pergamon Press, 1977, pp. 93–105.
4. Vincent, J. H., and Mark, D., Applications of blunt sampler theory to the definition and measurement of inhalable dust. In Walton, W. H., ed., Inhaled Particles V. Oxford, Pergamon Press, 1982, pp. 3–19.
5. Armbruster, L., and Breuer, H., Investigations into defining inhalable dust. In Walton, W. H., ed., Inhaled Particles V. Oxford, Pergamon Press, 1982, pp. 21–32.
6. Vincent, J. H., Mark, D., Miller, B. G., Armbruster, L., and Ogden, T. L., Aerosol inhalability at higher windspeeds. J. Aerosol Sci., 21, 577, 1990.
7. International Standards Organisation, Air Quality—Particle Size Fraction Definitions for Health-Related Sampling. Technical Report ISO/TR/7708–1983 (E). Geneva, International Standards Organisation, 1983.
8. American Conference of Governmental Industrial Hygienists, Particle Size-Selective Sampling in the Workplace. Report of the ACGIH Technical Committee on Air Sampling Procedures. Cincinnati, American Conference of Governmental Industrial Hygienists, 1985.
9. Soderholm, S. C., Proposed international conventions for particle size-selective sampling. Ann. Occup. Hyg., 33, 301, 1989.
10. Rappaport, S. M., Assessment of long-term exposures to toxic substances in air. Ann. Occup. Hyg., 35, 61, 1990.
11. Walton, W. H., Theory of size classification of airborne dust clouds by elutriation. Br. J. Appl. Phys., 5 (Suppl.), S29, 1954.

12. Mark, D., Vincent, J. H., and Gibson, H., A new static sampler for airborne total dust in workplaces. Am. Ind. Hyg. Assoc. J., 46, 127, 1985.
13. Mark, D., and Vincent, J. H., A new personal sampler for airborne total dust in workplaces. Ann. Occup. Hyg., 30, 89, 1986.
14. Dunmore, J. H., Hamilton, R. J., and Smith, D. S. G., An instrument for the sampling of respirable dust for subsequent gravimetric assessment. J. Sci. Instrum., 41, 669, 1964.
15. Courbon, P., Wrobel, R., and Fabries, J. -F., A new individual respirable dust sampler: the CIP10. Ann. Occup. Hyg., 32, 129, 1988.
16. Johnston, A. M., Jones, A. D., and Vincent, J. H., The influence of external aerodynamic factors on the measurement of the airborne concentration of asbestos fibres using the membrane filter method. Ann. Occup. Hyg., 26, 309, 1982.
17. Asbestos International Association, Recommended Technical Method No. 1: Reference Method for the Determination of Airborne Asbestos Fibre Concentrations at Workplaces by Light Microscopy (Membrane Filter Method). London, Asbestos International Association Health and Safety Publication, 1979.
18. Prodi, V., Belosi, F., and Mularoni, A., A personal sampler following ISO recommendations on particle size definitions. J. Aerosol Sci., 17, 576, 1986.
19. Mark, D., Borzucki, G., Lynch, G., and Vincent, J. H., The Development of a Personal Sampler for Inspirable, Thoracic and Respirable Aerosol. Presented at the Annual Conference of the Aerosol Society, Bournemouth, UK, March 1988.
20. Vincent, J. H., and Mark, D., Inhalable dust spectrometers as versatile samplers for studying dust-related health effects. Ann. Occup. Hyg., 28, 117, 1984.
21. Mark, D., Vincent, J. H., Gibson, H., Aitken, R. J., and Lynch, G., The development of an inhalable dust spectrometer. Ann. Occup. Hyg., 28, 125, 1984.
22. Vincent, J. H., Joint Investigations of New Generations of Dust Measuring Instruments for the Mining Industry. Synthesis Report of a Five-Nation Research Project Carried Out on Behalf of the European Coal and Steel Community. Luxembourg, Commission of European Communities, 1991.
23. Rubow, K. L., Marple, V. A., Loin, J., and McCawley, M. A., A personal cascade impactor: design, evaluation and calibration. Am. Ind. Hyg. Assoc. J., 48, 532, 1987.
24. Gibson, H., Mark, D., and Vincent, J. H., A personal inspirable dust spectrometer for applications in occupational hygiene research. Ann. Occup. Hyg., 31, 463, 1987.
25. Hodkinson, J. R., The optical measurement of aerosols. In Davies, C. N., ed., Aerosol Science. London, Academic Press, 1966.

10

Brian Boehlecke

Respiratory Protection

■

In workplace situations in which available environmental control technology cannot reduce airborne concentrations of toxic materials to safe levels, the use of personal respiratory protective devices (respirators) may be necessary. Respirators are especially useful for protection during brief or unusual exposures, such as may occur during accidental release of toxic agents or short-term work in an area with unavoidably high concentrations of an inhalant. The use of respirators should not be considered an acceptable alternative to engineering control measures that prevent atmospheric contamination, such as enclosure of operations, exhaust ventilation, or substitution of less toxic materials, when these measures are feasible.[1] This chapter will present some basic considerations in providing an effective personal respiratory protection program. More comprehensive discussions can be found elsewhere.[2-5]

Determination of the need for a respirator program must be based on a thorough assessment of the potential respiratory hazards of the workplace. The information to be reviewed includes the toxicological effects of all airborne contaminants, the relationship of airborne concentrations to established permissible exposure levels, and the projected duration of exposure. Work practices and engineering controls should be reviewed to determine if changes could reduce worker exposure to toxic materials to acceptable levels without the use of respirators. If this is not possible, an appropriate type of respirator should be sought. Selecting a respirator requires detailed information on the toxic agents involved and the legal requirements of governmental agencies that regulate the use of respiratory protective devices.[6, 7]

SELECTION OF A RESPIRATOR

Types of Respirators

The first step in developing an adequate respiratory protection program is to identify the type of respirator that, if used properly, is capable of reducing exposure to toxic materials to acceptable levels. Air-purifying respirators simply remove contaminants from ambient air, usually by filtration or adsorption, while atmosphere-supplying respirators provide a separate source of breathable gas. Clearly, if the ambient air is deficient in oxygen, only atmosphere-supplying respirators provide sufficient protection. Various agencies concerned with respiratory protection have defined oxygen deficiency differently, with oxygen contents of from 16.5% to 19.5% used as the lower limit for nonoxygen-deficient air. Even if the legal limit for oxygen deficiency in the applicable regulation is not exceeded, if the *potential* for reduced oxygen content exists, a medical judgment on the risk to the worker is necessary. The factors to be considered include the duration of exposure, the physical exertion required during exposure, and medical conditions present. Atmosphere-supplying respirators should be used if a risk of adverse health consequences is judged to be present due to reduced oxygen content. If oxygen deficiency is not present, air-purifying respirators may provide adequate protection, depending on the nature of the contaminant and its concentration.

Air-purifying respirators remove contaminants by passing inhaled air either through a fibrous filter to remove particulates, through a chemical sorbent to remove gaseous substances, or through a combination of both. Particulate removal depends upon the deposition of the particles on the filter by impaction, interception, or diffusion. The efficiency of entrapment is increased by using smaller diameter fibers more densely packed, but this increases resistance to air flow and thus makes inhalation more difficult. Excessive inspiratory efforts can be avoided by using powered respirators in which air is forced through the filter by a blower. Electrostatically charged resin coating of the fiber can also increase efficiency, but high temperatures and humidity or liquid aerosols (mists) destroy the effectiveness of this type of filter. Clearly, the size distribution and concentration of particles, as well as the volume of air inhaled per minute, influence the amount of particulate contaminant that passes through the filter. The removal efficiency of filters usually increases as the particulate load on the filter increases, but this also increases the resistance to air flow. Gases can be removed by chemical reaction, absorption, or adsorption. Activated charcoal is a commonly used sorbent, and other materials may be added to increase the removal of specific contaminants (e.g., iodine to remove mercury vapor). The ability of sorbents to remove gases and vapors diminishes as saturation occurs, and eventually the contaminant "breaks through." Sorbent canisters containing drying agents to protect the sorbent may have indicators which change color to warn of saturation of the drying agent, but the sorbent may become saturated before the drying agent. Warning of a breakthrough may occur if the worker notices an odor, a taste, or an irritative effect of the contaminant being inhaled. A contaminant is considered to have adequate warning properties if it can be detected in concentrations not greater than the permissible exposure limit (PEL). In the United States, federal regulations prohibit the use of air-purifying respirators for protection from organic vapors if the threshold concentration for warning is greater than three times the PEL.[7] For compounds with warning thresholds between one and three times the PEL, air-purifying respirators are acceptable only if it is determined that serious or irreversible adverse health effects do not occur from undetected exposure.

Performance Specifications

The efficiency of contaminant removal by filters and sorbents is measured directly as part of standardized certification testing of respirators performed by the National Institute for Occupational Safety and Health (NIOSH) at its Appalachian Laboratory for Occupational Safety and Health in Morgantown, West Virginia. For example, filters designed to provide protection from relatively nontoxic dusts must remove 99% of the suspended mass from 2.88 m^3 of air containing 50 mg/m^3 of silica dust, with particles averaging approximately 0.5 micron in aerodynamic diameter. High-efficiency filters for more toxic dusts must remove 99.97% of a test aerosol, with an average diameter of 0.3 micron at a concentration of 100 $\mu g/m^3$. Sorbents are tested with single or multiple gases, depending on their intended use. For example, cartridges to remove organic vapors must allow penetration of less than 5 parts per million (ppm) of carbon tetrachloride for at least 50 minutes when air containing 1000 ppm is passed through the cartridge at 32 L/min. This certification provides a basis for judging the effectiveness of the filters and sorbents under specific conditions but does not imply that the measured level of removal efficiency applies to all possible conditions under which the contaminants of concern may be encountered. Limitations of the NIOSH testing program and the problems that occur when a respirator is assumed to be equally effective under varying conditions have been described.[8]

To reduce the inhaled concentrations of a contaminant, a respirator must exclude nonfiltered air from being inhaled. Respirators may have quarter masks (covering the nose and mouth, but not extending below the chin), half masks (extending below the chin), or full masks (covering the entire face). Leakage of ambient air between the mask and face seal or through the one-way expiratory valve may occur during inspiration when pressure inside the mask is below ambient pressure. The amount of leakage depends on the effectiveness of the mask-to-face seal, the seating of the expiratory valve, and the pressure gradient across the mask. This gradient will be increased if resistance to inspiratory flow through the filter or sorbent cartridge is increased (e.g., because of dust loading or the use of more densely packed sorbent) or if the inspiratory flow rate is increased, as it may be during exertion. Even paint coating the exhalation valve can interfere with seating.[9] Leakage can thus be minimized by maintaining low inspiratory flow resistance, maintaining proper expiratory valve seating, and fitting respirator masks as closely as possible to individual users. Since masks are manufactured in a limited variety of sizes and shapes, a good match for the facial features of a given individual is not always possible. Crude but rapid-fit testing can be done each time a respirator is used by having the wearer inhale gently with the inlet of the respirator occluded to detect gross leakage. With appropriate sorbents in place, qualitative fit testing can also be done by exposing the wearer to vapors from isoamyl acetate (banana oil) or aerosols of stannic chloride which form by sublimation when this material is exposed to air. Detection of the characteristic odor of the former or the irritative effects of the latter indicates leakage. NIOSH also performs fit testing as part of the certification testing procedure and publishes lists of equipment meeting the current standards.[10, 11]

The same considerations concerning inspiratory leakage of ambient air apply to supplied atmosphere–type respirators. These respirators may use a continuous flow of air from the source or air may be supplied on demand through a valve that opens when pressure inside the mask drops at the onset of inspiration. Theoretically, inspiratory leakage can be eliminated in these types of respirators by providing a continuous flow that exceeds the maximal inspiratory flow of the wearer or by using a pressure-demand valve that maintains a positive pressure inside the mask at all times. However, with heavy exertion, the inspiratory flow may exceed the system's capacity to maintain a positive pressure, thereby creating the potential for inward leakage.[12] These methods of maintaining positive pressure inside the mask require more air from the source per minute than lower flow continuous or demand-type systems. If the source is a compressed cylinder, the useful life of the cylinder is thus reduced.

Protective Factors

The overall protective factor of a respirator is defined as the ratio of the concentration of an airborne contaminant outside the respirator mask to that inside the respirator. This factor reflects both filter or sorbent efficiency and the effectiveness of exclusion of ambient air by valves and the mask-to-face seal. Quantitative fit testing and measurement of the protection factor achieved can be done by sampling from within the mask of specially adapted respirators during exposure to a known concentration of a test aerosol, such as sodium chloride, in a test chamber or hood. Protection factors have been measured directly for different types of respirators with the various mask configurations by using a panel of persons to represent the variety of facial configurations in the work force.[13]

Protection factors representative of various types of respirators are listed in Table 10–1. These factors should be considered only approximate guidelines for the capabilities of a given class of respirator. Some respirators have achieved desired protection factors in only 61% of male and 22% of female subjects when

Table 10–1

■

Representative Respirator Protection Factors

Type of Respirator	Protection Factor
I. Air-purifying type	
A. For protection from particulates	
1. Single-use dust or quarter-mask dust	5
2. Half-mask dust or high efficiency	10
3. Full facepiece, high efficiency	50
B. For protection from gases or vapors	
1. Half-mask	10
2. Full facepiece	50
II. Atmosphere-supplying type	
1. Demand valve with half-mask	10
2. Demand valve with full facepiece	50
3. Pressure-demand valve with half-mask	1000
4. Pressure-demand valve with full facepiece	2000

Modified from Pritchard, J. A.; A Guide to Industrial Respiratory Protection. NIOSH 76-189. Washington, D.C., U.S. Department of Health, Education, and Welfare, 1976.

tested under laboratory conditions.[14] Protection in a laboratory setting and true protection in a work situation may not be comparable.[15] Other workers have found that certain demand-type atmosphere-supplying respirators performed poorly, giving protection factors less than 5 in some individuals.[16] Because the protection provided was less than that of air-purifying respirators for most of the respirators tested, the authors recommended that demand-type atmosphere-supplying respirators not be used.

Consideration of important factors in selecting the appropriate respiratory protective equipment for a given workplace condition can be done in a systematic manner by using the decision logic approach developed jointly by the Occupational Safety and Health Administration (OSHA) and NIOSH.[2] Current OSHA regulations should be consulted for applicable legal requirements, and detailed technical considerations are also available in the latest American National Standards Institute document on respiratory protection.[1, 5, 6] A draft generic Respiratory Protection Standard has been prepared by OSHA but has not yet been issued. Important factors already discussed include the chemical and physical form of the hazard, its relative toxicity and warning properties, and the expected or measured workplace concentration.

A determination of whether the hazard poses an immediate danger to life or health (IDLH) must also be made. An immediate danger is present if an unprotected worker is at risk to suffer death, immediate or delayed irreversible adverse health effects, or severe eye or respiratory tract irritation that could hamper escape with less than 30 minutes of exposure.[7] Regardless of their protection factors, air-purifying respirators are not considered acceptable for use in IDLH conditions. The need for protection from less severe eye irritation or cutaneous absorption of systemic toxins should also be considered. Also important is the worker's activity while wearing the respirator. Will respirator use be continuous or only for emergency escape? What is the duration of use, and what type of physical exertion and mobility is required? Once this information is available, the decision logic referred to earlier can be used to assist in the selection of an appropriate type of respirator.

RESPIRATORY PROTECTION PROGRAM

Merely providing workers with respirators does not constitute an adequate respiratory protection program. Individual fitting should be done to be sure that facial deformities, eyeglasses, or facial hair does not prevent a proper mask-to-face

Table 10–2

■

Components of Worker Training for Use of Respirators

I. Explanation of the need for respirators
A. Nature of the respiratory hazard
B. Reasons that environmental controls are not sufficient
C. Risks if protection not used properly
D. Details of when respirators are to be used
II. Instruction in use
A. Bases for selection and capabilities of respirator used
B. Limitations and detection of inadequate protection
C. Basic operation and maintenance
D. Fitting and periodic fit testing
E. Recognition and procedures for emergencies
F. Administrative structure for surveillance of the respiratory protection program

seal. Conducting a training program, as outlined in Table 10–2, is important to achieve a high degree of worker acceptance, without which adequate protection cannot be achieved.

In situations in which the risk is from the cumulative effects of chronic exposure, the percentage of workers who use the respirators issued to them tends to be low.[17] Workers' beliefs about associated discomfort and co-workers' attitudes toward respirator wearers may be important factors affecting use.[18] Even in more immediately threatening conditions, use may be intermittent, with little or no actual protection achieved.[19] Worker compliance with procedures for use should be monitored and equipment periodically inspected. Monitoring of working conditions to detect changes that might necessitate an alteration in respiratory protection should also be done continuously. Important factors include changes in workplace concentrations of airborne contaminants, the addition of new contaminants, and changes in work practices, such as longer durations of exposure or increased exertion during exposure. Naturally, these measures do not obviate the need for medical surveillance to detect adverse health effects indicating that protection is insufficient despite an apparently adequate respiratory protection program.

MEDICAL EFFECTS OF RESPIRATOR USE

Wearing respiratory protective equipment is itself an added stress for the worker, and OSHA regulations require that a worker not be assigned to a task requiring a respirator unless the individual is physically able to perform the work and use the equipment.[1] However, it is left to the responsible physician to decide what health and physical conditions are pertinent and the criteria for the ability to use a respirator. The physiological consequences of wearing industrial respirators have been reviewed elsewhere,[20, 21] but it is clear that physicians making these decisions must still rely on overall clinical judgment.

The added resistance to breathing that results from wearing a respirator is likely to prolong the duration of the obstructed phase of respiration and decrease the minute ventilation of the wearer, both at rest and during exercise.[22–25] Whether this in turn leads to significant gas exchange abnormalities probably depends on the amount of added resistance to flow, the duration and intensity of exertion, the wearer's underlying respiratory capacity, and the functioning of the respiratory drive control system.[22–34] Transient reductions in arterial blood oxygen tension and more persistent elevations in arterial carbon dioxide content have been observed in normal subjects exercising with added external resistance to breathing. Maximal allowable levels for resistance to air flow are set forth in the NIOSH certification criteria for respirators.[7] Measured at a steady flow of 85 L/min, acceptable inspiratory resistance (measured as pressure) ranges from 5.0 cm H_2O for dust respirators to 8.5 cm H_2O for pesticide respirators. Expiratory resistance must be less than 2.0 cm H_2O for all types of air-purifying respirators. Requirements for atmosphere-supplying respirators are similar, but the pressure-demand type may have an expiratory resistance of 5.1 cm H_2O at 85 L/min. The pressure flow characteristics of respirators are such that higher flows cause a steep nonlinear increase in pressure drop (i.e., the resistance to flow increases at higher flows). Thus, higher flow rates, such as those used during heavy exertion, may be difficult to achieve wearing a respirator, even though breathing seems little affected at rest or with mild exertion. This is especially true for persons with airflow obstruction who have decreased expiratory flow rates and thus require more expiratory time during each breathing cycle to achieve the same tidal volume. As the respiratory rate is increased, the relative time for inspiration must be decreased. Thus, the inspiratory flow rates must be increased even more than would occur in a healthy person for the same total minute ventilation. This could result in a violation of the assumptions which have been used to determine acceptable levels of resistance for respiratory protective devices.[35] Adding external resistance has been shown to reduce the maximal voluntary ventilation (MVV) more for persons with airflow limitation than for healthy persons.[36] The percentage reduction in ventilation during exercise caused by added resistance has been shown to be similar to the percentage reduction in MVV at rest with the same added resistance.[25] Reductions in MVV of 18% to 32% have been demonstrated, with respirator resistances of 8.5 cm H_2O for inspiration and 2.5 cm H_2O for expiration at 85 L/min, and this test was suggested as the test of choice for determining a worker's capability for wearing an industrial respirator.[37] While possibly useful, this test is not likely to be sufficient by itself and was only weakly predictive of maximum work performance while wearing a respirator.[38] The physiological adaptations during exercise with added resistance are likely to be dependent on many factors, including respiratory drive, which may not be directly related to the ventilation achievable by a voluntary maximal effort.

Pulmonary Impairment and Respiratory Equipment

Federal regulations state that the wearer of a respirator "shall not experience undue discomfort because of airflow restriction. . . ."[7] The mechanism for unpleasant awareness of breathing is not clearly understood, but 10% of men who exercised with added inspiratory resistance experienced this symptom when peak inspiratory pressure exceeded 14 cm H_2O.[39] This is higher than would be likely to occur with most respirators in use, unless very high inspiratory flow rates were necessary. Only 2 of 41 coal miners older than the age of 45 years experienced respiratory symptoms while exercising for 15 minutes at moderately heavy workloads (6 to 7 times resting oxygen consumption), with added resistance equivalent to 20 cm H_2O at a flow of 85 L/min.[40] No symptoms occurred in 16 persons with "moderate" obstructive lung disease (ratio of forced expiratory volume in 1 second [FEV_1] to forced vital capacity [FVC] less than 0.70, but otherwise not specified) while exercising up to 63% of their maximal capacity wearing an industrial respirator with an inspiratory resistance of 8.5 cm H_2O at a flow of 85 L/min.[41] However, symptoms have not been found to be sensitive indicators of gas exchange alterations during exercise with added resistance.[23, 29] Twelve subjects with a mean FEV_1/FVC ratio of 60% showed small but statistically significant reductions in minute ventilation and elevations of end-tidal carbon dioxide concentration during mild exercise (3 to 4 times resting oxygen consumption), with an inspiratory resistance of approximately 5.6 cm H_2O at a flow of 85 L/min, but none reported unpleasant respiratory sensations when asked standardized questions after the exercise.[42] A small study of women with mild restrictive pulmonary impairment showed expected trends but no significant changes in respiratory or cardiac variables during exercise with resistive loading compared with the unloaded state, except for increased mouth pressure swings.[43] The impaired subjects rated exercise with added resistance as detectably different from the unloaded condition but not uncomfortable. Thus, it appears that slight alterations in ventilation and gas exchange may occur as a consequence of wearing currently available industrial respirators, but even persons with mild pulmonary impairment are not expected to experience respiratory symptoms during short periods of exercise using this equipment.

Other potential effects which may limit a worker's ability to wear respiratory protective equipment have not been as well studied.[20] The added dead space of respirators may lead to carbon dioxide retention, especially at high work rates and in persons with a blunted respiratory drive. However, added dead space appeared to have little effect on the subjective response of normal subjects while added resistance, especially inspiratory, correlated with discomfort.[44] Cardiovascular effects caused by altered intrathoracic pressures have been less well documented. Invasive monitoring failed to document impairment of cardiac output during heavy exercise with a positive pressure apparatus.[45] Generally, heart rates have been similar during exercise with and without added respiratory resistance,[41-43] but some researchers have reported higher rates with added resistance.[20] Systolic blood pressure has been reported to increase approximately 12 mm Hg both at rest and during exercise, when subjects wore respirators, with lesser effects on diastolic pressure.[41] Metabolic effects caused by decreased oxygen uptake or alterations in blood pH have not been documented. Increased thermal stress is an adverse consequence which is more likely with a full facepiece or more complete enclosures and impermeable clothing. Claustrophobia may be produced even by disposable single-use masks. Skin irritation can occur from any device that forms a tight seal with the face.

Personal psychological and psychophysiological characteristics may be important determinants of the perceived stress of wearing a respirator. The subjective response to added respiratory loads appears to vary widely among individuals.[7] One study found "trait anxiety" determined from questionnaire responses to be highly predictive of respiratory distress while wearing a self-contained breathing apparatus during heavy exertion,[46] but this has not been confirmed for other situations. Workers' beliefs about discomfort and other unpleasant consequences of respirator use may be more important determinants in actual workplace settings.[18] One study suggested that adaptation may develop over 3 days of use, resulting in increased endurance at a heavy workload while wearing the respirator.[47] However, there was little change in respiratory pattern or subjective assessment of discomfort or difficulty in performing the exertion over the 6 days of the study.

Several reviews have described approaches to the evaluation of workers for respirator use,[48-50] and the Committee on Occupational Medical Practice of the American Occupational Medicine Association has reported guidelines.[51] Unfortunately, no simple all-inclusive criteria can be given for deciding who can safely wear a respirator or for who will tolerate it under actual workplace conditions. The worker's ability to perform the job itself should be a primary consideration, with respirator wear considered to add additional physiological and psychological stress. Some elevation in blood pressure and a reduction in minute ventilation may occur. Alterations in gas exchange, with reduced arterial oxygen pressure and elevated carbon dioxide pressure, may occur in some individuals, especially those with impaired pulmonary function. The physician must use his or her overall medical judgment in determining whether workers with conditions such as chronic airflow limitation, hypertension, ischemic heart disease, diabetes, epilepsy, or psychological problems can safely tolerate the stress of respirator use. Workers assigned jobs requiring respirators should be given adequate training and monitored closely for signs of adverse reactions. Job pressures or inappropriate beliefs may prevent them from readily volunteering problems, and ineffective intermittent use may result.

In summary, respirators are useful in providing adequate protection from respiratory hazards when engineering controls cannot reduce worker exposure to acceptable levels. Proper selection requires careful consideration of the nature of the hazard and the type of work to be performed while wearing the respirator. An adequate respiratory protection program must also include administrative and technical procedures to ensure proper training of the workers and continued medical and industrial hygiene surveillance. Information on the medical consequences of respirator use is incomplete but suggests that current respirators can be worn for brief periods of moderate exertion without causing undue distress or adverse physiological effects in healthy persons and those with only mild respiratory impairment. Use for longer durations, with more severe exertion, or by persons with psychological or other chronic medical conditions requires more thorough evaluation.

REFERENCES

1. U.S. Code of Federal Regulations, Title 29, Part 1910.134(a)(1), Respiratory Protection.
2. Pritchard, J. A., A Guide to Industrial Respiratory Protection. NIOSH 76–189. Washington, D.C., U.S. Department of Health, Education, and Welfare, 1976.
3. Douglas, D., Respiratory protective devices. *In* Clayton, G. D., and Clayton, F. E., eds., Patty's Industrial Hygiene and Toxicology. New York, John Wiley & Sons, 1985.
4. Lundin, A., Respiratory protective equipment. *In* Olishifski, J. B., ed., Fundamentals of Industrial Hygiene. Chicago, National Safety Council, 1979.
5. Standard Practices for Respiratory Protection. ANSI 88.2–1980 DRAFT (1988). New York, American National Standards Institute, 1988.
6. U.S. Code of Federal Regulations, Title 29, Part 1910.1000(e), Air Contamination Standards.
7. U.S. Code of Federal Regulations, Title 30, Part II, Respiratory Protective Devices; Tests for Permissibility; Fees.
8. Moyer, E. S., Review of influential factors affecting the performance of organic vapor air-purifying respirator cartridges. Am. Ind. Hyg. Assoc. J., 44, 45, 1983.
9. Bellin, P., and Hinds, W. C., Aerosol penetration through respirator exhalation valves. Am. Ind. Hyg. Assoc. J., 51, 555, 1990.
10. NIOSH Certified Equipment List. NIOSH 80–144. Washington, D.C., U.S. Dept. of Health and Human Services, 1980.
11. Supplement to NIOSH Certified Equipment List. NIOSH 82–106. Washington, D.C., U.S. Dept. of Health and Human Services, 1981.
12. Dahlback, G. O., and Novak, L., Do pressure-demand breathing systems safeguard against inward leakage? Am. Ind. Hyg. Assoc. J., 44, 336, 1983.
13. Hack, A. L., Hyatt, E. C., Held, B., et al., Selection of respirator test panels representative of U.S. adult facial sizes. Los Alamos Scientific Laboratory Report, #LA-5488. Los Alamos, NM, March 1974.
14. Hyatt, E. C., Respirator protection factors. Los Alamos Scientific Laboratory Report, #LA-6084-MS, January 1976.
15. Myers, W. R., Lenhart, S. W., Campbell, D., and Provost, G., Letter to the editor. Am. Ind. Hyg. Assoc. J., 44, B25, 1983.
16. Hack, A. L., Bradley, O. D., and Trujillo, A., Respirator protection factors: Part II—protection factors of supplied air respirators. Am. Ind. Hyg. Assoc. J., 41, 376, 1980.
17. Cotes, J. E., Advances in respiratory protection (conference report). Ann. Occup. Hyg., 22, 189, 1979.
18. White, M. C., Baker, E. L., Larson, M. B., and Wolford, R., The role of personal beliefs and social influences as determinants of respirator use among construction painters. Scand. J. Work Environ. Health, 14, 239, 1988.
19. Levine, M., Respirator use and protection from exposure to carbon monoxide. Am. Ind. Hyg. Assoc. J., 40, 832, 1979.
20. Raven, P. B., Dodson, A. T., and Davis, T. O., The physiologic consequences of wearing industrial respirators: a review. Am. Ind. Hyg. Assoc. J., 40, 517, 1979.
21. Harber, P., Brown, C. L., and Beck, J. G., Respirator physiology research: answers in search of the question. J. Occup. Med., 33, 38, 1991.
22. Zechman, F., Hall, F. G., and Hull, W. E., Effects of graded resistance to tracheal air flow in man. J. Appl. Physiol., 10, 356, 1957.
23. Gee, J. B. L., Burton, G., Vassallo, C., and Gregg, J., Effects of external airway obstruction on work capacity and pulmonary gas exchange. Am. Rev. Respir. Dis., 98, 1003, 1968.
24. Cerretelli, P., Sikand, R. S., and Farhi, L. E., Effect of increased airway resistance on ventilation and gas exchange during exercise. J. Appl. Physiol., 27, 597, 1969.
25. Tabakin, B. S., and Hanson, J. S., Lung volume and ventilatory response to airway obstruction during treadmill exercise. J. Appl. Physiol., 20, 168, 1965.
26. Tabakin, B. S., and Hanson, J. S., Response to ventilatory obstruction during steady-state exercise. J. Appl. Physiol., 15, 579, 1960.
27. Demedts, M., and Anthonisen, N. R., Effects of increased external airway resistance during steady-state exercise. J. Appl. Physiol., 35, 361, 1973.
28. Flook, V., and Kelman, G. R., Submaximal exercise with increased inspiratory resistance to breathing. J. Appl. Physiol., 35, 379, 1973.

29. Silverman, L., and Billings, C. E., Pattern of airflow in the respiratory tract. *In* Davis, C. N., ed., Inhaled Particles and Vapours. New York, Pergamon Press, pp. 9–46.
30. Thompson, S. H., and Sharkey, B. J., Physiological cost and air flow resistance of respiratory protective devices. Ergonomics, 9, 495, 1966.
31. Cherniack, R. M., and Snidal, D. P., The effect of obstruction of breathing on the ventilatory response to CO_2. J. Clin. Invest., 35, 1286, 1956.
32. Milic-Emili, J., and Tyler, J. M., Relation between work output of respiratory muscles and end-tidal CO_2 tension. J. Appl. Physiol., 18, 497, 1963.
33. Clark, T. J. H., and Cochrane, G. M., Effect of mechanical loading on ventilatory response to CO_2 and CO_2 excretion. B.M.J., 1, 351, 1972.
34. Flenley, D. C., Pengelly, L. D., and Milic-Emili, J., Immediate effects of positive-pressure breathing on the ventilatory response to CO_2. J. Appl. Physiol., 30, 7, 1971.
35. Cooper, E. A., Suggested methods of testing and standards of resistance for respiratory protective devices. J. Appl. Physiol., 15, 1053, 1960.
36. Zwi, S., Theron, J. C., McGregor, M., and Becklake, M. R., The influence of instrumental resistance on the maximum breathing capacity. Dis. Chest, 36, 361, 1959.
37. Raven, P. B., Moss, R. F., Page, K., et al., Clinical pulmonary function and industrial respirator wear. Am. Ind. Hyg. Assoc. J., 42, 897, 1981.
38. Wilson, J. R., and Raven, P. B., Clinical pulmonary function tests as predictors of work performance during respirator wear. Am. Ind. Hyg. Assoc. J., 50, 51, 1989.
39. Bentley, R. A., Griffin, O. G., Love, R. G., et al., Acceptable levels for breathing resistance of respiratory apparatus. Arch. Environ. Health, 27, 273, 1973.
40. Love, R. G., Muir, D. C. F., Sweetland, K. F., et al., Acceptable levels for breathing resistance of respiratory apparatus: results for men over the age of 45. Br. J. Ind. Med., 34, 126, 1977.
41. Raven, P. B., Jackson, A. W., Page, K., et al., The physiologic responses of mild pulmonary impaired subjects while using a ''demand'' respirator during rest and work. Am. Ind. Hyg. Assoc. J., 42, 247, 1981.
42. Hodous, T., Petsonk, E. L., Boyles, C., et al., Effects of added resistance to breathing during exercise in obstructive lung disease. Am. Rev. Respir. Dis., 128, 943, 1983.
43. Hodous, T. K., Boyles, C., and Hankinson, J., Effects of industrial respiratory wear during exercise in subjects with restrictive lung disease. Am. Ind. Hyg. Assoc. J., 47, 176, 1986.
44. Shimozaki, S., Harber, P., Barrett, T., and Loisides, P., Subjective tolerance of respiratory loads and its relationship to physiologic effects. Am. Ind. Hyg. Assoc. J., 49, 108, 1988.
45. Arboreluis, M., Dahlback, G. O., and Data, P. C., Cardiac output and gas exchange during heavy exercise with a positive pressure respiratory protective apparatus. Scand. J. Work Environ. Health, 9, 471, 1983.
46. Morgan, W. P., and Raven, P. B., Prediction of distress for individuals wearing industrial respirators. Am. Ind. Hyg. Assoc. J., 46, 363, 1985.
47. Epstein, Y., Keren, G., Lerman, Y., and Shefer, A., Physiological and psychological adaptation to respiratory protection devices. Aviat. Space Environ. Med., 53, 663, 1982.
48. Harber, P., Medical evaluation for respirator use. J. Occup. Med., 26, 496, 1984.
49. Hodous, T. K., Screening prospective workers for the ability to use respirators. J. Occup. Med., 28, 1074, 1986.
50. Beckett, W. S., Certifying the worker for respirator use. Semin. Occup. Med., 1, 119, 1986.
51. Committee on Occupational Medical Practice–American Occupational Medicine Association, Guidelines for respirator users. J. Occup. Med., 28, 72, 1986.

Basic Mechanisms in Occupational Lung Diseases Including Lung Cancer and Mesothelioma

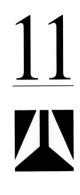

J. Bernard L. Gee

Brooke T. Mossman

This chapter addresses important basic biological mechanisms in two groups of occupational disorders. The first is the "interstitial" disorders primarily involving the alveolocapillary units, even though they affect alveolar ducts and bronchioles and the relevant lymphoid system is largely extra-alveolar. We will not address primary airway disorders except insofar as our second concerns are mechanisms of lung cancer and mesothelioma. Cellular and molecular mechanisms of asbestos- and silica-associated diseases are emphasized here based on our clinical and basic research expertise and interests.

INTERSTITIAL DISEASES

These disorders may entail or include acute lung injuries, pulmonary edema, chronic inflammatory processes, and granulomatous and fibrous lung disorders. The approach is based on the general principle that much pathology derives from subversion of both the normal lung defenses and the healing mechanisms, resulting in injury cascades and disordered repair. We focus on cellular and matrix mechanisms and on the inflammatory cellular processes. To understand these mechanisms, it is necessary to understand the recent advances in our knowledge of surface molecules, on both cells and matrix, and the way in which these and other cellular products orchestrate specific functions. These adherence molecules and interleukins are particularly important in regulating inflammatory and healing processes. There are many excellent texts on pulmonary disorders, but for our purposes perhaps the most useful are the two volumes edited by Crystal and West,[1] which include much information on lung cell biology.

Alveolocapillary Unit: Injury and Repair

Structural Cells

One may, somewhat artificially, divide lung tissue cells into primarily structural (mesenchymal) and primarily immunoinflammatory subgroups. While this may be convenient, all cells are obviously biochemically active, and we address later the inflammatory and repair processes mediated by such structural lung cells as endothelial cells and fibroblasts.

Figure 11–1 depicts the structure of the alveolocapillary units by electron microscopy. The alveolar surface is lined by type I epithelial cells, which are flattened and have a large surface area, thus providing a suitable framework for gas exchange. Little is known about the biochemistry of these epithelial cells, which do not undergo mitosis. Tight junctions between neighboring type I cells and also with

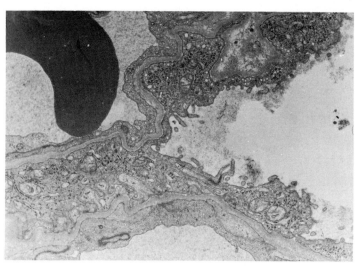

Figure 11–1. Structure of alveolocapillary unit as shown by electron microscopy.

a subjacent second lung cell type (type II) occur. Review of the nature of these junctions and their role in water solute exchange may be found elsewhere. The junctions between type I and type II cells are a common location for the migration from capillary to lung air spaces of polymorphonuclear neutrophils (PMNs) following intra-alveolar inflammatory states.

The second cell type mentioned, the type II cell, tends to occur in the alveolar corners. When these cells mature, they are characterized by the presence of lamellar bodies (Fig. 11–2). Type II cells derive from a primitive cuboidal epithelium which invades the mesenchyme at an early embryological stage. The mesenchyme is necessary for the next type II maturation step: when near term, the type II cells both mature and differentiate. This maturation is characterized by the appearance initially of glycogen and later of lamellar bodies with surfactant secretion. The maturation is promoted by corticosteroids, thyroxine, and other substances, but depressed by androgens via a fibroblast (FB) pneumocyte factor[2] and by the mullerian inhibiting substance, a glycoprotein derived from the testicular Sertoli cells.[3] These type II cells also differentiate into type I cells. Both maturation and differ-

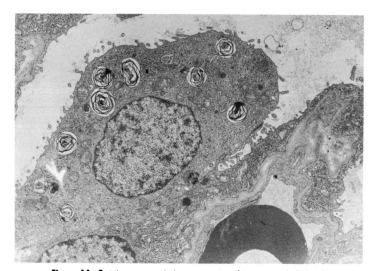

Figure 11–2. Ultrastructural characteristics of type II epithelial cell.

entiation are partly controlled by a fibroblast-derived peptide. These later embryological developments form the basis for one function of type II cells in the adult
lung, where they also serve to regenerate type I cells. This process is relatively
slow in normal lungs but provides a rapid repair mechanism following alveolar
injury. Studies employing low levels of toxic gases such as nitrogen dioxide[4] have
shown that injury to type I cells following inhalation of oxidants leads to hyperplasia and proliferation of type II cells with their subsequent differentiation into type
I cells (Fig. 11–3). These studies have employed tritiated thymidine as a tracer to
show that differentiation and complete type II cell turnover occurs within 2 to 4
days following acute airspace injury. Type II cell hyperplasia also occurs with
ozone (O_3), hyperoxia, asbestos, and silica.[5, 6]

Some *in vitro* studies have demonstrated that type II cells only retain normal
morphology when grown on basement membranes and do not function well when
grown on a collagenous stroma lacking a basement membrane. Among the affected
functions are the production of surfactant, organization into a monolayer, and
probably the production by type II cells of a basement membrane. Much remains
to be done to define the surface characteristics that best serve these type II cell
functions, but it is already clear that repair following injury critically depends on
the cell–basement membrane surface relationship.

Endothelial cells (ECs) form the equivalent in the capillaries of the air surface
type I cells. They constitute 40% of all pulmonary cells. In healthy lungs, about
1% of endothelial cells turn over each day. Following injury, these cells rapidly
proliferate and can readily repopulate the basement membrane and synthesize its
materials. Pure lines of such cells are available from a number of larger blood
vessels, including pulmonary vasculature and umbilical cords. Thus, much more is
known about them; for instance, they synthesize clotting factor VIII.[7] While these
cells have an extensive surface area with flattened cytoplasm, as do type I cells,
they additionally increase their surface area by the presence of small almost spherical indentations termed caveolae on the blood surface of the cell. Studies by Ryan
and Ryan[8] have demonstrated the caveolae to be the site of many surface ectoen-
zymes, such as those responsible for the degradation of serotonin, prostaglandins,
and adrenergic compounds. Additionally, angiotensin converting enzyme (ACE) is
also localized at this site and degrades both angiotensin I (to angiotensin II) and
bradykinin. Both actions involve the removal of two C-terminal amino acids from
oligopeptides, and hence this enzyme is a generalized dipeptidyl peptidase. The
large surface area and cell surface enzymes enhance not only alveolocapillary gas

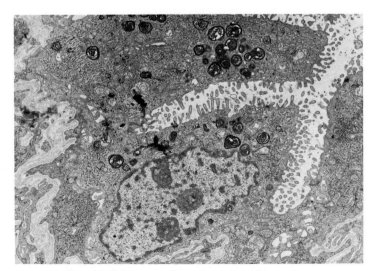

Figure 11–3. Depiction of type II epithelial cell hyperplasia.

exchange but also vascular clearance of chemical mediators of inflammation. ECs also play key roles in inflammatory reactions, which are discussed later. Pericytes with contractile properties are associated with ECs.

The alveolocapillary interstitium contains such mesenchymal cells as fibroblasts and smooth muscle cells (SMCs). The cells are part of the connective tissue system and are a source of matrix materials, which is described later. The fibroblast is paradoxically capable of generating both collagen and a specific collagenase[9] which attacks collagen types I and III. Fibroblasts are also phagocytic cells. Uptake of particles (e.g., latex) promotes the release of collagenase and other proteases. Fibroblast function is regulated by the interleukins (ILs) (see later discussion). Both cell types proliferate in interstitial pulmonary fibrosis. Additionally, myofibroblasts, cells with contractile properties and probably related to SMC, also proliferate in idiopathic pulmonary fibrosis (IPF).

These cells and their response to injury have been succinctly reviewed.[2, 10] In certain acute-onset occupational lung diseases, both type I epithelial cells and endothelial cells are injured. For instance, they are damaged by oxidant gases (NO_2, O_3), paraquat, chlorine, phosgene, acid mists, and such materials as sublimates of cadmium and mercury. This damage is manifest as a capillary leak pulmonary edema. When the damage is not fatal, the repair processes often lead to complete recovery, but an obliterative fibrosing terminal bronchiolitis and alveolitis can also result.

Studies have also emphasized that the alveolocapillary units also leak in the early phases of such chronic diseases as asbestosis.[11] In a sheep model, intratracheal asbestos instillation causes transudation of albumin and transferrin from blood to air spaces. This can readily be demonstrated with intravenous radioactive gallium scanning. Gallium largely binds to transferrin. Following its appearance in the air space, the gallium is sequestered in the alveolar macrophage (AM); a similar phenomenon occurs in both idiopathic and asbestos-induced pulmonary fibrosis.

Type II cells are more resistant to injury; their role in tissue repair is discussed in detail later. In some patients with silicosis, bronchoalveolar lavage (BAL) has shown many type II cells to be present. The significance of this observation is unclear, but there are reports of a proliferative type II cell response and alveolar proteinosis in acute experimental silicosis.

Matrix Components

The extracellular matrix of the lung parenchyma consists of a basement membrane on which alveolar epithelial cells rest, a second basement membrane on which endothelial cells reside, and a collagenous interstitium separating these two membranes. In certain regions, known as the thin segments of the capillary loop, these two membranes fuse. These structural components form a scaffold on which normal cell function is maintained and an architectural framework for normal repair after injury.

The extracellular matrix of the alveolar wall consists of four broad classes of structural macromolecules: (1) collagen types I, III, IV, and so on; (2) noncollagenous glycoproteins (e.g., laminin and fibronectin); (3) elastin; and (4) proteoglycans.

COLLAGENS

There are fourteen genetically distinct varieties of collagen, all of which contain hydroxyproline.[12] Types I and III collagens form triple helix fibrils and are located in the interstitium of the lung. Types IV and V do not form fibrils and contain helical collagenous, as well as noncollagenous, globular domains. The fibrillar character of collagen, in general, requires the preservation of a glycine occurring as every third amino acid in the collagen molecule sequence. In type IV collagen, the glycine content constitutes less than one third of the amino acids, and there are interruptions in the tertiary repetition of glycine. Type IV collagen is exclusively found in the basement membrane. Type V has both a basement membrane and interstitial localization. Type II collagen is found only in cartilaginous tissues and therefore is not a component of the alveolar wall.

Collagen makes up about 65% of the normal lung connective tissue. There is a 2.5-fold increase in the collagen content of fibrotic lungs when compared to normal ones. In IPF, there are profound changes in the distribution of the various collagens. There is an increase in type I collagen in thickened alveolar septa and a concomitant disappearance of type III collagen from that location. Type V collagen content is increased and found around smooth muscle cell clusters. Only type IV collagen in the basement membrane appears unchanged in both location and extractable amounts. No measurements of collagen composition are available in such occupational lung fibroses as asbestosis.

NONCOLLAGENOUS PROTEINS: LAMININ AND FIBRONECTIN

These two proteins are important in that they can interact with both collagens and cell surfaces and thereby function as adhesive agents. Laminin, a large protein of molecular weight 1 million, spontaneously forms aggregations.[13] The molecule has a cruciate shape with irregular arms, and its amino acid composition is known. These arms serve as cross-linking agents to other proteins and cell surfaces. Laminin has an exclusive basement location, where it has been demonstrated to play a role in the attachments of such cells as liver epithelial cells. FBs have both laminin receptors and fibronectin receptors. The precise role of laminin in the lung is presently unclear.

The fibronectins are somewhat smaller than laminin. Fibronectin in its dimeric, near-linear form has a molecular weight of 450,000. It has been found in both the interstitium and the basement membrane, as well as in plasma. Several molecular domains exist within this linear molecule, with separate binding sites for collagen, heparin, fibrin, and other fibronectin molecules and for cell surfaces. Fibronectin is produced by endothelial cells, platelets, fibroblasts, and macrophage lines. While fibronectins from various sources may exist in several minor molecular variations, a number of general functions are becoming clear. For instance, fibronectin in plasma serves as a general opsonin for phagocytosis by promoting nonspecific ''sticking'' of particulates to phagocyte cell surfaces. It thus differs from such immunospecific opsonic immunoglobulins as those produced in response to specific bacterial materials. Additionally, fibronectin has been shown to play a role in cell attachment, cellular shape, and differentiation of many mesenchymal cell lines. Fibronectin provides a surface upon which FBs can migrate; it also provides a FB chemotaxin. Additionally, fibronectin is itself a true chemoattractant for FBs which migrate toward increasing fibronectin concentration. Employing various proteolytic enzymes, one may separate fibronectin-fibroblast binding sites from those responsible for collagen-fibronectin interactions. Thus, as the name suggests, fibronectin can serve as a nexus relating cells to structural proteins.

Enhanced production of fibronectin by rodent AM occurs following the ingestion of certain forms of asbestos. The fibronectin content of BAL fluid is increased in IPF but does not appear to correlate with clinical progression in that disorder.[1] Fibronectin is a major component of the ''fibrous'' material of the lungs of patients with progressive massive fibrosis.[14]

ELASTIN

Electron microscopic observation of mature elastic fibers reveals two distinct components.[15] There is a microfibrillar tubular structure whose most important component is the 50-kD glycoprotein fibrillin. The molecule contains growth factor amino acid sequences, and the fibrillin gene on chromosome 15 is abnormal in Marfan's syndrome. The second component is amorphous under electron microscopy, appears to fill the spaces between the microfibrils, and contains the protein elastin. Elastin is difficult to solubilize, owing to its unusually high content of nonpolar amino acids and particularly to the presence of certain cross-linking amino acids, demosine and isodemosine. This cross-linking depends on the activity of a Cu^{2+}-containing enzyme, lysyl oxidase. The cellular origin and factors determining the architectural arrangement of lung elastin are poorly understood. Presumably, as in other tissues, lung elastin is generated by FBs and SMCs. Elastin is found in the noncapillary blood vessel linings and also in the basement membrane and lung interstitium. Elastinolysis and loss of elastic recoil are usually regarded as hallmarks of emphysema. The individual contributions of elastin and other matrix proteins to stress-strain lung mechanics are poorly understood, but it appears likely that elastin confers high extensibility and excellent recoil but low tensile strength. Fibrillar collagens probably confer limits to lung distensibility. Elastin degradation peptides are chemotactic for FBs.

PROTEOGLYCANS

These proteins have one or more attached, often large, glycosoaminoglycan chains, e.g., hyaluronate, heparan sulfate, heparin, and so on.[16-19] In the extracellular matrix, proteoglycans retain water, which they draw by osmosis from surrounding areas. Their linkages organize the matrix coating fibrous proteins. In the connective tissue matrix secreted *in vitro* by SMCs, removal of this coat is a prerequisite for specific enzymes to act on such fibrous proteins as elastin. In the basement membrane they act as charge-dependent filtration mechanisms. A family of proteoglycans, the syndecans, are an integral part of the cell membrane. They have a large, complex proteoglycan extracellular domain and a proteinase-sensitive region just outside the cell membrane, and the transmembrane domain ends intracellularly with three conserved tyrosine residues. These occur on epithelial cells and human lung fibroblasts and are subject to modulation by growth factors and cytokines. Syndecans, a family of integral membrane proteins, possess heparan and chondroitin sulfate chains. Syndecans bind cells to many fibrous proteins, forming a stable cohesive matrix, and probably play a role in cellular signal transduction via their tyrosine residues. Certain growth factors, e.g., epidermal and FB growth factors, bind to syndecans. For instance, endothelial cells release complexes of fibroblast growth factor heparan sulfate under the influence of plasminogen activator–mediated proteases. This may have two consequences. First, these complexes provide a surface-bound local growth factor reservoir which may be directly presented to other cells (e.g., FBs). Second, heparin (not heparan) released in acute inflammation causes mast cell mobilization and degranulation and also displaces heparan sulfate–bound growth factors. These features provide a matrix-derived focal repair mechanism.

Betaglycan is another proteoglycan found on mammalian cell membranes, where it functions as one of the beta-transforming growth factor (TGF_β) receptors. Other cell membrane proteoglycans include the descriptively termed thrombomodulin and the integrin family CD44 (see later discussion). The latter is important in lymphocyte homing and confers a "recognition signal" between lymphocytes and the high endothelial venule of lymphoid structures. CD_{44}, *inter alia*, is regulated by IL-5.

Inflammatory Cells

The sterility of the normal human lung requires many mechanisms, which include airway ciliary clearance, local humoral immune mechanisms (e.g., secretory IgA), and the native ability of AM to kill microorganisms in the lung air spaces. Additional factors maintaining lung sterility are the immunological responsiveness to previously encountered microorganisms as mediated by local lymphocyte populations, AM activation, and the recruitment of polymononuclear neutrophils (PMNs) into air spaces under acute inflammatory reactions associated with bacterial invasion. Detailed considerations of these defense mechanisms may be found elsewhere. This discussion will emphasize the inherent ability of the "normal" activities of these three cell types (PMNs, AMs, and lymphocytes) to cause lung injury. This potential is readily apparent in many lung diseases and is relevant to certain occupational disorders. The pathogenetic potential of the normal physiology of each of these three cell types will be described together with some of the roles of the mast cell. Discussion of the regulation of their cell functions by soluble mediations and surface molecules follows.

POLYMONONUCLEAR NEUTROPHILS (PMNs)

PMNs are professional phagocytes.[20, 21] They are normally rare in the lung parenchyma, uncommon in normal airways, and infrequently found in BAL fluid from normal nonsmoking subjects. In human BAL fluid, PMNs constitute about 1% and from 1% to 5% of nucleated cells in normal nonsmoking and smoking subjects, respectively. However, neutrophils are sequestered in the pulmonary microcirculation, where they form a large pool adherent to the vascular surface of endothelial cells—a phenomenon known as margination. Following a number of inflammatory responses in the lung, chemotaxins and adherence molecules readily mobilize PMNs to cross into air spaces by the process known as diapedesis. PMNs have a relatively short circulating half-life of 2 days and a tissue life of a few hours. They provide a powerful antibacterial defense mechanism. Two physiological and pathogenetic features of these cells are the release of oxidants and the release of degradative enzymes.

Oxidants. PMNs contain few mitochondria, and their resting respiration is relatively low. However, there is a brisk rise in oxygen consumption following either phagocytosis of particles or the exposure of the cells *in vitro* to stimulants such as complement factors (C5a), chemotactic factors, leukotrienes, aggregated immunoglobulins, bacterial peptides, and cytokines (see later discussion). This brisk rise in oxygen consumption depends upon a cyanide-insensitive, flavoprotein-containing nicotinamide adenine dinucleotide phosphate (NADPH) oxidoreductase whose complex structure involves surface receptors with membrane integral hemes and cytosol regulatory proteins.[21] Several genetic disorders affect various components of this enzyme complex and manifest defective O_2 production and poor resistance to bacterial infections. During phagocytosis, this external surface of the cell membrane becomes internalized with the invagination of the fully enclosed phagocytic vacuole. Oxidant products are released extracellularly both following nonparticulate stimulation and during the process of internal vacuole formation during phagocytosis. The major biological products resulting from reduction of molecular oxidants are highly reactive oxidants listed in Figure 11–4. Of these, the immediate and most important product is superoxide anion, which can undergo

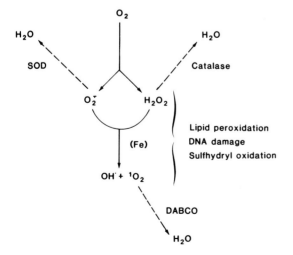

Figure 11–4
Diagram of generation of oxygen free radicals and some naturally occurring (catalase, superoxide dismutase [SOD]) and synthetic 1,4-diazobicyclo(2.2.2.) octane scavengers.

spontaneous or enzymatic dismutation (by superoxide dismutase) to form hydrogen peroxide. Additionally, in the presence of halides present in normal extracellular fluid, a highly reactive hypohalide ion may be formed (e.g., HOCl −). One particular enzyme, myeloperoxidase, which constitutes 5% of the dry weight of the PMN, is important in the production of hypohalide ions and also subserves the oxidation of many substrates.

There is ample evidence that such oxidant materials are powerful microbicidal agents. However, for our purposes, such oxidants are highly injurious to the lung. For instance, in a number of experimental models of inflammatory lung disease[21] in which PMN mobilization and activation is produced by such agents as C5a, protection occurs when antioxidants such as superoxide dismutase are employed. Fibroblasts and umbilical vessel ECs are damaged by activated PMNs by an oxidation-dependent mechanism. Likewise, matrix materials such as hyaluronic acid can be oxidized by superoxide anion.

An important effect of oxidants is on alpha-1-antiprotease.[21] This specific protein, normally present in the circulating blood and in BAL fluid, is an important constituent of the antiprotease screen. It combines in a molar ratio with a number of important proteases discussed later. At its active site is a methionine molecule containing a reduced sulfhydryl group. This group may be oxidized by superoxide anion, hydrogen peroxide, and a number of other oxidizing materials, probably including cigarette smoke, rendering the alpha-1-antiprotease incapable of inhibiting certain serine proteases, notably PMN elastase. Oxidation of alpha-1-antiprotease is greatly enhanced by myeloperoxidase, which is also liberated by PMN degranulation. This effect is preventable by catalase. Direct oxidant damage to endothelial cells, direct injury of matrix proteoglycans, and indirect damage to matrix proteins resulting from impairment of antiproteolytic mechanisms all combine to injure the alveolocapillary unit. Such injury may be manifest on an acute basis as a capillary leak and subsequent pulmonary edema or as more chronic tissue injury.

Asbestos fibers[22] and coal dust evoke oxidant generation by phagocytes, although this appears to be a general response to a number of particulates.

Proteases. PMNs contain a wide range of enzymes capable of degrading lipid, proteinaceous, and carbohydrate-containing molecules. Many such enzymes are localized within the two types of neutrophil granules that may properly be termed lysosomes. Aside from the substrate specificity, there are two distinct groups of degradative enzymes characterized by the relative pH optima. Those with acid pH optima tend to be more strictly granule associated and probably operate when the lysosomal granule fuses with a phagocytic vacuole to produce a phagolysosome in which the pH is about 6.0. The second group is more important with respect to matrix injury, and includes certain neutral proteases whose pH optima is in the range of 7.4 to 8.0. These enzymes are released from PMN into the extracellular fluid and can attack native, insoluble, cross-linked structural matrix materials in the extracellular environment whose pH is presumed to be approximately 7.4. Two of the best studied of these enzymes are elastase and collagenase, both of which are stored pre-formed in the PMN granules. Other proteases include cathepsin G. These enzymes are released by the same factors that promote oxidant activity by PMN. Proteolytic tissue injury depends on an initial attack on insoluble matrix materials in the extracellular environment, followed by partial degradation of such molecules which are subsequently either further degraded by other proteases or ingested and exposed to intralysosomal acid proteases.

There is an important distinction, however, between the release of oxidants and proteases. The latter require functioning cytoplasmic microtubular structures for granule movement and hence protease exteriorization. Oxidant release, however, is in part a surface phenomenon and does not require such microtubule-directed cytoplasmic granule migration. Thus, colchicine, an inhibitor of microtubule reassembly, will diminish lysosomal degranulation and protease release but has little or no effect on oxidant responses by PMN.

Two key PMN enzymes in matrix digestion are collagenase and elastase.[23] These enzymes are biochemically well characterized, and their molecular actions are relatively well defined. PMN elastase attacks elastin, type IV collagen, laminin, fibronectin, various proteoglycans, and blood clotting factors. As such, it is a more general protease than its name suggests. PMN elastase activity against elastin is enhanced by a platelet product (PF$_4$), thus indirectly involving platelets in tissue injury. PMN elastase reacts on a molar basis with alpha-1-antiprotease in its reduced form and also with alpha-2-macroglobulin to form protease-antiprotease complexes. Such complexes with alpha-1-antiprotease are inactive against native elastin. Those with alpha-2-macroglobulin have been reported to be active against elastin and certainly attack certain low-molecular-weight elastin residues and oligopeptides. Once these complexes are formed, they can be subsequently ingested by macrophages. There are other elastase inhibitors: mucus protease inhibitor, a secretory leukoprotease inhibitor formed by airway epithelial cells, and elafin, which is generated by type II cells.

Neutrophil collagenase is a more specific enzyme for collagen and fibronectin. It has no effects on elastin. It attacks native insoluble collagen fibrils (type I but not type III), cleaving collagen molecules at a single point. Such cleavage permits unfolding of the collagen helical structure and its subsequent attack by other less specific proteolytic enzymes active both at neutral and acid pH. Collagenase also differs from elastase in that it does not have a serine group at its active site, is a zinc-containing metalloproteinase, and is not inhibited by alpha-1-antiprotease. Some collagenases, e.g., type IV human 92 and 72 kD, are also elastinolytic.

Both of these enzymes are implicated in the pathogenesis of a number of nonoccupational lung diseases.[20] The currently accepted theory of the pathogenesis of emphysema states that this disorder largely results from the digestion of structural proteins including elastin as a result of an imbalance between proteases and antiproteases. The digestion of elastin and other matrix proteins leads to a loss of elastic recoil. Elastase may also play an important role in more acute diseases such as the adult respiratory distress syndrome (ARDS), in which large numbers of PMNs, high concentrations of free elastase, and significant oxidation of alpha-1-antiprotease all have been demonstrated in BAL fluid. While there are no known occupational diseases that parallel generalized emphysema, focal emphysema-like changes and bronchiolar dilatation are features of certain pneumoconioses, e.g., coal workers' pneumoconiosis. Some occupational disorders resemble ARDS. Among these are paraquat inhalation, polyethylene fume fever, and exposure to sublimates of metals. PMN mobilization to the lung has been demonstrated in paraquat exposure, and paraquat itself is a powerful oxidizing substance.

There are two chronic diseases in which both BAL leukocytosis and free collagenase in BAL fluid occur, idiopathic pulmonary fibrosis (IPF) and asbestosis.[22]

MONONUCLEAR PHAGOCYTES (MPs)

Mononuclear phagocytes derived from maturation of bone marrow stem cells differentiate first into circulating blood monocytes and subsequently into tissue macrophages including alveolar macrophages (AMs). A few AMs normally arise by *in situ* division. AMs are easily recovered from human lungs by BAL, and their biochemistry and other functions can be readily examined, though there are suggestions that interstitial lung macrophages have different properties. In the normal nonsmoking person, BAL cellular yield is around 10 million cells, of which approximately 80% are AMs. Lavage of otherwise healthy smokers' lungs yields 5 to 10 times more cells, of which 95% are AMs with multiple inclusion materials. When studied in tissue culture, the cells from smokers are more adherent to tissue culture vessels and show enhanced secretory activity, particularly of such enzymes as lysozyme (muramidase).

Adaptive and Biosynthetic Activity. The differentiation of circulating monocytes into tissue phagocytes varies with local organ conditions. For instance, macrophages found within the peritoneum are characteristically anaerobic in their energy metabolism, whereas AMs, which reside at the relatively high oxygen tension in the lung, preferentially use aerobic metabolism as a source of adenosine triphosphate (ATP) generation. Both animal and human AMs are relatively rich in mitochondria and show brisk oxidative phosphorylation. In addition to adaptations specific for the tissue in which the macrophage resides, other adaptations to local perturbations of the chemical environment in the lung occur. Such specific intrapulmonary adaptations include the production of aryl hydrocarbon hydroxylase by human AMs derived from cigarette smokers exposed to such polycyclic hydrocarbons as benzpyrene. Additionally, tissue-cultured rabbit AMs grown in the presence of red cells develop a hemoxidase which is not present in the normal cell. There are over 50 known products of AM.[20] Most importantly, MPs are an important source of interleukins (see later discussion). Such interleukins and other AM-derived PMN chemotaxins are key regulators of PMN activity and migration. AM products also inhibit FB secretory activities.

Oxidant Responses. As previously indicated, PMNs generate highly toxic free radicals from molecular O_2. Monocytes and tissue macrophages, including human AM, also generate oxidants[24] that are probably important in intracellular antimicrobial factors, e.g., against mycobacteria. However, they release smaller amounts of such materials into the tissue culture medium and presumably into the extracellular fluid *in vivo*. During the differentiation of monocytes into tissue macrophages, there is an increase in the activity of a number of systems that detoxify these oxidants within the cell, thereby limiting their extracellular oxidant release. Phagocytes contain several forms of superoxide dismutase, which generates hydrogen peroxide from superoxide anion. Catalase, present in high concentrations in rabbit and human AMs, causes the oxidoreduction of hydrogen peroxide to water and molecular oxygen. More importantly, a cytoplasmic glutathione system similar to that present in the red cells exists in AMs. This pathway is quantitatively the single most important antioxidant defense system of the cell.[25] Regeneration of NADPH by the pentose shunt and glutathione reductase are responsible for maintenance of high levels of reduced glutathione, which in turn maintains normal microtubular and other cell functions. The glutathione system is important in the detoxification not only of O_2 products but also lipid hydroperoxides generated by the oxidation of unsaturated fatty acids.[26, 27] Lipid hydroperoxides initiate self-perpetuating chain reactions that irreversibly impair cell membrane function and structures. These reactions are preventable by lipid soluble vitamins A and E and related compounds. All three of these antioxidant enzyme systems are largely intracellular, though catalase release follows phagocytosis by PMN and AM. There are two other important antioxidants: the acute phase-reactant copper-containing protein ceruloplasmin, whose role in lung diseases is largely uninvestigated, and the water-soluble ascorbic acid.

A second group of oxidant products plays many physiological and pathological roles. Nitric oxide has recently passed from the realm of air pollution into a cellular product influencing such diverse functions as relaxing vascular muscle tone, central nervous system (CNS) oxygen toxicity, platelet aggregation, and host defense.[28–30] Nitric oxide is generated as a gaseous rapidly diffusible free radical, $NO^{\bullet}$, from a five-electron oxidation of a guanido N_2 in L-arginine catalyzed by the dioxygenase nitric oxidase synthase (NOS). In this reaction, L-arginine, molecular O_2, and NADPH function as co-substrates yielding $NO^{\bullet}$ and citrulline. The enzyme is present in activated macrophages, PMNs, brain cells, FBs, ECs, and so on. NOS contains flavin groups and requires a biopterin as co-factor. There are homologies with cytochrome P450. Many cytokines enhance NOS activity (e.g., TNF, IL-1, and others). NO activates soluble guanate cyclase by nitrosation of its heme. (An analogy exists with meat curing by reacting nitrite to myoglobin.) Thus, cyclic guanosine monophosphate (cGMP)–dependent processes are affected (e.g., vasodilation). NO affects $O_2^{\bullet-}$ toxicity in a complex fashion but clearly diminishes PMN

$O_2^{\overline{\cdot}}$ generation, largely by a direct action on the NADPH oxidase.[31] Cytoplasts, mobile anucleate fragments artificially prepared from PMN whose normal microbicidal agents are thereby largely excluded, manifest NO-dependent killing of *Staphylococcus aureus*. Cytotoxicity also occurs. For instance, the lung injury and dermal vasculitis induced by immune complexes are attenuated by the NOS inhibitor, N^G monomethyl-L-arginine, even though the PMN tissue accumulation is unaffected.[32] The attenuation is reversed stereospecifically by L-arginine but not D-arginine. While the above aspects are clear, the relation between these two highly reactive free radicals, $O_2^{\overline{\cdot}}$ and $NO^{\cdot}$, is complex, involving the generation of other radicals such as $OH^{\cdot}$ and $ONOO^-$ (peroxynitrite anion). The latter generates toxic lipid peroxides, attacks respiratory enzymes, and damages DNA.

The toxic effects of oxidants include EC damage, disruption of proteoglycans, and damage to DNA by strand breaking, hydroxylation, and impairment of the DNA repair enzyme, polyadenosine diphosphate (ADP) ribose polymerase. Intracellular and permeable oxidants damage ATP generation, attack the reduced sulfhydryl groups of the glycolysis enzyme, glyceraldehyde-3-phosphate dehydrogenase, and impair endoplasmic reticulum-associated biosynthesis.[33] Cell surface or nonpermeable oxidants such as oxidation products of unsaturated lipids (e.g., linoleic hydroperoxide) damage cell membranes, impair phagocytosis in AM, and so on.[27]

It is evident therefore that antioxidant systems are essential under both pathological and host defense conditions.

Degradative Enzymes. AMs contain a wide range of lysosomal enzymes. Some of these, including such proteolytic enzymes as the cathepsins, are stored in pre-formed lysosomes. In addition, beta-glucuronidase, beta-galactosidase, and a number of lipid-splitting enzymes are also present. One important enzyme, lysozyme (muramidase), is partially stored in the cytoplasm but requires relatively continuous synthesis for its secretion into the external medium, a process enhanced in smokers.[34] Lysozyme is weakly microbicidal and exerts an interesting antichemotactic effect on PMN.

In mononuclear phagocytes, there is considerable species variation in the presence of the two important neutral proteases described in PMN, collagenase and elastase. Collagenase is certainly present in rabbit AM, where it is in turn activated by another neutral protease. Neither of these enzymes is stored in the cell, and both require continuous protein synthesis. Rat AMs produce an elastase with similar properties to those of the mouse peritoneal macrophage, a metalloproteinase capable of attacking native elastin. Human monocytes contain a nonsecreted serine protease elastase. Activation of peritoneal macrophages evokes the secretion of a metalloproteinase elastase, which attacks native elastin and also degrades alpha-1-antiprotease. In human AM there is considerable debate concerning the presence of such an elastase, but collagenase has not been detected in human AM. As regards elastase, there are reports[34] claiming the presence of a metalloenzyme based on assays employing three substrates: a chromophore-like elastin peptide (succinyl-trialanine-paranitrophenyl-phosphate), solubilized elastin, and tritium-labeled native elastin. Conclusive proof that this is true in extracellular elastase is lacking. However, human AMs can ingest complexes of PMN elastase with either alpha-1-antiprotease or alpha-2-macroglobulin. In addition, human PMN elastase can bind to human AM cell membranes and be subsequently ingested without precomplexing with either of the antiproteases. Some of this PMN elastase can be released as an active elastase. Thus, the role of AM in regulation of elastinolysis is a complex one and exhibits much species variation.

The distinction between the two types of elastase has been shown by studies employing inhibitors. The macrophage enzyme, a metalloproteinase, is inhibited by chelating agents, whereas the PMN enzyme (serine protease) is inhibited by a group of relatively specific oligopeptide chloromethylketone inhibitors and also by alpha-1-antiprotease.

Human umbilical cord ECs, activated by TNF_L or IL-1B (see later discussion), release a product which trypsin converts to a collagenolytic protease.[35] This, in turn, degrades several collagen species, notably type I, cleaving at Gly-Leu or Gly-Ile bonds of the triple helix. This enzyme, designated matrix metallo-proteinase 1 (MMP-1), is generated by FBs, SMCs, mononuclear phagocytes, but not by human AMs or by PMN where its collagenase appears to be a specific gene product. Most importantly, MMP-1 also inhibits a group of antiproteases, the serpins, which include α_1-antiprotease, anti-chymotrypsin, α_2-antiplasmin, and an inhibitor of plasminogen activator. However, α_2-macroglobulin irreversibly binds MMP-1. Somewhat similar behavior occurs with bacterial metalloelastases (e.g., from *Pseudomonas*), which attack both elastin and α-antitrypsin. Human stromelysin (MMP-3), a human FB product, has similar action to antiproteases and is an "omnivorous" matrix protease. In addition to the counterpoised activities on both the insoluble matrix substrates and the soluble antiproteases, these sepinases have an additional counterpoised action. For instance, α_1-antiprotease products from cleavage of its active site are PMN chemotaxins at nanomolar concentrations, and MMP-antiprotease complexes bind to MP membranes prior to endocytosis.

Mouse peritoneal macrophages, human monocytes, and human AMs also exhibit another neutral protease, plasminogen activator,[36, 37] which catalyzes the formation of plasmin from plasminogen (a circulating enzyme). Plasmin, in turn, lyses fibrin and activates complement factors (C_1 and C_3) and Hageman factor, thus releasing several inflammatory mediators. Plasmin also degrades tissue matrices, including glycosaminoglycans. This action may be important in exposing fibrillar proteins to the action of collagenases and elastases. These actions are potentiated by direct surface contact between macrophages and the matrix.[38] Additionally, there is a positive feedback loop inherent in these enzyme activities, since their products, complement and collagen cleavage fragments, are macrophage chemoattractants.

Mononuclear phagocytes are important in such diverse processes as skin wound healing, postpartum uterine involution, and bone destruction in periodontal disease. Macrophages are primary promoters of angiogenesis acting at several stages of EC cell transition into vessels.[39] They modify matrices, degrade fibrin by plasmin and other substances, induce EC migration largely by IL-8, and via heparin-binding growth factors promote tube formation by EC cells. For this, macrophages need "activation" as part of an inflammatory state or perhaps by hypoxia. Perversely, under other conditions they also suppress angiogenesis. Monocytes and AMs may play similar roles in repairing and inducing lung injury by the foregoing proteolytic mechanisms. Suppression of macrophage protease secretion by corticosteroids and lymphocyte-activated protease secretion have been demonstrated to date only in animal studies; determination of the factors affecting human AM function requires further study.

RESPONSE TO INHALED MATERIALS

In occupational lung disease, activities of macrophage focus partly on its scavenger function. The ultimate response of the macrophage depends on the nature of the particle scavenged.[40, 41] For instance, in occupational infectious diseases the macrophage plays an antimicrobial role and can kill and digest bacteria. For nonbiodegradable particles, the AMs sequester and transport such materials as coal dust, hematite, and a number of other minerals. Neither of the first two particles causes any long-term change in macrophage function. A third type of particle, silica, is readily ingested by phagocytes but produces major cellular dysfunction. Morphological and biochemical evidence of macrophage lysosomal membrane injury is well documented, but the precise mechanism for this remains uncertain. Two mechanisms are generally proposed: (1) hydrogen bonding of silica to lysosomal membranes with subsequent fragility of that membrane, and (2) activation of a lysosomal membrane phospholipase, thus degrading the lipids of the membrane. However, silica ultimately causes cell autolysis by lysosomal digestion of the cytoplasm. Thus, silica particles can be recycled through a series of macrophages. Silica (quartz) causes *in vitro* lipid peroxidation in guinea pig macrophages.[42]

Vitamin E has been reported to prevent lung fibrosis following quartz exposure *in vivo*. These impaired macrophages exhibit deficient antimycobacterial activity.

Asbestos fibers produce different effects.[22, 40, 41] In general, asbestos fibers are relatively nontoxic for macrophages. Fibers longer than 10 to 20 μm are not completely ingested by macrophages, which presumably transport them poorly. Fibers of these or greater lengths, when deposited in the lung, are thought to be more fibrogenic than smaller ones. The action of asbestos fibers may depend on sialic acid groups in cell membrane glycoproteins and be mediated by the surface charge of the fiber.[43] Asbestos fibers release lysosomal enzymes, cause variable changes in the secretion of neutral proteases, and activate a cell membrane phospholipase, with resulting release of arachidonic acid, the precursor of both prostaglandins and such lipoxygenase products as the leukotrienes. However, there is little or no cell autolysis seen morphologically or suggested biochemically by the release of cytosol lactate dehydrogenase (LDH) into tissue culture media. Asbestos also stimulates macrophages to release fibronectin. Ingestion of crocidolite by AM increases the number of surface receptors for complement (C3) and the Fc component of IgC. This and other observations on AM are of uncertain significance but could imply a heightened immune responsiveness.

Finally, in immunological occupational lung diseases such as farmer's lung, pigeon breeder's lung, and beryllium disease, the presentation of antigens to lymphocytes requires processing either by macrophages or perhaps more importantly by the neighboring dendritic cells. In sarcoidosis, experimental studies show enhanced processing of an exogenous antigen, tetanus toxoid, by human AM.

MAST CELLS (MCs)

Basophil staining cells occur in many locations, notably gut and lung. The taxonomy of these cells is incomplete. However, the involvement of mast cells in asthma is recognized widely. Their role in immunoregulation, their control by lymphocytes, and their relation to mesenchymal cell function and IPF are now becoming evident.

Most of these cells are normally found in the lung parenchyma, below the basement membrane of the epithelial cells of the airway lumen, but a small number of these cells may also be found in the airways. Their granules are sources of a number of inflammatory mediators and smooth muscle constrictive agents, including histamine, serotonin (5-hydroxytryptamine [5HT]), eosinophil chemotactic factors, heparin, proteases (e.g., chymase),[44] and arachidonic acid products.

The involvement of 5HT in delayed hypersensitivity reaction, at least in mice, has been established by a number of pharmacological studies, notably those by Askenase et al.[45] For instance, reserpine, a 5HT-depleting agent, diminishes these reactions. The effect of reserpine can be abrogated by preventing the oxidation of monoamines such as 5HT with the monoamine oxidase inhibitor (pargyline). Cyproheptadine, a competitive antagonist of both 5HT and histamine, also modifies these reactions. Morphological and autoradiographic (with tritiated 5HT) studies of mast cell degranulation confirm this effect. In contrast with anaphylaxis, massive degranulation of mast cells does not occur in delayed hypersensitivity reactions. However, in delayed reactions, pseudopodial movement, fusion of some granules with the cell membrane and accompanying release of 5HT, causes gaps to be formed between vascular ECs. Colloidal carbon and PMN move from the circulation to tissue spaces through these gaps. In this manner, tissue mast cells regulate both vascular integrity and the inflammatory effects of PMN on tissues.[45]

Pharmacological and immunological manipulations in this system demonstrate that the function of mast cells is regulated by T lymphocytes in both immediate (IgE mediated) and delayed hypersensitivity reactions. Whether histamine, another major mediator produced by mast cells, terminates the immune responses by reacting with the type 2 histamine receptor on T_s cells needs further study.

The relation among mast cells, T lymphocytes, PMNs, and vascular ECs provides an integrated feedback circuit between inflammatory, immunological, and structural cells. Another example of this type of cellular cooperation between inflammatory and structural cells involves FBs and mast cells.[46] In tissue culture, a single FB can phagocytose many extruded mast cell granules, a phenomenon also microscopically observable in skin biopsies. Thereby, the proteolytic actions of such granule-associated materials as chymotrypsin are terminated. In turn, these granules influence FB behavior. Depending on the number of granules ingested, the enzymes beta-hexosaminidase and collagenase are released by the FBs. Such collagenase is capable of injuring matrix proteins.

In idiopathic pulmonary fibrosis (IPF), lung biopsies show excess numbers of mast cells, some of which are partially degranulated.[47] Haslam et al. showed an average twofold rise in the histamine content of BAL fluid from patients with IPF.[48] Histamine levels correlated with the neutrophil and eosinophil counts from the BAL fluid in these patients. While there was no statistical correlation with the biopsy mast cell counts, both the BAL leukocytosis and histamine levels appeared to be related to a measurement of fibrosis in these biopsies. These clinical studies, although suggestive, do not define a pathogenetic sequence which is implied by the foregoing cell biology studies. A role for mast cells in fibrosis[49] and occupational lung disease is therefore suggested in asbestosis[50] and delayed hypersensitivity disorders, particularly since a monocyte chemotactic and activating factor releases histamine from basophils.[51]

Interleukins

In past decades, many cell-derived factors (e.g., endogenous pyrogen, lymphotoxin) have been identified with certain specific actions. Human monocytes secrete the pyrogen (now known to be an interleukin), a process enhanced in monocytes derived from sarcoidosis patients.[52] The last decade has extended our knowledge of these soluble factors so that several families of proteins produced by and regulating cells have been identified.[53–56] These are termed interleukins (ILs) or cytokines. At least thirteen ILs and other cytokines are known. Information on their structure, genetic bases, biosynthesis, secretion, regulation, and responding cell receptor is being rapidly clarified. They may act via the circulation (endocrine), on neighboring cells (paracrine), or importantly on the source cell itself (autocrine). They fall, with some overlap, into two general groups: the mitogenic cytokines (e.g., growth factors), and the proinflammatory cytokines (e.g., IL-1, IL-6, IL-8, and so on) and tumor necrosis factor. The subject is fully reviewed elsewhere, and we will focus on a few of them and on their complex networking interactions. A caveat: while they are clearly very important and can be studied in humans (both chemically and histochemically), much of the data derive from tissue culture studies with the limits those techniques impose, particularly when evaluating interactions *in vivo*. For instance, one agent, TGF_β (see later discussion), produces opposite effects when operating locally or systemically.[57]

INTERLEUKINS 1, 6, AND 8

IL-1, IL-6, and IL-8 are produced by MPs, AMs, PMNs, ECs, FBs, SMCs, MCs, lymphocytes, and other substances. Their release is promoted by IL-1 itself (autocrine effect) and by endotoxin, asbestos, silica, viruses, and other cytokines and is suppressed *inter alia* by corticosteroids. The effects are transduced by protein kinase C, a unique phospholipase pathway, and G protein. IL-1 endocrine effects include acute phase effects, fever, acute phase protein syntheses (α_1AT, ACTH release), and so on; various procoagulant and hematopoietic responses, hyaluronate production by human FBs; and even increased slow wave sleep. Most importantly, they exert effects on neighboring cells, a paracrine effect. Particularly where derived from MPs or AMs, they provide a second signal in the T cell–AM antigen presentation reaction by the binding of IL-1 to its T cell receptor. IL-1 also provokes other cytokine releases and activates B cell mitosis and immunoglobulin synthesis.

IL-5, a distinct protein from IL-1, has many similar actions. IL-8 is a basic protein relatively resistant to proteolysis. It exerts chemotactic effects on PMN, MP, and lymphocytes at nanomolar concentrations and evokes the activation of PMN at millimolar concentrations.

TUMOR NECROSIS FACTOR (TNF)

TNF was named for the action of a factor developed in the serum of mycobacterium-primed, endotoxin-challenged mice. The β form was originally known as lymphotoxin. This and the α form have similar pro-inflammatory actions, notably by activating lymphocytes, monocytes, and PMNs and by inducing both the adhesion molecules and chemotactic cytokines derived from endothelial, mesothelial, and FB cells. TNF also evokes angiogenesis and fibrosis. In the lung, the AMs are the major source of TNF_α, a constitutive process enhanced by endotoxin and other factors, including asbestos and silica. In murine silicosis,[58] TNF_α mRNA in lung disease is enhanced. The silica-induced collagen production (assessed as hydroxyproline lung content) is almost completely prevented by anti-TNF antibody and enhanced by continuous pump infusion of recombinant TNF. This effect was associated with silver stain evidence of less fibrils around the silicotic nodules whose number and size were unaffected by the TNF manipulations. Mast cells are also involved in experimental silicosis since mast cell–deficient mice receiving intratracheal silica develop only small lung inflammatory responses and diminished alveolar lymphocyte and PMN responses. Among the mechanisms for this are deficient TNF_α production in these mast cell–deficient mice.[59]

TNF has also been implicated in immune-complex lung injury, where AMs are again the main TNF source, and activated PMNs are a feature of these models. Pulmonary vascular ECs are injured by oxidants, as judged by monolayer permeability studies, an effect enhanced by TNF_β, which depletes these cells of reduced glutathione (GSH) by enhanced oxidation to oxidized glutathione (GSSG). The involvement of oxidants produced by xanthine oxidase present in ECs,[32] perhaps in peroxisomes,[60] is shown by the amelioration both of cytotoxicity and of GSH depletion with allopurinol. This cascade effect is enhanced by PMN secretion of a serine protease elastase which converts the pre-formed xanthine dehydrogenase present in pulmonary ECs into the oxidant-generating xanthine oxidase. This effect requires cell contact since, in addition to the inhibition of this conversion by soluble chromophore elastase inhibitors and α_1-antiprotease, xanthine oxidase production is diminished by antibodies to a particular PMN—an endothelial cell adherence glycoprotein (CD11b). Thus, PMN migration and EC injury, two features of many ARDS-like disorders, represent reasons to term this disorder "gout lung." This disorder, which certainly occurs in several acute occupational exposure disorders (e.g., sublimates, paraquat,) is a cascading multicellular interactive proteolytic and oxidant injury process. Human AMs release tumor necrosis factor (TNF_α) when exposed to coal mine dust.[61]

The mitogenic cytokines include platelet-derived FB growth factors (PDGF) and transforming growth factors (TGF).

PLATELET-DERIVED GROWTH FACTOR (PDGF)

Initially discovered in platelet-α granules, this cationic glycoprotein, which exists in three dimeric isoforms, is secreted by a wide variety of cells. The target cells include the structural cells, FBs, epithelial cells, and ECs. It is primarily a mitogen acting on a group of "competence" genes, including the proto-oncogenes c-*myc*, c-*fos*, and c-*jun*. These genes set the stage for a "progression factor" which leads to mitosis. Platelets, FBs, AMs, ECs, and mesothelial and epithelial cells generate PDGF. Certain nonbiodegradable substances (e.g., ceroid in Hermansky-

Pudlak syndrome, asbestos) evoke AM secretion of PDGF. This factor is an important mediator of asbestos-induced fibroses in experimental animals.[22, 62]

TRANSFORMING GROWTH FACTORS (TGF)

TGF was recognized first as an agent inducing FB phenotypic transformation. Historically, TGFs were initially named for this common attribute, namely promoting the growth of cells cultured in a soft medium—i.e., without substratum attachment. The α and β forms, however, are distinct proteins.

TGF$_\beta$. TGF$_\beta$ represents a ubiquitous complex multifunctional group of proteins capable of regulating matrix turnover and immune function. They are members of a supergene family of dimeric proteins linked by disulfide bonds. Most tissues produce such materials, and there is much homology both interspecies and across tissue types. Initially secreted as a 390 amino acid precursor, TGF$_\beta$ is cleaved by plasmin and cathepsin G—its biosynthesis is regulated at the post-translation stage of the macromolecule whose activity is subject to several regulatory sites. Most importantly, the TGF$_\beta$ gene expression exhibits autoregulation by the biologically unusual forces of positive feedback, i.e., an autocrine function. The activation of the macromolecular form probably occurs at the cell surface of human monocytes and PMNs mediated by their proteases, an effect some consider to be enhanced by oxidant also generated at the cell surface by these cell lines. Additionally, antiproteases diminish this activation. These α_1-antiproteases act on the proteases, whereas α_2-macroglobulin binds TGF$_\beta$. The TGF$_\beta$ receptors are complex but exist in many cell lines and matrix proteins. The secondary signaling pathway includes the guanine nucleotide–binding regulatory proteins and cyclic nucleotides cAMP or cGMP. TGF$_\beta$ causes cell division directly by effects on the cell, and indirectly both by modulating other cytokines and by changing the extracellular matrix. These are enhanced by its autocrine function. In some cells, TGF$_\beta$ is cytostatic. Generally, lymphocyte functions are diminished, whereas mononuclear phagocytes, PMNs, are activated. Both mast cells and platelet granules also contain TGF$_\beta$.

TGF$_\beta$ is important in tissue injury and repair.[57, 63] It can initiate injury mechanisms by the chemoattraction of macrophages (MPs) and PMNs and by interactions with other cytokines. Second, it can cause matrix deposition, stimulating the synthesis of fibronectin, collagens, proteoglycans, tenascin, and so on. This enhanced biosynthesis is augmented by the simultaneous diminution of protease and enhancement antiprotease production. These matrix activities, together with angiogenesis, are important in tissue repair. However, as with lung defenses, this repair process can lead to disorganized tissue scarring, a process possibly reinforced by TGF$_\beta$'s autocrine activity. TGF$_\beta$ levels are elevated in the lungs of persons with idiopathic pulmonary fibrosis (IPF) and in experimental bleomycin fibrosis, in which TGF$_\beta$ mRNA levels rise before the appearance of an augmented gene expression for procollagens, fibronectin, and laminin. The cellular sources of TGF$_\beta$ in such fibroses need more exploration but include the above-mentioned cells and bronchial epithelial cells and ECs. In other systems, following vascular endothelial injury, TGF$_\beta$ evokes, *inter alia,* smooth muscle cell migration. Such cells are a rich source of matrix materials and are conspicuous in IPF. Since TGF$_\beta$ activity can be blocked by antibodies affecting receptor binding and by certain specific proteoglycans (decorin and biglycan), therapeutic modulation of unregulated pulmonary fibrosis appears possible. TGF$_\beta$ also has important immunosuppressive effects. Using picryl chloride dermally to induce experimental murine, mast-cell mediated, immediate and delayed hypersensitivity, systemic TGF$_\beta$ diminished both phases of the skin responses when given simultaneously with re-exposure to picryl chloride.[64] Part of this result is mediated by an effect, directly or otherwise, on mast cell serotonin release. An excellent review[57] stresses the importance of two factors influencing the effects of TGF$_\beta$, namely, the source of TGF$_\beta$ and the activity state of the responding cells. First, local, matrix-bound TGF$_\beta$ initiates a gradient promoting directional inflammatory cell recruitment and subsequent activation of the more immature cells and initiating a cascade of inflammatory responses. However, systematically administered TGF_β suppresses these responses in part by offsetting these local TGF_β chemotactic gradients and also by suppressing cell proliferation as indicated earlier in delayed hypersensitivity responses. Second, the cell receptor state determines the response. Thus, monocytes with full TGF_β receptor expression are activated by TGF_β, but the experimentally demonstrated loss of receptor when they become tissue cells renders them unresponsive. The opposite phenomenon recurs with T lymphocytes, where T cell differentiation by antigenic or mitogenic stimulation leads to *enhanced* lymphocyte TGF_β receptors, rendering these cells more subject to growth inhibition.

TGF_α. This family of transmembrane proteins is solubilized by two cleavage steps, releasing a 52 amino acid residue homologous with epidermal growth factor and with fibrillin in the elastic fiber. The latter reacts with receptors on epithelial, endothelial, and mesenchymal cells. By this process, TGF_α is important in fetal lung development, affecting both airway and parenchymal cells. Interestingly, non-small cell lung cancers frequently contain TGF_α, whose vaso-active and angiogenic effects together with the promotion of mesenchymal stroma formation processes further tumor development. Finally, AMs generate TGF_α, particularly when activated, a process also evident in skin wound healing. Thus, effects on epithelialization structural cells following lung injury also seem to be TGF_α dependent.

Adhesion Molecules, Chemotaxins, and Diapedesis

These materials, families of transmembrane glycoproteins, determine cell-matrix and cell-cell interactions. Various cells and matrix components express such glycoproteins, which (1) serve as attachment recognition mechanisms, (2) react with other ligands on participating cells, and (3) are subject to induction in maturing cell lines or to varying degrees of surface expression, often under the influence of cytokines. They profoundly influence cell shape, differentiation, proliferation, and secretory activities. They also play key roles in PMN and eosinophil diapedesis and in the homing of lymphocytes.[65–68] For the first, a three-step process is now envisaged. The first step is EC cell tethering. One protein family, the L-selectins, are surface-expressed in most circulating nucleated cells. P-selectins are present in the α granules of platelets and Weibel-Palade bodies of ECs. Various agents, IL-1, TNF, and endotoxin, induce surface selectin expression on vascular ECs. PMNs thereby rapidly (in seconds) develop a labile tethering to the endothelial surface of blood vessels. They then develop a rolling action prior to firm adhesion and subsequent diapedesis (transendothelial migration) through the intercellular tight junctions.

Chemoattractants involved in the second step were described much earlier than the adhesion molecules.[20] These include leukotrienes, formylated peptides, C_5a, and macrophage-derived products, including IL-8. The last is chemotactic for PMNs, basophils, and T cells. PMNs also respond to most chemotaxins by exocytosis; oxidant generation and their migration then may result in vascular wall damage and edema. The various chemotaxins have different PMN surface receptors but share common signal transduction, namely, a G protein and protein kinase C pathways. PMNs can sense as little as 1% chemotaxin concentration gradients across their diameter. Since intravascular chemotaxins would be rapidly diluted, it appears that the labile selectin adherence provides the first migratory step which may well be enhanced by the "focusing" effect of chemotaxin-matrix binding, which achieves high local concentrations of chemotaxins.

The integrins are so named for their capacity to integrate the extracellular matrix.[69] The cytoplasmic domain of these transmembrane glycoproteins connects with the intracellular contractile proteins, e.g., α-actinin. The much larger extracellular domain comprises two subunits which can bind (1) to tissue matrix proteins—fibronectin, laminin, collagens, tenascin, thrombospondin, and so on; (2) to various intercellular adhesion molecules (ICAMs); and (3) to fibrin, Von Willebrand's factor, and so on. The tripeptide Arg-Gly-Asp is a common recognition sequence in these reactions. The hereditary disorder leukocyte adhesion deficiency (LAD) manifests the lack of an integrin functional subunit by failed PMN migration, lack of pus formation, and poor resistance to infection. Appropriate antibodies to specific integrins inhibit the response to chemotaxins and also both the stable PMN adherence to the vasculature and subsequent PMN migration. However, the rolling action of circulating PMN is unaffected. The integrins and their corresponding ligating molecules are rapidly regulatable by cytokines, and so on. They play roles in experimental immune complex lung disease.[70] Hypoxia can induce IL-1 production and subsequent induction of an endothelial leukocyte adhesion molecule (ELAM-1).[71] Other intercellular adhesion molecules (ICAM-1) occur in type I alveolar cells.[72] ICAM-1 is a natural ligand for the lymphocyte adhesion protein (LFX-1), also found on the surface of ECs and FBs. ICAM-1 was not present in rat type II cells cultured on artificial surfaces, but at 48 hours the ICAM-1 was readily detectable by immunofluorescence microscopy. This was associated with the transition to type I cells as judged by cell morphology, lectin responsiveness, and other surface markers. Double staining techniques show ICAM-1 to be present in rat type I cells *in vivo*. The presumptive importance of these findings lies in showing cell localizing differentiation patterns in lung epithelial cells. Type I cell membrane ICAM-1 is able to bind activated T lymphocytes, thus providing one mechanism for attracting and retaining lymphocytes in close proximity to the alveolar air space. Such T cells serve in antigen presentation to resident/mobilized AM in the alveoli but also confer a risk of type I cell damage from cytotoxic T lymphocytes.

Senior et al.[73] pointed out an important feature of the specific basement membrane 150 kD sulfated glycoprotein, called entactin. This protein not only binds to the structural proteins collagen IV and laminin but also has both adhesive and chemoattractant (at subnanomolar concentrations) effects on PMN. Both of these latter effects require interactions between the single Arg-Gly-Asp sequence at the 672-4 amino acid residues of entactin, with a recently described PMN response integrin. A mutant entactin, with the single substitution of glutamic acid for aspartic acid at amino acid 672, did not display these effects. Entactin also evokes the release by PMN of a specific granule metalloproteinase which can degrade matrix materials. Entactin appears important therefore in transmembrane migration, but whether the proteinase is required is not certain.

Lymphocytes show similar adhesion features. For instance, naive and memory lymphocytes traffic differently through both lymphoid and nonlymphoid tissue influenced by surface molecules.[65] Specific antigen-induced lymphocyte accumulation is mediated by the induction of integrins and/or selectins on vascular endothelia within the lymph nodes. For instance, the high endothelial venules in lymph nodes can express one of a family of addressins, which bind to the selectins present in certain circulating lymphocytes. Since lymphocytes migrate poorly *in vitro*, chemotaxins are not yet defined. However, pertussis toxin blockade of a G protein inhibits the last step of lymphocyte arrest in and migration into Peyer's patches. Parenthetically, the same mechanisms are involved in promoting tumor metastases, tumor cell proliferation, local spread, and vascular invasion, the last being the obverse of PMN diapedesis. Materials related to the Arg-Gly-Asp tripeptide will diminish tumor cell migration in *in vitro* invasion assays.

Specific Disorders

Acute Lung Injury

This group of disorders, characterized by airway dysfunction and pulmonary edema, has many causes: metal sublimates, paraquat, toxic fumes and gases, immune complex deposition, among others. The lung responses include (1) direct toxic effects on type I cells and ECs; (2) complement activation; (3) coagulation factors activation; and (4) EC biochemical responses and PMN recruitment and activation that release proteases and oxidants, which, together with the initial insult, amplify the injury. Interleukin responses are little studied in humans, but the presence of fever as in welders' ague and other fume fevers suggests release of IL-1 and/or IL-6. Aside from recruited PMNs, EC cells are a rich source of interleukins themselves and also of TNF and a group of chemotaxins characterized by the so-called cys-tandem, cys-x-cys, where x is a variable amino acid.[74]

Patients with this first group of disorders, even when severe, frequently make a complete recovery, and lung fibrosis is not the rule.

Pulmonary Fibroses

The term *pulmonary fibrosis* focuses on the end result. Scadding's term, *fibrosing alveolitis*, seems more accurate, since it emphasizes the disease origin from inflammatory alveolar disease—a term that includes the air space and the alveolocapillary unit. This seems particularly appropriate for occupational causes, since the alveoli are clearly the initial site of injury, and the response to dusts and inhalants is mobilization of phagocytes into both alveolar structures and air spaces. This response is initially one of PMNs and later of AMs. Depending on the insult, these phases may resolve with little or no sequelae or involvement of other lung cells. Alternatively, acute or chronic inflammatory responses supervene with involvement of most if not all of the cell types, matrix materials, and humoral factors, notably the interleukins and products of arachidonic acid (leukotrienes and prostaglandins). We indicate the evidence for alveolitis, the factors in repair, and what is known about the basis of the disordered repair that underlies the irreversibly stiff lung characteristic of the disease group. The role of ILs and growth factors in lung disease was reviewed by Elias and colleagues.[55, 56]

Histologically, at least in IPF and asbestosis, the sequence is as follows. The initial alveolitis is predominantly mononuclear, though a transient PMN migration may occur first, before the fibrosing features are evident. Alveolar cells, including macrophages, fibroblasts, and so on, show marked proliferation. Smooth muscle cells increase some tenfold in IPF. Some eosinophils may appear. The next stage involves structural damage and fibrotic alveolar wall thickening. At this stage, PMNs accumulate in the alveoli and lung interstitium. Finally, irreversible architectural distortion occurs. In IPF, and particularly in asbestosis, the units involved include the terminal bronchioles and the alveolar ducts. Basement membranes are frequently damaged, and both ECs and type I cells disappear. A number of factors influence the development of this process, which is essentially a subversion of normal growth and repair mechanisms. First, an inflammatory process occurs, as judged by persistent oxidant radical generation and protease release. The oxidants are derived from AMs and PMNs and are manifest by low BAL fluid reduced glutathione (GSH) levels. Free active collagenase and elastase-related products can be detected in BAL fluid.[75, 76] BAL fluid for IPF patients exerts toxic effects on cultured lung epithelial cells. Eosinophils, also seen at least in IPF lungs, also damage lung tissue. This is apparent from the disorders, including lung pathology associated with the massive blood and tissue eosinophilia associated with the recent episodes caused by the toxic product of L-tryptophan manufacture. Certainly eosinophils can injure lung epithelial cells, and their cationic protein is present in IPF.[77]

A second factor is basement membrane injury, which affects cell behavior, since it constitutes a biochemically active scaffolding with cell-adhesive and cell-activating properties. While ECs do make basement membrane components, preservation of this membrane is important. Thus, as classical anatomical pathologists have for many years insisted, pulmonary fibrosis is seen only in disorders in which there is significant damage to the basement membranes upon which endothelial and type I cells reside. They have thus emphasized that cellular renewal following injury requires a preservation at least of this component of the normal lung architecture. For the lung, the first experimental support for this view was provided by

Vracko,[78] who employed oleic acid to produce an ARDS model. Where the basement membrane was preserved, type II cells regenerated a normal lung architecture. Destruction of the basement membrane resulted in fibrosis. This view is consistent with the evidence presented earlier, which suggested the critical importance of the matrix cellular interactions in the differentiation and normal function of lung cells. However, the matrix itself is synthesized by epidermal and mesenchymal cells, including type II cells, FBs, and smooth muscle cells. Thus, there is a complex interplay between the effects of matrix on the cell function and the effects of cell function on matrix formation.

Third, matrix injury occurs at point of contact between macrophages and the matrix surface. Campbell et al.[79] examined the relative importance of cell-surface contact and oxidative inactivation of protease inhibitors. They employed PMNs layered to provide direct contact with ^{125}I-labeled fibronectin surfaces. They showed that PMN-derived oxidants did not protect secreted elastase from inhibition by alpha-1-antiprotease. Additionally, they demonstrated that under these conditions, both alpha-1-antiprotease and alpha-2-macroglobulin did not inhibit PMN elastase as effectively as they could inhibit PMN elastase in solution. This and other observations[80] suggest that cell-surface contact zones may exclude various soluble phase materials, including antiproteases and antioxidants, such as ceruloplasmin. Matrix injury is even more complicated than the degradation of a single material such as elastin and involves several enzymes in sequence, e.g., plasmin and elastase. Finally, the matrix has profound effects on platelets, which can release powerful mediators. For instance, exposed ''collagen'' activates platelets. Exposure of collagen can readily occur following basement membrane injury, thus amplifying an already injurious cascade.

Fourth, the involvement of fibronectin, ILs, and growth factors systems has been described. TGF$_\beta$ may well be the most important component. Its continuous local production sustains inflammatory and fibrogenic cell behavior. Blockade of TGF$_\beta$ by either certain matrix proteoglycans[63] or by appropriate TGF$_\beta$ antibodies inhibits many fibrosing inflammatory diseases, e.g., glomerulonephritis, arthritis, and experimental encephalomyelitis.[57]

Fifth, proliferation and differentiation of type II cells have already been mentioned. Even in the presence of a normal basement membrane, following some inflammatory or toxic destruction of type I cells, the factors affecting the differentiation of type II cells assume considerable importance. These factors are being elucidated, and their importance is apparent in some important experiments by Witschi et al.[81] This group employed a number of injury mechanisms, including hyperoxia, chemical compounds, and radiation, to investigate the effects of a second injury applied 3 days after an initial injury—for example, the application of hyperoxia following radiation. They showed that, under certain circumstances, impaired type II cell proliferation was associated with subsequent fibrosis. Under these circumstances, FB proliferation replaces the normal type II cell differentiation. This may lead to a disorderly excessive deposition of matrix proteins, rather than an organized re-epithelialization by type II–derived type I cells. Alternatively, the cuboidal epithelium, often seen lining the air spaces in IPF, may arise because type II cells fail to repopulate the basement membrane. The cuboidal cells morphologically resemble those present in the early embryonic stage of lung development or those from primitive airways. They may redevelop in the face of type II cell failure.

Sixth, it is often assumed that cells casually die of old age. In fact, cell death is a highly programmed process termed apoptosis, which presumably modulates both inflammation and repair. The process primarily involves nuclear events, partly influenced by cytokines and interestingly affected by nicotine.

Seventh, there is an important consequence of this chronic inflammatory process, namely the risk of neoplasia. IPF and asbestosis are associated with increased lung cancer risks. In asbestos workers, bronchial squamous metaplasia is associated with BAL fluid evidence of an inflammatory process in BAL fluid.[82] The early stage of IPF or asbestosis is manifest by enhanced mitosis under the influence of growth factors and faces the mutagenic risks of oxidizing radicals. These mitogenic factors promote cell division, matrix invasion, and angiogenesis—all factors influencing tumorigenesis and both local and hematogenous tumor spread. Later, alveolar metaplasia occurs where the fibrosis ensues. For instance, where alveolar structures are damaged, bronchiolar or more primitive cuboidal cells come to line the air spaces. Epithelial cells become stacked, and squamous metaplasia occurs. The involvement of terminal airways is a feature of IPF, asbestosis, and the bronchiolar organizing pneumonias.

Beryllium Lung Diseases

Beryllium lung diseases, which include an acute lung injury and chronic changes simulating sarcoidosis, cause lung fibrosis. The fibrosis is mediated by proliferation of CD4 positive helper/inducer T cells under the influence of lung tissue Be and Be-specific T cell clones. This provides the basis for immunological tests for Be disease performed on BAL lymphocytes.[83, 84] Of greater interest is the genetic factors now known to play a discriminant role. The presentation of the Be antigen requires the presence of the major histocompatibility complex II (MHCII) molecules, which are subject to genetic variation among individuals.[85] Evaluation of the MHC class II genes in 33 cases of chronic Be disease and 44 controls by Richeldi et al.[86] showed statistical association with certain HLA gene types. They show that Be susceptibility is conferred by an HLH-DP type in which a glutamic acid change has occurred. These components of MHCII are known to be involved in the susceptibilities to such autoimmune disorders as rheumatoid arthritis, insulin dependent diabetes, and so on, and also in T cell responses to nickel and gold.

Thus, Be disease is now an example of a pharmacogenetic disease, and an individual's risk can be predicted. This is important since, while acute berylliosis may be prevented by setting Be exposure limits, Be sensitivity remains a problem. Thus, genetic screening holds promise of prevention, as do BAL lymphocyte tests, in the diagnosis of Be sensitivity.

Parenthetically, as regards MHCII, there is now good evidence for its involvement in the formation of multinucleated giant cells from peripheral blood monocytes.[87] These cells are features of several disorders, Be disease, hard metal disease, and nonoccupational disorders.

Therapeutic Considerations in Interstitial Diseases

These complex interactive mechanisms indicate both the difficulties and potential approaches to therapy. There are several possibilities.

Anti-inflammatory drugs have roles. While neither nonsteroidal nor steroidal agents are effective in established fibrosis, the latter suppress the injuries of immediate and delayed hypersensitivity and immune-complex disorders. Colchicine probably has no effect. Mepacrine has several anti-inflammatory actions, impairing PMN migration, O_2 generation, and degranulation. It ablates PMN migration in a rat silica instillation model.[88] The analogue chloroquine diminishes skin sarcoid granulomata and rheumatoid joint inflammation. MC product antagonists need exploration. Tyrosine kinase antagonists are available and may have a role in diminishing the second messenger stage of growth factor actions.[89] Manipulation of interleukins will prove complex, but TGF_β antibodies clearly abrogate fibrosing models in animals.[58, 63] Angiotensin converting enzyme inhibitors, e.g., captopril, diminish fibrosis and granuloma size in experimental schistosomiasis.[90] Antioxidants and retinols (vitamin A–like compounds) may also be effective in prevention and treatment of both fibrotic lung disease (asbestosis)[91] and lung cancer, primarily by reversing abnormal differentiation of epithelial cells.[92]

LUNG CANCER AND MESOTHELIOMA

As emphasized in the preceding section, this discussion will focus on the mechanisms of carcinogenesis by asbestos fibers in lung and pleura and limited data on how inflammation and fibrogenesis by silica may contribute to lung cancers in smokers. Since many carcinogens in the workplace (i.e., nickel, chromium, and so on) may act through similar and common pathways, particularly those invoking oxidative stress,[93] analogies and critical references will be supplied throughout the text. Here we focus on a general overview of mechanisms of carcinogenesis, hypotheses concerning the roles of chronic inflammation and cell proliferation in the development of tumors by pathogenic and nonpathogenic inhaled particles in rodents, and the controversial question of whether oxidants mediate the proliferative and genotoxic effects of asbestos and crystalline silica observed in some cell types. Because asbestos and crystalline silica constitute distinct families of chemically and physically diverse minerals, it should be kept in mind that one cannot directly compare studies from laboratories using different cell types or reference standards of these minerals.

Mechanisms of Carcinogenesis

Carcinogenesis is a multistage process occurring in humans over a long latency period. During this extremely protracted period, which can be more than 40 years in some asbestos-related mesotheliomas,[94] cells acquire multiple genetic and phenotypic changes as they progress from normality to malignancy. One unresolved question is whether the complex genetic alterations observed in frank tumors are integrally related to the development of neoplasms or to nonspecific changes reflecting a general genetic instability of rapidly dividing cells. In the past, we have regarded most carcinogens as genotoxic, as they frequently cause gene mutations or chromosomal changes in cells. However, a recent review of the 23 group 1 carcinogens classified by the International Agency for Research on Cancer as exhibiting carcinogenic effects in both rodents and humans shows that both asbestos and conjugated estrogens are nongenotoxic (i.e., epigenetic) in bacterial mutagenicity tests and rodent bone marrow assays.[95] This observation, and the fact that many nongenotoxic agents cause chronic inflammation and proliferation at high doses in rodent models, has led to the hypothesis that "mitogenesis induces mutagenesis," or transformation of cells by elicitation of oxidative stress during the inflammatory process.[96] It is well known that oxidants can cause breakage and oxidative lesions in DNA as well as proliferation of cells which makes them more susceptible to a variety of chemical carcinogens.[93] Moreover, a body of information suggests that uncontrolled cell division is a cause of many human cancers.[97]

Several classes of genes, including oncogenes (both those with and without genomic similarity to oncogenic viruses) may be molecular targets in carcinogenesis.[98] Searches for oncogenes that may be activated (or tumor suppressor genes such as p53 or Rb that are inactivated) during tumor development have yielded over 50 often homologous candidates in a number of tumor types. Gene products may act as modified receptors for growth factors (c-*sis*, c-*erB-2*), in cell signaling pathways controlling cell replication (c-*fos*, c-*jun*), and/or on phosphorylation of proteins governing cell cycle control *(raf-1)*. Other oncogenes (c-*myc*) may be causally related to late events in progression of tumor development.

In lung cancers, multiple genetic deletions and amplifications affecting a number of chromosomes (e.g., 1, 3, 11, 13, 17) may be required for transformation and selection of differentiation pathways unique to certain tumor types.[99] Although oncogenes may be expressed differentially in certain classifications of tumors (i.e., small cell vs. non–small cell cancers), there is no unique chromosomal or gene marker represented in all lung tumors or individual tumor types. These observations undoubtedly reflect the complex etiology of lung cancers and the myriad of carcinogens affecting the lungs.

Several reports indicate nonrandom chromosomal aberrations in human mesotheliomas, the majority of which were associated with occupational exposure to asbestos. These include losses of chromosomes 4, 22, and 9p, increases in chromosomes 5, 7, and 20, and deletions of chromosomes 3p and 17p.[100–102] Thus, these changes do not suggest a cytogenetic alteration common to all mesotheliomas. An initial study indicated mutational changes in the p53 gene in three of four mesotheliomas examined,[103] but a follow-up study of 20 human mesothelioma cell lines showed p53 abnormalities in only three lines.[104] Moreover, *Ki-ras* activation, a frequent event in small cell lung tumors in humans, was not observed. Other studies have shown differences in expression of oncogenes regulating growth factor production in normal mesothelial cells as compared to mesotheliomas.[105–107] For example, in human, but not in rat, mesotheliomas, increased expression of c-*sis*, an oncogene encoding platelet-derived growth factor (PDGF), is observed. Moreover, transfection of the PDGF gene into a human mesothelial cell line immortalized with SV40 T antigen causes transformation to malignancy, suggesting a role of PDGF in carcinogenesis.[108]

Cellular Mechanisms of Carcinogenesis by Asbestos

The cellular mechanisms of asbestos-associated lung cancers and mesotheliomas may be different, reflecting unique pathways of interaction with asbestos or repair from injury by target cells. For example, the mesothelial cell is a hybrid cell type, exhibiting properties of both epithelial cells and fibroblasts such as expression of vimentin and keratins and growth factor receptors common to both cell types.[109] On the other hand, common cellular responses, such as inflammation and cell proliferation, may be causally related to the development of both mesothelioma and lung cancer. The dissection of critical events occurring in asbestos-induced lung cancers is particularly difficult owing to the confounding and overwhelming contribution of smoking to the development of tumors. For example, epidemiological data suggest that asbestos may be noncarcinogenic in lung, acting primarily as a cofactor in combination with chemical carcinogens in cigarette smoke.[110, 111]

Plausible mechanisms of interaction between asbestos fibers and carcinogens in smoke have been suggested in experimental studies using rodent cells. For example, asbestos fibers may act as vehicles for adsorption of polycyclic aromatic hydrocarbons (PAHs) in smoke, thus increasing their availability to AMs or epithelial cells of the respiratory tract after inhalation.[112, 113] Asbestos also prolongs the uptake of PAHs by tracheal epithelial cells and adduct formation with DNA. Fibers may also catalyze, through oxidative mechanisms, the formation of carcinogenic derivatives from PAH.[114] Clearance of fibers is also impaired by smoking, resulting in their increased uptake by epithelial cells.[115, 116] Some evidence suggests that oxidants derived from cigarette smoke enhance smoke-mediated transport of fibers into tracheobronchial epithelium.[117]

The elicitation of chronic cell inflammation and epithelial cell proliferation by asbestos in lung as documented by histopathology, morphometric analyses, and increased incorporation of tritiated thymidine in many studies[22] may facilitate the transformation of these cell types by chemical carcinogens in smoke, as rapidly dividing cells are more susceptible to DNA damage by carcinogens. In both mesothelial and epithelial cells, cell replication may also favor an expanding population of genetically altered cells and render these sensitive to subsequent genetic instability and genetic errors occurring during tumor progression (Fig. 11–5). We are now just beginning to unravel the molecular mechanisms of cell proliferation by asbestos as well as the cell signaling events initiating various pathways of cell proliferation.[118]

One mechanism of cell proliferation by asbestos that appears to be oxidant-mediated is induction of ornithine decarboxylase (ODC), an enzyme which is rate-limiting in the biosynthesis of polyamines.[119, 120] Polyamines must be increased in cells for cell division to occur, and inhibition of ODC using specific inhibitors or

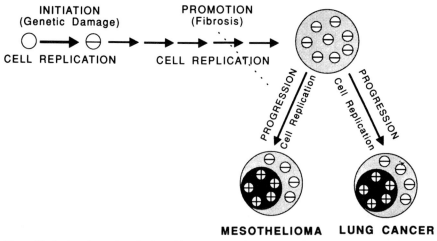

Figure 11–5. The relationship of cell proliferation to the development of asbestos-associated diseases. (From Mossman, B.T., and Gee, J.B.L., Pulmonary reactions and mechanisms of toxicity of inhaled fibers. In Gardner, D.E., Crapo, J.D., and McClellan, R.O., eds., Toxicology of the Lung, New York, Raven Press, 1993.)

other steps in the pathway of polyamine biosynthesis has been used as an approach in cancer chemotherapy.[121] Both crocidolite and chrysotile asbestos, as well as chemical generating systems of activated oxygen species (AOS), increase steady-state mRNA levels of ODC in tracheal epithelial cells within a 4-hour period, indicating that asbestos and AOS cause transcriptional activation of this gene. Moreover, scavengers of AOS and antioxidants inhibit asbestos-induced ODC mRNA and enzyme activity. α-Difluoromethylornithine, which competitively inhibits ODC, abrogates increased squamous metaplasia and hyperplasia occurring in hamster tracheal organ cultures after addition of crocidolite asbestos, an indication of the importance of polyamines in aberrant cell proliferation.[122] Since a number of nonasbestos fibers of similar size also cause increases in ODC activity in tracheal epithelial cells, and longer fibers are more potent than shorter fibers or nonfibrous particles (no induction of ODC), geometry and size of particles appear to be intrinsic to this pathway of cell proliferation.

Asbestos also appears to increase gene expression of "early response genes" such as c-*jun* and c-*fos* that are critical to the initiation of DNA synthesis and transit of cells into the S phase of the cell cycle.[123] These proto-oncogenes are activated through complex cell signaling pathways involving protein kinases. Their protein products then form a heterodimer or transcription factor (AP-1) which binds to the promoter region of a number of genes causally linked to initiation of DNA synthesis. Unlike growth factors (i.e., PDGF, and so on) or soluble hyperplastic chemicals (i.e., phorbol esters, and so on) which cause immediate and transient increases in gene expression of c-*fos* and c-*jun*, gene induction is delayed and persistent after exposure to crocidolite and chrysotile asbestos in mesothelial cells, undoubtedly reflecting the fact that fibers persist in cells after phagocytosis *in vitro*. These patterns are also observed in tracheal epithelial cells, although only c-*fos* is expressed in this cell type after exposure to asbestos.[123] In both cell types, increases in AP-1 protein binding to DNA are seen with asbestos, indicating that the protein products of these proto-oncogenes are able to induce DNA synthesis in these cell types.

Demonstration of a consistent molecular response to asbestos which is linked to a biological end point (i.e., cell proliferation) critical to the pathogenesis of both cancers and fibrosis has allowed dose-response studies to explore the important question of whether a threshold exists at the molecular level in response to various types of fibers. Results show that both crocidolite and chrysotile cause induction of proto-oncogenes in a dose-responsive fashion with no increases at lowest concentrations of minerals and distinct differences in responses to fiber types.[123] At equal fiber numbers, crocidolite is more active than chrysotile asbestos. Moreover, induction of c-*fos* and c-*jun* by erionite, a more potent mesotheliomagenic agent in humans and rats,[124] is more striking in comparison to a number of particulates tested to date.[125] As has been observed in experiments examining ODC gene induction,[119, 120] particles such as polystyrene beads and riebeckite (a nonfibrous dust chemically similar to crocidolite asbestos) do not stimulate proto-oncogene expression in mesothelial or tracheobronchial epithelial cells. Thus, fibrous geometry and type are important in elicitation of "early response" genes.

The persistent activation of proto oncogenes by asbestos suggests a model of chronic cell proliferation that may be relevant to the progression of both lung cancers and mesotheliomas as well as asbestosis (see Fig. 11–5). In addition, compensatory hyperplasia following cell damage by asbestos at the high concentrations normally used in chronic rodent inhalation studies may contribute to increases in genetic instability and proliferative potential of tumor cells commonly observed in tumor development. An intriguing possibility is that carcinogenic potential is directly related to the durability of inhaled fibers which persist in lung and pleura, giving rise to chronic inflammation (accompanied by mutagenic oxidant production) and cell proliferation. This may then explain the increased pathogenicity of the amphiboles, crocidolite and amosite, in comparison to chrysotile, a more soluble fiber, in humans.[126]

A topic of debate is whether asbestos-induced cell damage, proliferation, and interaction with isolated DNA *in vitro*[127] are mediated by direct interaction of fibers with cells or through the formation of oxidants. For example, several laboratories have reported that cell damage and hyperplasia, particularly by amphiboles, are inhibited in a number of cell types *in vitro* by the addition of naturally occurring or synthetic antioxidants.[92, 93] We have also learned that asbestos causes increased generation of oxidants from AMs and neutrophils, presumably during phagocytosis[127, 128] and by redox reactions occurring on the surface of fibers.[129] A mechanism which might be interrelated to increased reactivity of amphiboles such as crocidolite or amosite (which contain as much as 36% iron in weight) is the mobilization of iron from these fibers over time in the lung or pleura.[130] Iron catalyzes the formation of the potent hydroxyl radical from superoxide and hydrogen peroxide. If iron is chelated from asbestos, subsequent cytotoxicity, lipid peroxidation, and DNA breakage *in vitro* are inhibited.[131–133] The compendium of data presented above suggests that certain asbestos-associated cellular events are mediated by active oxygen species. Other reviews stress the linkages between oxidant stress and carcinogenesis by ultraviolet and ionizing radiation, nickel, and chromium.[93, 134, 135]

Mechanisms of Pathogenicity by Crystalline Silica

As discussed in other chapters, evidence for carcinogenicity of silica is weak in some occupational cohorts and absent in others. Moreover, carcinogencity studies in rodents have demonstrated the development of tumors in only one species, the rat, after inhalation of quartz.[136, 137] The appearance of these tumors is a late phenomenon, and lung fibrosis is a prominent feature in tumor-bearing animals. Conversely, not all species exhibiting fibrosis exhibit tumors. Certain caveats also should be acknowledged when interpreting chronic inhalation studies in rats, including the frequent appearance of benign lesions such as adenomas and adenomatosis and differences in tumor types when compared to lesions observed in humans.[138] Rats also have a propensity for tumor development after exposure to a number of noncarcinogenic particles (titanium dioxide, carbon black, talc) which may reflect the uniqueness of the rat lung in responding to widespread chronic damage and pulmonary fibrosis.[139]

Like asbestos, silica particles are nonmutagenic in bacterial mutagenicity assays of mammalian cells;[140] but freshly crushed preparations may cause the generation of oxidants,[141] which may then cause chemical bonding to DNA and DNA breakage *in vitro*.[142, 143] Silica or silica-mediated oxidant generation may influence metabolism of chemical carcinogens which may influence their deactivation and/or metabolism to derivatives interacting with DNA.[144] In cell transformation systems, α-quartz shows low transforming activity in comparison to asbestos and does not cause chromosomal aberrations in cells.[145] Moreover, we have been unable to demonstrate induction of proto-oncogenes by cristobalite silica in cultures of mesothelial or tracheal epithelial cells (unpublished data).

Type II epithelial cell hyperplasia and proliferation of lung fibroblasts are common features of quartz dusts in the rat lung.[136] As suggested by Saffiotti and Stinson,[146] differences in the intensity of epithelial cell responses in different species of rodents may correlate directly with their predilection to silicosis and lung cancers. That the processes of carcinogenesis and fibrosis are functionally and causally related in asbestos workers has been espoused by Kushner[147] and others,[94] and that may be true in lung cancers occurring in silicotics as well. Several mechanisms appear feasible. First, nidi of fibrosis in the lung may serve as favorable sites for transformation of surrounding epithelial cells mediated by growth factors released by fibroblasts or attendant AMs.[148, 149] Lymphocytes and neutrophils may also release cytokines, influencing proliferation of both lung fibroblasts and epithelial cells.[150–152] Moreover, cytokines released by epithelial cells and fibroblasts may also stimulate proliferation by each other, events critical to the progression of fibrosis and/or development of tumors. Lastly, proteases and oxidants generated by inflammatory cells in silicotic and asbestotic lesions may create a favorable environment for progression and metastases of lung cancers by facilitating invasion of tumor cells. The issue of carcinogenicity of silica can only be finally settled by well-controlled epidemiological studies.

Acknowledgments

We thank Mr. Bernie Ravenelle for his excellent technical assistance.

REFERENCES

1. Crystal, R.G., and West, J.B., eds.-in-chief, The Lung: Scientific Foundations, Vols. 1 and 2. New York, Raven Press, 1991.
2. Panos, R.J., Cytokines and alveolar type II cells. *In* Kelley, J., ed., Cytokines of the Lung. Lung Biology in Health and Disease, Vol. 61. New York, Marcel Dekker, Inc., 1992, p. 417.
3. Cate, R.L., Donahoe, P.K., and MacLaughlin, D.T., Mullerian inhibiting substance. *In* Sporn, M.B., and Roberts A.B., eds., Peptide Growth Factors and Their Receptors II. New York, Springer-Verlag, 1990, p. 179.
4. Adamson, I.Y.R, and Bowden, D.H., Type 2 cell as a progenitor of alveolar epithelial regeneration. A cytodynamic study in mice after exposure to oxygen. Lab. Invest., 30, 35, 1974.
5. Panos, R.J., Voekel, N.F., Cott, G.R., et al., Alterations in eicosanoid production by rat alveolar type II cells isolated after silica-induced lung injury. Am. J. Cell Mol. Biol., 6, 430, 1992.
6. Suwabe, A., Panos, R.J., and Voelker, D.R., Alveolar type II cells isolated after silica-induced lung injury in rats have increased surfactant protein A (SP-A) receptor activity. Am. J. Respir. Cell Mol. Biol., 4, 264, 1991.
7. Carvalho, A.C.A., Bellman, S., Saullo, J., et al., Altered plasma factor VIII antigen: A sensitive indicator of endothelial damage. Am. Rev. Respir. Dis., 123, 98, 1981.
8. Ryan, U.S., and Ryan, J.W., Correlations between the fine structure of the alveolar-capillary unit and its metabolic activities. *In* Bakhle, Y.S., and Vane, J.R., eds., Metabolic Functions of the Lung. New York, Marcel Dekker, 1977, p. 197.
9. Kelman, J., Brin, S., Horwitz, A., et al., Collagen synthesis and collagenase production by human lung fibroblasts. Am. Rev. Respir. Dis., 115, 343, 1977.
10. Smith, B.T., and Post, M., Fibroblast-pneumocyte factor. *In* Kelley, J., ed., Cytokines of the Lung. Lung Biology in Health and Disease, Vol. 61. New York, Marcel Dekker, Inc., 1992, p. 403.
11. Begin, R., Rola-Pleszczynski, M., Sirois, P., et al., Early lung events following low-dose asbestos exposure. Environ. Res., 26, 535, 1981.
12. Reiser, K., McCormick, R.J., and Rucker, R.B., Enzymatic and nonenzymatic cross-linking of collagen and elastin. FASEB J., 6, 2439, 1992.
13. Martin, G.R., and Sank, A.C., Extracellular matrices, cells, and growth factors. *In* Sporn, M.B.,

and Roberts, A.B., eds, Peptide Growth Factors and Their Receptors II. New York, Springer-Verlag, 1990, p. 463.

14. Wagner, J.C., Burns, J., Munday, D.E., et al., Presence of fibronectin in pneumoconiotic lesions. Thorax, 37, 54, 1982.

15. Rosenbloom, J., Abrams, W.R., and Mecham, R., Extracellular matrix 4: the elastic fiber. FASEB J., 7(13), 1208, 1993.

16. Knudson, C.B., and Knudson, W., Hyaluronan-binding proteins in development, tissue homeostasis, and disease. FASEB J., 7 (13), 1233, 1993.

17. Raghu, G., and Kinsella, M., Cytokine effects on extracellular matrix. In Cytokines of the Lung. Lung Biology in Health and Disease, Vol. 61. New York, Marcel Dekker, Inc., 1992, p. 491.

18. Hardingham, T.E., and Fosang, A.J., Proteoglycans: many forms and many functions. FASEB J., 6, 861, 1992.

19. Laurent, T.C., and Fraser, J.R.E., Hyaluronan. FASEB J., 6, 2397, 1992.

20. Sibille, Y., and Reynolds, H.Y., Macrophages and polymorphonuclear neutrophils in lung defense and injury. Am. Rev. Respir. Dis., 141, 471, 1990.

21. Jesaitis, A.J., and Dratz, E.A., eds., Molecular Basis of Oxidative Damage by Leukocytes. Boca Raton, FL, CRC Press, 1991.

22. Rom, W.N., Travis, W.D., and Brody, A.R., Cellular and molecular basis of the asbestos related diseases. Am. Rev. Respir. Dis., 143, 405, 1991.

23. Havemann, K., and Janoff, A., Neutral Proteases of Human Polymorphonuclear Leukocytes. Baltimore, Urban & Schwartzenberg, 1978.

24. Gee, J.B.L., Vassallo, C.L., Bell, P., et al., Catalase-dependent peroxidative metabolism in the alveolar macrophage during phagocytosis. J. Clin. Invest., 49, 1280, 1970.

25. Vogt, M.T., Thomas, C., Vassallo, C.L., et al., Glutathione-dependent peroxidative metabolism in the alveolar macrophage. J. Clin. Invest., 50, 401–410, 1971.

26. Mason, R.J., Stossel, T.P., and Vaughn, J., Lipids of alveolar macrophages, polymorphonuclear leukocytes, and their phagocytic vacuoles. J. Clin. Invest., 51, 2399, 1972.

27. Khandwala A., and Gee, J.B.L., Linoleic acid hydroperoxide: impaired bacterial uptake by alveolar macrophages, a mechanism of oxidant lung injury. Science, 182, 1364, 1973.

28. Gaston, B., Drazen, J.M., Loscalzo, J., and Stamler, J.S., The biology of nitrogen oxides in the airways. Am. J. Respir. Crit. Care Med., 149, 538, 1994.

29. Nathan, C., Nitric oxide as a secretory product of mammalian cells. FASEB J., 6, 3051, 1992.

30. Oury, T.D., Ho, Y-S., Piantadosi, C.A., et al., Extracellular superoxide dismutase, nitric oxide, and central nervous system O_2 toxicity. Proc. Natl. Acad. Sci. U.S.A., 89, 9715, 1992.

31. Clancy, R.M., Leszczynska-Piziak, J., and Abramson, S.B., Nitric oxide, an endothelial cell relaxation factor, inhibits neutrophil superoxide anion production via a direct action on the NADPH oxidase. J. Clin. Invest., 90, 1116, 1992.

32. Ward, P.A., and Mulligan, M.S., Leukocyte oxygen products and tissue damage. In Jesaitis, A.J., and Dratz, E.A., eds., Molecular Basis of Oxidative Damage by Leukocytes. Boca Raton, FL, CRC Press, 1991, p. 139.

33. Cochrane, C.G., Mechanisms of cell damage by oxidants. In Jesaitis, A.J., and Dratz, E.A., eds., Molecular Basis of Oxidative Damage by Leukocytes. Boca Raton, FL, CRC Press, 1991, p. 149.

34. Hinman, L.M., Stevens, C.A., Matthay, R.A., and Gee, J.B.L., Elastase and lysozyme activities in human alveolar macrophages: effects of cigarette smoking. Am. Rev. Respir. Dis., 121, 263, 1980.

35. Desrochers, P.E., Jeffrey, J.J., and Weiss, S.J., Interstitial collagenase (matrixmetalloproteinase-1) expresses serpinase activity. J. Clin. Invest., 87, 2258, 1991.

36. Gordon, S., The secretion of lysozyme and a plasminogen activator by mononuclear phagocytes. In Van Furth, R., ed., Mononuclear Phagocytes in Immunity, Infection, and Pathology. Oxford, Blackwell Scientific Publications, 1975, p. 463.

37. Sitrin, R.G., Plasminogen activation in the injured lung: pulmonology does not recapitulate hematology. Am. J. Respir. Cell Mol. Biol., 6, 131, 1992.

38. Werb, Z., Vainton, D.F., and Jones, P.A., Degradation of connective tissue matrices by macrophages. J. Exp. Med., 152, 1537, 1980.

39. Sunderkotter, C., Steinbrink, K, Boebeler, M., et al., Macrophages and angiogenesis. J. Leukoc. Biol., 55, 410, 1994.

40. Gee, J.B.L., and Khandwala, A.S., Motility, transport and endocytosis in lung defense cells. In Brain, J.D., Proctor, D.F., and Reid, L.M., eds., Respiratory Defense Mechanisms. New York, Marcel Dekker, 1977, p. 927.

41. Allison, A.C., Mechanisms of macrophage damage in relation to the pathogenesis of some lung diseases. In Brain, J.D., Proctor, D.F., and Reid, L.M., eds., Respiratory Defense Mechanisms. New York, Marcel Dekker, 1977, p. 1075.

42. Gabor, S.Z., Anca, Z., Sugravu, E., et al., In vitro and in vivo quartz-induced lipid peroxidation. In Brown, R.C., Chamberlain, M., Davies, R., and Gormley, I.P., eds., The In Vitro Effects of Mineral Dusts. London, Academic Press, 1980, p. 131.

43. Light, W.G., and Wei, E.T., Surface charge and asbestos toxicity. Nature, 265, 537, 1977.

44. Caughey, G.H., The structure and airway biology of mast cell proteinases. Am. J. Respir. Cell Mol. Biol., 4, 387, 1991.

45. Askenase, P.W., Metzler, D.M., and Gershon, R.K., Localizations of leukoytes in sites of delayed-type hypersensitivity and in lymph nodes: dependence of vasoactive amines. Immunology, 47, 239, 1982.

46. Rao, P.V.S., Friedman, M.M., Atkins, F.M., et al., Phagocytosis of mast cell granules by cultured fibroblasts. J. Immunol., 130, 341, 1983.
47. Kawanami, O., Ferrans, V.J., Fulmer, J.D., et al., Ultrastructure of pulmonary mast cells in patients with fibrotic lung disorders. Lab. Invest., 40, 717, 1979.
48. Haslam, P.L., Cromwell, O., Dewar, A., et al., Evidence of increased histamine levels in lung lavage fluids from patients with cryptogenic fibrosing alveolitis. Clin. Exp. Immunol., 44, 587, 1981.
49. Jordana, M., Mast cells and fibrosis—who's on first? Am. J. Respir. Cell Mol. Biol., 8, 7, 1993.
50. Wagner, M.M.F., Edwards, R.E., Moncrieff, C.B., et al., Mast cells and inhalation of asbestos in rats. Thorax, 39, 539, 1984.
51. Alam, R., Lett-Brown, M.A., Forsythe, P.A., et al., Monocyte chemotactic and activating factor is a potent histamine-releasing factor for basophils. J. Clin. Invest., 89, 723, 1992.
52. Bodel, P.T., Major, P.T., and Gee, J.B.L., Increased production of endogenous pyrogen and lysozyme by blood monocytes in sarcoidosis. Yale J. Biol. Med., 52, 247, 1979.
53. Sporn, M.B., and Roberts A.B., eds., Peptide Growth Factors and Their Receptors II. New York, Springer-Verlag, 1990.
54. Kelley, J., ed., Cytokines of the Lung. Lung Biology in Health and Disease, Vol 61. New York, Marcel Dekker, Inc., 1992.
55. Rochester, C., and Elias, J.A., Cytokines and cytokine networking in the pathogenesis of interstitial and fibrotic lung disorders. Semin. Respir. Med., 14(5), 389, 1993.
56. Elias, J.A., and Zitnik, R.J., Cytokine-cytokine interactions in the context of cytokine networking. Am. J. Respir. Cell Mol. Biol., 7, 365, 1992.
57. McCartney-Francis, N.L., and Wahl, S.M., Transforming growth factor B: a matter of life and death. J. Leukoc. Biol., 55, 401, 1994.
58. Piguet, P.F., Collart, M.A., Grau, G.E., et al., Requirement of tumour necrosis factor for development of silica-induced pulmonary fibrosis. Nature, 344, 245, 1990.
59. Suzuki, N., Horiuchi, T., Ohta, K., et al., Mast cells are essential for the full development of silica-induced pulmonary inflammation. Am. J. Respir. Cell Mol. Biol., 9, 475, 1993.
60. Kinnula, V.L., Whorton, A.R., Chang, L-Y., et al., Regulation of hydrogen peroxide generation in cultured endothelial cells. Am. J. Respir. Cell Mol. Biol., 6, 175, 1992.
61. Gosset, P., Lassalle, P., Vanhee, D., et al., Production of tumor necrosis factor-a and interleukin-6 by human alveolar macrophages exposed in vitro to coal mine dust. Am. J. Respir. Cell Mol. Biol., 5, 431, 1991.
62. Brandt-Rauf, P.W., Smith, S., Hemminki, K., et al., Serum oncoproteins and growth factors in asbestosis and silicosis patients. Int. J. Cancer, 50, 881, 1992.
63. Roberts, A.B., and Sporn, M.B., The transforming growth factor-Bs. In Sporn, M.B., and Roberts, A., eds., Peptide Growth Factors and Their Receptors. New York, Springer-Verlag, 1990, p. 419.
64. Meade, R., Askenase, P.W., Geba, G.P., et al., Transforming growth factor-B inhibits murine immediate and delayed type hypersensitivity. J. Immunol., 149, 521, 1992.
65. Springer, T.A., Traffic signals for lymphocyte recirculation and leukocyte emigration: the multistep paradigm. Cell, 76, 301, 1994.
66. Smith, C.W., Rothlein, R., Hughes, B.J., et al., Recognition of an endothelial determinant for CD18-dependent human neutrophil adherence and transendothelial migration. J. Clin. Invest., 82, 1746, 1988.
67. Hughes, B.J., Hollers, J.C., Crockett-Torabi E., et al., Recruitment of CD11b/CD18 to the neutrophil surface and adherence-dependent cell locomotion. J. Clin. Invest., 90, 1687, 1992.
68. Mulligan, M., Polley, M.J., Bayer, R.J., et al., Neutrophil-dependent acute lung injury. J. Clin. Invest., 90, 1600, 1992.
69. Ruoslahti, E., Integrins. J. Clin. Invest., 87, 1, 1991.
70. Mulligan, M.S., Varani, J., Dame, M.K., et al., Role of endothelial-leukocyte adhesion molecule 1 (ELAM-1) in neutrophil-mediated lung injury in rats. J. Clin. Invest., 88, 1396, 1991.
71. Shreeniwas, R., Koga, S., Karakurum, M., et al., Hypoxia-mediated induction of endothelial cell interleukin-1a. J. Clin. Invest., 90, 2333, 1992.
72. Christensen, P.J., Kim, S., Simon, R.H., et al., Differentiation related expression of ICAM-1 by rat alveolar epithelial cells. Am. J. Respir. Cell Mol. Biol., 8, 9, 1993.
73. Senior, R.M., Gresham, H.D., Griffin, G.L., et al., Entactin stimulates neutrophil adhesion and chemotaxis through interactions between its arg-gly-asp (RGD) domain and the leukocyte response integrin. J. Clin. Invest., 90, 2251, 1992.
74. Mantovani, A., Bussolino, F., and Dejana, E., Cytokine regulation of endothelial cell function. FASEB J., 6, 2591, 1992.
75. Cantin, A.M., North, S.L., Fells, G.A., et al., Oxidant mediated epithelial cell injury in idiopathic pulmonary fibrosis. J. Clin. Invest., 79, 1665, 1987.
76. Sibille, Y., Martinot, J.B., Polomski, L.L., et al., Phagocyte enzymes in bronchoalveolar lavage from patients with pulmonary sarcoidosis and collagen vascular disorders. Eur. Respir. J., 3, 249, 1990.
77. Hallgren, R., Bejermer, L., Lundgren, R., et al., The eosinophil component of the alveolitis in idiopathic pulmonary fibrosis: signs of eosinophil activation in the lung are related to impaired lung function. Am. Rev. Respir. Dis., 139(2), 373, 1989.
78. Vracko, R., Significance of basal lamina for regeneration of injured lung. Virchows Arch. (Path. Anat.), 355, 264, 1972.

79. Campbell, E.J., Senior, R.M., McDonald, J.A., et al., Proteolysis by neutrophils. Relative importance of cell-substrate contact and oxidative inactivation of proteinase inhibition in vitro. J. Clin. Invest., 70, 845, 1982.

80. Sibille, Y., Lwebuga-Mukasa, J., Polomski, L., et al., An *in vitro* model for polymorphonuclear leukocyte-induced injury to an extracellular matrix. Relative contribution of oxidants and elastase to fibronectin release from amnionic membranes. Am. Rev. Respir. Dis., 134, 134, 1986.

81. Witschi, H.R., Haschek, W.M., Klein-Szanto, A.J.P., et al., Potentiation of diffuse lung damage by oxygen: determining variables. Am. Rev. Respir. Dis., 123, 98, 1981.

82. Merrill, W., Carter, D., and Cullen, M.R., The relationship between large airway inflammation and airway metaplasia. Chest, 100, 131, 1991.

83. Rossman, M.D., Kern, J.A., Elias, J.A., et al., Proliferative response of bronchoalveolar lymphocytes to beryllium. Ann. Intern. Med., 108, 687, 1988.

84. Saltini, C., Winestock, K., Kirby, M., et al., Maintenance of alveolitis in patients with chronic beryllium disease by beryllium-specific helper T cells. N. Engl. J. Med., 320, 1103, 1989.

85. Todd, J.A., Acha-Orbea, H., Bell, J.I., et al., A molecular basis for MHC class II-associated autoimmunity. Science, 240, 1003, 1988.

86. Richeldi, L, Sorrentineo, R., and Saltini, C., HLA-DPB-1 glutamate 69: a genetic marker of beryllium disease. Science, 262, 242, 1993.

87. Orentas, R.J., Reinlib, L., and Hildreth, J.E.K., Anti-class MHC antibody induces multinucleated giant cell formation from peripheral blood monocytes. J. Leukoc. Biol., 51, 199, 1992.

88. Mikes, P.S., Polomski, L.L., and Gee, J.B.L., Mepacrine impairs neutrophil response after acute lung injury in rats: effects on neutrophil migration. Am. Rev. Respir. Dis., 138, 1464, 1988.

89. Livitzki, A., Pyrphostins: tyrosine kinase blockers as novel antiproliferative agents and dissectors of signal transduction. FASEB J., 6, 3275, 1992.

90. Weinstock, J.V., Boros, D.L., Gee, J.B.L., et al., The effect of SQ14225, an inhibitor of angiotensin I converting enzyme, on the granulomatous response to *Schistosoma mansoni* eggs in mice. J. Clin. Invest., 67, 931, 1981.

91. Mossman, B.T., Marsh, J.P., Sesko, A., et al., Inhibition of lung injury, inflammation and interstitial pulmonary fibrosis by polyethylene glycol-conjugated catalase in a rapid inhalation model of asbestosis. Am. Rev. Respir. Dis., 141, 1266, 1990.

92. Mossman, B.T., Craighead, J.E., MacPherson, B.V., Asbestos-induced epithelial changes in organ cultures of hamster trachea: inhibition by the vitamin A analog, retinyl methyl ether. Science, 207, 311, 1980.

93. Janssen, Y.M.W., Van Houten, B., Borm, P.J.A., et al., Biology of disease: cell and tissue responses to oxidative damage, Lab. Invest., 69, 261, 1993.

94. Mossman, BT., and Gee, J.B.L., Asbestos-related diseases. N. Engl. J. Med., 320, 1721, 1989.

95. Shelby, M.D., The genetic toxicity of human carcinogens and its implications. Mutat. Res., 204, 3, 1988.

96. Ames, B.N., and Gold, L.S., Mitogenesis increases mutagenesis. Science, 249, 970, 1990.

97. Preston-Martin, S., Pike, M.C., Ross, R.K., et al., Increased cell division as a cause of human cancer. Cancer Res., 50, 7415, 1990.

98. Pitot, H.C., The molecular biology of carcinogenesis. Cancer, 72, 962, 1993.

99. Bergh, J.C.S., Gene amplifications in human lung cancer. Am. Rev. Respir. Dis., 142, S20, 1990.

100. Gibas, Z., Li, F.P., Antman, K.H., et al., Chromosome changes in malignant mesothelioma, Cancer Genet. Cytogenet., 20, 191, 1986.

101. Hagemeijer, A., Versnel, M.A., Van Druen, E., et al., Cytogenetic analysis of malignant mesothelioma. Cancer Genet. Cytogenet., 47, 1, 1990.

102. Popescu, N.C., Chahanian, A.P., and DiPaolo, J.A., Nonrandom chromosome alterations in human malignant mesothelioma. Cancer Res., 48, 142, 1988.

103. Cote, R.J., Jhanwar, S.C., Novick, S., et al., Genetic alterations of the p53 gene area feature of malignant mesotheliomas. Cancer Res., 51, 5410, 1991.

104. Metcalf, R.A., Welsh, J.A., Bennett, W.P., et al., p53 and Kirsten-ras mutations in human mesothelioma cell lines. Cancer Res., 52, 2610, 1992.

105. Gerwin, B.I., Lechner, J.F., Reddel, R.R., et al., Comparison of production of transforming growth factor-B and platelet-derived growth factor by normal human mesothelial cells and mesothelioma cell lines. Cancer Res., 47, 6180, 1987.

106. Versnel, M.A., Hagemeijer, A., Bouts, M.J., et al., Expression of c-sis (PDGF-B) chain and PDGF-a chain in ten human malignant mesothelioma cell lines derived from primary and metastatic tumors. Oncogene, 2, 601, 1988.

107. Walker, C., Bermudez, E., Stewart, W., et al., Characterization of platelet-derived growth factor and platelet-derived growth factor receptor expression in asbestos-induced rat mesothelioma. Cancer Res., 52, 301, 1992.

108. Van der Meeren, A., Seddon, M.B., Betsholtz, C.A., et al., Tumorigenic conversion of human mesothelial cells as a consequence of platelet-derived growth factor-A overexpression. Am. J. Respir. Cell Mol. Biol., 8, 214, 1993.

109. Jaurand, M.C., Bignon, J., and Brochard, P., eds., Mesothelial cell and mesothelioma. Past, present and future. Eur. Respir. Rev., 3, 1990.

110. Mossman, B.T., Bignon, J., Corn, M., et al., Asbestos: scientific developments and implications for public policy. Science, 247, 294, 1990.

111. Miller, G.H., The toxicity of asbestos and its relation to smoking and lung cancer. The Chemist, January/February, 13, 1994.
112. Eastman, A., Mossman, B.T., and Bresnick, E., Influence of asbestos on the uptake of benzo(a)pyrene and DNA alkylation on hamster tracheal epithelial cells. Cancer Res., 43, 1251, 1983.
113. Mossman, B.T., Eastman, A., Landesman, J.M., et al., Effects of crocidolite and chrysotile asbestos on cellular uptake, metabolisms and DNA after exposure of hamster tracheal epithelial cells to benzo(a)pyrene. Environ. Health Perspect., 51, 331, 1983.
114. Graceffa, P., and Weitzman, S., Asbestos catalyzes the formatation of the 6-obenzo(a)pyrene radical from 6-hydroxybenzo(a)pyrene. Arch. Biochem. Biophys., 253, 481, 1987.
115. McFadden, D., Wright, J., Wiggs, B., et al., Cigarette smoke increases the penetration of asbestos fibers into airway walls. Am. J. Pathol., 123, 95, 1986.
116. McFadden, D., Wright, J., Wiggs, B., et al., Smoking inhibits asbestos clearance. Am. Rev. Respir. Dis., 133, 372, 1986.
117. Churg, A., Hobson, J., Berean, K., et al., Scavengers of active oxygen species prevent cigarette smoke-induced asbestos fiber penetration in rat tracheal explants. Am. J. Pathol., 135, 599, 1989.
118. Mossman, B.T., Asbestos: An update. Cancer Prevention, October, p. 1, 1992.
119. Marsh, J.M., and Mossman, B.T., Mechanisms of induction of ornithine decarboxylase activity in tracheal epithelial cells by asbestiform minerals, Cancer Res., 48, 709, 1988.
120. Marsh, J.M., and Mossman, B.T., Role of asbestos and active oxygen species in activation and expression of ornithine decarboxylase in hamster tracheal epithelial cells. Cancer Res., 51, 167, 1991.
121. Pegg, A.E., Polyamine metabolism and its importance in neoplastic growth and as target for chemotherapy. Cancer Res., 48, 759, 1988.
122. Cameron, G., Woodworth, C.D., Edmondson, S., et al., Mechanisms of asbestos-induced squamous metaplasia in tracheobronchial epithelial cells. Environ. Health Perspect., 80, 101, 1989.
123. Heintz, N., Janssen, Y.M.W., and Mossman, B.T., Persistent induction of c-fos and c-jun protooncogene expression by asbestos. Proc. Natl. Acad. Sci. U.S.A., 90, 3299, 1993.
124. Artvinli, M., and Baris, Y.I., Malignant mesothelioma in a small village in the Anatolian region of Turkey: an epidemiologic study. J. Natl. Cancer Inst., 63, 17, 1979.
125. Janssen, Y.M.W., Marsh, J.P., Heintz, N., et al., Induction of c-fos and c-jun protooncogenes in target cells of the lung and pleura by carcinogenic fibers. Am. J. Respir. Cell Mol. Biol. (in press).
126. Wagner, J.C., The discovery of the association between blue asbestos and mesotheliomas and the aftermath. Br. J. Ind. Med., 48, 399, 1991.
127. Lund, L.G., and Aust, A.E., Iron mobilization from crocidolite asbestos greatly enhances crocidolite-dependent formation of DNA single strand breaks in oX174 RFI DNA. Carcinogenesis, 13, 637, 1992.
128. Hansen, K., and Mossman, B.T., Generation of superoxide (O2) from alveolar macrophages exposed to asbestiform and nonfibrous particles. Cancer Res., 47, 1681, 1987.
129. Weitzman, S.A., and Graceffa, P., Asbestos catalyzes hydroxyl and superoxide radical generation from hydrogen peroxide. Arch. Biochem. Biophys., 228, 373, 1984.
130. Lund, L.G., and Aust, A.E., Iron-catalyzed reactions may be responsible for the biochemical and biological effects of asbestos. Biofactors, 3, 83, 1991.
131. Goodglick, L.A., Pietras, L.A., and Kane, A., Evaluation of the causal realtionship between crocidolite asbestos-induced lipid peroxidation and toxicity to macrophages. Am. Rev. Respir. Dis., 139, 1265, 1989.
132. Turver, C.J., and Brown, R.C., The role of catalytic iron in asbestos-induced lipid peroxidation and DNA-strand breakage in C3H10T1/2 cells. Br. J. Cancer, 56, 133, 1987.
133. Weitzman, S.A., and Weitberg, A.B., Asbestos-catalyzed lipid peroxidation and its inhibition by desferrioxamine. Biochem. J., 225, 259, 1985.
134. Kasprzak, K.S., The role of oxidative damage in metal carcinogenicity. Chem. Res. Toxicol., 4, 604, 1991.
135. Costa, M., Molecular mechanisms of nickel carcinogenesis. Annu. Rev. Pharmacol. Toxicol., 31, 321, 1991.
136. Holland, L.M., Crystalline silica and lung cancer: recent experimental evidence. Regul. Toxicol. Pharmacol., 12, 224–237, 1990.
137. Saffiotti, U., Lung cancer induction by silica in rats, but not in mice and hamsters. In Seemayer, N.H., and Hadnagy, W., eds., Environmental Hygiene II. New York, Springer-Verlag, 1990, pp. 235–238.
138. Craighead, J.E., Do silica and asbestos cause lung cancer? Arch. Pathol. Lab. Med., 116, 16–20, 1992.
139. Davis, J.M.G., In vivo assays to evaluate the pathogenic effects of minerals in rodents. In Guthrie, G.D., and Mossman, B.T., eds., Health Effects of Mineral Dusts. Reviews in Mineralogy, Mineralogical Society of America, 28, 471–488, 1993.
140. IARC: International Agency for Research on Cancer, Silica and Some Silicates, Vol. 42. Lyon, France, International Agency of Research on Cancer, 1987.
141. Vallyathan, V., et al., Generation of free radicals from freshly fractured silica dust. Am. Rev. Respir. Dis., 138, 1213–1219, 1988.
142. Daniel, L.N., Mao, Y., and Saffiotti, U., Oxidative DNA damage by crystalline silica. Free Radic. Biol. Med., 14, 463–472, 1993.

143. Saffiotti, U., Daniel, L.N., Mao, Y., et al., Biological studies on the carcinogenic mechanisms of crystalline silica. *In* Guthrie, G.D., and Mossman, B.T., eds., Health Effects of Mineral Dusts. Reviews in Mineralogy, Mineralogical Society of America, 28, 523–544, 1993.

144. Miles, P.R., Bowman, L., and Miller, M.R., Alterations in the pulmonary microsomal cytochrome P-450 system after exposure of rats to silica. Am. J. Respir. Cell Mol. Biol., 8, 597–604, 1993.

145. Oshimura, M., Hesterberg, T.W., Tsutsui, T., et al., Correlation of asbestos-induced cytogenetic effects with cell transformation of Syrian hamster embryo cells in culture. Cancer Res., 44, 5017, 1984.

146. Saffiotti, U., and Stinson, S.F., Lung cancer induction by crystalline silica: relationships to granulomatous reactions and host factors. Env. Carcinoma Revs. (J. Environ. Sci. Health) C6(2), 197–222, 1988.

147. Kushner, M., The effects of MMMF on animal systems: some reflections on their pathogenesis. Ann. Occup. Hyg., 31, 791, 1987.

148. Driscoll, K.E., Lindenschmidt, R.C., Maurer, J.K., et al., Pulmonary response to silica or titanium dioxide: inflammatory cells, alveolar macrophage-derived cytokines, and histopathology. Am. J. Cell Mol. Biol., 2, 381–390, 1990.

149. Lugano, E.M., Dauber, J.H., Elias, J.A., et al., The regulation of lung fibroblast proliferation by alveolar macrophages in experimental silicosis. Am. Rev. Respir. Dis., 1239, 767–771, 1984.

150. Lesur, O., Melloni, B., Cantin, A.M., and Begin, R., Silica-exposed lung fluids have a proliferative activity for type II epithelial cells: a study on human and sheep alveolar fluids. Exp. Lung Res., 18, 633–654, 1992.

151. Li, W., Kumar, R.K., O'Grady, R., and Velan, G.M., Role of lymphocytes in silicosis: regulation of secretion of macrophage-derived mitogenic activity for fibroblasts. Int. J. Exp. Pathol., 73, 793–800, 1992.

152. Sjostrand, M., Absher, P.M., Hemenway, D.R., et al., Comparison of lung alveolar and tissue cells in silica-induced inflammation. Am. Rev. Respir. Dis., 143, 47, 1991.

12

Anthony Seaton

Silicosis

■

HISTORICAL ASPECTS

Silicosis is the name given to the fibrotic disease of the lungs caused by inhalation of dust containing crystalline silicon dioxide. As this compound forms the greater part of the earth's crust, the possibilities of exposure to the dust are numerous and have been since humans first took to making tools and weapons from flint. Since almost any occupation involving the mining into or the cutting, shaping, or polishing of rock involves a risk of silicosis, it is curious that little mention of lung disease among such workers was made in classical times. Pliny the Elder, in his *Natural History* written in the 1st century AD, mentions the dangers to miners of fumes and vapors, but not those of dust. Not until Agricola's major work on the mining and production of metals, *De re metallica,* was published in 1556[1] was an account given of the fatal effects of dust. In the sixth book, Agricola writes: "It remains for me to speak of the ailments and accidents of miners, and of the methods by which we can guard against them, for we should always devote more care to maintaining our health, that we may freely perform our bodily functions, than to making profits."

Unhappily the advice given here has not always been heeded, and the drive for profit both by individual miners and by their employers has over the succeeding four centuries resulted, by the neglect of safety precautions, in the production of untold ill health and premature death. Even in recent times, early widowhood has been the common lot of the women of mining areas, as it was in Agricola's day.

Agricola described the machinery necessary for ventilation of mines, though the emphasis was more on the removal of stale air that would not support combustion and of the fumes of fires used to crack the rocks than on the reduction of dust. Moreover, he described the responsibilities of the various mine officials in ensuring the safety of the workings.

A hundred and fifty years after Agricola, Ramazzini published *De Morbis Artificum Diatriba,* describing in the first chapter the diseases afflicting miners.[2] He emphasized the unpleasant and dangerous nature of mining by pointing out that the occupation was still, in the 18th century, considered a suitable punishment for malefactors, as it had been in Pliny's time. While Ramazzini mentioned cough and asthma as being recorded among miners by previous authors, he attributed most of their ill health to the absorption of the metals they were mining. He later mentions the use of powdered flint in pottery, but records that morbidity in this trade was due to lead poisoning. Finally, in his chapter on stonecutters, he records the inhalation of splinters leading to asthmatic afflictions, consumption, and cough. He quotes the pathological work of Diemerbroeck, who in studying the lungs of stonecutters who had died of asthma had found them full of sand. Ramazzini was aware that in this trade very small particles were suspended in the air, and he quoted a master stonecutter who had told him of finding a handful of very fine sand inside an ox bladder hung in his workshop.

During the 18th century there was a gradual realization of the hazards to health associated with work on millstones and grinding wheels in Europe, though the resultant disease was always assumed to be tuberculosis. Johnstone[3] in 1796 gave a paper to the Medical Society of London in which he described the frequency of premature death of needle pointers from phthisis, attributing this to irritation of the lungs by inhaled particles of iron and stone. He advised the use of a gauze helmet to limit dust inhalation. He also noted that the work was so well known to be fatal that there was difficulty in employing labor and that the high wages paid to attract workers contributed to ill health by allowing them intemperance. By the time of the publication of Thackrah's great work on occupational health in 1831,[4] lung disease was known to cause premature death in knife grinding, the quarrying and cutting of sandstone as opposed to limestone, and the filing of cast iron as opposed to wrought iron. This work is particularly interesting because Thackrah made measurements of vital capacity on the workers he studied, comparing one group with another. While such tests form one of the bases of all studies of occupational lung disease nowadays, Thackrah's use of the technique antedated the development of the spirometer by Hutchinson in 1846.

In 1860, Peacock[5] produced an early example of a controlled mortality study when he compared the normal life span of wire basket makers with the typical 40-year life span of the makers of French burr millstones, though both groups were employed in the same factory and working conditions in terms of temperature, dampness, and light were, if anything, worse for the basket makers. He suggested the use of water and ventilation for dust suppression and the wearing of respirators. He examined the lungs by a technique of ashing and treatment with hydrochloric acid and described the finding of siliceous matter similar to that found in the workshop. This technique was taken a little further by Greenhow,[6] who in 1865 published an investigation of a grinder's lung which contained small black crystalline masses. These were not soluble in hydrochloric acid, so they were not iron. The tissue was ashed and dissolved in hydrochloric acid and the residue examined. It included small angular masses that transmitted polarized light and dissolved in hydrofluoric acid, and thus seemed to be silica. The same author also described this disease in potters,[7] enumerating the particular aspects of that trade in which inhalation of silica and alumina could occur.

Silicosis made its appearance in the medical literature of the United States in the last quarter of the 19th century in isolated case reports, described as a "chronic disease of the air passages" among employees of a cutlery factory.[8] Early in the present century the disease was recognized among miners and rock crushers, and with the development of mechanization and the consequent increase in the prevalence of silicosis and silicotuberculosis, public concern began to be generated. In a survey by the United States Public Health Service in 1913 to 1915, 60% of 720 lead and zinc miners in Missouri were found to have these diseases.[9] Subsequent studies showed a very high prevalence of silicosis among Vermont granite workers and New York tunnellers, and by the 1930s the disease had been described in most of the trades in which it was known to occur in Europe.

The turning point in the history of silicosis in the United States came in the 1930s. Methods of dust suppression and dust avoidance were developed and their application spread, largely owing to the impetus of legal action for negligence taken against employers by many of the, by then, large population of silicotics. Public opinion was aroused particularly by the appalling episode at Gauley Bridge in southern West Virginia. In order to produce hydroelectric power, a tunnel was driven through a sandstone mountain. Cheap labor, largely brought in from the South, was used and no precautions were taken to diminish exposure to dust. Vigorous attempts were made to prevent the effects of this becoming public knowledge, but congressional hearings revealed that 476 workers had died in the course of the construction and some 1500 more had contracted silicosis.[10, 11] Today a plaque celebrates the engineering achievement.

During the 1930s and 1940s, the states began to introduce laws providing for compensation of victims of silicosis, and many also established programs of industrial hygiene. Methods of dust control became more widely applied as the hazards became more fully known, though the application of these measures was slow, particularly in smaller industries and companies. The introduction of antituberculosis chemotherapy in the 1950s further revolutionized the management of that most serious complication of the disease, and there is little doubt that silicosis is much less prevalent now than a few decades ago. Interest in the problem, however, has been rekindled by the suggestion that quartz may be carcinogenic, a matter which will be discussed later. Moreover, silicosis remains an important risk of stone and mine workers in the developing and underdeveloped world (Fig. 12–1).

SILICA AND INDUSTRY

Forms of Silica

Silicon dioxide, or silica, is one of the most abundant materials in the earth's crust. The silica atoms usually occur at the center of tetrahedra formed by four oxygen atoms. These interlink at their apices in a variety of ways to produce the silica polymorphs (pure SiO_2) and, when combined with other elements, the silicate minerals. The various arrangements of these atoms in space produce the crystalline, microcrystalline, and amorphous polymorphs. The commonest naturally occurring form of crystalline silica is quartz, a component of many rock types (Fig. 12–2). While quartz is almost pure silicon dioxide, it often contains traces of other elements that are responsible for the range of colors that it can assume and that give certain varieties, such as amethyst or smoke quartz, value as gems or ornamental

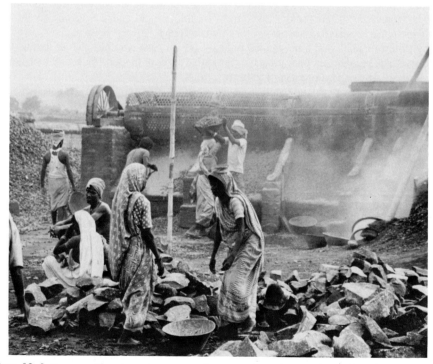

Figure 12–1. Young and female workers at a small stone crushing plant in India. Such workers are at high risk of silicosis if stone contains significant amounts of quartz.

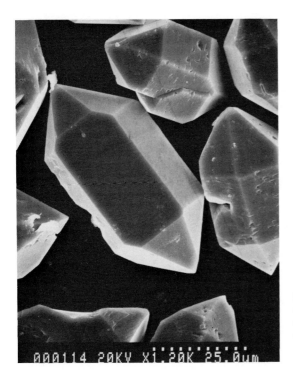

Figure 12–2
Quartz crystals, in this case extracted from limestone. Scanning electron microscope (SEM) photograph; marker indicates 25 μm. (Courtesy of Mr. John Addison.)

materials. Other crystalline forms of silica are cristobalite and tridymite, which occur naturally in volcanic rocks, for example in Colorado and California, but which may also be produced by heating quartz or amorphous silica in industrial situations. There is some evidence that these forms are even more toxic than quartz itself. Of two other naturally occurring forms of crystalline silica, stishovite and coesite, the former with an octahedral structure appears in experimental studies to be less toxic.

Microcrystalline, or cryptocrystalline, silica consists of minute crystals of cristobalite bonded together by amorphous silica as in flint, agate, or chert. Amorphous silica, which is noncrystalline and relatively nontoxic, occurs as diatomite (kieselguhr) and vitreous silica. The former consists of the skeletons of prehistoric marine organisms. Its usefulness largely depends on its being calcined, that is heated either alone or with alkali flux. This process converts most of the amorphous silica to cristobalite, which is probably responsible for its toxicity. Vitreous silica is formed when crystalline silica is melted then cooled quickly. Again, heating above about 1200°C will ensure that vitreous silica contains cristobalite. All these forms of silicon dioxide may be referred to as free silica, to distinguish them from the silica combined with other elements in the silicate minerals. These latter compounds, which include asbestos, micas, and talc, present different hazards to health and are discussed in Chapters 13 and 14.

It can thus be seen that free silica occurs in a wide range of rocks, though it is not always the main component. For example, sandstone may contain almost 100% quartz, slate and shale up to 40%, and granite between 10% and about 30%. Flints consist of almost 100% amorphous or cryptocrystalline silica, while certain smectite clays (e.g., fuller's earth or bentonites) may contain up to 10% of quartz or cristobalite. Usually very low levels occur in the carbonate rocks, limestone, dolomite, or marble, though cases of silicosis have occurred in workers exposed to dusts from these materials presumably contaminated with quartz. A hazard to health should always be suspected whenever dust containing free silica is likely to be liberated into the air, but the magnitude of the hazard can only be estimated by measurement of the dust levels and analysis of the content and type of free silica present.

Analysis of Silica

The standard methods used for the analysis of quartz in respirable dust samples are infrared spectophotometry (IR) and x-ray diffractometry (XRD). Either the direct, on-filter IR method or the indirect potassium bromide disk IR method can be used for analysis, provided that care is taken to ensure that the standard reference minerals used for calibration are properly prepared. The XRD method is usually restricted to direct on-filter analysis when limited amounts of dust are available for analysis.

Exposure to Silica

The importance of silica as a health hazard today relates to its ubiquity and to the fact that, though its risks are well known, protective measures may be ignored. While this may be excusable in underdeveloped countries with unsophisticated or absent medical services, it is clearly negligent in the Western democracies. Thus, while the occurrence of rapidly progressive silicosis in Nigerians carving sandstone grinding wheels[12] or in Indians making slate pencils[13] may occasion little surprise, the same disease in oil rig sandblasters and silica flour workers in the United States[14, 15] and in government-employed stonemasons and coal miners in Britain[16, 17] comes as a shock. Such outbreaks of fatal disease occur through neglect of preventive measures and often of legal obligations, sometimes through ignorance but sometimes from an incorrect balancing of costs of preventive measures against perceived benefits. Thus, the use of quartz-containing sand was banned for metal blasting in Britain in 1949 and in the European Community in 1955, yet persists in the United States. The occurrence of fatal silicosis in two British stonemasons recently might have been prevented had equipment for exhaust ventilation not been considered too costly. Such disregard of knowledge is almost universally to be found when silicosis occurs.

A complete list of all industries in which silicosis may occur would not only be impracticable but meaningless in the absence of the sort of detail obtained in a careful occupational history. However, the major groups of industries in which a risk of exposure to silica dust may be suspected are as follows.

Quarrying, Stone Cutting, Mining, and Tunneling

Sandstone and granite are extensively used in building, as is slate, though now to a lesser extent. These materials may also be used in a ground or crushed form as fillers and abrasives and in road building. While they are usually obtained by quarrying, slate may be mined. Exposure to silica in these industries depends on the amount of water suppression and the adequacy of ventilation, particularly in the sheds where the stones are shaped or crushed (Fig. 12–3). The trades involved in the cutting, engraving, and polishing of these stones are clearly at risk, especially where sandblasting is used. Similarly, the cleaning and repair of stone public buildings, when not carried out as a wet process, may generate a dust hazard. Excavation, such as digging graves in sandstone, preparing foundations for buildings, and removing silica-containing overburden in open-cast, or strip, mining for other minerals may also entail a silicosis risk.

Mining for metals usually involves the removal of quartz-rich ores, and silicosis may occur in gold, tin, iron, copper, nickel, silver, tungsten, and uranium mining. Other useful minerals, such as asbestos, mica, shales, barytes, fireclays, and fluorite, are also mined in such a way that the dust may contain silica. It is important to remember that while tin refining and barium sulphate production produce the benign pneumoconioses, stannosis, and baritosis (see Chapter 16), mining for these minerals involves a risk of silicosis.[18, 19] Coal mining may involve exposure to silica in hardheading, driving shafts and tunnels, roof bolting, and

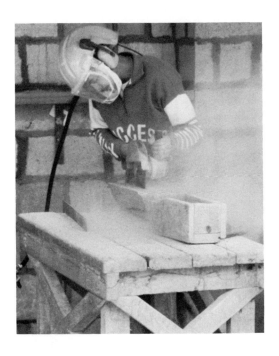

Figure 12–3
Stonemason at work in a yard in which two fatal cases of silicosis occurred. Note dependence on inadequate respiratory protection and use of powered cutting tools.

using sand as a friction material on rails, and when intrusions of roof and floor are cut with the coal seam.

Tunneling through sandstone or granite constitutes an obvious risk, especially with the use of modern machinery and the difficulties of providing effective ventilation. However, tunneling through limestone and the use of limestones with a low silica content to prevent explosion in coal mines (commonly called rock-dusting) do not entail a risk of silicosis. A note of warning should be sounded here. Silicosis has been described in limestone workers exposed to high levels of dust containing quartz as well as calcium carbonate.[20] The author has recently seen two severe examples of this (Fig. 12–4).

Foundry Work

Foundries are the places where castings of iron, steel, and nonferrous materials such as bronze are made. The process involves the production of a mold into which the molten metal is cast. A core may also be used to produce a hollow casting. The solidified casting is then knocked out of the mold. Silica, predominantly cristobalite, and other contaminants from the mold that have burnt onto the surface of the casting need to be cleaned off. Exposure to silica can potentially occur in the production of the molds and cores, which are made of quartz sand bonded by clays or resins, in the knocking out of castings, and especially in the process of cleaning and polishing of the product. This is often known as fettling or dressing, and may be done with hammers, grinding wheels, mills, or abrasive blasting. Silicosis has resulted from the continued use of sandblasting in the southern United States in the production of large-scale castings for shipbuilding and oil platforms.[15] Foundry workers may also be responsible for knocking out the linings of furnaces, which may include quartz and crocidolite.

Workers in foundries are therefore exposed to a wide range of possible hazards, including silica, iron oxides, and fumes from molten metals and from the bonding resins. These resins may include isocyanates, and occupational asthma is not unknown among such workers. Fettlers and those involved in furnace lining are at greatest risk of silica exposure, though true silicosis with progression to massive fibrosis is probably rare except when sandblasting is used (Fig. 12–5). The radiographic abnormalities in these workers usually represent a more benign mixed dust

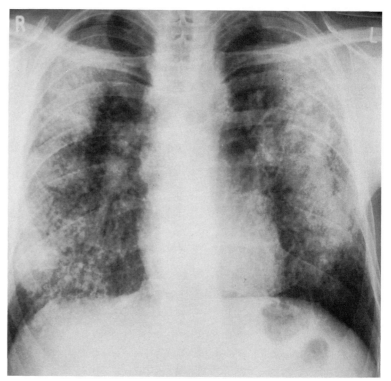

Figure 12–4. Chest radiograph of 40-year-old man with bilateral massive fibrosis resulting from exposure to quartz dust at the crushing plant of a limestone quarry.

pneumoconiosis, the principal cause of radiographic shadowing often being iron oxide.

Other possible sources of exposure to silica in foundries include the cleaning and repairing of furnaces lined with silica brick (see later) and the general contamination of the workplace by dusty processes.

Ceramics

Powdered flint and clays containing free silica have traditionally been used in the manufacture of china and earthenware, and some of these may contain relatively

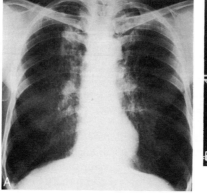
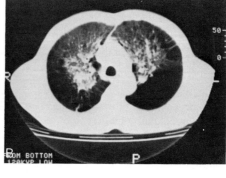

Figure 12–5. Chest radiograph (A) and computed tomography (CT) scan (B) of patient with massive fibrosis and surrounding bullous emphysema, resulting from 30 years of work polishing iron castings with an abrasive tool in a foundry.

high proportions of quartz.[21] China clay itself usually contains a relatively small proportion (less than 5%) of silica, but crushed, calcined flint or other siliceous clays need to be added, usually in a wet process, prior to shaping and firing. The unfinished articles are then polished or fettled and may subsequently be glazed with a mixture also containing silica. Risks of exposure occur chiefly among those involved in crushing flint and in fettling. Significant exposure can occur from contaminated clothing. In the past, articles were baked in kilns on a bedding of powdered flint, and workers were exposed to this. More recently, this has been replaced by alumina, while other substitutes for flint and siliceous clays in the clay mixture are being introduced. Thus, the hazards of silicosis in this industry, which used to be appreciable, are now very much reduced. Historically, this used to be one of the very few industries in which women contracted silicosis. However, the increasing employment of women in jobs traditionally held by men has also widened their opportunities of getting this disease.

Production of refractory brickware for lining kilns, furnaces, boilers, and other places where fire resistance is required involves the crushing, shaping, and baking of sandstone. Exposure may occur in the initial mining, crushing, and milling processes; in shaping and laying the bricks; and especially in stripping, cleaning, and repairing of the linings of boilers and similar plants. It should be noted that boilermakers or repairers may be exposed to a number of hazards, often in very confined spaces—silica from brick linings, asbestos from lagging, cement and occasionally filling between bricks, and, in the case of work on oil-fired boilers, vanadium from oil residues. The fly-ash residue of coal burning is probably not hazardous, since it has a low silica content, though there has been one rather dubious report of "fly-ash pneumoconiosis."[22]

Other Industries

Silicosis may also be encountered in a wide range of other trades. The use of finely ground quartz in sandblasting has already been referred to; it is to be hoped that substitution of other materials such as shot, slag, grit, and silicon carbide will soon eliminate this hazardous material. The abrasive properties of silica are also still made use of in some scouring powders, polishes, toothpastes, and sandpaper, although adequate and less toxic substitutes are available. Silica flour, or finely milled crystalline silica, is used in many of these products, and also as a filler in paints, woods, surfacing materials, rubbers, and plastics. Not only is it potentially very toxic, but it may be marketed and labeled incorrectly as amorphous silica.[23] Rapidly progressive silicosis has been described in the production of silica flour in the United States[14] and Australia.[24, 25]

Diatomaceous earth, being amorphous silica, is thought not to entail a great hazard; however, when calcined, it is converted largely into cristobalite and tridymite. Extensive deposits occur in the western United States, where it is strip mined, crushed, and calcined. It is used in filters, abrasives, insulation materials, and absorbents. Exposure may therefore occur in many different and unexpected situations. It is probably only when exposure to calcined material occurs that there is a significant risk of silicosis.[26]

Other uses of silica in industry include glassmaking, where sand may be used both for polishing and as a component, and enameling, where quartz and other materials are crushed and melted together. Other small industries employing stone containing silica, such as in the use of slate in the manufacture of table mats, billiard tables, and ornaments, and the manufacture of semi-precious stones from colored forms of quartz, survive in industrialized nations, while traditional crafts such as the manufacture of slate pencils and sandstone grinding wheels may still be found in less industrially developed countries.

EPIDEMIOLOGY

Measuring the Effects of Silica on Populations

Many problems beset those who wish to study the epidemiology of silicosis. The population at risk is constantly changing, mobile, and almost impossible to measure. Since the disease occurs as a consequence of cumulative exposure over years, and since the industries that provide the risk are those most likely to be affected by the economic health of the nation, the size of the population from which cases are drawn is likely to be very different at the time the disease occurs from that when exposure first started. Moreover, conditions of dust exposure may well have changed, though not necessarily for the better. And then definition of silicosis may not be as straightforward as it appears. Even if the International Labor Organization (ILO) classification is used (and this is still not universal), the category for case definition may vary for different purposes, and different readers may vary widely in their interpretation of films. Finally, it is usually impossible to obtain anything other than a very rough estimate of the exposures to quartz of individuals in any study. It is perhaps worth posing the question, why do we need to study the epidemiology of silicosis? The answers are two: first, in order to measure as accurately as possible the relationships between exposure to quartz and risk of disease and, second, in order to assess the efficacy of preventive measures. For the first objective, knowledge of the exposure history of individuals in the study population is necessary, while for the second all that is required is a standard measure of response. Both are of course specific to the population being studied; even exposure-response relationships may not be generalizable because workers in different industries are rarely exposed to quartz dust that is the same in toxicological or mineralogical terms. Thus, reports of studies of the epidemiology of silicosis need to be read with caution.

Risks Associated with Different Types of Silica

Almost all the silica to which workers are exposed in industry is quartz, usually mixed with other minerals. The proportion of quartz may vary from very low levels, as in some limestones and coal mine dusts, to almost 100%, as in silica flour and some hard sandstones. Many mineral dusts, such as those generated by cutting granite and slate, contain a variable amount of quartz from workplace to workplace and even within the same workplace. Even apparently innocuous dusts, such as from limestone, may occasionally contain relatively high proportions of quartz. In general, it appears that the rapidity with which silicosis appears and progresses depends on the total amount of quartz to which workers are exposed, the time over which that exposure occurs, and the presence of other minerals, especially clays, that may interfere with the toxicity of the quartz. It also seems likely that the surface properties of the quartz particles may be important and that recently fractured crystals, produced for example by the use of powered cutting tools, may be more toxic than unfractured particles. Rapidly progressive fatal silicosis has been described in workers milling silica flour,[14] drilling the overburden of surface coal mines,[27] cutting hard sandstone with powered tools,[16] sandblasting,[28] and producing pottery.[29] All these episodes have been characterized by relatively short exposures to extremely high levels of quartz, in the case of the stonemasons up to 20 mg/m^3. Slightly less progressive silicosis, affecting a high proportion of the work force and proving fatal over the course of about 10 years, has been reported in Indian slate pencil workers.[13, 30] Levels of respirable quartz measured in the breathing zone of cutters in this trade have been shown to range between 2 and 10 mg/m^3. Similar patterns of disease have been described among sandblasters in Louisiana, where mean levels of exposure were recorded around 5 mg/m^3,[31] among jade polishers in Hong Kong exposed to silica flour (around 0.7 mg/m^3),[32] and among workers making abrasive soaps and exposed to silica flour in Ontario.[33]

The clinical effects of exposures to other forms of silica are less well documented. Calcined or heated silica-containing minerals may be anticipated to contain cristobalite. Thus, workers exposed to dust in furnace relining and fettling, where silica has been heated to high temperatures, and in the production of diatomaceous earth may be exposed in part to this mineral. A study of workers exposed to diatomaceous earth has shown that silicosis occurred in some 25% of workers with more than 5 years' exposure in 1953;[26] 10% of this population had massive fibrosis, indicating a severe and often progressive form of the disease. Follow-up surveys in 1974 and 1979, after the introduction of effective dust control measures, showed the prevalence to have fallen considerably, all cases occurring in workers with greater than 15 years' exposure.[34, 35] In all these surveys, disease occurred almost exclusively in workers exposed to the calcined diatomaceous earth, which contained between 20% and 60% cristobalite.

The effects of amorphous silica have been investigated in the diatomaceous earth industry as well as in the production of silicon metal and of submicron silica. In the former industry, workers in quarries have been and are exposed to uncalcined diatomaceous earth, though there is no good evidence in the literature of their exposure levels. Since the work is in the open air, they may not be very high. Nevertheless, in a 26-year follow-up of men who took part in a study in 1953, low categories of pneumoconiosis were found in at least two quarry workers.[35] Similarly, a study of 26 Italian diatomaceous earth quarry workers has shown two with category 1 and one with category 2 pneumoconiosis.[36] These men were said to have been exposed to dust that contained less than 2.35% quartz and was primarily amorphous silica. The risk of serious disease, as opposed to minor radiologic changes, in such workers appears to be very small.

In the silicon metal industry, quartz is heated above its boiling point (2350°C). Workers may be exposed to a fume consisting of very small (0.05 to 0.75 μm) spherical particles of silica. Two papers have reported changes consistent with pneumoconiosis in these workers. In 1977, 11 of 40 United States men exposed to this process were said to have abnormal radiographs, and convincing evidence of radiographic abnormality was presented for three of these.[37] In two, lung biopsies had been carried out and showed a process of fibrosis and histiocytosis unlike classical silicosis and similar to that found in experimental animals exposed to the same dust. However, the authors noted that this dust contained crystalline silica, and the experimental study indicates that it consisted of cristobalite surrounded by a layer of amorphous silica. The second paper, from France in 1980, records finding irregular and nodular radiologic shadows in 10 people working in a silicon foundry.[38] Biopsies in two confirmed interstitial fibrosis associated with amorphous silica; fewer than 1% of the pulmonary particles were crystalline silica.

Clinical studies of workers exposed to submicron amorphous silica with particle sizes in the region of 0.02 μm have reported no radiologic changes.[39, 40] However, these studies were based on clinical radiologic readings by one observer, and the lengths of exposure of the workers were relatively short. The results can therefore be taken only as suggesting that exposures in this industry may not be particularly dangerous.

From these and other studies, it can be concluded that quartz and cristobalite are capable of causing silicosis in humans, and there is no epidemiological evidence that one is more toxic than the other. Calcined diatomaceous earth is similarly harmful, and there is some evidence that the uncalcined mineral occasionally has caused pneumoconiosis. There is insufficient evidence to state with confidence that amorphous silica is nontoxic; this material may exist in different forms with potentially differing toxicities. For example, animal studies have shown that diatomaceous earth heated to 800°C but containing no crystalline silica is more fibrogenic than unheated material.[41] By the same token, there is little clinical doubt that quartz dust from different sources may differ considerably in toxicity depending on how it has been generated and which other minerals it is mixed with.

Exposure-Response Relationships

In order to prevent silicosis with surety, it is necessary to have information on the likely risks to health of exposures to known concentrations of dust. The difficulties of obtaining such information are enormous, especially when it is necessary to take account of different toxicities of silica in its different forms and combinations, as discussed in the previous section. It is not surprising, therefore, that there is no study available that gives sufficiently clear information of exposure-response relationships to allow administrations to be confident of the level at which a preventive dust standard should be set. Having said this, there is sufficient information available from a number of publications, all of which have some flaws, to give general guidance on levels of risk. The most important studies have been those of Ontario gold and uranium miners, Vermont granite workers, North Carolina dusty trades workers, South Africa gold miners, English gypsum workers, and Scottish coal miners; but many other studies have provided useful additional information.

Vermont Granite Workers [42–49]

In the early years of this century, severe and progressive silicosis was commonplace among these workers, and studies in the 1930s showed that those exposed to concentrations of above 40 million particles per cubic foot (mppcf) suffered rapid progression. Those exposed to between 10 and 20 mppcf developed silicosis, and these workers probably also had a progressive disease and a high mortality from the complicating tuberculosis. Following these studies, dust control measures were introduced, and a recommended dust limit of 10 mppcf was set. Surveys thereafter appear to confirm that this limit was generally adhered to, mean levels being around 5 mppcf, and that the quartz content of the airborne dust approximated 25%. Subsequent x-ray surveys showed little if any pneumoconiosis among workers (ex-workers were not included), and this apparent absence of new cases was the main reason that it has been recommended that the United States quartz standard be set at 50 $\mu g/m^3$, the approximate gravimetric equivalent of 5 mppcf. More recent analyses of the Vermont data, with up-to-date gravimetric samples, have been carried out, and have shown no clear evidence of classical silicosis in men exposed after dust levels were reduced but who remained working in the industry. These survivors showed a low prevalence of mostly irregular opacities, which related to exposure both to granite dust and to cigarette smoke.[49]

North Carolina Dusty Trades Workers [50, 51]

This state has provided comprehensive medical and hygiene services to workers in dusty trades, allowing the accumulation of data on radiologic change (through using 100-mm films, classified as silicosis or normal) and estimates of quartz exposure. From case-control studies it has been concluded that exposures over 40 years to 1 mppcf (roughly equivalent to 0.1 mg/m^3) entailed no significant risk of silicosis, whereas those to 2.5 mppcf did so.

South Africa Gold Miners [52–54]

Studies of a cohort of these miners, exposed to dust containing approximately 30% quartz, are said to have shown a clear relationship between dust exposure and probability of developing silicosis, assessed by comparison with ILO standard films. However, it is difficult with the information given to be sure how the exposure units compare with levels in mg per mg/m^3.

English Gypsum Miners [55, 56]

A cross-sectional study of radiographs of such workers, linked to estimates of lifetime dust exposure, showed a relationship between the latter and presence of small rounded opacities. In these workers, the authors estimated a risk of category 1/0+ radiologic change of about 50% following 20 years' exposure to 0.1 mg/m³ quartz.

Scottish Coal Miners [17, 57]

One Scottish colliery was associated, because of geological problems, with relatively high levels of quartz in the dust in the early 1970s. A number of men showed rapidly progressive changes of pneumoconiosis, likely as a result of these quartz exposures. Figure 12–6 shows the cumulative quartz exposures of these men

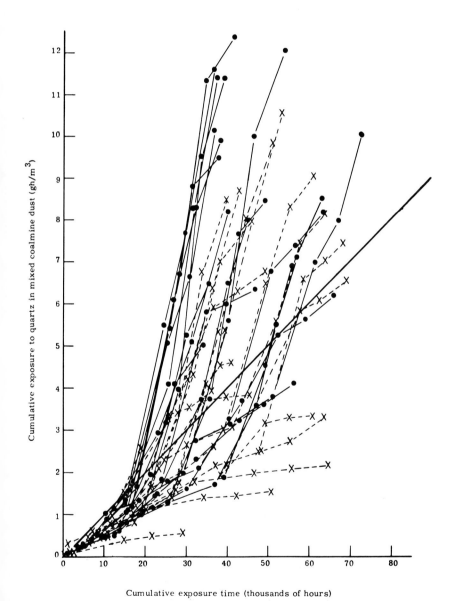

Figure 12–6. Cumulative exposure to quartz (gh/m³) of a group of British coal miners over 80,000 working hours. Men who showed rapid radiologic progression of pneumoconiosis (●——●) had received doses around or above the level, represented by a continuous 45° line, of an average exposure to 0.1 mg/m³. Control subjects (x–––x) without rapid progression at the time of study had received a wide range of doses. (From Seaton, A., Dick, J. A., Dodgson, J., and Jacobsen, M., Quartz and pneumoconiosis in coal miners. Lancet, 2, 1272, 1981. © by The Lancet, Ltd., 1981.)

in relation to that of a hypothetical man exposed to 0.1 mg/m³ over his working life. Most men with rapid progression (and several control subjects) had received exposures above this level, but three progressors fell just below the line. Further follow-up studies and detailed analyses of these dust exposure data are now under way.

In a separate study, coal miners from the British coalfield who showed rapid progression of simple pneumoconiosis were compared with control subjects from the same collieries who had shown no progression. Those with rapid progression had had significantly higher exposures to quartz, the proportion in the inhaled dust averaging 6% as compared with 2% in control subjects.

Ontario Gold and Uranium Miners [58-60]

Perhaps the most careful and detailed study of the effects of quartz exposure comes from an analysis of radiographs of over 2000 Ontario miners, their detailed working histories, and estimates of their lifetime exposures to respirable quartz. The films were read independently by five readers, and the end point was taken to be category 1/1 change. Dust counts made by konometer were converted, after careful comparisons and some reconstruction of past mining methods, to gravimetric measurements. The estimates of risk are illustrated in Figure 12–7 for increasing levels of reader agreement and provide a good basis for setting standards. It should be noted that, in general, quartz exposures were in the range below 0.1 mg/m³ and therefore of direct relevance to standard setting without the need for downward extrapolation. However, this was also the range within which conversion of dust counts was least reliable. Moreover, the study was of working miners and was not able to take account of likely progression to category 1/1 after exposure ceased—a common occurrence in true silicosis as opposed to mixed dust pneumo-

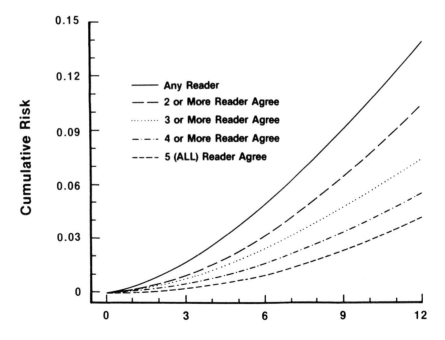

Cumulative Respirable Silica Exposure (mg/m³-years)

Figure 12–7. Risks of category 1/1 + silicosis in hardrock miners in Ontario in relation to cumulative exposure to respirable silica, lagged 5 years. The different curves represent different levels of agreement between the five film readers. (From Muir, D. C. F., Julian, J. A., Shannon, H. S., et al., Silica exposure and silicosis among Ontario hardrock miners: III. Analysis and risk estimates. Am. J. Ind. Med., 16, 29, 1989. Reprinted by permission of John Wiley & Sons, Inc.)

coniosis. Nevertheless, these results give the most useful information so far obtained on exposure-response relationships in silicosis.

Other Groups of Workers

Many other studies hint at an exposure-response relationship between quartz and radiologic silicosis, without giving adequate quantitative information. Studies of pottery workers,[61, 62] slate miners,[63] and foundry workers[64] all have shown increasing risk with increasing exposure. A study of tungsten miners in China reported a clear relationship leading to a suggested exposure limit of 0.24 mg/m^3; it failed, however, to report the criteria for diagnosis of silicosis.[65] Studies of Indian slate pencil workers showed a high risk of severe silicosis in workers exposed to between 2 and 10 mg/m^3,[13, 30] while studies of sandblasters in Louisiana and jade polishers in Hong Kong have shown similar effects at around 5 mg/m^3 and 0.7 mg/m^3, respectively.[31, 32] In the latter case, the exposure was to silica flour.

CLINICAL FEATURES

Because of its relative rarity, silicosis is often initially misdiagnosed. This is facilitated by the wide spectrum of radiologic features, most of which appear before any symptoms. The key to diagnosis is to take an occupational history—any patient with strange diffuse radiologic changes who has worked for several years in an environment where stone dust could get into the air should be suspected of having the disease. The type of presentation depends on the length and intensity of exposure. Long-term exposure to dust containing relatively little quartz is likely to be associated with a slowly progressive nodular appearance on the chest film, in a few cases progressing to massive fibrosis. Exposures to higher concentrations can cause a more rapidly progressive nodular change with a high risk of massive fibrosis, while even higher exposures may present with irregular upper zone fibrosis, diffuse irregular fibrosis, or diffuse alveolitis on the x-ray film. These patients have symptoms early, usually also have concomitant emphysema, and deteriorate rapidly. Most true silicosis, as opposed to mixed dust pneumoconiosis, progresses even after exposure ceases.[17, 66] That progression may, however, cease after several years, and it is not at present possible to predict who will progress and who will not. As a general rule, those who have had intense but relatively short exposures are those most likely to progress.

In the sections that follow, the disease is described as three different types: chronic, accelerated, and acute. It is important to remember that these may merge and that confusing radiologic and pathologic appearances may result.

Chronic Silicosis

The most usual form of silicosis is that which occurs after many years of exposure to relatively low levels of dust. This disease resembles coal workers' pneumoconiosis in that the simple nodular form is not associated with any symptoms or physical signs. Such subjects may complain of cough, sputum, or breathlessness, but these symptoms are likely to be related to accompanying disease of the airways. However, simple radiologic silicosis is more usually a progressive disease, even in the absence of further dust exposure, and will frequently develop into progressive massive fibrosis unless the exposure has been predominantly to mixed dust (as in foundrymen) or has been relatively limited.

When progressive massive fibrosis occurs, the patient develops symptoms related to reduction of lung volumes, distortion of bronchi, and, though to a lesser extent than in coal workers' pneumoconiosis, bullous emphysema. The main symptom is shortness of breath, though cough and sputum production are also common. The breathlessness is progressive and ultimately disabling. The final episode in the life of the silicotic patient is the development of cardiorespiratory failure. If the physiological effect of the silicosis has been predominantly restrictive, as is most usually the case, it tends to be of the hypoxic type, with electrocardiographic evidence of pulmonary hypertension but without overt cardiac failure. However, with the predominantly obstructive type of functional defect associated with bullous emphysema or complicating airways disease, clinical cor pulmonale may occur. The classical description of complicated silicosis, and one that was still accurate in many respects in the potteries of England when the author worked there in the 1960s, came from J.T. Arlidge, a distinguished physician who studied occupational medicine in that region during the latter half of the nineteenth century. His book, *The Hygiene, Diseases and Mortality of Occupations,* published in 1892, contains the following description of complicated silicosis, a description which is applicable to the disease in whatever occupation it occurs.

The pulmonary mischief from the dust of potter's clay is slow but sure in its occurrence. The siliceous character of the clay lends it more potency for harm than almost any other dust. . . . It is much more irritant than coal dust and stands on a par with the worst kinds of stone dust. . . . When uncomplicated by tubercles, the potter's disease advances imperceptibly. Haemoptysis does not usher in the malady, and more frequently than not never makes its appearances. . . . There is no febrile reaction, no accelerated pulse, no hectic, and no rapid emaciation. . . . The cough is more paroxysmal and violent than that of phthisis, and the urgency of dyspnoea greater, and out of proportion to the ascertained extent of consolidated lung. The signs of condensation are not so specially limited to the infraclavicular spaces as in tuberculous lesions, and hence the sinking below the clavicles is not marked.

Areas of dullness on percussion are often distributed at different parts particularly in the scapular region near the base of the lungs. Between these an emphysematous condition is discoverable; a phenomenon more common along the anterior margin of the lungs. There is not an equal shrinking and contraction of the thoracic cavity at large. . . . As might be foreseen from the increased strain on the pulmonary circulation, the heart gets frequently involved, the right side becomes dilated and the valves inefficient. Hence anasarca in prolonged cases is no infrequent occurrence before the scene closes. I would add that the general aspect and physiognomy differ from those of tubercular phthisis . . . the lustrous eye, the often pink and transparent skin of phthisis, the clubbed finger ends, and the incurved nails are wanting. But in looking for these distinctive signs we must never forget how frequently tubercular deposit modifies the picture of fibrosis.

This description of a progressive disease causing breathlessness but few physical signs—no finger clubbing or crackles in particular—cannot be bettered. While this end point in the disease is now rare and, in general, chronic silicosis develops only after a prolonged period of exposure, this very rarity may lead to complacency about the need to take preventive measures, and cases are still occurring even in the developed world.

Accelerated Silicosis

In some occupations, exposure to high concentrations of silica over a period of as little as 5 years results in a more rapidly progressive form of the disease. The symptom of breathlessness presents early, and the patient deteriorates rapidly to hypoxic respiratory failure. Again, physical signs are few and related to the presence of complicating emphysema rather than the fibrosis. Radiologic features, described later, may be confusing, but the history is characteristic in that the patient has worked in a job where high concentrations of finely divided silica have escaped into the air and no or inadequate respiratory protection has been provided. Such rapidly progressive and fatal cases have been described in sandblasting,[15] production of silica flour,[14] and stonemasonry using powered tools on high-quartz sandstone.[16]

There is no effective treatment for this condition, other than lung transplantation. This operation, however, has now become a reality, and all such patients, faced as they are with remorseless deterioration and death, should be considered for such surgery.

Acute Silicosis

An acute form of silicosis occurs in subjects exposed to very high concentrations of silica over periods of as little as a few weeks. This disease was first described by Middleton in 1929 as an occupational hazard for those involved in the production of abrasive soap powders.[67] The first cases in the United States were described by Chapman, also in workers involved in the mixing of alkali and finely ground crystalline silica to produce abrasive soap powders.[68] In spite of its dramatic course and general knowledge of the dangers of silica, acute silicosis has been described repeatedly even in recent decades, for example, in sandblasters,[69] flint crushers,[70] ceramic workers,[29] silica flour workers,[24] workers in abrasive manufacture,[25] and open-cast coal miners.[43] The history is typically one of progressive dyspnea, fever, cough, and weight loss after a heavy but relatively short exposure to silica. The exposure may vary from a few weeks to 4 or 5 years. Death occurs in hypoxic respiratory failure, and the fatal course of the disease is probably not influenced by steroids, bronchial lavage, or any other treatment, though there are anecdotal reports of temporary alleviation of symptoms by steroids. It is likely that such patients will also be suitable candidates for lung transplantation, which should be considered in all cases.

COMPLICATIONS OF SILICOSIS

Mycobacterial and Opportunist Infections

The major complication of silicosis is pulmonary tuberculosis. Early description of lung disease in dusty industries did not distinguish between pneumoconiosis and tuberculosis, and undoubtedly before chemotherapy most fatal cases of silicosis were complicated by that disease. Although tuberculosis has come under increasing control in the developed world, reactivation of an old primary infection still remains a risk of silicotic patients. In endemic areas and among poorer people in the United States and other advanced countries, the danger of tuberculosis in silicosis is very real. In South Africa, a necropsy series of gold, coal, and asbestos miners has shown a greater proportion of silicotic patients to have active tuberculosis than those without silicosis.[71] Previous studies in that country showed than 20% of silicotic gold miners had active disease even in the 1960s, though the overall prevalence of silicosis had fallen sharply following the introduction of dust controls.[72] Over the same period, tuberculosis was found to occur 30 times more frequently in silicotic than in nonsilicotic copper miners in Northern Rhodesia.[73] In United States metal miners in the early 1960s, 5.3% of silicotics and 0.6% of nonsilicotics showed radiographic evidence of active or quiescent disease, while 0.5% of British slate miners studied in the 1950s had bacteriologically proven active disease.[74] A more recent study of these men has shown almost half to have radiologic evidence of healed tuberculosis.[75] Even studies from Sweden in the 1960s and Switzerland in the 1950s have reported that 9% and 21%, respectively, of silicotics were found to have active disease.[76, 77]

It seems likely that tuberculosis is an even more frequent complication of accelerated and acute silicosis, though this is based on clinical observation of selected individuals rather than epidemiological study. Of 83 silicotic sandblasters in New Orleans, 10 had tuberculosis, while nine had infection with *Mycobacterium kansasii* and three with *Mycobacterium avium–intracellulare*. These two organisms have been reported as complications of silicosis in other studies,[78, 79] and probably occur whenever disease caused by them is endemic, as in New Orleans. In Scotland, *Mycobacterium malmoense* is the most frequent atypical mycobacterial pathogen, and the author has seen one patient with silicosis infected by this organism.

Other opportunistic infections may occur in patients with accelerated or acute silicosis—nocardiosis, sporotrichosis, and cryptococcosis have been described,[15] and aspergillomata may complicate cavitating massive fibrosis.

The development of tuberculosis in a silicotic patient must result either from reactivation of an old primary infection or from recent infection in the presence of impaired lung defenses. Since silica is extremely toxic to macrophages and macrophages are the lung's main defense against *Mycobacterium tuberculosis,* the connection between the two diseases is not surprising.

Tuberculosis usually supervenes in a patient with chronic silicosis fairly late in the course of the disease. There may be no symptoms, but loss of weight, increased cough, hemoptysis, and rapid radiologic change should alert the physician. In accelerated and acute silicosis, diagnosis may be even more difficult, and repeated sputum culture is often the only reliable method.

Pneumothorax

Pneumothorax is a recognized complication of diffuse pulmonary fibrosis and bullous disease. It is therefore not likely to occur in excess in simple silicosis but may be anticipated in massive fibrosis complicated by bullous emphysema. It occurs frequently in accelerated and acute silicosis, in which it may prove a fatal complication.[15]

Rheumatoid and Other Collagen Diseases

Patients with silicosis show an increased prevalence of antinuclear antibodies,[80] though these probably reflect tissue damage rather than play a pathogenic role. Rheumatoid nodules, which may either calcify or cavitate, may appear in the lungs of silicotics with rheumatoid disease or with rheumatoid factor in their blood,[81] and a Finnish study of a cohort of granite workers has shown them to have had an increased incidence of rheumatoid arthritis, predominantly a severe seropositive type.[82] Both the skin and visceral manifestations of systemic sclerosis or scleroderma have been described frequently in silicotics,[83] however; and there is little doubt that this disease occurs more commonly in individuals with silicosis than in the general population. Indeed, it was first described as a common disease in stonemasons in 1914.[84] Sandblasters with accelerated silicosis have been reported to have scleroderma, rheumatoid disease, or systemic lupus erythematosus in about 10% of cases.[85] This suggests that there is a real connection between the tissue damage of silicosis, the production of antinuclear antibodies, and the development of autoimmune disease, though the mechanisms remain a matter for speculation. In such cases, some authors have observed an accelerated progression of the lung lesions and have suggested a therapeutic role for steroids.[85]

Renal Disease

Several case reports have recorded the coincidence of silicosis with renal disease, and both mild focal proliferative glomerulonephritis and proximal tubular lesions have been described.[86–90] Most of these patients were exposed to very high, but unmeasured, levels of quartz, sufficient to cause acute or accelerated silicosis. No studies of the prevalence of renal disease in quartz-exposed workers appear to have been carried out, although one study of 15 patients with silicosis found normal function in all,[91] while, in contrast, another of 20 patients found renal impairment in nine.[92] One study of renal biopsies showed high levels of elemental silicon, though whether these were higher than would have been found in quartz-exposed workers without renal disease is not known.[93] More recently, a study of silicotics and silica-exposed workers showed them to have significantly higher urine protein excretion than age-matched nonexposed subjects.[94] The evidence seems to indicate a relationship between heavy exposure to quartz and renal failure characterized by minimal histological change in the kidneys, perhaps mediated by toxic damage from circulating quartz particles. The evidence, however, remains anecdotal, and epidemiological studies of quartz-exposed workers are required.

Lung Cancer

There is some experimental evidence that quartz inhalation may cause epidermoid carcinoma in rats if the animals survive sufficiently long.[95, 96] This evidence is relatively new, applies predominantly to female rats, and is somewhat surprising in view of the many previous studies of quartz inhalation that preceded it. Interestingly, hamsters, which have macrophages resistant to quartz damage, do not show the same effects.

It is conceivable that quartz may be a human carcinogen, acting either directly or as a co-carcinogen promoting the effects of other carcinogens such as tobacco smoke or radon, or through the production of scar cancers. If it were a human carcinogen, there would need to be an explanation of why this had not been commented on previously by clinicians. In fact it has. The classic description of a cause of lung cancer was in the silica-exposed Schneeberg miners,[97] though we now believe that the cause was likely to have been radiation, and a pathologist in Liverpool drew attention to anaplastic lung cancer in two silicotic patients in 1934.[98] However, in general the possibility of an association between silicosis and cancer escaped the attention of doctors until quite recently.

Interest in the subject has been rekindled by a number of epidemiological studies which have pointed to an association between quartz exposure and risk of lung cancer. Some of these have been based on mortality of patients registered for disability benefits for silicosis, and it is relatively easy to point to a possible bias, in that such individuals, being disabled, are likely to have included large excesses of smokers and others exposed to pollutants likely to have increased their risks of cancer. Many studies have not provided information on the subjects' smoking habits. In the case of underground miners, radon exposures have often not been controlled for; while in the case of foundry workers, allowance has not been made for exposure to polyaromatic hydrocarbons and other possible carcinogens. Furthermore, there is the publication bias to be considered, whereby positive results tend to be published and negative not.

Bearing these problems in mind, there is now evidence of an association that is becoming more difficult to dispute. Several studies, from Canada, South Africa, Italy, Singapore and Finland, have taken account of the effects of smoking and found an increased risk of lung cancer either in silicotics or in workers exposed to silica.[99–103] In the South African study, there was not only evidence of an exposure-response relationship but also a suggestion of a synergistic effect with smoking. A study of North Carolina dusty trades workers, controlling for smoking, age, and exposure to other occupational carcinogens, has demonstrated a significantly increased risk of lung cancer in silicotics.[104] However, other studies, for example of United States granite workers and Italian silicotics, have failed to find a significant effect.[105, 106] In an effort to resolve this problem, the International Agency for Research on Cancer (IARC) has encouraged a series of important studies in which the main confounders were taken account of. The publication of the results of these studies, from several different countries and occupational groups, has given strong and consistent support to the hypothesis that exposure to quartz is carcinogenic in humans, particularly in those exposed to sufficient amounts to develop silicosis.[107]

In summary, it seems likely that exposures to certain types of silica may increase the risk of individuals' developing lung cancer, most probably through synergism with tobacco and other carcinogens. The effect is clearly a weak one, not to be compared with, for example, that of asbestos, and indeed at this stage the hypothesis cannot be said to have been proved. It seems possible, indeed likely, that there are also substantial differences between quartz in different circumstances, relating to its surface activity and to the presence or absence of other modifying minerals. From a medicolegal point of view, it seems to the author that an employer who takes appropriate steps to protect workers from silicosis would be unlikely to be found negligent if one of them subsequently developed lung cancer. In Britain, where a no-fault compensation scheme for industrial disease operates (see Chapter 4), lung cancer has been prescribed as an occupational disease in subjects with silicosis. Readers interested in this subject are referred to two monographs[107, 108] and a review.[109]

RADIOGRAPHIC CHANGES

Chronic Silicosis

The earliest signs of silicosis are usually nodular shadows in the upper zones of the lungs. These are often quite sparse and are easily disregarded as being insufficient even to be classified as category 0/1. Moreover, they are often indistinguishable from similar shadows in people with healed minimal tuberculosis. Subsequently, the course of silicosis differs markedly from that of other pneumoconioses. The individual nodules become more profuse with increasing dust exposure, and they also increase in size.[17, 110] Thus, when first seen, the nodules often correspond most closely to a q lesion in size, but after several years the predominant opacity size is r (Fig. 12–8). Even after exposure has ceased, this progression in size and profusion is likely to occur, and it is not unknown for workers to have left the industry with category 0 films and then develop progressive changes of simple silicosis and even progressive massive fibrosis several years later, assuming that they had been exposed to sufficient dust in the later years of their work.

One occasional feature of silicosis is eggshell calcification of the hilar and intrapulmonary lymph nodes (Fig. 12–9). While this only occurs in a minority of exposed subjects, it is almost pathognomonic of quartz exposure (it is said to be seen, exceedingly rarely, in sarcoidosis or after mediastinal radiotherapy for lymphoma). It may occur in the absence of pulmonary silicosis, and the radiographic changes of silicosis are usually unaccompanied by eggshell calcification. Even more uncommonly, the silicotic nodules themselves may calcify. This may occur in rheumatoid pneumoconiosis or sometimes in very long-standing nonprogressive small nodules (Fig. 12–10).

Complicated silicosis occurs as a consequence of aggregation of small nodules. Its occurrence may be predicted where there is an increased profusion of such small lesions, usually in middle and upper zones. When it occurs, it usually progresses, other similar lesions appear, and frequently emphysematous bullae develop around the masses (Fig. 12–11). Cavitation is relatively unusual in silicosis, as opposed to coal workers' pneumoconiosis, and when it occurs, complicating mycobacterial infection should always be suspected (Fig. 12–12).

While complicated silicosis usually occurs on a background of simple silicosis, it may occasionally occur in isolation. In such circumstances, it may easily be mistaken for a bronchial carcinoma. However, its shape is rarely as spherical as that of a peripheral carcinoma, its outline is usually smooth, and it is often surrounded by emphysematous bullae (Fig. 12–13). Clearly each case must be judged on its clinical merits, and often such patients need to be referred for surgery. The uncertainties surrounding the relationships of quartz exposure and lung cancer, and the possible development of scar cancer, make this often the wiser course of action.

Caplan's syndrome, or large nodular pneumoconiosis in someone with a rheumatoid diathesis, occurs occasionally in silicosis, as in coal workers' pneumoconiosis. This frequently occurs on a background of sparse or no simple nodules and may antedate the development of rheumatoid lesions in the joints. The nodules may calcify and larger ones frequently cavitate.

Text continued on page 246

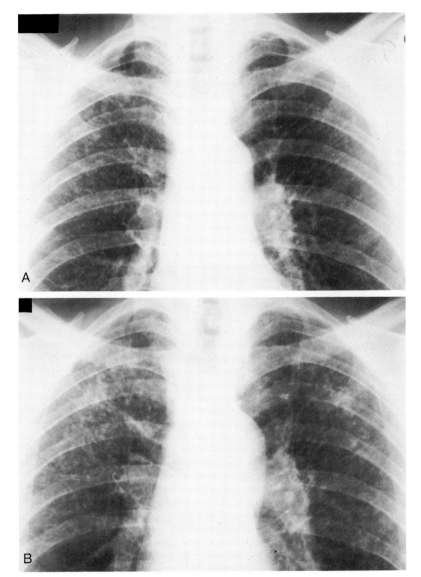

Figure 12–8. *A,* Coal miner exposed to high proportion of quartz in mixed coal mine dust. Radiograph shows few dense p- and q-size nodules in upper lobes in 1974. *B,* Same subject 4 years later, showing increase in both size and profusion of nodules, with early bilateral conglomeration. (From Seaton, A., Dick, J. A., Dodgson, J., and Jacobsen, M., Quartz and pneumoconiosis in coal miners. Lancet, 2, 1272, 1981. © by The Lancet, Ltd., 1981.)

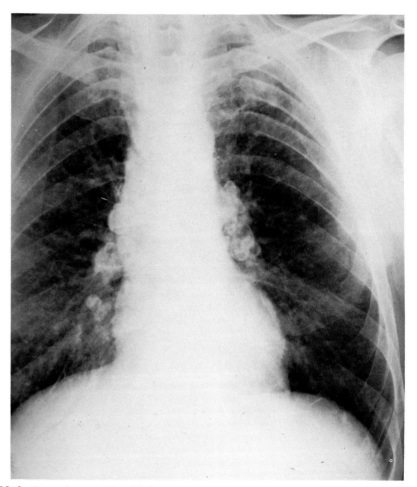

Figure 12–9. Chest radiograph of Welsh slate quarry worker showing category 1/2 simple silicosis with well-marked eggshell calcification of hilar lymph nodes. (Courtesy of the late Dr. J. Lyons.)

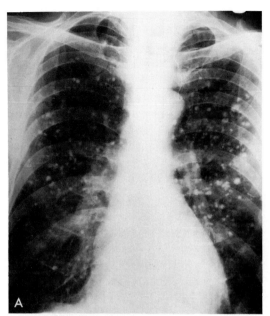

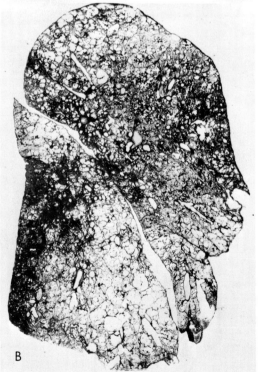

Figure 12–10
Calcified nodules in lungs of a
Scottish granite quarry worker. At
autopsy, those nodules were shown to
be of the Caplan type. *A*, Chest
radiograph. *B*, Gough paper section,
showing lesions distributed particularly
around the oblique fissure. (Courtesy
of the late Dr. J. Lyons.)

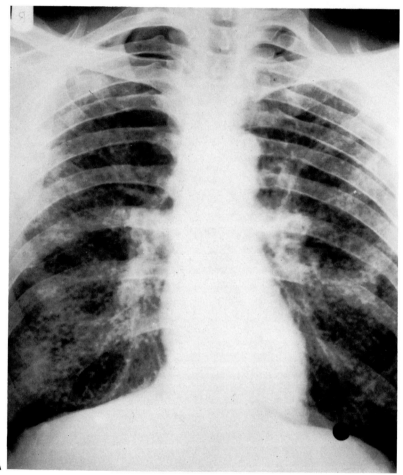

A

Figure 12–11. *A,* Chest radiograph of Welsh lead miner with heavy exposure to silica dust. Radiograph taken in 1952, showing category 3/3 simple silicosis. At this stage the man left the industry.

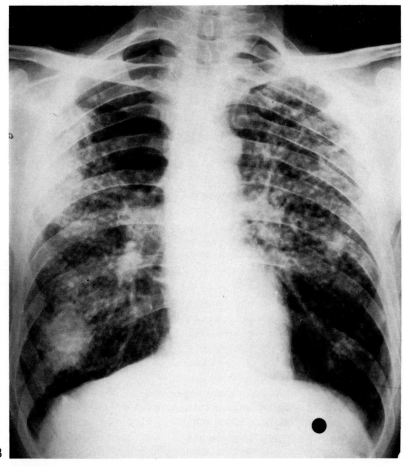

B

Figure 12–11 *Continued B,* Radiograph of the same patient, taken in 1958. Category B complicated silicosis has developed in right upper and lower zones.

Illustration continued on following page

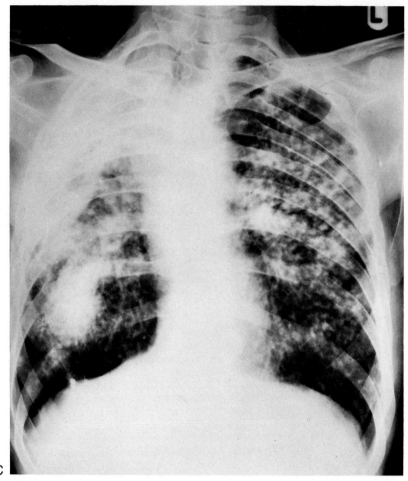

C

Figure 12–11 *Continued C,* By 1964, the same patient has stage C complicated disease, and conglomeration is beginning in the left lung. Marked fibrosis is present over the right upper lobe, and there is bullous change at the right base. (Courtesy of the late Dr. J. Lyons.)

Pleural fibrosis is a usual accompaniment of massive fibrosis in silicosis. It is usually diffuse and bilateral and may occasionally calcify, though it is rarely as impressive radiologically as in asbestos exposure. There has been one report at least of pleural effusion complicating silicosis.[111]

As mentioned before, pneumothorax and tuberculosis may complicate silicosis. The former occurs usually as a result of a ruptured bulla. The latter may be very difficult to appreciate radiologically, but should be suspected if there is rapid change in the size of lesions, cavitation develops, or new softer or streaky lesions develop. The cornerstone of diagnosis is clinical and bacteriological, rather than radiologic.

Accelerated Silicosis

In accelerated silicosis, the changes may be the same as in chronic silicosis, but occur earlier and progress more rapidly. They may present as upper zone nodularity that progresses both to massive lesions and to irregular fibrosis and contraction of the upper lobes (Fig. 12–14). They make their first appearance within 5 or 6 years of first exposure and progress to massive fibrosis over a similar period. Bullous emphysema is a usual accompaniment of the massive lesions.

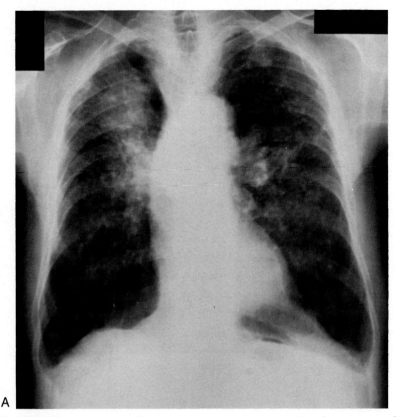

A

Figure 12–12. *A*, Radiograph of coal miner exposed to silica in tunneling, showing massive fibrosis and eggshell calcification of hilar nodes.

Illustration continued on following page

Acute Silicosis

Acute silicosis presents the most confusing appearance, since the nodular pattern is missing (except in those cases where the acute pattern is superimposed on pre-existing chronic disease). The lungs show a ground-glass appearance, similar to that of pulmonary edema. The condition may simply become more extensive or may consolidate into appearances more characteristic of massive fibrosis over the short period before death (Fig. 12–15).

Radiologic Classification and Diagnosis

In the author's experience, physicians often become confused about the processes involved in reading chest films of people exposed to dust. The following remarks apply generally to x-ray reading for pneumoconiosis and are not specific to silicosis. They are of particular importance, however, in studies of silicosis and coal workers' pneumoconiosis occurring in parts of the world where tuberculosis, pulmonary eosinophilia, and other diseases causing pulmonary shadowing are endemic.

In any epidemiological study using radiographs, the film must always first be read clinically, in order to detect any disease which requires prompt investigation and treatment. In such reading, the physician is wearing a clinical hat and should take account of any other factors such as history of ill health, microscopy of the sputum, blood eosinophil count, and so on. The balance of diagnostic probability should normally be tipped toward suspecting the treatable, nonpneumoconiotic condition, and appropriate action should be taken.

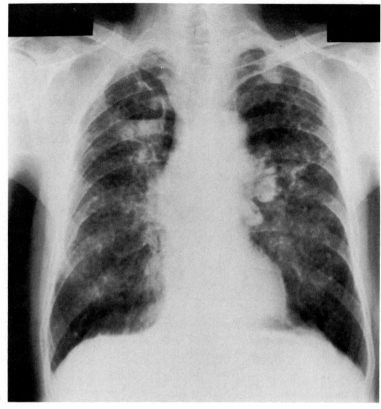

Figure 12–12 *Continued B,* Same man as in *A,* showing cavitation of massive lesion in right upper lobe. Sputum culture proved positive for tubercle bacilli.

Confusion most often arises when a physician then reads the films for pneumoconiosis using the ILO classification. Here, strictly speaking, the reader is acting like a machine, simply recording the appearances in accordance with the standard films and the ILO guidance notes. In other words, the physician is wearing an epidemiological hat. There is however one proviso—the reader must first decide whether or not the appearances are consistent with pneumoconiosis. If they are, and this is in fact a clinical decision which depends very much on the reader's experience, then the next step is to classify the film. It is this step, deciding on whether the appearances are consistent with pneumoconiosis, that causes most difficulty. Illustrated are two films (Fig. 12–16), one of which was of a patient with extensive tuberculosis who had never been exposed to dust, while the other was of a man with cavitating silicotic massive fibrosis but who had no evidence of tuberculosis. The causes are essentially indistinguishable radiologically, although the clinical differentiation was very easily made.

Other difficulties arise from ignorance of the range of appearances of pneumoconiosis. For example, irregular upper zone fibrosis (see Fig. 12–14) may be due to silicosis, though most radiologists would dismiss this as healed tuberculosis in the developing world or as possible chronic sarcoidosis, chronic allergic alveolitis, or ankylosing spondylitis lung in the West. The coarse irregular fibrosis of berylliosis, which resembles chronic sarcoidosis or cystic fibrosis radiologically, is not well represented on the standard ILO films, and the diffuse appearances of acute silicosis or acute allergic alveolitis are not classifiable by the ILO scheme at all.

The pragmatic solution to these problems when classifying films epidemiologically is simply to record all appearances that could be due to pneumoconiosis and

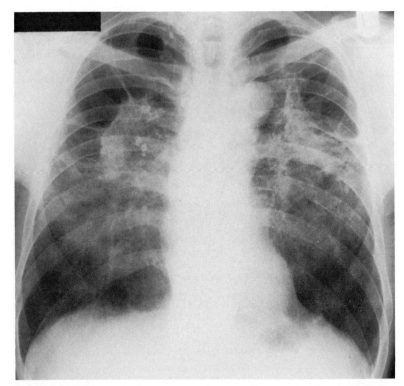

Figure 12–13. Radiograph of stonemason with massive fibrosis and well-marked bullous emphysema surrounding the lesions.

that are represented in the standard films. If it is felt, on the basis of experience, that an alternative cause, such as tuberculosis, may be responsible, this can be recorded as a comment, so that allowance can be made for the possibility during the analyses.

A final point should be made concerning low category (1/0 and 0/1) appearances, especially when these are predominantly irregular in shape. The mistake should not be made of assuming that all such shadows are due to pneumoconiosis. There is clear evidence that small irregular opacities of low profusion occur in relation to aging and cigarette smoking as well as to dust exposure.[112, 113] In epidemiological studies, such interrelationships may be investigated by appropriate multivariate statistical analyses; but in making a clinical comment on an individual film, it is unwise to diagnose pneumoconiosis on the sole basis of less than 1/1 small opacities taken in conjunction with a history of appropriate dust exposure.

Silicosis and Mixed Dust Pneumoconiosis

The radiologic appearances described above apply to people exposed to dust containing predominantly quartz as the pathogenic substance. In general, this means dusts containing more than about 10% quartz, the residue being mainly other silicates. If the dust contains coal, iron oxides, or a number of other minerals, the appearances may differ with predominantly smaller, less well-defined opacities and less tendency for progression. Furthermore, foundry workers, who are often at risk of classic silicosis, may sometimes be exposed to less fibrogenic dust containing iron oxides and develop radiologic changes of mixed dust pneumoconiosis rather than silicosis. In most circumstances, these individuals are labeled clinically as having silicosis, though the disease may be much more benign.

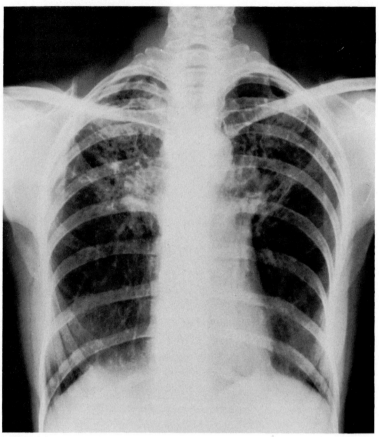

Figure 12–14. Radiograph of woman exposed to high levels of calcined diatomaceous earth in operating xerox camera, showing upper lobe fibrosis and lower lobe emphysema due to accelerated silicosis.

LUNG FUNCTION

In all studies of the lung function of people with pneumoconiosis, account should be taken of a number of different and confounding influences. While the disease itself may cause deterioration in function, so also may the dust or some of its components acting independently. For example, silicotic nodules may cause a general reduction of lung volumes, while the silica and silicate-containing dust may separately affect small airways or alveoli and contribute toward airflow obstruction.[114] In addition, the effects of smoking, which is usually widespread among industrial populations, and of other lung disease such as healed tuberculosis need to be taken into account. And, finally, studies of the effects of silicosis need to ensure that the disease in question is indeed silicosis and not the more benign mixed dust fibrosis.

Consideration of the pathological features of simple silicosis would lead one to expect that this disease *per se* would have no appreciable effect on lung function except perhaps at the category 3 stage. This has been borne out by published studies when account has been taken of smoking habits, where minor reductions in diffusing capacity, lung volumes, compliance, and ventilatory function have been recorded only in people with advanced simple silicosis.[112–117] Similarly, as expected, subjects with complicated silicosis show on average a reduction in ventilatory capacity, lung volumes, and compliance. The presence of bullous emphysema in these patients would of course be expected to result in a more obstructive pattern of lung function.

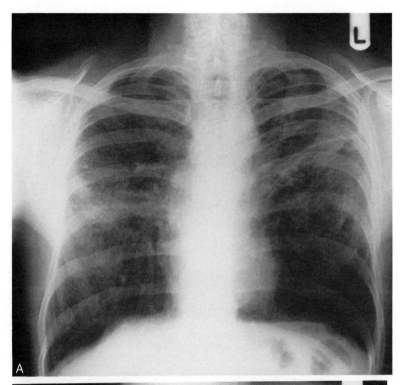

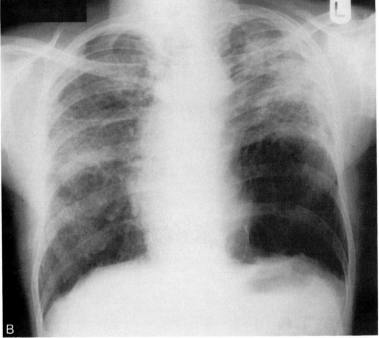

Figure 12–15
A, Chest radiograph of stonemason, showing diffuse bilateral shadowing of acute silicosis. *B,* Radiograph of same patient a year later, shortly prior to death, showing progression of the shadowing and emphysema well developed in left lower zone.

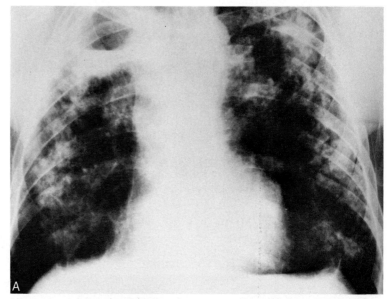
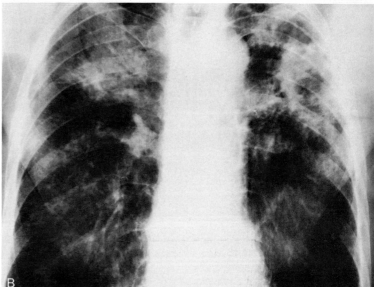

Figure 12–16
A, Radiograph of man with extensive tuberculosis who had never been exposed to dust, showing what appear to be massive and small nodular lesions, with cavitation on the right. B, Radiograph of man with massive fibrosis due to mining, showing cavitation on the left but no tuberculosis.

Studies of change in ventilatory capacity in patients with silicosis have shown a wide range of decline, in general related to progression of the radiologic disease and previous dust exposure. The FEV_1 and vital capacity usually decline at roughly the same rate, indicating a predominantly restrictive pattern.[110]

How far such changes are due to the pathological process of silicosis and how far they are due to other effects of dust exposure have been thrown into question by a series of studies of South African gold miners. One study has shown no difference in function between miners with and without silicosis when matched for dust exposure.[117] A large longitudinal study has shown that dust exposure is related to excess loss of FEV_1 in these miners, and that the effects of dust exposure added to those of smoking.[118] In this study, the average dust exposure was estimated to have been about 14 gh/m^3, the dust containing roughly 30% quartz, and the effect of this exposure on FEV_1 was approximately half that of smoking 20 cigarettes a day for 30 years.

On balance, it seems likely that dust exposure (together of course with cigarette smoking) is responsible for the decrement in ventilatory capacity seen in workers exposed to silica-containing dusts, usually independently of the effect of any nodular silicosis. Only in very extensive simple silicosis or when massive fibrosis supervenes does the fibrosis make a substantial contribution.

In contrast, and not unexpectedly, accelerated silicosis and acute silicosis are associated with marked restriction of lung volumes, fall in diffusing capacity, oxygen desaturation, and rapid decline to death from hypoxic respiratory failure.[28, 119, 120]

DIFFERENTIAL DIAGNOSIS

Normally the diagnosis of silicosis should present no problems, though unfamiliarity with the manifestations of the disease can lead to mistakes, and the author has discovered several cases of advanced disease recently misdiagnosed as sarcoidosis or cryptogenic interstitial fibrosis. The finding of diffuse radiographic shadowing in a patient known to have been exposed to quartz, or to a dust that could contain it, is usually sufficient to suspect the disease. Nonindustrial causes of diffuse pulmonary mottling are almost always associated with defects of gas diffusion on lung function testing. Such conditions, including sarcoidosis, cryptogenic fibrosing alveolitis, rheumatoid lung, carcinomatous lymphangitis, and pulmonary hemosiderosis, may of course occur in subjects who have been exposed to silica. If this is the case, the existence of previous radiographs is of great help. Moreover, the finding of restrictive lung function abnormalities and physical signs of pulmonary fibrosis (clubbing and basal crackles) suggests nonindustrial disease.

Difficulties commonly arise at the onset of progressive massive fibrosis, or less frequently with Caplan's syndrome, in excluding carcinoma or tuberculosis. Tuberculosis must always be suspected, and regular bacteriological testing of sputum is necessary. Carcinoma can usually be excluded by inspection of serial radiographs and, often, by the finding of several opacities. Very occasionally diagnosis of a newly arisen single peripheral opacity is impossible without lung biopsy or thoracotomy. Generally, however, a neoplasm is a better defined and more rapidly growing lesion than early massive fibrosis, and the distinction can be made radiographically.

The diagnosis of accelerated or acute silicosis may give rise to confusion if a careful industrial history is not taken. The former may progress to an irregular upper zone fibrosis that can be mistaken for tuberculosis, chronic sarcoidosis, chronic allergic alveolitis, or rare conditions such as ankylosing spondylitis lung (which may occur in the absence of clinical spondylitis) or histiocytosis X. The acute disease may resemble pulmonary edema, alveolar proteinosis, or acute allergic alveolitis. In all these cases the occupational history is paramount in leading to the diagnosis, and confirmation will often result from some quick inquiries at the workplace. As discussed in Chapter 3, further investigation of the patient is generally not necessary.

PATHOLOGY

For a detailed description of the pathology of silicosis, the reader is referred to reference 121.

Chronic and Accelerated Silicosis

Macroscopic Appearance

Inspection of the lungs commonly shows fibrous adhesions in the pleural cavity, with silicotic plaques (candlewax lesions) visible over the pleural surfaces. The lungs tend to be more pigmented than usual. The hilar lymph nodes are often enlarged, containing fibrotic nodules, and sometimes are calcified. When the lung is cut, grayish fibrotic nodules are seen, more profuse in the apical and posterior parts of upper and lower lobes (Fig. 12–17). These vary both in size, from a few millimeters to large conglomerate masses occupying most of a lobe, and in profusion. They are hard and occasionally calcified. Nodules that have been cut across show a characteristic whorled appearance both in the lung and in the lymph nodes. Several of these nodules may appear to have become confluent to produce very large lesions. These areas of massive fibrosis may show cavitation (Fig. 12–18), either in relation to ischemic central necrosis or, more commonly in silicosis, in association with tuberculous infection. In the latter instance, caseation may be seen in the nodules. Emphysematous bullae often surround the areas of massive fibrosis. Enlargement of the right side of the heart occurs not uncommonly in advanced complicated silicosis, but evidence of congestive failure is less frequent in the absence of chronic airways obstruction.

Silica may be transferred by lymphatics into the blood, and fine particles may then be deposited in other organs, such as spleen or bone marrow, where typical silicotic nodules may be found.[122, 123]

Microscopic Appearance

The silicotic nodule characteristically arises in the region of the respiratory bronchiole, around the pulmonary arterioles, and in paraseptal and subpleural tissues. The nodule consists of hyalinized collagen fibers centrally and reticulin fibers peripherally, the whole having a concentric arrangement and showing some fibroblastic activity at the edges in early lesions (Fig. 12–19). The respiratory bronchioles and small pulmonary vessels are involved in the progressing fibrosis and destroyed, and the elastic laminae of pulmonary arteries may sometimes be seen in the midst of a collagenous mass. In this respect, the silicotic nodule differs markedly from the coal macule described in Chapter 15.

Particles of silica may be demonstrated in the nodules, occasionally by staining with toluidine blue to show metachromasia,[124] but more reliably by viewing the sections under polarized light when the birefringent particles can be seen (Fig. 12–20). Microincineration techniques, with hydrochloric acid treatment and dark-ground illumination, result in the best demonstration of these particles and allow those smaller than 1 micron to be seen. Such methods have demonstrated that the amount of silica is variable and bears no relationship to the extent of the collagenous reaction. Indeed, reliance on seeing doubly refractile particles may be positively misleading, as in some cases recently seen by the author when extremely high quartz levels in the lung were accompanied by little visible refractile material.[16] In such cases, it is likely that the quartz particles are too small to refract polarized light. Final proof of the presence and quantity of quartz must therefore rely on x-ray diffraction and electron microscopic techniques.

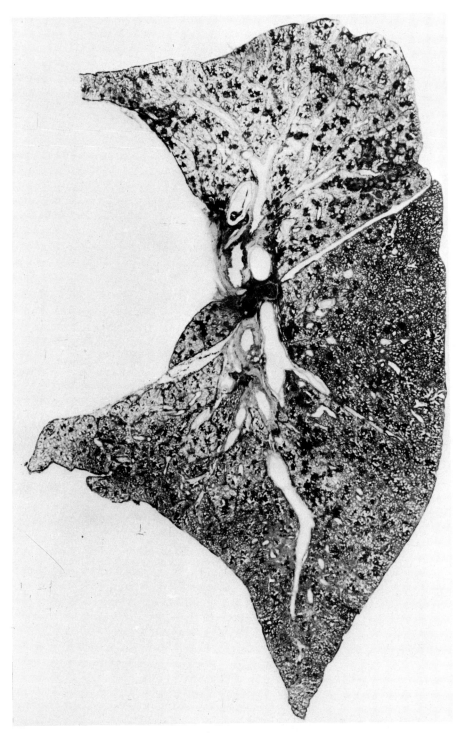

Figure 12–17. Whole lung (Gough) section of silicotic lung from North Wales slate quarry worker, showing eggshell hilar calcification and silicotic nodules predominantly in the apical and posterior parts of both upper and lower lobes.

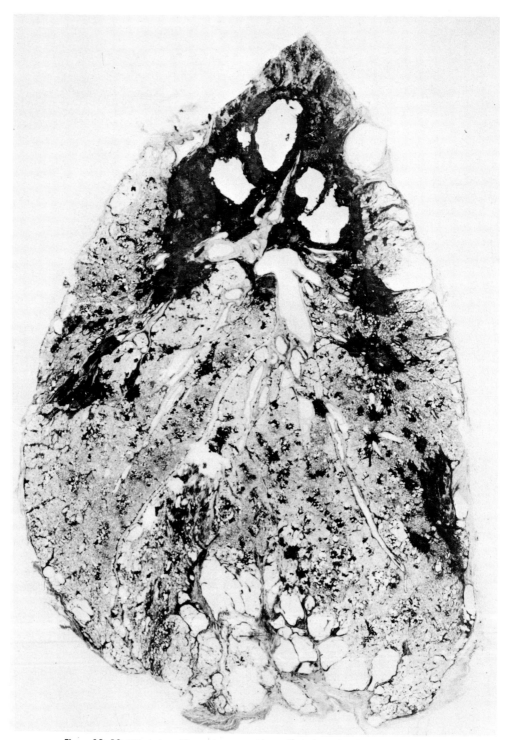

Figure 12–18. Whole lung (Gough) section of lung of North Wales slate worker, showing massive fibrosis with ischemic necrosis and cavitation. The massive lesion can be seen to be composed of smaller silicotic nodules that have become confluent.

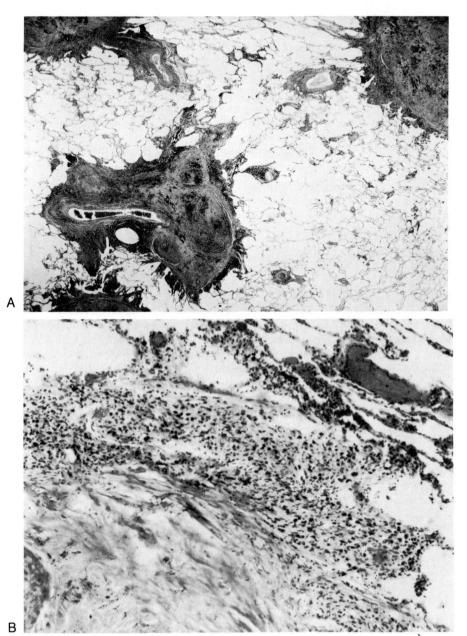

Figure 12–19. *A,* Lower power photomicrograph of silicotic lung, showing the perivascular location of the nodules and their whorled appearance. *B,* Higher power photomicrograph of the edge of the large lesion in *A,* showing dense acellular collagen *(bottom left)* surrounded by a rim of fibroblasts and macrophages.

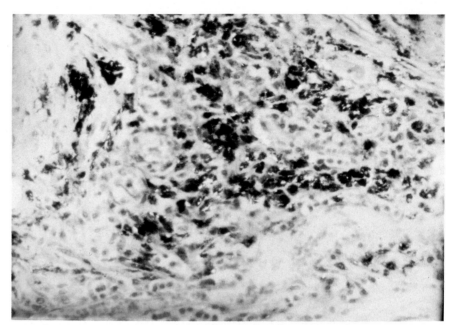

Figure 12–20. High-power photomicrograph, under polarized light, taken from the peripheral rim of tissue in Figure 12–19B, showing doubly refractile silica particles contained within macrophages.

The lesions of massive fibrosis consist of dense hyalinized collagen, often with necrosis in the center. The lesions are avascular and may not show the typical whorled appearance. These masses destroy the normal pulmonary architecture, and the elastin ghosts of pulmonary vessels may again be demonstrated within them. Tuberculous infection may be detected by the finding of acid-fast bacilli and caseation in the center of nodules and by finding the characteristic tubercles of epithelioid cells and Langhans giant cells. Sometimes, however, the presence of this infection may be difficult to detect microscopically, since the histological appearance may be altered by the coexistence of silicosis.

The accelerated form of silicosis differs from chronic silicosis only in degree, the differentiation being clinical rather than pathological. However, descriptions of the pathology of what would be regarded as accelerated silicosis, for example, in diatomaceous earth workers and sandblasters,[28, 125] indicate that in addition to silicotic nodules and massive fibrosis, diffuse thickening of alveolar walls with proliferation of type II alveolar cells may be found. This was a feature in one case described by the author (Fig. 12–21). In addition, a granulomatous reaction with occasional giant cells may be a prominent feature. These cases typically show extensive upper zone fibrosis and lower zone emphysema.

Acute Silicosis

The pathology of acute silicosis is quite unlike that of the chronic form of the disease. The lungs are firm and edematous, and the pleural cavities may contain fibrinous adhesions. Microscopically, there is infiltration of the alveolar walls with plasma cells, lymphocytes, and fibroblasts with some collagenization. The alveoli themselves are filled with an eosinophilic coagulum that is positive to periodic acid-Schiff staining (Fig. 12–22). Electron microscopy shows widening of alveolar walls with some collagen and clusters of type II cells. The alveolar spaces contain degenerating cells that are probably type II alveolar cells and macrophages.[24] The presence of the interstitial pneumonitis differentiates this disease from pulmonary alveolar proteinosis. Although silica particles may be demonstrated in the lungs and lymph nodes, silicotic nodules are few or absent. The lesions of acute silicosis

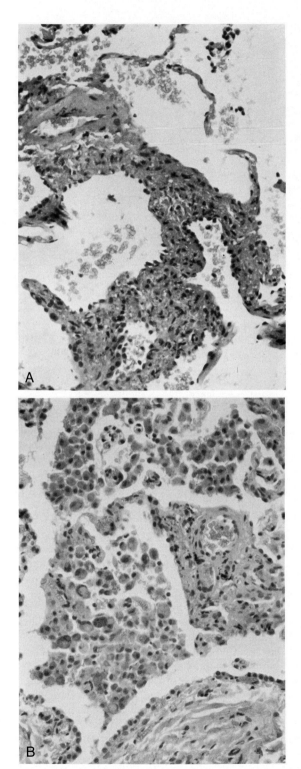

Figure 12–21
Section of lung from patient with accelerated silicosis, showing alveolar wall fibrosis and inflammatory cell infiltration (A), and proliferation of alveolar type II cells (B).

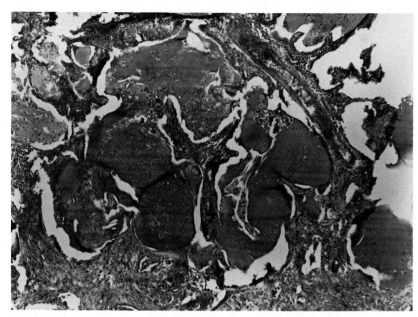

Figure 12–22. Section of lung from patient with acute silicosis, showing interstitial fibrosis and alveoli containing macrophages and PAS-positive eosinophilic material. (Courtesy of Dr. N. L. Lapp.)

may be produced in experimental animals, usually by causing them to inhale concentrations of finely particulate quartz[126, 127] (Fig. 12–23).

PATHOGENESIS

The study of the mechanisms of silicosis has attracted the attention of pathologists over many decades, in a search more for a convenient model of fibrosis than for a means of bettering the lot of quartz-exposed workers. But silicosis is at best a poor model of clinical lung fibrosis, which is generally diffuse in contrast to the discrete nodular nature of silicosis. Furthermore, the typical intratracheal injection method of dosing animals is far from the means whereby humans have been exposed. Nevertheless, useful lessons have been, and continue to be, learned from these studies.

There is good evidence that the type of quartz and the other components of the dust with which it is mixed are important in modulating the fibrotic response. The fine particles, generally less than 10 microns in diameter, that reach the alveoli and are retained in the interstitial tissues have the potential to damage alveolar or interstitial macrophages, alveolar lining cells and any other phagocytes attracted to the area of inflammation. Freshly fractured quartz seems to be more toxic than unfractured, and the larger the total surface area of quartz to which cells are exposed, the greater will be the damage. Certain clay minerals, aluminum salts, and polyvinyl pyridine-*N*-oxide (PNO) inhaled simultaneously will reduce toxicity.

The observable phenomena occurring in experimental studies are that, after phagocytosis, the quartz-filled phagosomes are surrounded by lysosomes which pour their enzymes into them.[128–130] The phagosome is then disrupted and the quartz is liberated into the cytoplasm with subsequent cell death. It is believed that the reaction between the silica and the cell membrane results from peroxidation of the membrane lipids. However, it is possible that the events leading to fibrosis result from reactions occurring while the macrophage is still alive rather than from products of its disruption. Several studies have demonstrated *in vitro* and *in vivo* the release of factors capable of mediating an inflammatory and fibrogenic re-

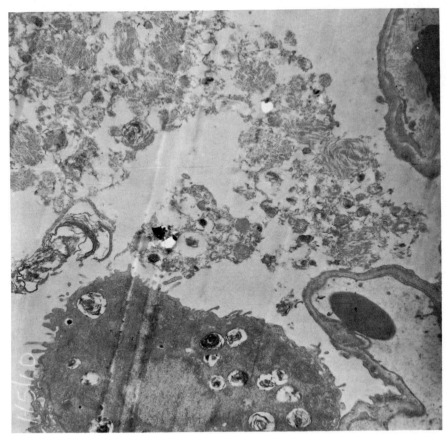

Figure 12–23. Electron micrograph of rat lung following exposure of the animal to quartz dust for 20 hours daily over 6 weeks. The cell at bottom left is a type II alveolar cell, showing lamellar bodies. Sphingomyelin inclusions from these structures are also present free in the air space, giving rise to the so-called proteinaceous material. Also present are small quartz particles with associated tearing of the tissue.

sponse, including interleukin-1, macrophage derived growth factors, the neuropeptide bombesin, tumor necrosis factor, and the fibroblast chemoattractant fibronectin.[131–134] Evidence has been adduced that the fibrotic reaction occurs as a response to stimulation of the interstitial macrophage rather, or to a greater extent, than the free alveolar macrophage.[135] The mechanism of transport of the silica across the alveolar membrane may be by migration of alveolar macrophages or by endocytosis by alveolar lining cells[136]—probably both mechanisms play a part.

It is clear from the distribution of fibrotic lesions that inhaled silica is transported widely in the lungs, and predominantly along lymphatic pathways. Thus, compared to experimental animals, in the human inhaling relatively low concentrations of quartz, the small amount that is actually retained in the lung is usually cleared by a macrophage transport system from interstitial lymphatics to pulmonary and hilar nodes, where usually the greatest concentrations of quartz may be found. The inflammatory reaction is centered on these sites—the alveolus, where attraction of macrophages and neutrophils can be demonstrated by alveolar lavage in experimental animals,[137, 138] around the lymphatics, and in the nodes. But it is in the last two sites rather than in the alveoli that the fibrosis occurs.

Finally, it should be made clear that studies of the pathogenicity of silica depend critically on the type that is used, and that naturally occurring dusts collected in a workplace may have widely different effects depending on their surface properties and the other substances with which they are mixed. Even with pure silica, different crystal structures produce different effects, with cristobalite being probably more toxic than quartz, and quartz more than the octahedral stishovite or amorphous silica.

In summary, the liability of silica to cause fibrosis depends on its particle size, which determines its ability to reach alveoli; its surface properties, which affect its ability to induce an inflammatory response and to stimulate macrophages to produce fibrogenic factors; and the presence in the inhaled dust of other substances capable of interfering with its toxicity.

PREVENTION

Prevention of silicosis depends on recognition of the risk; currently, the chief danger lies in those industries in which silica appears in some disguise. This has been the case with abrasive soap powders and bentonite milling. Once the presence of particles of silica of respirable size has been recognized, the general measures of enclosure of processes, suppression of dust by water and ventilation, and protection of the worker by efficient respirators must be applied. Where heavy concentrations of silica occur, as in sandblasting, tunneling, or stripping of furnace linings, the only adequate protection is for the worker to be isolated from the dust by a protective helmet and suit with its own positive-pressure air supply. The importance of this measure has been emphasized by studies of sandblasters, in which high levels of silica were found *inside* respirators. Moreover, these individuals often worked without respirators when sandblasting had finished but while dust levels were still extremely high.[139] As previously stated, suitable alternatives to silica should be introduced wherever possible.

In all industries in which a dust hazard is recognized, regular monitoring of levels of respirable dust should be carried out, and usually this is required by law. The current standard for silica-containing dusts in the United States is

$$\frac{10}{\% \text{ quartz} + 2} \text{ mg/m}^3$$

For dust containing tridymite and cristobalite, this value is divided by 2, whereas dusts with very low quartz levels (around 1%) are controlled by a nuisance dust standard of 10 mg/m^3. In Britain, a new 8-hour time-weighted maximum exposure limit (MEL) of 0.4 mg/m^3 has been set for all forms of respirable crystalline silica. The law requires employers to keep levels as low as reasonably practicable below this figure (see Chapter 2). Apart from careful control of the environment, workers exposed to silica should undergo chest radiography on a regular basis. A film every 4 to 5 years should be sufficient if silica levels are kept below the hygiene standard, but it should be remembered that radiographs will not help the work force if they are exposed to excessive dust levels.

MANAGEMENT

Once simple silicosis has developed, it is undesirable that the worker should continue to be exposed to the dust, since this will increase the likelihood of massive fibrosis occurring. The exception is foundry work, where this complication is very rare. However, in most cases nowadays, silicosis occurs toward the end of an individual's working life, and this advice may be modified in relation to the known risks in the particular industry.

Symptomatic measures in advanced disease include the provision of oxygen, antibiotics for acute respiratory infections, and cardiac drugs when cor pulmonale supervenes. It is not known whether steroids are of any use, either in preventing progression or in treating the disease at a late stage, as no controlled trials have been carried out. However, there is a possibility that they may slow down the accelerated form of the disease, and if they are to be used, prophylactic antituberculous drugs should also be given.

More specific measures that have been suggested for the treatment of silicosis include inhalation of aluminum powder and treatment with D-penicillamine or polyvinyl pyridine-*N*-oxide. The former has been shown in a careful controlled trial to be ineffective in the treatment of established silicosis when given over a 3-year period.[140] D-Penicillamine is a drug originally introduced for chelating copper in Wilson's disease (hepatolenticular degeneration) that has been found to have a favorable action in severe rheumatoid arthritis.[141] One of its actions is to inhibit collagen synthesis and to allow soluble rather than insoluble collagen to be formed. It is possible that this action might be of use in the management of massive fibrosis and Caplan's syndrome, though clinical evidence so far is sparse. Moreover, D-penicillamine has troublesome side effects on the stomach, skin, kidney, and blood that will inevitably limit its use.

Polyvinyl pyridine-*N*-oxide is a polymer that carries a strong negative charge. It probably forms hydrogen bonds with polymerized silicic acid, thus preventing the latter forming these bonds with the constituents of phagosomal membranes. Given by inhalation or by injection, it protects animals from the toxic effects of silica.[142] However, because it has proved carcinogenic in animals, a search is under way for an effective but nontoxic related chemical that could be used in humans.

Studies of the management of acute silicosis have been confined to case reports. By analogy with alveolar proteinosis, it would seem worthwhile to try bronchopulmonary lavage. The most practicable method of management now is lung transplantation, which should be considered in all such patients of appropriate age. One such patient survived 10 months after transplantation as long ago as 1970;[143] the prospects now are very much better.

Tuberculosis in silicotics should be treated along standard lines, commencing with quadruple therapy until sensitivities are known. Standard triple therapy worked adequately in the past,[144, 145] and the author's experience is that new 6-month regimens using four drugs are sufficient to cure the complicating disease. The other mycobacterial infections, *M. kansasii*, *M. avium–intracellulare*, and *M. malmoense*, would also be expected to respond, or fail to respond, in silicosis as they do in other patients. The treatment of these infections is discussed in standard textbooks of respiratory medicine.[146]

REFERENCES

1. Agricola, G., De re Metallica, 1556. Hoover, H. C., and Hoover, L. H., trans., The Mining Magazine (London), 1912.
2. Ramazzini, B., De Morbis Artificum Diatriba, 1713, Wright, W. C., trans., New York, Hafner Publishing Co., 1964.
3. Johnstone, J., Some account of a species of phthisis pulmonalis, peculiar to persons employed in pointing needles in the needle manufacture. Mem. Med. Soc. London, 5, 89, 1799.
4. Thackrah, C. T., The Effects of Principal Arts, Trades and Professions and of Civic States and Habits of Living on Health and Longevity; With a Particular Reference to the Trades and Manufactures of Leeds. London, Longman, Rees, Orne, Brown and Green, 1831.
5. Peacock, T. B., On French millstone maker's phthisis. Br. Foreign Med. Chir. Rev., 25, 214, 1860.
6. Greenhow, E. H., Specimen of diseased lung from a case of grinder's asthma. Trans. Path. Soc. Lond., 16, 39, 1865.
7. Greenhow, E. H., Specimen of potter's lung. Trans. Path. Soc. Lond., 17, 36, 1866.
8. Trasko, V. M., Silicosis: a continuing problem. U.S. Public Health Reports, 73, 839, 1958.
9. Lanza, A. J., and Childs, S. B., Miners' consumption: a study of 433 cases of the disease among zinc miners in southwestern Missouri. Public Health Bulletin No. 85, Washington, D.C., U.S. Government Printing Office, 1917.
10. U.S. Congress House Committee on Labor Sub-Committee. An investigation relating to health conditions of workers employed in the construction and maintenance of public utilities. H. J. Res. 449, 74th Congress. Washington, D.C., U.S. Government Printing Office, 1936.
11. Cherniak, M., The Hawk's Nest Incident: America's Worst Industrial Disaster. New Haven, CT, Yale University Press, 1986.

12. Warrell, D. A., Harrison, B. D. W., Fawcett, I. W., et al., Silicosis among grindstone cutters in the north of Nigeria. Thorax, 30, 389, 1975.

13. Saiyed, H. N., Parikh, D. J., Ghodasara, N. B., et al., Silicosis in slate pencil workers: I. An environmental and medical study. Am. J. Ind. Med., 8, 127, 1985.

14. Banks, D. E., Morring, K. L., Boehlecke, B. A., et al., Silicosis in silica flour workers. Am. Rev. Respir. Dis., 124, 445, 1981.

15. Bailey, W. C., Brown, M., Buechner, H. A., et al., Silico-mycobacterial disease in sandblasters. Am. Rev. Respir. Dis., 110, 115, 1974.

16. Seaton, A., Legge, J. S., Henderson, J., and Kerr, K. M., Accelerated silicosis in Scottish stone-masons. Lancet, 337, 341, 1991.

17. Seaton, A., Dick, J., Dodgson, J., and Jacobsen, M., Quartz and pneumoconiosis in coalminers. Lancet, 2, 1272, 1981.

18. Fox, A. J., Goldblatt, P., Kinlen, L. J., A study of the mortality of Cornish tin miners. Br. J. Ind. Med., 38, 378, 1981.

19. Seaton, A., Ruckley, V. A., Addison, J., and Brown, W. R., Silicosis in barium miners. Thorax, 41, 591, 1986.

20. Doig, A. T., Disabling pneumoconiosis from limestone dust. Br. J. Ind. Med., 12, 206, 1955.

21. Rees, D., Cronje, R., and du Toit, R. S. J., Dust exposure and pneumoconiosis in a South African pottery. 1. Study objectives and dust exposure. Br. J. Ind. Med., 49, 459, 1992.

22. Golden, E. B., Warnock, M. L., Hulett, L. D., and Church, A. M., Fly ash lung: a new pneumoconiosis? Am. Rev. Respir. Dis., 123, 108, 1982.

23. Banks, D. D., Morring, K. L., and Boehlecke, B. E., Silicosis in the 1980s. Am. Ind. Hyg. Assoc. J., 42, 77, 1981.

24. Xipell, J. M., Ham, K. N., Price, C. G., and Thomas, D. P., Acute silicolipoproteinosis. Thorax, 32, 104, 1977.

25. Zimmerman, P. V., and Sinclair, R. A., Rapidly progressive fatal silicosis in a young man. Med. J. Aust., 2, 704, 1977.

26. Cooper, W. C., and Cralley, L. J., Pneumoconiosis in diatomite mining and processing. Public Health Service Publication No. 601. Washington, D.C., Government Printing Office, 1958.

27. Banks, D. E., Bauer, M. A., Castellan, R. M., and Lapp, N. L., Silicosis in surface coal mine drillers. Thorax, 38, 275, 1983.

28. Suratt, P. M., Winn, W. C., Brody, A. R., et al., Acute silicosis in tombstone sandblasters. Am. Rev. Respir. Dis., 115, 521, 1977.

29. Roeslin, N., Lassabe-Roth, C., Morand, G., and Batzenschlager, A., La silico-proteinose aigue. Arch. Mal. Prof., 41, 15, 1980.

30. Saiyed, H. N., and Chatterjee, B. B., Rapid progression of silicosis in slate pencil workers: II. A follow-up study. Am. J. Ind. Med., 8, 135, 1985.

31. Samini, B., Ziskind, M., and Weill, H., The relation of silica dust to accelerated silicosis. Ecotoxicol. Environ. Safety, 1, 429, 1978.

32. Ng, T. P., Allan, W. G. L., Tsin, T. W., and O'Kelly, F. J., Silicosis in jade workers. Br. J. Ind. Med., 42, 761, 1985.

33. Nelson, H. M., Rajhans, G. S., Morton, S., and Brown, J. R., Silica flour exposures in Ontario. Am. Ind. Hyg. J., 39, 261, 1978.

34. Cooper, W. C., and Jacobson, G., A 21-year radiographic follow-up of workers in the diatomite industry. J. Occup. Med., 19, 563, 1977.

35. Cooper, W. C., and Sargent, E. N., A 26-year radiographic follow-up of workers in a diatomite mine and mill. J. Occup. Med., 26, 456, 1984.

36. Franzinelli, A., Sartorelli, E., LoMartire, N., and Carini, R., A contribution to the study of fossil flour pneumoconiosis. Med. Lav., 62, 258, 1971.

37. Vitinus, V. C., Edwards, M. J., Niles, N. E., et al., Pulmonary fibrosis from amorphous silica dust, a product of silica vapour. Arch. Env. Health, 32, 62, 1977.

38. Brambilla, A., Brambilla, C., Rigaud, D., et al., Pneumoconiosis due to amorphous silica fume—mineralogical and ultrastructural study of six cases. Rev. Fr. Mal. Respir., 8, 383, 1980.

39. Volk, H., The health of workers in a plant making highly dispersed silica. Arch. Environ. Health, 1, 125, 1960.

40. Plunkett, E. R., and de Witt, B. J., Occupational exposure to Hi-Sil and Silene. Report of an 18-year study. Arch. Environ. Health, 5, 469, 1962.

41. Svensson, A., Glomme, J., and Bloom, G., On the toxicity of silica particles. Arch. Ind. Health, 14, 482, 1956.

42. Russell, A. E., Britten, R. H., Thomson, R. L., and Bloomfield, J. J., The health of workers in dusty trades. II. Exposure to siliceous dust (Public Health Bulletin 187). Washington, D.C., U.S. Treasury Department, Public Health Service, 1929.

43. Russell, A. E., The health of workers in dusty trades. VII. Restudy of a group of granite workers (Public Health Bulletin 269). Washington, D.C., U.S. Federal Security Agency, Public Health Service, 1941.

44. Theriault, G. P., Peters, J. M., and Johnson, W. M., Pulmonary function and roentgenographic changes in granite dust exposure. Arch. Environ. Health, 28, 23, 1974.

45. Theriault, G. P., Burgess, W. A., Diberadinis, L. J., and Peters, J. M., Dust exposure in the Vermont granite sheds. Arch. Environ. Health, 28, 12, 1974.

46. Theriault, G. P., Peters, J. M., and Fine, L. J., Pulmonary function in granite shed workers in Vermont. Arch. Environ. Health, 28, 18, 1974.

47. Ashe, H. B., and Bergstrom, D. E., Twenty-six years' experience with dust control in the Vermont granite industry. Ind. Med. Surg., 73, 23, 1964.

48. Davis, L. K., Wegman, D. H., Monson, R. R., and Froines, J., Mortality experience of Vermont granite workers. Am. J. Ind. Med., 4, 705, 1983.

49. Graham, W. G. B., Ashikaga, T., Hemenway, D., et al., Radiographic abnormalities in Vermont granite workers exposed to low levels of granite dust. Chest, 100, 1507, 1991.

50. Rice, C., Harris, R. L., Lumsden, J. C., and Symons, M. J., Reconstruction of silica exposure in the North Carolina dusty trades. Am. Ind. Hyg. J., 45, 689, 1984.

51. Rice, C. H., Harris, R. L., Checkoway, H., and Symons, M. J., Dose-response relationships for silicosis from a case-control study of North Carolina dusty trades workers. In Goldsmith, D. F., Winn, D. M., and Sly, C. M., eds., Silica, Silicosis and Cancer. New York, Praeger, 1986, p. 77.

52. Beadle, D. G., The relationship between the amount of dust breathed and the development of radiological signs of silicosis: an epidemiological study in South African gold miners. In Walton W. H., ed., Inhaled Particles III. Old Woking, Unwin Bros., 1971, p. 953.

53. Beadle, D. G., Harris, E., and Sluis-Cremer, G. K., The relationship between the amount of dust breathed and the incidence of silicosis. In Shapiro H. A., ed., Pneumoconiosis: Proceedings of the International Conference, Johannesburg, 1969. Cape Town, South Africa, Oxford University Press, 1970, p. 473.

54. Sluis-Cremer, G. K., Silica exposure and silicosis in Witwatersrand gold mines in South Africa. In Goldsmith, D. E., Winn, D. M., and Shy, C. M., eds., Silica, Silicosis and Cancer. New York, Praeger, 1986, p. 67.

55. Oakes, D., Douglas, R., Knight, K., et al., Respiratory effects of prolonged exposure to gypsum dust. Ann. Occup. Hyg., 26, 833, 1982.

56. McDonald, J. C., and Oakes, D., Exposure-response in miners exposed to silica. In VI International Pneumoconiosis Conference, 1983, Bochum, Bergbau-Berufsgenossenschaft, 1984, p. 114.

57. Jacobsen, M., and Maclaren, W. M., Unusual pulmonary observations and exposure to coalmine dust: a case-control study. In Walton, W. H., ed., Inhaled Particles V. Oxford, Pergamon Press, 1982, p. 753.

58. Muir, D. C. F., Shannon, H. S., Julian, J. A., et al., Silica exposure and silicosis among Ontario hardrock miners: I. Methodology. Am. J. Ind. Med., 16, 5, 1989.

59. Verma, D. K., Sebestyen, A., Julian, J. A., et al., Silica exposure and silicosis among Ontario hardrock miners: II. Exposure estimates. Am. J. Ind. Med., 16, 13, 1989.

60. Muir, D. C. F., Julian, J. A., Shannon, H. S., et al., Silica exposure and silicosis among Ontario hardrock miners: III. Analysis and risk estimates. Am. J. Ind. Med., 16, 29, 1989.

61. Fox, A. J., Greenberg, M., Ritchie, G. L., and Barraclough, R. N. J., A survey of respiratory disease in the pottery industry. London, Her Majesty's Stationery Office, 1975.

62. Rees, D., Steinberg, M., Becker, P. J., and Solomon, A., Dust exposure and pneumoconiosis in a South Africa pottery. 2. Pneumoconiosis and factors influencing reading of radiographic opacities. Br. J. Ind. Med., 49, 465, 1992.

63. Glover, J. R., Bevan, C., Cotes, J. E., et al., Effects of exposure to slate dust in North Wales. Br. J. Ind. Med., 37, 152, 1980.

64. Lloyd Davies, T. A., Respiratory disease in foundrymen. Report of a survey. London, Her Majesty's Stationery Office, 1971.

65. Pang, D., Fu, S. C., and Yang, G. C., Relation between exposure to respirable silica dust and silicosis in a tungsten mine in China. Br. J. Ind. Med., 49, 38, 1992.

66. Ng, T-P., Chan, S-L., and Lam, K-P., Radiological progression and lung function in silicosis: a ten year follow up study. Br. Med. J., 295, 164, 1987.

67. Middleton, E. L., The present position of silicosis in industry in Britain. Br. Med. J., 2, 485, 1929.

68. Chapman, E. M., Acute silicosis. J.A.M.A., 98, 1439, 1932.

69. Buechner, H. A., and Ansari, A., Acute silico-proteinosis. A new pathologic variant of acute silicosis in sandblasters, characterised by histologic features resembling alveolar proteinosis. Dis. Chest, 55, 274, 1969.

70. Scott, G. A., Acute silicosis. Ulster Med. J., 33, 116, 1964.

71. Sluis-Cremer, G. K., Active pulmonary tuberculosis discovered at post-morten examination of the lungs of black miners. Br. J. Dis. Chest, 74, 374, 1980.

72. Chatgidakis, C. B., Silicosis in South African white gold miners. A comparative study of the disease in its different stages. Med. Proc., 9, 383, 1963.

73. Paul, R., Silicosis in Northern Rhodesia copper mines. Arch. Environ. Health, 2, 96, 1961.

74. Jarman, T. F., Jones, J. G., Phillips, J. H., and Seingry, H. E., Radiological surveys of working quarrymen and quarrying communities in Caernarvonshire. Br. J. Ind. Med., 14, 95, 1957.

75. Glover, J. R., Bevan, C., Cotes, J. E., et al., Effects of exposure to slate dust in North Wales. Br. J. Ind. Med., 37, 152, 1980.

76. Bruce, T., Silicotuberculosis. Scand. J. Respir. Dis., 65 (Suppl.), 139, 1968.

77. Burckhardt, P., Die Silikotuberkulose und uhre Prophylaxe. Schw. Med. Woch., 97, 980, 1967.

78. Dworski, M., Schepers, G. W. H., Wilson, G. E., et al., Fatal pulmonary disease in an industrial worker caused by an atypical acid-fast bacillus. Ind. Med. Surg., 26, 536, 1957.

79. Schepers, G. W., Smart, R. H., Smith, C. R., et al., Fatal silicosis with complicating infection by an atypical acid-fast photochromogenic bacillus. Ind. Med. Surg., 27, 27, 1958.

80. Jones, R. N., Turner-Warwick, M., Ziskind, M., and Weill, H., High prevalence of antinuclear antibodies in sandblasters' silicosis. Am. Rev. Respir. Dis., 113, 393, 1976.
81. Gambini, G., Agnoletto, A., and Magistretti, M., Tre casi di sindrome di Caplan. Med. Lav., 55, 261, 1964.
82. Klockars, M., Koskela, R-S., Jarvinen, E., et al., Silica exposure and rheumatoid arthritis: a follow-up study of granite workers 1940–81. Br. Med. J., 294, 997, 1987.
83. Rodnan, G. P., Benedek, R. G., Medsger, T. A., and Cammarata, R. J., The association of progressive systemic sclerosis (sideroderma) with coal miners' pneumoconiosis and other forms of silicosis. Ann. Int. Med., 66, 323, 1967.
84. Bramwell, B., Diffuse sclerodermia: its frequency; its occurrence in stone-masons; its treatment by fibrolysin-elevations of temperature due to fibrolysin injections. Edin. Med. J., 12, 387, 1914.
85. Ziskind, M., Jones, R. N., and Weill, H., State of the art—Silicosis. Am. Rev. Respir. Dis., 113, 643, 1976.
86. Saldhana, L. F., Rosen, V. J, and Gonick, H. C., Silicon nephropathy. Am. J. Med., 59, 95, 1975.
87. Giles, R. D., Sturgill, B. C., Suratt, P. M., and Bolton, W. K., Massive proteinuria and acute renal failure in a patient with acute silicoproteinosis. Am. J. Med., 64, 336, 1978.
88. Hauglustaine, D., Van Damme, B., Daenens, P., and Michielsen, P., Silicon nephropathy: a possible occupational hazard. Nephron, 26, 219, 1980.
89. Bolton, W. K., Suratt, P. M., and Sturgill, B. C., Rapidly progressive silicon nephropathy. Am. J. Med., 71, 823, 1981.
90. Banks, D. E., Milutinovic, J., Desnick, R. J., et al., Silicon nephropathy mimicking Fabry's disease. Am. J. Nephrol., 3, 279, 1983.
91. Capazzuto, A., La functionalita renale nei silicotici. Folia. Med., 46, 679, 1963.
92. Saita, G., and Zavagilia, O., La functionalita renale nei silicotici. Med. Lav., 42, 41, 1951.
93. Kolev, K., Doitschinov, D., and Todorov, D., Morphologic alterations in the kidneys by silicosis. Med. Lav., 61, 205, 1970.
94. Ng, T. P., Ng., Y. L., and Phoon, W. H., Further evidence of human silica nephrotoxicity in occupationally exposed workers. Br. J. Ind. Med., 50, 907, 1993.
95. Dagle, G. E., Wehner, A. P., Clark, M. L., and Buschbom, R. L., Chronic inhalation exposure of rats to quartz. *In* Goldsmith, D. F., Winn, D. M., and Shy, C. M., eds., Silica, Silicosis and Cancer. Controversy in Occupational Medicine. New York, Praeger, 1986, p. 255.
96. Holland, L. M., Wilson, J. S., Tillery, M. I., and Smith, D. M., Lung cancer in rats exposed to fibrogenic dusts. *In* Goldsmith, D. F., Winn, D. M., and Shy, C. M., eds., Silica, Silicosis and Cancer. Controversy in Occupational Medicine. New York, Praeger, 1986, p. 267.
97. Harting, F. H., and Hesse, W., Der Lungenkrebs, die Bergkrankheit in der Schneeberger Gruben. Vjschr. Gerichtl. Med., 31, 102, 1879.
98. Dible, J. H., Silicosis and malignant disease. Lancet, 2, 982, 1934.
99. Infante-Rivard, C., Armstrong, B., Petitclerk, M., et al., Lung cancer mortality and silicosis in Quebec 1938–85. Lancet, 2, 1504, 1989.
100. Hnizdo, E., and Sluis-Cremer, G. K., Silica exposure, silicosis and lung cancer: a mortality study of South African gold miners. Br. J. Ind. Med., 48, 53, 1991.
101. Mastrangelo, G., Zambon, P., Simonato, L., and Rizzi, P., A case-referent study investigating the relationship between exposure to silica dust and lung cancer. Int. Arch. Occup. Environ. Health, 60, 299, 1988.
102. Ng, T. P., Chan, S. L., and Lee, J., Mortality of a cohort of men in a silicosis register: further evidence of an association with lung cancer. Am. J. Ind. Med., 17, 163, 1990.
103. Kurppa, K., Gudbergsson, H., Hannunkari, I., et al., Lung cancer among silicotics in Finland. *In* Goldsmith, D. F., Winn, D. M., and Shy, C. M., eds., Silica, Silicosis and Cancer. Controversy in Occupational Medicine. New York, Praeger, 1986, p. 311.
104. Amandus, H. E., Shy, C., Wing, S., et al., Silicosis and lung cancer in North Carolina dusty trades workers. Am. J. Ind. Med., 20, 57, 1991.
105. Steenland, K., and Beaumont, J., A proportional mortality study of granite cutters. Am. J. Ind. Med., 9, 189, 1986.
106. Carta, P., Cocco, P. L., and Casula, D., Mortality from lung cancer among Sardinian patients with silicosis. Br. J. Ind. Med., 48, 122, 1991.
107. Simonato, L., Fletcher, A. C., Saracci, R., and Thomas, T. L., Occupational exposure to silica and cancer risk. IARC Sci. Publ., No. 97, 1990.
108. Goldsmith, D. F., Winn, D. M., and Shy, C. M., Silica, Silicosis and Cancer. Controversy in Occupational Medicine. New York, Praeger, 1986.
109. Pairon, J. C., Brochard, P., Jaurand, M. C., and Bignon, J., Silica and lung cancer: a controversial issue. Eur. Respir. J., 4, 730, 1991.
110. Ng, T. P., Chan, S. L., and Lam, K. P., Radiological progression and lung function in silicosis: a ten year follow up study. Br. Med. J., 295, 164, 1987.
111. Al-Kassimi, F. A., Pleural effusion in silicosis of the lung. Br. J. Ind. Med., 49, 448, 1992.
112. Weiss, W., Cigarette smoking and small irregular opacities. Br. J. Ind. Med., 48, 841, 1991.
113. Seaton, A., Cigarette smoking and small irregular opacities. Br. J. Ind. Med., 49, 453, 1992.
114. Churg, A., Wright, J. L., Wiggs, B., et al., Small airways disease and mineral dust exposure. Prevalence, structure and function. Am. Rev. Respir. Dis., 131, 139, 1985.
115. Teculescu, D. B., Stanescu, D. C., and Pilat, L., Pulmonary mechanics in silicosis. Arch. Environ. Health, 14, 461, 1967.

116. Teculescu, D. B., and Stanescu, D. C., Carbon monoxide transfer factor for the lung in silicosis. Scand. J. Respir. Dis., 41, 150, 1970.
117. Irwig, L. M., and Rocks, P., Lung function and respiratory symptoms in silicotic and nonsilicotic gold miners. Am. Rev. Respir. Dis., 117, 429, 1978.
118. Hnizdo, E., Loss of lung function associated with exposure to silica dust and with smoking and its relation to disability and mortality in South Africa gold miners. Br. J. Ind. Med., 49, 472, 1992.
119. Buechner, H. A., and Ansari, A., Acute silico-proteinosis. Dis. Chest, 55, 274, 1969.
120. Jones, R. N., Weill, H., and Ziskind, M., Pulmonary function in sandblasters' silicosis. Bull. Physiopath. Respir., 11, 589, 1975.
121. Silicosis and Silicate Diseases Committee. Diseases associated with exposure to silica and nonfibrous silicate materials. Arch. Path. Lab. Med., 112, 673, 1988.
122. Langlois, S. L. E. P., Sterrett, G. F., and Henderson, D. W., Hepatosplenic silicosis. Austr. Radiol., 21, 143, 1977.
123. Slavin, R. E., Swedo, J. L., Brandes, D., et al., Extrapulmonary silicosis: a clinical, morphologic and ultrastructural study. Hum. Path., 16, 393, 1985.
124. Curran, R. C., Observations on the formation of collagen in quartz lesions. J. Pathol. Bact., 66, 271, 1953.
125. Vigliani, E. C., and Mottura, G., Diatomaceous earth pneumoconiosis. Br. J. Ind. Med., 5, 148, 1945.
126. Gross, P., and de Treville, R. T. P., Alveolar proteinosis: its experimental production in rodents. Arch. Pathol., 86, 255, 1968.
127. Heppleston, A. G., Atypical reaction to inhaled silica. Nature, 213, 199, 1967.
128. Allison, A. C., Harrington, J. S., and Birbeck, M., The examination of the cytotoxic effect of silica on macrophages. J. Exp. Med., 124, 141, 1966.
129. Allison, A. C., Harrington, J. S., Birkbeck, M., and Nash, T., Observations on the cytotoxic action of silica on macrophages. In Davies, C. N., ed., Inhaled Particles and Vapours II. Oxford, Pergamon Press, 1967, p. 121.
130. Davis, G. S., Pathogenesis of silicosis: current concepts and hypotheses. Lung, 164, 139, 1986.
131. Schmidt, J. A., Oliver, C. N., Lepe-Zuniga, J. L., et al., Silica-stimulated monocytes release fibroblast proliferation factors identical to interleukin 1. J. Clin. Invest., 73, 1462, 1984.
132. Wiedermann, C. J., Adamson, I. Y. R., Pert, C. B., and Bowden, D. H., Enhanced secretion of immunoreactive bombesin by alveolar macrophages exposed to silica. J. Leukoc. Biol., 43, 99, 1988.
133. Piguet, P. F., Collart, M. A., Grau, G. E., et al., Requirement of tumour necrosis factor for development of silica-induced pulmonary fibrosis. Nature, 344, 245, 1990.
134. Driscoll, K. E., Maurer, J. K., Lindenschmidt, R. C., et al., Respiratory tract responses to dust: relationships between dust burden, lung injury, alveolar macrophage fibronectin release, and the development of pulmonary fibrosis. Toxicol. Appl. Pharmacol., 106, 88, 1990.
135. Bowden, D. H., Hedgecock, C., and Adamson, I. Y. R., Silica-induced pulmonary fibrosis involves the reaction of particles with interstitial rather than alveolar macrophages. J. Path., 158, 73, 1989.
136. Brody, A. R., Roe, M. W., Evans, J. N., et al., Deposition and translocation of inhaled silica in rats. Lab. Invest., 47, 533, 1982.
137. Kusaka, Y., Donaldson, K., and Cullen, R. T., Lymphocyte modulation by inflammatory bronchoalveolar lymphocytes. FEMS Microbiol. Immunol., 64, 9, 1990.
138. Adamson, I. Y. R., and Bowden, D. H., Role of polymorphonuclear leukocytes in silica-induced pulmonary fibrosis. Am. J. Pathol., 117, 37, 1984.
139. Samini, B., Neilson, A., Weill, H., and Ziskind, M., The efficiency of protective hoods used by sandblasters to reduce silica dust exposure. Am. Ind. Hyg. J., 36, 140, 1975.
140. Kennedy, M. C. S., Aluminium powder inhalations in the treatment of silicosis of pottery workers and pneumoconiosis of coal-miners. Br. J. Ind. Med., 13, 85, 1956.
141. Andrews, F. M., Golding, D. N., Freeman, A. N., et al., Controlled trial of D-penicillamine in severe rheumatoid arthritis. Lancet, 1, 175, 1973.
142. Barhad, B., Rotarn, G., Lazarescu, I., et al., Experience in polyvinyl pyridin-N-oxide action on experiment lung silicosis. 4th International Pneumoconiosis Conference, Bucharest, 1971, p. 315.
143. Derom, F., Barbier, F., Ringoir, S., et al., Ten month survival after lung homotransplantation in man. J. Thorac. Cardiovasc. Surg., 61, 835, 1971.
144. Medical Research Council Miners' Chest Diseases Treatment Centre. Chemotherapy of pulmonary tuberculosis with pneumoconiosis. Tubercle, 48, 1, 1967.
145. Dubois, P., Gyselen, A., and Prignot, J., Rifampicin-combined chemotherapy in coalworkers' pneumoconio-tuberculosis. Am. Rev. Respir. Dis., 115, 221, 1977.
146. Seaton, A., Seaton, D., and Leitch, A. G., Crofton & Douglas's Respiratory Diseases, 4th ed. Oxford, Blackwell's, 1989, p. 439.

13

Silicates and Lung Disease

W. Keith C. Morgan

■

Silicates are formed from the combination of silicon dioxide with other elements, in particular, potassium, aluminum, iron, magnesium, and calcium.

Most rocks contain silicon either in the form of free silica (silicon dioxide) or combined as various silicates. The three most commonly occurring groups of rocks are classified as igneous, sedimentary, and metamorphic. Igneous rocks are the primary rocks found on the earth's surface and are formed by the cooling of the earth's crust. The crystalline structure of the rocks is determined by the rate of cooling of the various molten minerals. Sedimentary rocks are formed by slow weathering from sun, wind, and ice or by the deposition of marine life in the sea or lake bottom. Metamorphic rocks result from the action of heat; from movements of the earth's crust with its shearing effects; or by percolation of hot fluids, steam, and gases through the various defects on the earth's surface. The more free silica present in the rock, the more acid it is. The more base that is present (i.e., potassium, magnesium, calcium, and others), the more alkaline is the rock.

Silicates exist in fibrous and nonfibrous forms. At this juncture, however, it is important to emphasize that there is much disagreement concerning the use of the term *fiber*. The Occupational Safety and Health Administration (OSHA) has chosen to define a fiber by its aspect ratio (i.e., any particle that is three times as long as it is broad is regarded as a fiber).[1] Many other regulatory agencies in other countries use the same definition. However, most geologists and mineralogists maintain that it is nonspecific and imprecise and that a better definition would also include a statement to the effect that a fiber is a structure that can be woven.[2, 3] In this connection, it is relevant to bear in mind how the term fiber became common usage in industrial hygiene. The first practical and reliable method of measuring airborne fibers was the British membrane filter. This was used predominantly for determining the number of fibers present in the air of asbestos factories and in other situations where it was justifiable to assume that most elongated airborne particles present were composed of asbestos. The method is, however, nonspecific and includes other fibers in the counts, in particular, cotton. When used in other situations where asbestos is not the major airborne contaminant, other long thin particles will be detected and counted. Should they be nonasbestiform fibers, clearly, they do not have the same sinister significance.

The most important fibrous mineral is asbestos, and this is dealt with in Chapter 14. Other silicates exist in leaf- or plate-like forms and are often referred to as "phyllosilicates" (from the Greek *phyllon*, or leaf).[4] These include talc, mica, kaolin, and other clays (Table 13–1). Some clays and other minerals, in particular, wollastonite, attapulgite, certain zeolites, and sepiolite, have a fibrous or acicular configuration, at least as far as their aspect ratio is concerned (Table 13–2). Similarly, certain of the phyllosilicates may appear as fibers when examined under a microscope, especially when viewed from the edge or the side of the particle. When

Table 13–1
■
More Common Disease-Inducing Silicates

	Chemical Composition
Phyllosilicates	
Talc	$Mg_3Si_4O_{10}(OH)_2$
Mica	K Na Al silicate
Kaolin	$Si_2O_5Al_2(OH)_4$
Fullers' earth (montmorillonite)	Variable amounts of Ca, K, Fe_2, Fe_3, and Mg and Si dominant
Attapulgite and palygorskite	15% Al_2 in palygorskite
Chain Silicates	
Wollastonite	$CaSiO_3$
Orthosilicates	
Mullite	Al silicate
Framework Silicates	
Feldspar	Al silicate with K, Na, or Ca
Zeolites (fibrous erionite)	Al silicate with Na or Ca

seen from a frontal aspect, they have an entirely different appearance that is more aptly referred to as acicular. When describing such particles, most geologists and mineralogists prefer to designate such particles as acicular, thereby avoiding the term *fibrous* since the latter has an entirely different connotation in regard to health effects.

TALC

Talc is a hydrated silicate with an approximate formula of $Mg_3Si_4O_{10}(OH)_2$.[4] It is produced by the metamorphosis of either dolomite or quartzose rocks or by hydrothermal alteration of ultramafic and mafic rocks. Talc occurs as sheet-like crystals which cleave into thin leaf-like structures. These thin slices are soft and have the capacity to smooth surfaces on which they are deposited.

Talc has many uses and is often added to cosmetic powders. One form of talc, which is known as soapstone because of its slippery feeling, is often used for smoothing surfaces and is frequently applied to the rubber inner tubes of tires. Soapstone is a less pure form of talc; steatite is a more dense purer talc that can be machined. French talc is often used by tailors and by welders for marking. The greatest demand for talc comes from the ceramic industry in which it is essential for the manufacture of kiln furniture, sanitary enamel wear, floor and wall tile, crockery, and dinnerware. A second major use is as a filler for paints and pigments. It is also used in the manufacture of paper, as a ''carrier'' for agricultural chemicals, in asphalt shingles, and as a constituent of floor and shoe polish.

The United States is the major world producer of talc, which is mined in Oklahoma, Vermont, California, Montana, and upstate New York. Large deposits

Table 13–2
■
Phyllosilicates*

Nonfibrous Phyllosilicates	Fibrous Phyllosilicates
Kaolin	Serpentine
Talc	Sepiolite
Vermiculite	Attapulgite
Mica	Palygorskite

*''Phyllo'' from *phyllon* or leaf (Greek)

also exist in Italy, France, Ontario, and other parts of Canada. The mining of talc is mostly carried out in open cast operations, but a fair number of underground mines exist. Underground mining involves the drilling of the rock and its excavation by blasting operations. Talc is often found in compact seams; therefore, contact with nearby rock strata that contain silica is limited. Once the talc seam has been identified and mining commenced, exposure to silica is generally minimal, and the seam may be worked for many years. The rock from which the talc is removed is relatively stable and hard. As a consequence, roof falls are rare. Little in the way of roof support is needed.

Although talc is often referred to as a fibrous silicate, this is a misnomer since the terminology depends on how a fiber is defined. Talc, as mentioned, consists of ultrathin plate-like forms, except in rare cases in which it is pseudomorphic, but it may contain other minerals that can, under certain circumstances, have an aspect ratio that conforms to the OSHA definition of a fiber. Thus, many deposits of talc are associated with tremolite, actinolite, or anthophyllite, but it needs to be remembered that these minerals exist both as asbestiform and nonasbestiform variants.[3, 5] Similarly, crocidolite, amosite, and chrysotile have their asbestiform and nonasbestiform counterparts (Table 13–3). The asbestiform and nonasbestiform minerals can be distinguished without difficulty by competent mineralogists (Fig. 13–1).[3–5] The asbestiform forms of tremolite, actinolite, and amosite are carcinogenic in both humans and animals, but the overwhelming body of evidence indicates that their nonasbestiform variants are noncarcinogenic.

Talc Pneumoconiosis

The inhalation of talc has been known to be associated with radiographic abnormalities since the early 1930s. Thus, Merewether reported on 11 subjects who worked in a tire factory and who had abnormal chest radiographs, suggesting diffuse fibrosis of the lungs.[6] He ascribed the changes to the inhalation of fine powdered talc dust. Additional cases were described by him later. Postmortem studies were carried out, and it was evident that, at that time, the workers were exposed to an inordinately high level of dust, often above 100 million particles per cubic foot (mppcf). Later, Porro et al. described 15 subjects with what he and his colleagues termed ''talc pneumoconiosis.''[7] In five of these subjects, postmortem examinations were carried out. The employees examined by Porro et al. were drawn from two companies who had been surveyed and studied previously by Dreesen and Dalla Valle.[8] The highest dust level recorded was 1444 mppcf, with an average concentration of 52 mppcf. These levels are unbelievably high compared with present-day conditions in which the average concentration in most North American mines is around 5 to 10 mppcf. Nondisabling fibrosis was found in nearly all workers. Dreesen and Dalla Valle had found no free silica in the ambient air of the facilities they studied, but large amounts of silicates, tremolite (whether asbestiform or nonasbestiform was and is unknown), and soapstone were detected.

Although Porro et al. described the postmortem findings in several of these subjects, it is clear that the separation of the effects of dust inhalation from other

Table 13–3
■
Asbestiform Minerals and Their Nonasbestiform Counterparts

Asbestiform	Nonasbestiform
Chrysotile	Antigorite
Crocidolite	Riebeckite
Amosite	Cummingtonite-grunerite
Tremolite	Tremolite
Actinolite	Actinolite
Anthophyllite	Anthophyllite

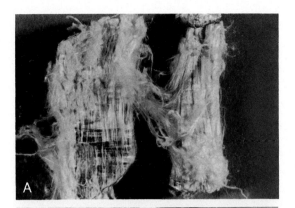

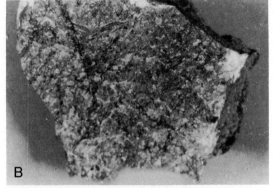

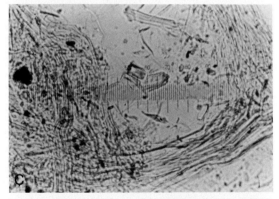

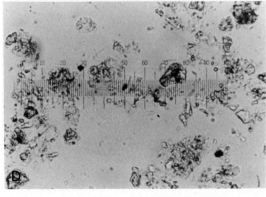

Figure 13–1
Specimens of chrysotile (A) and
antigorite (B). Photomicrographs of
chrysotile (C) and antigorite (D), to
illustrate different configurations of
fibers and cleavage products (265
× 2.75 μm/division).
*Illustration continued
on following page*

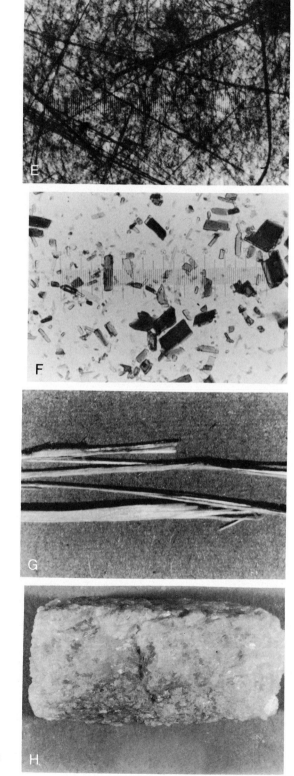

Figure 13–1 *Continued*
Photomicrographs of crocidolite
fibers *(E)* and riebeckite cleavage
products *(F)* (265 × 2.75
μm/division). Specimens of
asbestiform *(G)* and nonasbestiform
(H) tremolite.

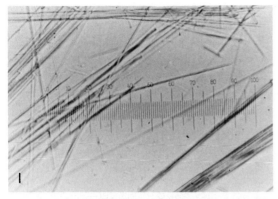

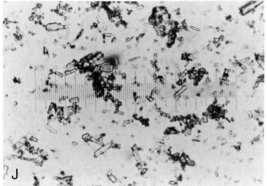

Figure 13–1 *Continued*
Asbestiform *(I)* and nonasbestiform
(J) tremolite showing different
configuration of fibers and cleavage
products (265 × 2.75
μm/division). (*A* to *G*, Courtesy of
John Kelse. *H* to *J*, From Kelse, J.
W., and Thompson, C. S., The
regulatory and mineralogical
definitions of asbestos and their
impact on amphibole dust analysis.
Am. Ind. Hyg. Assoc. J., 50(11),
616, 1989.)

naturally occurring diseases, such as tuberculosis, was not always either easy or possible.[7] Three of the five subjects who had undergone postmortem examinations were found to have had tuberculosis, and some subjects also had had exposure to free silica. Nevertheless, it seems reasonable to attribute at least a part of the fibrosis to the inhalation of talc. Many subjects had complicated pneumoconiosis. Asbestos-like bodies were found in the lungs in all five subjects who had a necropsy. The radiographic appearances were described as reticular in certain instances and nodular in others. However, most of those with nodular lesions had been exposed to silica or iron oxide. It was interesting to note that Gardner had previously described bodies similar to those seen in asbestos workers in talc workers.[9] Clearly, we now know that these would have been better termed "ferruginous bodies," and the term *asbestos bodies* is incorrect when applied to the bodies found in talc workers.

Siegal et al. investigated the talc mining and milling industry in upstate New York.[10] They found almost no free silica in the talc. In 221 subjects, 32 men were found with advanced fibrosis, all of whom had worked for 10 or 12 years or longer. The fibrosis was described as fine and diffuse. Some nodulation was also recorded. Dust counts ranged from 6 to 5000 mppfc in mining and from 20 to 215 mppfc in milling. The average dust counts for some activities were in excess of 1000 mppcf.

In 1955, Kleinfeld et al.[11] conducted a follow-up study of the 32 workers previously examined by Siegal et al.[10] Radiographic progression and increasing impairment had occurred over the period of observation, but progression was slow. Disabling impairment was only found in the older workers. The presence of asbestos-like bodies was noted in those whose lungs were examined. Pleural plaques and pleural calcification were found frequently in the chest radiographs. A further study of the clinical, radiographic, and lung function of workers exposed to granular and "fibrous" talc was carried out in 1964.[12] The photomicrographs in this article of the fibrous talc, however, appear to be elongated cleavage fragments of amphiboles. Lung function abnormalities were more frequent in those exposed to fibrous talc. Those subjects who developed talcosis and who had been exposed to fibrous talc had been exposed for 11 or more years to dust levels that far exceeded the maximal allowable concentration for most of their working days in the year. The predominant radiographic abnormality was reticulonodulation in the lower zones. Those workers who were exposed only to granular talc had less severe effects.

In 1965, Kleinfeld et al. studied the lung function of 43 workers employed in a talc mill.[13] The mean duration of exposure was 19.3 years, and the time-weighted average exposure to particles was 62 mppcf. This article seems to be an elaboration of the prior study and describes the same subjects but adds some dust exposure data. Interstitial infiltrates were noted in the middle and lower zones, but in a few instances, the infiltrates were described as nodular. It is clear from the use of the terms "nodular" and "interstitial" that they had different connotations then to what they have at present. The investigators found no correlation between symptoms and radiographic findings. Progression of radiographic findings was still occurring at the time of the follow-up study, but it was much slower than in the original Kleinfeld et al. study.[11] This was attributed to better industrial hygiene.

A mortality study was performed of the talc miners who were employed between 1940 and 1965 and who had 15 or more years of exposure to talc dust.[14] The cohort included 220 workers. Of the 91 deaths that had occurred, nine were presumed to be due to carcinoma of the lung, and the 10th was attributed to a fibrosarcoma of the lung. Clearly, consideration must be given to the possibility that this latter death may have been due to a pleural mesothelioma. There were, however, no excess deaths caused by gastrointestinal cancer. The observed death rate for lung cancer was four times the expected death rate for white men. However, smoking histories were taken in only a minority of subjects. Moreover, it was known that several subjects had exposures to other harmful agents, including asbestos, before starting their work in the talc industry. The average age at which death occurred in the talc workers was greater than might have been expected (mean age at death, 60.4 years). The comparable figure for white male workers in the United States as a whole was 54.4 years.

Kleinfeld et al. also described six talc workers who underwent a postmortem examination.[15] They all had huge dust exposures which exceeded the then dust standards by 100 to 1000 times. Although many showed evidence of talc pneumoconiosis or pleural plaques, some also had other conditions that were unrelated to talc exposure, including bronchiectasis, emphysema, tuberculosis, and lymphatic leukemia.

A further clinical and environmental study of workers employed in the manufacture of commercial talc indicated that, despite a mean exposure of 16.2 years (range, 11 to 22 years), only one worker showed any abnormality on chest radiograph.[15a] Thirty-nine workers examined were miners or millers, and the highest dust levels were found in those involved in the primary crushing of the ore. Although the authors claimed that the workers included in the study were exposed to asbestiform minerals, this statement is unlikely to be accurate. They were probably exposed to cleavage products from the breakdown of nonasbestiform tremolite and anthophyllite.[16] It was pointed out that although the latency period for the development of talcosis had increased, workers were still contracting the disease. No subjects were found with malignancies.

Radiographic Appearances

Pure talc is far less fibrogenic than silica, and a much greater amount needs to be deposited in the lungs before fibrosis and radiographic abnormalities appear.

Two distinct radiographic appearances may be seen following long exposure to talc (Figs. 13–2 and 13–3). The first is a nodular pattern affecting the middle and upper zones of both lungs. It resembles silicosis and, indeed, in some instances,

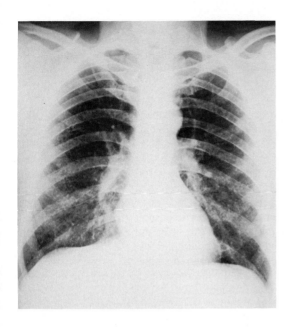

Figure 13–2
Radiograph of subject with simple talcosis showing small rounded nodules in the upper and mid zones of the lungs with scanty irregular opacities in the lower zones. (Courtesy of Dr. P. Leophonte.)

is indistinguishable. This is not surprising because high concentrations of silica have been reported in around 40% of samples of talc, and some of the fibrosis is a response to silica rather than talc.[17] In those patients with a nodular pattern, the opacities are rounded and of the "q" or "r" type.

Pure talc, when it causes pneumoconiosis, leads to a mixture of rounded (q and r) and irregular (t and u) opacities, which appear in the middle zones and are often perihilar in distribution (see Figs. 13–2 and 13–3). The opacities slowly spread both up and down from their perihilar distribution.[18]

Occasionally, the predominant opacities are of the irregular type (i.e., reticulonodulation) and are located in both lower zones with a mixture of t and scanty u opacities. The presence of irregular opacities seems to be more common in talc workers who are smokers and who have cough and sputum. One must also bear in mind that, during the early stages of *en face* pleural plaque formation, plaques can easily be mistaken for parenchymal infiltrates, especially when they occur in the

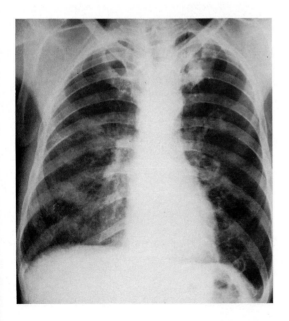

Figure 13–3
Irregular opacities in the lower and mid zones with predominant involvement of the right side. Early large shadows are present at the left apex and in the left mid zone. (Courtesy of Dr. P. Leophonte.)

middle and lower zones. Overt parenchymal pneumoconiosis caused by talc is currently a relative rarity in North America. Large opacities may be found but are now seldom seen in North America or Europe (Fig. 13–4).

Lung Function

Although a large number of studies of lung function in talc workers have been carried out, most have taken little account of the various confounding factors.[11–16] This is particularly true of many of the early studies in the upstate New York workers. Besides being exposed to levels of dust often 100 to 1000 times greater than the maximal allowable concentration, the frequent and concomitant presence of other chest diseases, such as tuberculosis, bronchiectasis, and emphysema, along with the fact that some of the workers had other exposures (in particular, to free silica and asbestos in prior jobs), obscured the true effects of exposure to pure talc. Some recent studies have purported to show abnormalities in the ventilatory capacity in the absence of talc pneumoconiosis. Most such studies have been carried out in either rubber workers or talc miners. In the case of the former, exposure to soapstone and other forms of talc was frequent.

Fine et al. carried out a number of studies related to the respiratory status of a group of rubber workers.[19, 20] The workers were selected according to their job and as to whether they had potentially harmful exposures. Included were 123 curing workers, 46 workers exposed to talc, and 30 processing workers. The curing workers were exposed to a number of irritant fumes but not to talc.[19] It was calculated that the ventilatory capacity of the most heavily exposed curing workers would show an annual decrement in the forced expiratory volume in 1 second (FEV_1) of 173 ml/year. Since the men were around 40 years of age, they would have an expected working life of at least a further 20 years. Were this projected decrement correct, the workers' FEV_1 would decrease on average by 3.46 L over the period. Since the mean FEV_1 at the time of the study was 3.56 L, clearly, such a projection could not be valid. Unfortunately, the complex regression analyses used by the investigators did not take into account the problems associated with collinearity.

In a second study in those exposed to talc, the same investigators used the same statistical method and claimed that exposure to talc caused an excess decre-

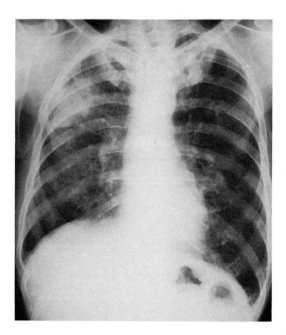

Figure 13–4
Talcosis with conglomerate shadows on a background of mixed opacities. (Courtesy of Dr. P. Leophonte.)

ment in the FEV_1 of 26 ml/year.[20] However, the mean FEV_1 of the talc-exposed group compared with that of the controls differed by less than 200 ml. Moreover, the cigarette smoking data showed a number of anomalies in that, among the talc workers, the most exposed had smoked for a mean of 14.8 years while the less exposed were 11 years younger and had smoked for 12.5 years. This indicates that there was some selection bias at least as far as smoking habits were concerned. Were projected decrements in the FEV_1 of these rubber workers valid, then not only the curing workers but also the talc workers would have shown an increased death rate from respiratory disease. This was not the case, and rubber workers have a relatively normal life expectancy and no increased death rate from respiratory disease.[21, 22]

A follow-up study of the respiratory effects of talc was carried out by Wegman et al.[23] In this study, 103 of 116 subjects who had been studied had pulmonary function tests repeated 1 year later. Although there was said to be an increased rate of decline in the FEV_1 and forced vital capacity (FVC), there was no demonstrable relationship between the decline in these indices and dust exposure or, if it comes to that, pack-years. The authors state that the annual loss of FEV_1 in the heavy smokers ranged between 25 and 51 ml/year. This is an extraordinarily small decrement since smokers may lose up to 300 to 400 ml/year, as shown by Fletcher et al. (Charts F3 to F8).[24] Once again, the authors had difficulty separating the effects of dust exposure from cigarette smoking because they were both collinearly related.

Gamble et al. conducted an epidemiological study of a cohort of talc miners and millers.[26] Ninety-three subjects had worked with talc only, and of the total work force of 156, 121 participated. The average duration of exposure was 10.2 years. The lung function values of the talc miners were compared with those in a reference population of 1077 potash miners. The potash mine, however, was located in the southwestern United States, whereas the talc mine was located in the northeastern United States. Moreover, potash ores are soluble and, for the most part, are deposited in the upper respiratory tract where they dissolve and produce irritation. This is not true of talc particles, which are insoluble and are deposited anywhere in the respiratory tract according to their size. The investigators found an increased prevalence of small irregular opacities which increased with age, cigarette smoking, and with dust exposure in both the dust and potash workers. The prevalence of such irregular opacities after adjustment for these various factors was somewhat higher in the talc workers than in the potash workers. Pleural thickening was much more common in the talc workers than in the potash workers and was associated with a decrement in the FEV_1 and FVC but was not separated into diffuse or localized. Although those with more pleural thickening had worked about 3 years longer than did those without pleural thickening, they were 7 years older and may also have been appreciably heavier. The latter could have led to some false-positive readings for pleural thickening. There was also a concomitant decline in the $FEV_1/FVC\%$ which would indicate obstructive rather than restrictive impairment. Were the reduced FEV_1 and FVC a consequence of pleural thickening, these indices would have been reduced to roughly the same extent when expressed as a percentage of the predicted value.

A further study was conducted in which 299 miners and millers exposed to talc derived from Montana, Texas, and North Carolina underwent radiographic examinations, lung function tests, and the administration of a questionnaire.[26] The Montana talc was free of elongated particulates (i.e., asbestiform fibers), and respiratory symptoms were unrelated to years worked. Pleural thickening was noted in all three mines, with 7%, 16%, and 14% of the workers affected in Montana, Texas, and North Carolina, respectively. Bilateral pleural thickening was associated with a reduction of lung function and was more common in workers 40 years of age or older. The entire population of those exposed to talc showed no difference in lung function as far as the FEV_1 and FVC were concerned, according to the location of the talc mines, or when compared with potash miners and other blue collar workers.

The most reliable study of lung function in talc workers is probably that of

Leophonte and Didier.[18] They studied 39 workers with talc pneumoconiosis and 39 controls matched for age and smoking habits. The pneumoconiotic subjects showed mild restriction compared with the nonexposed subjects. No excess obstruction was noted. A greater effect on ventilatory capacity was noted in six workers who had large opacities on a higher background of simple talc pneumoconiosis. The FVCs for the nonexposed group, those with pneumoconiosis, and those with large opacities were 103%, 96.8%, and 87%, respectively, of the predicted values. The comparable figures for the talc workers were 100%, 94.2%, and 86%, respectively. Thus, large opacities tend to be associated with greater restrictive impairment.

Bronchoalveolar lavage in talc workers with pneumoconiosis shows hypercellularity, with a significant increase in neutrophils and eosinophils.[18] Numerous talc particles are usually visible in the macrophages, and there are often atypical ferruginous bodies present in the lung parenchyma (Fig. 13–5).

Pathological Findings

The interpretation of many earlier reports of the pathological changes found in talc pneumoconiosis is difficult, if not impossible, because of the attention given to the concomitant and, we now know, fortuitous association with other diseases, such as tuberculosis, lung cancer, and emphysema. It is apparent that talc, with or without nonasbestiform amphibole content, is far less fibrogenic than is crystalline silica. In this, it resembles kaolin, mica, and other phyllosilicates.

Talc induces pleural thickening and calcification. The histological appearance of the pleural thickening is identical to that seen in asbestos-induced pleural plaques and consists of relatively acellular collagenous connective tissue.

Long continued inhalation of talc may also produce a mild alveolitis, which does not tend to be severe since the talc is continuously being removed from the alveoli by macrophages and the lungs' defense mechanisms.[18] As time goes by, granulomata may develop. Subsequently, small nodules appear in the interstitial tissue in roughly the same site where the typical silicotic nodule develops, i.e., in the peribronchial and perivascular zones (Fig. 13–6). The histological appearances differ, however, from those of the typical whorled nodule characteristic of silicosis. The granulomata that form from the inhalation of talc resemble foreign body granulomata and consist of foreign body giant cells, macrophages, and epitheloid cells. The macrophages often contain doubly refractile bodies. The typical vasculitis that develops following the intravenous use of talc is not seen when talc is inhaled. Later, some of the granulomata undergo collagenous fibrosis, but the deposition of collagen is not as extensive as that which occurs in typical silicosis. Conglomerate talcosis appears to be a result of the aggregation of many nodules into a larger mass. As mentioned earlier, ferruginous bodies are often present.

Talc as a Carcinogen

There have been a number of early studies in which it was suggested that talc, when contaminated by tremolite, leads to an increased incidence of lung cancer.[14, 27]

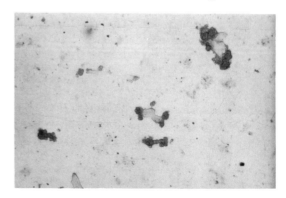

Figure 13–5
Bronchoalveolar lavage specimen showing ferruginous bodies formed from talc. (Courtesy of Dr. P. Leophonte.)

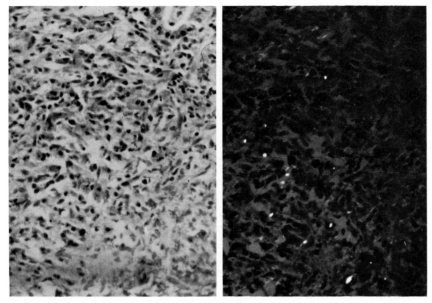

Figure 13–6. Area of fibrosis in lung of patient who inhaled contents of medicinal capsules before performance as a punk rock musician. View on right shows talc particles visible by their transmission of polarized light.

We now know that most of these workers were not exposed to asbestiform tremolite but to its nonasbestiform counterpart.

It is probably appropriate to discuss briefly what is known about the manner in which various mineral fibers induce mesothelioma and lung cancer. The precise mechanisms leading to tumorigenesis are still not understood, but Wagner showed that mesothelioma could be induced by the intrapleural instillation of free fibers in animals.[28] These early experiments shed no light on the biological activity of nonasbestiform tremolite. Subsequently, Wagner et al. showed that asbestiform tremolite, when injected into the pleural cavity of rats, induced mesotheliomata, whereas an equal dose of two nonasbestiform tremolites did not.[29] Several nonasbestiform fibers, including glass, were found to be capable of inducing mesothelioma, providing the diameter of the fibers was less than 0.5 μm, but nonasbestiform actinolite, biotite, and talc did not produce tumors. The relationship between fiber size and the development of mesothelioma was demonstrated. It was concluded that the fiber structure was the pre-eminent influence in the induction of malignant tumors of the pleura.

Later, Stanton and Wrench carried out experiments using various forms of asbestiform and nonasbestiform fibers, including fibrous glass and various fibrous clays, such as attapulgite and sepiolite.[31] It became apparent that carcinogenicity was related to the dimensional distribution of those fibers which were longer than 8 μm and of a width less than 0.25 μm. Stanton et al. also reported on further studies in rats in which both asbestiform and nonasbestiform minerals were included in samples of talc that contained nonasbestiform tremolite.[31] Asbestiform tremolite induced tumors in virtually 100% of the treated rats, but nonasbestiform tremolite was noncarcinogenic. Additional studies yielding similar results have been carried out by various investigators.[32]

A thorough study of the toxicology and carcinogenesis of tremolite in animals was carried out by the United States Public Health Service National Toxicology Program.[33] The latter study included the administration of tremolite by various methods and, in particular, studies of the ingestion of tremolite. No tumors were found following the ingestion of talc.

When we turn from animal studies, there have been a number of investigations carried out among workers exposed to nonasbestiform amphibole minerals found in talc and other mineral deposits. Thus, McDonald et al. evaluated the mortality rate of gold miners exposed to cummingtonite-grunerite, the nonasbestiform analogue of amosite.[34] Although there were more deaths caused by pneumoconiosis and tuberculosis than expected, no such trend was seen for cancers of the respiratory system. Brown et al. studied gold miners who had worked underground in the same mine for at least 1 year and found similar results.[35] Cooper et al. studied taconite miners employed for at least 3 years and found no association between respiratory cancer and tenure of work or latency.[36]

Of paramount importance to the issue of the carcinogenicity of asbestos analogues are the studies on talc miners and millers in New York. A proportionate mortality study of talc workers was published by Kleinfeld et al. in 1967[14] and a further study on the same workers in 1974.[27] The study group consisted of all talc workers employed in 1940 with 15 or more years of exposure. There were 108 deaths, including 12 attributed to lung cancer, one to fibrosarcoma of the pleura (possibly a mesothelioma), and one to peritoneal mesothelioma. The proportionate mortality rate for respiratory cancer was 12% compared with the 3% expected. Excess deaths appeared, however, only in the 60- to 79-year-old age group and mainly for the period before 1945 to 1969. There were, however, no adequate necropsy data; smoking and work histories were inadequate or rudimentary at best; and environmental information was lacking.

Brown et al. conducted a retrospective mortality study of 398 workers in one New York talc mine and mill from which bulk samples contained 30% to 60% nonasbestiform tremolite and 5% to 15% nonasbestiform anthophyllite.[37] The main findings were nine deaths caused by lung cancer (standardized mortality rate [SMR], 270). Here again, no smoking histories were available, and five of the nine workers who died of lung cancer had been employed for 1 year or less.

The best designed and most important study was that of Gamble, who updated the original cohort of talc workers from upstate New York. His analysis[38] added 8 more years of follow-up to the study of Brown et al.,[37] an exposure latency analysis, and a nested case-control study to account for possible confounding factors by smoking and other occupational exposures. The case-control study focused on 22 cases of lung cancer, each matched with three controls on birth and date of hire. When the data were stratified by smoking, the odds ratio decreased with tenure. No relationship was seen between death from lung cancer and length of talc employment. Numerous other studies have been carried out, some of which were reviewed in some detail in an editorial entitled, ''On talc, tremolite, and tergiversation.''[16]

Most of the evidence at the present time suggests that there is no increased risk either of lung cancer or of mesothelioma in workers exposed to talc, providing there is no evidence of contamination by asbestiform tremolite, actinolite, or anthophyllite. The talc mined in Vermont, upstate New York, and most of the rest of the United States is free from contamination by asbestos.

There has been much argument about whether or not asbestiform and nonasbestiform tremolite can be distinguished with reasonable certainty by competent geologists and mineralogists. The American Thoracic Society issued a statement which suggested the distinction cannot be made reliably,[39] and their viewpoint was endorsed by Case[40] but subsequently rebutted.[41]

Finally, the most compelling argument against talc being a carcinogen is related to the fact that, of 210 patients who underwent a talc-induced pleurodesis, there was no increased incidence of lung cancer and not a single mesothelioma.[42]

KAOLIN (CHINA CLAY)

Kaolin is an aluminum silicate derived from igneous feldspar rocks by weathering or by sedimentation. The main constituent of china clay is kaolinite, the composition of which is $Al_2Si_2O_5(OH)_4$. Kaolinite occurs as microscopic leaf- or plate-like crystals with small quantities of quartz, iron, and titanium as contaminants.[43] In conditions of intense weathering, small amounts of iron enter into the crystalline structure. Halloysite (hydrated kaolinite) has a tubular lattice and expands after saturation with ethylene glycol.

Kaolin deposits are frequently found in sedimentary rocks and may be highly concentrated, as in Georgia. Under such circumstances, the mineral is often found in association with other phyllosilicates, such as mica and smectite (montmorillonite). Georgia china clay contains around 85% to 95% kaolinite, with very little free silica. In contrast, the Cornish china clay deposits found around St. Austell contain between 10% and 40% of kaolinite with a residue of quartz, mica, and feldspar.

In Georgia, the raw kaolin is removed from deposits by strip mining and is further processed by a wet or dry method.[44] In the former, clay is dispersed in an aqueous medium, and sand and other gross contaminants are removed by differential sedimentation. At the processing plant, the clay is classified by its size, and excess water is removed by vacuum infiltration and spray drying before the kaolin is shipped to end users as a rehydrated slurry or as dry clay. With dry or air-flow processing, the clay is dried and pulverized, and sand and gross contaminants are removed by differential air flotation. Processed Georgia kaolin has a particle size less than 10 μm. With filler clays, 50% of particles are less than 2 μm. In the finest grades of kaolin, 90% or more of particles are less than 2 μm. For certain purposes, processed china clay is calcined. This involves the removal of the water of hydration by heating to approximately 1000°C for 20 minutes or so. Calcined china clay contains alumina and silica in a leaf-like amorphous noncrystalline configuration that maintains the particle structure of hydrated kaolin. Workers whose jobs involve drying, bagging, and loading of the clay are exposed to the highest levels of respirable kaolin dust.

Cornish kaolin is mined from open pits by directing highly pressurized water jets onto the walls of the pit.[45, 46] Subsequently, the slurry is subjected to differential sedimentation so that any contaminants, such as grit, mica, and sand, are removed while the kaolin remains suspended. The water slurry is then removed by filter presses or by siphoning. The residue of kaolin is then transferred to drying kilns. From there, it is moved to storage hoppers on a conveyor belt where it is dried, usually by spray drying. The kaolin now contains only about 10% moisture. It is then bagged mechanically or loaded into railway trucks for transportation. Some residual quartz often persists in Cornish kaolin.

Some 40 countries produce in excess of 25 million tons/year of kaolin. The United States produces 7 million and the United Kingdom, 3 million. When refined, kaolin is used as a functional mineral filler in paper, plastics, rubber, ceramics, and in other industries.[47] The less pure product is used in ceramic bodies in which the nonkaolin content is important and in building materials, such as bricks and cement. An increasing amount of calcined kaolin is used in industry to whiten writing and other paper. Aside from the United States and Great Britain, kaolin is mined in Brazil, Spain, and Germany, and, to a lesser extent, in Canada and Australia.

Kaolin clays are divided into fire, flint, and ball and plastic clays. These contain varying amounts of kaolin, which contribute to the desired properties of the particular clay. Those with a fusion point about 1420°C are used as fire clays. Halloysite is a rare mineral which is related to kaolin and occurs in tubular form, owing to the curvature of the crystal lattice. It is mined commercially in Japan, South Korea, New Zealand, and in the western United States. The largest deposit is found in Matauri Bay, New Zealand. It is used in the manufacture of high-quality porcelain and bone china.

Kaolin Pneumoconiosis or Kaolinosis

Pneumoconiosis induced by exposure to china clay was first described in Cornish china clay workers in 1936.[48] A number of additional reports from the

British, North American, and Egyptian kaolin industries[49–55] have since been published. Most have involved relatively few subjects. The radiological and pathological features have been described.[50, 56, 57] Correlation of the incidence of pneumoconiosis with industrial hygiene measurements has, for the most part, been lacking.

As with most other pneumoconioses, the prevalence of kaolinosis is closely related to the duration of exposure and the dustiness of the job.[44, 52, 54, 55] The prevalence of radiographic abnormalities varies according to the series described, with a greater rate being present in workers in their 50s and 60s.[58] Both simple and complicated forms of kaolinosis occur.[44, 54, 55] As in silicosis and coal workers' pneumoconiosis, there usually needs to be a significant background of simple pneumoconiosis before the onset of the complicated form of the disease.[44, 58] Early changes of kaolin pneumoconiosis usually occur in the upper zones. Bulk loading, bagging, and kaolin preparation are the most dusty jobs, and workers in these jobs have the greatest prevalence of this condition.[44, 53] Dry processing is associated with a greater rate of pneumoconiosis than is wet processing.

For the most part, the radiographic opacities in Georgian kaolin workers are rounded and, as mentioned, usually develop first in the upper zones.[44, 50, 56] The opacities are usually of the q and r type and are less well defined than those that occur in silicosis or in coal workers' pneumoconiosis (Figs. 13–7 to 13–10). In a few instances, larger irregular opacities of the u type may be observed. In Cornish china clay workers, however, nodular opacities of the q and r type were usually associated with a high quartz content in the inhaled dust.[46, 57] Many of the men in whom radiographic appearances suggesting nodular fibrosis developed had worked with china stone, and their lungs were found to have a high quartz content.[46, 57] In

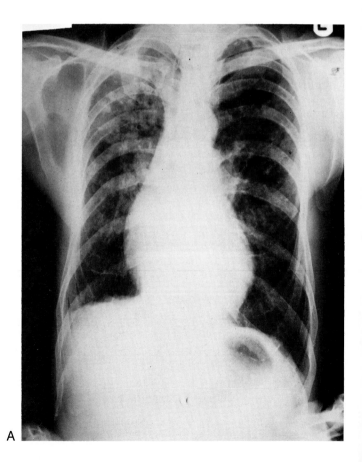

Figure 13–7

A, Chest radiograph of a Cornish china clay worker. His only industrial exposure, over 30 years, had been to china clay. He died of cor pulmonale. Radiograph shows pneumoconiosis with p and q type opacities and conglomerative changes in the right upper lobe with loss of volume in the right lung.

A

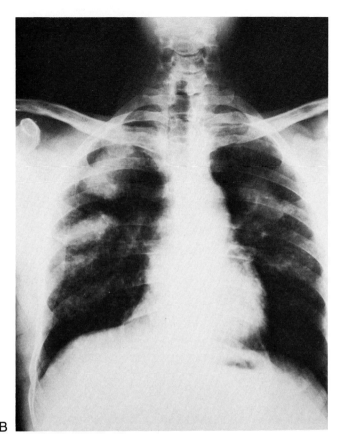

Figure 13–7 *Continued*
B, Conglomerate kaolinosis in a Georgian kaolin worker.

B

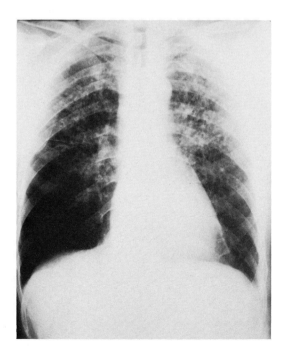

Figure 13–8
Simple kaolinosis in a bagger (category 2/3, mixture of r and u opacities).

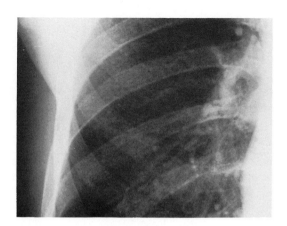

Figure 13–9
Simple kaolinosis. Magnified view
of mixture of p and q opacities (bulk
loader).

those who worked with relatively pure kaolinite, interstitial fibrosis was observed.
The pathological appearances were stated to correlate with the radiologic appearances. However, smoking histories were lacking, and it is well accepted that
cigarette smoking may induce irregular opacities in chest radiographs.[59]

A later study by Ogle et al. indicated that the improvement in dust control
lessened the likelihood of the development of pneumoconiosis and indicated that

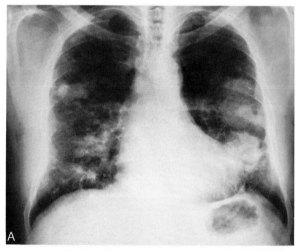

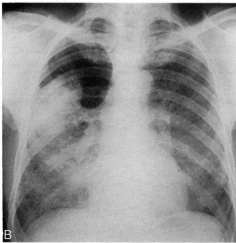

Figure 13–10
A, Large opacities in a Georgia kaolin worker.
Background of r opacities. Also has chronic airflow
limitation and emphysema. B, Complicated kaolinosis,
stage B, on a background of p-type opacities (category
3/3). There is a large emphysematous bulla in the right
upper lobe. This region has been spared, and no
opacities are present.

the incidence of pneumoconiosis as of 1971 was about one half what it was before that date.[58] The study also showed that the milling of china stone, a practice that ceased about 18 to 20 years ago, had the largest effect on the induction of radiographic abnormalities. Large opacities tend to be well delineated and occur in the upper, middle, and lower zones, although they seem marginally more common in the upper zones.[58] As the large opacities increase in size, they have a tendency to migrate toward the hila and lead to the development of compensatory emphysema in the adjacent lung parenchyma.

Lung Function

The first controlled epidemiological study was carried out by Oldham in the China clay industry of Cornwall.[54] Evidence of pneumoconiosis was found in 23% of workers, of whom 1.1% had a large shadow indicating complicated pneumoconiosis. An increasing category of pneumoconiosis was associated with a significant but small reduction in the FVC. The effect on the FVC was relatively mild and, in the case of the FEV_1, was barely evident. To use Oldham's words, "the loss of FEV_1, even if present, is of trivial magnitude."[54] In this regard, it must be remembered that an appreciable number of the Cornish china clay workers have been exposed to a significant concentration of silica. It might be inferred that the minor reduction in the FVC noted by Oldham was more likely a consequence of silica than of kaolin exposure.

Subsequently, Kennedy et al. studied a group of 459 Georgia kaolin workers and found that, for the most part, the workers with radiographic evidence of pneumoconiosis had a similar ventilatory capacity to that of workers with normal radiographs.[53] Clinical impairment of pulmonary function did not occur, except in advanced cases. At about the same time, Sepulveda et al. examined both active and retired workers and combined the groups for the purpose of the analysis.[60] The design of the study was flawed in that many of the ex-workers had been referred by the union and were selectively recruited.[61]

A large study of more than 2000 kaolin workers from East and Central Georgia was carried out later.[44] The workers were selected according to standard epidemiological principles, and the ventilatory capacity, radiographic findings, job, and type of impairment were investigated. Participation in this study was excellent, and the criteria for acceptability were measurements of the FEV_1 and FVC of 99% and 98%, respectively. The investigation confirmed that ventilatory impairment was related to the presence of complicated pneumoconiosis, the calcining of clay, and pre-eminently, to cigarette smoking. Those with simple pneumoconiosis had a ventilatory capacity which was similar to that of other nondust-exposed workers in the kaolin industry. In those working in the calcining of clay, there was an increased prevalence of abnormality of the FEV_1 but not the FVC compared with those of both wet and dry processors. The difference could not be explained by either cigarette smoking or the presence of pneumoconiosis. The magnitude of abnormality in the calcined clay workers was, however, unlikely to lead to disabling impairment. In workers with more than 3 years of tenure, there were 90 subjects with simple pneumoconiosis, and 18 with complicated pneumoconiosis, yielding an adjusted prevalence of 3.2% and 0.6%, respectively, in the sample examined. Dry processing was associated with a greater risk of developing pneumoconiosis than wet processing.

A later publication by Ogle et al. showed that, in china clay workers from Cornwall, the rate of decline in ventilatory capacity was related to the radiographic category and age.[58] However, the decline attributed to the change of radiographic category was relatively minor and appreciably less than that caused by cigarette smoking. Here again, some of the workers had been exposed to china stone, and the decline in ventilatory capacity may have been a silica effect. Variations in the lung function and the prevalence of kaolinosis have been noted in different plants, but neither their significance nor cause has been explained.[62]

Pathological Findings

An excellent review of the pathological effects of inhalation of kaolin in Cornish china clay workers has been published by Gibbs.[46] As mentioned earlier, many of these men had been exposed to china stone and kaolinite. The mineral dust analyses and exposure data suggested that separate responses occurred in the lung.[46, 57] As a result, it was possible to divide the subjects into three groups. The first consisted of the china clay group. In these subjects, the constituent of the lung showed (1) a kaolinite content greater than 90%, (2) a quartz content less than 1.1%, and (3) a feldspar content greater than 1%. The second group was the china clay and china stone group. In these subjects, the constituents of the lung showed (1) a kaolinite content less than 90%, (2) a quartz content greater than 0.9%, and (3) a feldspar content greater than 0.9%. In the third miscellaneous group, the lung dust did not conform to that in either of the first two groups.

Kaolin macules were found only in those working in the drying and loading areas. Most lesions were 2 to 3 mm in diameter but, occasionally, a little larger. They were of a grayish color (Figs. 13–11 and 13–12). Some were palpable, but others were not. Massive lesions measuring several centimeters in width were found predominantly in the upper zones of the lung. On gross examination, the massive lesions were fairly firm and had the consistency of putty. Occasionally, cavitation was present. In a few instances, there was interstitial involvement and honeycombing.

Microscopically, the early macules were located around the respiratory bronchioles. They consisted mainly of macrophages containing particulate brown matter. As the lesions increased in size, the macrophages infiltrated the lung interstitium and migrated along the alveolar walls. In some areas, the lesions aggregated, giving an appearance of linear fibrosis or stranding, but extensive fibrosis was uncommon. Most such macules showed only limited fine fibrosis (Fig. 13–13). A few larger macules showed a collagenous center surrounded by heavily dust-laden macrophages, many of which lined the alveolar walls. In the conglomerate large shadows, there was an irregular laying down of collagenous fibers, most of which were heavily admixed with large numbers of dust-laden macrophages. Many particles exhibited birefringence. The small vessels adjacent to the massive lesions often showed infiltration of their walls with macrophages, chronic inflammatory cells, and fine fibrosis. Cavitation appeared to be due to ischemic necrosis. Scanty ferruginous bodies were noted to be present and appeared to develop in leaf- or plate-like particulate matter.

An *in vitro* study of kaolin dust on mouse peritoneal macrophages showed that kaolinite was cytotoxic. The cytotoxicity was not related to particle morphology but appeared to be related to a silica-rich gel that coated the particle.[63]

Summary

The evidence suggests that kaolinite, in the absence of free silica, can induce a pneumoconiosis. This can be of the simple or complicated form. It is clear, however, that kaolin is far less fibrogenic than is quartz, and simple kaolinosis is not associated with significant ventilatory impairment. With better industrial hygiene, the incidence and prevalence of kaolin-induced pneumoconiosis has been declining rapidly.

FULLER'S EARTH

To full is to scour or beat, and this is a term usually applied to the finishing and thickening of woolens. Hence, a fuller is one who scours or fulls cloth or woolens. Fuller's earth was originally used in the cleaning and roughening of the surface of woolens to absorb any grease or oil that might be present. Unfortunately, the term is used differently in various parts of the world.

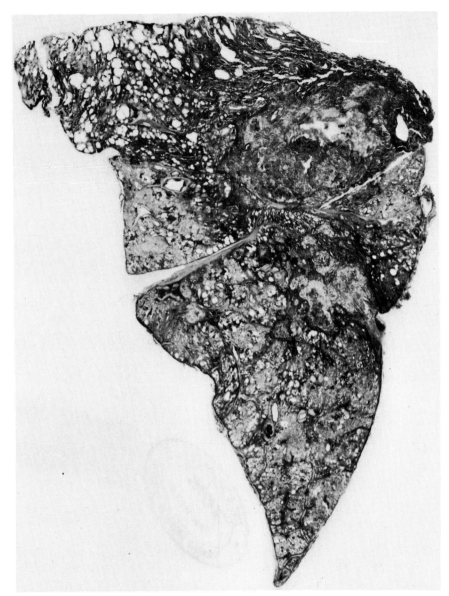

Figure 13–11. Whole-lung (Gough) section from a Cornish china clay worker showing massive fibrosis in posterior part of upper lobe and large nodules throughout the rest of the lung. Interstitial fibrosis and cystic change are present in the upper lobe.

The best fulling clays are composed mainly of montmorillonite, a mineral which contains loosely bound cations of either calcium or sodium.[47] Calcium montmorillonite is generally called fuller's earth in Europe, and sodium montmorillonite is known as bentonite. Large deposits of calcium montmorillonite are found in Surrey, in Bedfordshire, and near Bath in England. There are also some deposits in Illinois in the United States. Sodium montmorillonite originates from volcanic ash, is highly plastic, and often contains a high proportion of free silica. It is mined in the western part of the United States.

Montmorillonite has three important physicochemical properties. First, the extremely small, flexible, and leaf-like crystals provide a large surface area. Second, a negative excess electrical charge leads to the presence of exchangeable cations between the aluminosilicate layers of the mineral's structure. Third, it has the

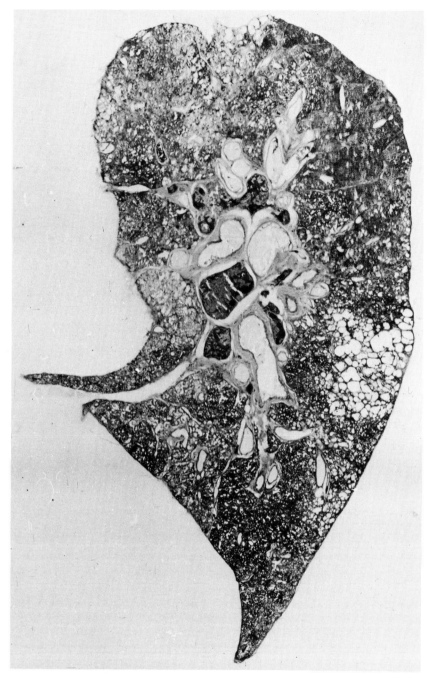

Figure 13–12. Whole-lung (Gough) section from Cornish china clay worker showing diffuse interstitial fibrosis and some cystic areas, most marked in posterior part of lower lobe.

intracrystalline capacity to swell and expand.[47] Calcium montmorillonite, when it absorbs water, increases its volume to a limited extent. In contrast, bentonite swells to several times its original volume.

In the United States, palygorskite, attapulgite, and sepiolite are also often referred to as fuller's earth since they have similar absorbent properties.

In the description of the disease known as fuller's earth pneumoconiosis, we are referring only to a condition produced by calcium montmorillonite. Sodium

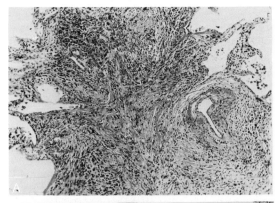

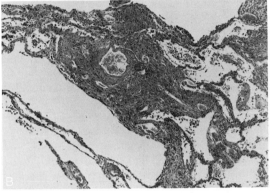

Figure 13-13
A, Lower power magnification. Nodular lesion containing numerous dust-laden macrophages around respiratory bronchioles and vessels. Fibrosis is present predominantly located centrally. B, Higher power magnification. Dust-laden macrophages arranged in a granulomatous nodular pattern in interstitium and around blood vessels. Interstitial fibrosis is present.

montmorillonite will be dealt with later, and the other clays will be treated separately.

Fuller's Earth Pneumoconiosis

Middleton originally drew attention to the occurrence of radiographic changes in workers exposed to fuller's earth in 1940.[64] Subsequently, McNally and Trostler studied the radiographs of 49 men engaged in the production and loading of the material and found an increase in the bronchovascular markings in most.[65] Two had advanced massive fibrosis and were unable to work because of shortness of breath. Unfortunately, no postmortem examinations were available.

It is evident that, like kaolin, fuller's earth is much less fibrogenic than free silica. However, heavy exposure, such as occurs in bagging and loading areas, may eventually produce pneumoconiosis, with radiographic changes similar to those seen in coal workers' pneumoconiosis and silicosis. In Illinois, it is likely that quartz plays some role in the induction of these radiographic alterations. In addition, this is probably the case in a small group of workers from Germany who were noted to have similar changes.[66]

The pathological findings of fuller's earth pneumoconiosis were described originally by Campbell and Gloyne in 1942.[67] They found irregular, black, soft patches located mainly in the upper lobes. Later, Tonning described a 79-year-old man who died of a stroke and who had fuller's earth pneumoconiosis.[68] Microscopically, the air spaces contained many dust particles surrounded by reticulin, although there was relatively little cellular reaction. His lungs likewise showed multiple black nodules, consisting of dust-laden macrophages surrounded by reticulin with some surrounding focal emphysema but little in the way of collagen formation. Foreign body giant cells were absent, and the smaller lesions tended to resemble those seen in kaolin pneumoconiosis. More recently, Sakula investigated fuller's earth workers and found two subjects with the radiographic changes of simple pneumoconiosis.[69] In one, an autopsy showed similar features to those described earlier. The lungs showed multiple birefringent crystals when examined with polarized light. X-ray and electron diffraction studies of Sakula's subjects showed the characteristic mineralogic patterns of montmorillonite but no significant quartz.

MICA

The micas are a group of industrial minerals that are used in the manufacture of plastics, in drilling, and in special paints.[47] Muscovite is the most commonly used mica. Phlogopite-biotite is darker and finds its use as a filler. Vermiculite is also a mica but will be dealt with separately. Since the micas are fire resistant, they are finding increasing use as fire retardants.

A strictly limited number of subjects with mica pneumoconiosis have been reported. Ferguson, in an unpublished article, which was quoted by Middleton in 1936, reported radiographic changes in 5 of 12 workers.[48] In 1985, Skulberg et al. could find only 66 cases of mica pneumoconiosis and concluded that, of that 66, only 26 could be attributed directly to the inhalation of mica alone.[70] Contamination by other minerals, in particular particles of quartz, was frequent.

A solitary case of mica pneumoconiosis was described by Pimentel and Menezes in 1978.[71] These authors claimed that the patient was exposed to pure mica. She developed severe restrictive impairment, and multiple granulomata were found in her lungs. Davies and Cotton have since described two subjects with disabling pneumoconiosis which occurred in a plant that processed muscovite.[72]

Three epidemiological studies have been carried out in mica workers. Two of the groups who were studied had been exposed to relatively pure mica.[73, 74] The third group was exposed to mica that was fairly heavily contaminated with crystalline silica.[75]

The first published study was that of Dreesen et al. who studied 109 subjects in North Carolina who were working with sheet mica.[73] They found that 1% had radiographic evidence of pneumoconiosis. A further 57 subjects who worked with ground mica dust were included, and 18% had pneumoconiosis. Most of the latter group had been exposed to more than 10 mppcf. In a second epidemiological study, Vestal et al. studied 79 subjects who were grinding and milling mica and found an 11% prevalence of pneumoconiosis.[74] These subjects also came from North Carolina. Later, Heimann et al. studied workers in Bihar, India and found more than 44 had radiographic abnormalities.[75] The hard mica which they were mining was thought to be heavily contaminated by quartz. Elsewhere, Li Weizu found no subjects with mica-induced pneumoconiosis in a survey of 302 Chinese mica workers[76] (quoted by Skulberg et al.[70]).

The radiographic appearances of mica-induced pneumoconiosis are a mixture of fine nodulation and linear shadows.[70, 72] Landas and Schwartz described a recent patient with mica pneumoconiosis who underwent high-resolution computed tomographic scanning. Diffuse fibrosis and focal honeycombing were noted.[77] Energy dispersive specroscopy analysis and electron diffraction studies confirmed the presence of mica. Pleural thickening has also been reported in workers exposed to mica.[78] Lung function tests show restrictive impairment and a reduction in the diffusing capacity.[70, 72, 77]

Gibbs recently published an excellent description of the pathological changes found in mica pneumoconiosis.[46] Microscopically, the lungs show the presence of gray, soft stellate lesions varying between 1 and 2 mm in size. Massive lesions also occur and likewise are gray. They are also softer than the massive fibrosis of silicosis. A fine interstitial fibrosis is often noted in the simple form of mica pneumoconiosis.

The earliest changes are noted along the walls of the respiratory bronchioles where dust-laden macrophages accumulate. Later, the macrophages extend along the wall of the alveolar ducts and the walls of the adjacent alveoli. Doubly refractile particles are extremely common. Ferruginous bodies have also been noted by Gibbs,[46] but others have not reported them. The ferruginous bodies develop on the plate-like particles of mica. Randomly oriented collagen is usually present in the massive lesions along with large quantities of dust.

A single case of a mica worker in whom peritoneal mesothelioma developed has been reported.[79] The clinical significance of a solitary case report such as this must remain dubious.

In summary, mica can induce both simple and complicated pneumoconioses. Both forms are associated with restrictive impairment and a diffusing capacity. However, the condition appears to be extremely uncommon.

VERMICULITE

Vermiculite is an alteration product of biotite (phlogopite mica), of which there are relatively limited deposits.[47] The term *vermiculite* is derived from the Latin *vermis*, or worm, and relates to the mineral's physical appearance. The major producers of vermiculite are South Africa and the United States, but Australia, Argentina, Brazil, and Malawi also have limited deposits that are mined. When heated to around 800°C, vermiculite expands to many times its original volume. At this temperature, the mineral exfoliates in a concertina-like fashion as a result of water escaping from the crystal lattice that prises the layers apart at right angles to the mineral's cleavage.[47]

After exfoliation, vermiculite is fire resistant and an effective insulator of low density. It also has uses in agriculture as a soil filler. In some instances, the natural deposits of vermiculite are contaminated by asbestiform tremolite and actinolite. Dust exposure occurs during mining, processing, bagging, and loading of the mineral. End users are also sometimes exposed and at risk.

Exposure to vermiculite dust probably does not lead to a pneumoconiosis; however, a significant number of subjects show the presence of small irregular opacities.[80, 81] These are usually relative scanty, and it is unusual to find a category above 1/1. Pleural thickening, both circumscribed and diffuse, had been reported to occur in workers exposed to vermiculite.[80] One study of both past and present Montana vermiculite miners found a prevalence rate of irregular opacities of 18.4%. The greatest prevalence was noted in the most exposed workers.[81] For pleural thickening, a prevalence rate of 28% was found; however, a rate of 8.5% was found in the radiographs of the nonexposed group (47 subjects) of whom 2.7% showed calcification. Lockey et al. studied end users and found 12 subjects who had a benign pleural effusion.[82]

A later study carried out by McDonald et al. involved 194 vermiculite miners from South Carolina.[83] Only a few subjects had irregular opacities. The examination of the sputum of those workers included in this group who had a productive cough showed a few specimens contained typical ferruginous bodies. Contamination of the South Carolina vermiculite with tremolite occurred but in very low concentrations, unlike that of the Montana deposits.

A study of a peculiar type of vermiculite found only in South Africa has recently been published.[84] A geological anomaly known as the Loolekop volcanic pipe is located about 260 miles northeast of Johannesburg in South Africa where there are two large open cast mines which produce around 20,000 tons of Palabora vermiculite each year. The mill dust of this vermiculite is said not to contain amphiboles, but scanty amphiboles have been found in the freshly mined product. A cross-sectional morbidity study showed no excess of symptoms in the Palabora miners compared with that in the control group. Significant radiographic abnormalities did not occur more frequently than in the reference population. The lungs of three deceased Palabora vermiculite miners showed scanty ferruginous bodies but no fibrosis. The core of the bodies was composed of crocidolite.

Mortality Studies

Three well-conducted studies of the respiratory mortality rate of vermiculite miners have been published.[83, 85, 86] In the Montana miners, where significant contamination of the vermiculite deposits by tremolite and actinolite occurred, the SMRs from malignant respiratory disease and also from nonmalignant respiratory disease were significantly elevated and were directly related to cumulative fiber exposure. In Enoree, South Carolina, no excess deaths were noted from respiratory malignancy or from nonmalignant respiratory causes.[83] Four mesothelioma cases occurred in the Montanan miners: three were pleural and one was peritoneal.[86]

In summary, it would seem that vermiculite, in itself, is not harmful, but since it is frequently contaminated with amphiboles, in those workers most exposed, there is an increased risk of lung cancer and mesothelioma.

FIBROUS SILICATES, INCLUDING PHYLLOSILICATES

A number of ''fibrous'' silicates are used commercially. Of these, the most important are the various forms of asbestos. Whether the term *fibrous silicates* should be applied to the clays is a moot point, and is discussed in Chapter 14. Other asbestiform fibers, i.e., tremolite, actinolite, and anthophyllite, while not commercially mined, may contaminate various commercially used minerals, such as mica and vermiculite. They have been dealt with earlier in this chapter. The nonasbestiform variants of chrysotile, amosite, and crocidolite have been described earlier, and the distinction between the asbestiform and the nonasbestiform forms of these minerals has been stressed. Although fulfilling the OSHA criteria for a fiber, at least as far as the aspect ratio is concerned, the nonasbestiform counterparts are usually not regarded as fibers by most mineralogists.

Attapulgite and Palygorskite

Attapulgite and palygorskite are often used synonymously. Although this is mainly correct as far as the chemical composition is concerned, it is incorrect when it comes to the physical structure of these two fibrous clays.[47] Both are silicates, with silicon and magnesium as the dominant cations. Lesser amounts of calcium, potassium, aluminum, and iron are present in variable amounts. Palygorskite may contain up to 15% aluminum. In general, attapulgite fibers from Georgia and Florida deposits are mostly less than 2 μm in length and are much shorter than the fibers of palygorskite, which are often longer than 5 μm.[87]

Attapulgite is mined mainly in northern Florida and southern Georgia, but deposits of attapulgite are found in Spain, Australia, South Africa, and Senegal.[47, 88] Attapulgite and palygorskite differ structurally from the nonfibrous silicates in that they are chain-type silicates and not layered. It is this structure that gives rise to their fine fibrous nature. Up to 1 million tonnes of attapulgite are mined annually. It is used in coatings, drilling muds, and cat litter and has similar uses to fuller's earth.

Published studies of humans exposed to attapulgite are uncommon. One case report of lung fibrosis was described in a 40-year-old engineer who was exposed to French attapulgite during processing operations.[89] Numerous attapulgite fibers were found in the alveolar lavage fluid (42,000/ml), but the patient may have had fibrosing alveolitis. The presence of the fibers may have been unrelated to his disease. Subsequently, Gamble et al. (1988) studied 785 attapulgite workers from two companies located in Georgia and Florida.[90] There was no significant association between attapulgite exposure and respiratory symptoms. They observed a statistically nonsignificant decrease of ventilatory capacity with increasing exposure. Small irregular opacities were noted in the radiographs of 6.4% of the subjects and increased with age and exposure. Most occurred in subjects who had worked for 15 or more years. The median ages of those employed in the two companies were 38.1 and 38.8 years, and prolonged exposure was uncommon. The methods used in the studies of the two companies were slightly different, and some of the disparate findings may have arisen from divergent methods.

Waxweiler et al. conducted a retrospective cohort mortality study among 2302 male workers who had been employed in one major American attapulgite mining and milling company.[91] They included workers who had been employed for at least 1 month between 1940 and 1975. A statistically significant excess of lung cancer was observed among whites but not among nonwhites. A dose-response relationship was noted among both the whites and the nonwhites exposed to high dust levels for more than 5 years. However, no account was taken of smoking habits. It must be remembered, however, that whites smoke significantly more cigarettes in this part of the world than do blacks, and this has been previously observed in Georgia kaolin workers.[44] One of the companies whose employees were studied owned both kaolin mines and an attapulgite mine. In some instances, men were transferred from the attapulgite to the kaolin mine and *vice versa*. In addition, there were a small number of deaths, i.e., 315, and there were many missing death certificates. Moreover, death rates were compared with the general population in the United States as a whole rather than with state or county death rates for Georgia and Florida. Animal experiments have shown attapulgite to be less fibrogenic than asbestos.[92]

Sepiolite

Sepiolite is a fibrous mineral that is a hydrated magnesium silicate closely related to meerschaum, and is a clay that is composed of elongated parallel fibers which are used for many of the same purposes as bentonite.[47] It has additional uses as a clarifying agent, in the manufacture of filters, as an absorbent, as a carrier for pesticides, and as an agent for suspension mixtures. It is more stable at higher temperatures than is attapulgite and can absorb 2.5 times its weight in water. It is the latter property that makes it useful in pet litters.

Sepiolite is mined in Spain, the United States, Turkey, France, Madagascar, Japan, China, and sundry other countries. The first three countries produce 90% of the world's production.

Present epidemiological data relating to occupational exposures to sepiolite are inadequate, and it is not known whether sepiolite can cause pneumoconiosis or respiratory symptoms. Similarly insufficient data are available to give a reliable opinion as to its carcinogenicity. Animal inhalation experiments with sepiolite showed granuloma formation but no tumors.[87] Nevertheless, it has been shown that the long fibers of sepiolite can induce malignant tumors following intrapleural or intraperitoneal inoculation.[93]

Nonoccupational exposure in humans results mainly from exposure to pet litters and from the inclusion of sepiolite in drugs. Some concern has been expressed about the health-related risks resulting from the inhalation and ingestion of sepiolite, but no definite risk has been noted. The aspect ratio of the fibers seems to be of prime importance when it comes to the development of tumors in animals.

One cross-sectional study of 218 Spanish sepiolite workers did not find any relationship between the duration of exposure and the prevalence of radiographic abnormalities. There was a relationship between the prevalence of small opacities and the workplace exposure; however, this was less than what was observed with age. No excess deaths from lung cancer were reported in these sepiolite workers.[94]

Further investigations of this cohort were carried out to ascertain the effects on the ventilatory capacity of exposure to sepiolite dust.[94a] After an allowance for smoking was made, it was shown that the workers most exposed to dry dust showed a significantly greater decline in FEV_1 than did those with less exposure. The FVC was similarly affected. There was, however, no evidence of any accompanying radiographic change in those who were most exposed to dust.

OTHER CLAYS

Shale

The shales split readily into laminae and consist of the arenaceous (sandy) shales, carbonaceous shales associated with coal deposits, and oil or bituminous shales. All contain various percentages of quartz. Pneumoconiosis has been described in Scottish shale miners.[95] This industry, once an important producer of mineral oil, has now closed down in Scotland. Shale oil was produced in France, and the industry survives in Estonia. A new industry with plans for massive oil production may come into existence in Colorado and the other mountain states. There are also large deposits of shale in Alberta, but whether this will be used commercially for the production of oil is debatable.

Scottish and Rocky Mountain shales differ. The former have a higher content of quartz and silicates, and the latter contain more limestone. In the Scottish subjects, radiological and pathological changes of both simple pneumoconiosis and massive fibrosis were described. The lesions resembled those of kaolin-induced pneumoconiosis (Figs. 13–14 to 13–16), but whether kaolin or other clay minerals in the shale are responsible for the induction of pneumoconiosis has not been established.

Two naturally occurring refined forms of bentonite are found: sodium bentonite and calcium bentonite.[47] Montmorillonite (sodium bentonite) is used in oil well drilling and in the manufacture of paper and chemicals. Calcium bentonite is often treated with organic acid to increase its surface area and to modify its properties. When treated with acids, it is changed into acid-activated montmorillonite. About

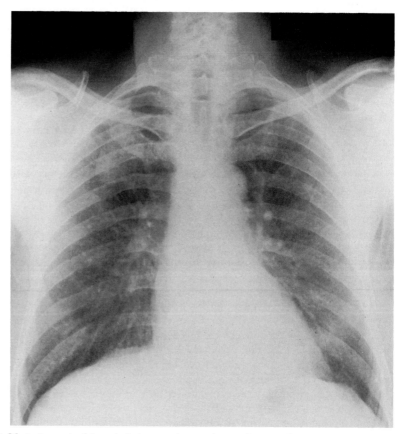

Figure 13–14. Radiograph of Scottish shale miner showing lesion of massive fibrosis in right upper zone.

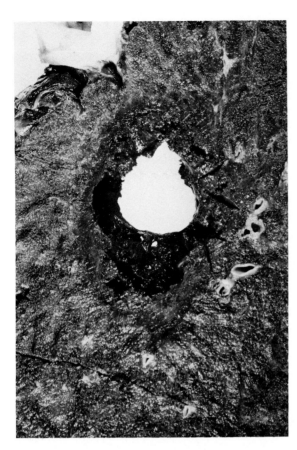

Figure 13–15
Resected right upper lobe from same patient as in Figure 13–14 showing cavitated massive fibrosis.

0.5 to 0.6 million tonne/year of acid-activated bentonite are produced. The products of acid-activated montmorillonite are used for the refining, decolorization, and purification of vegetable oils; the refining of sulfur; and as catalysts in the production of insecticides and fungicides.

Bentonite clay is formed from the deposition of airborne volcanic ash which is refined by sea and ground water. Virtually all deposits contain some impurities, including kaolin, cristobalite, and other forms of free silica. Mining is carried out by the open cast method, and the clay is then crushed and milled. Subsequently, the clay is dried in cylindrical barrels. A significant quantity of free silica is found in the mill dust with high concentrations of cristobalite.[96] Some of the larger deposits are found in Wyoming.

When pneumoconiosis occurs in bentonite millers, it is not related to the inhalation of bentonite itself but to the inhalation of contaminants such as cristobalite and other free silicas. Bentonite itself appears to be nonfibrogenic, but it may produce scanty reticulin fibrosis.[97] It has also been reported to have mild toxicity *in vitro* but does not appear to be fibrogenic in animal experiments.[98]

MISCELLANEOUS SILICATES

Sillimanite

Sillimanite is an anhydrous aluminum silicate with the formula of $Al_2O_3SiO_2$ and is related to kyanite and andalusite. It is found in metamorphic rocks in an acicular whiskery form with interlaced and interlocked quartz and other minerals.

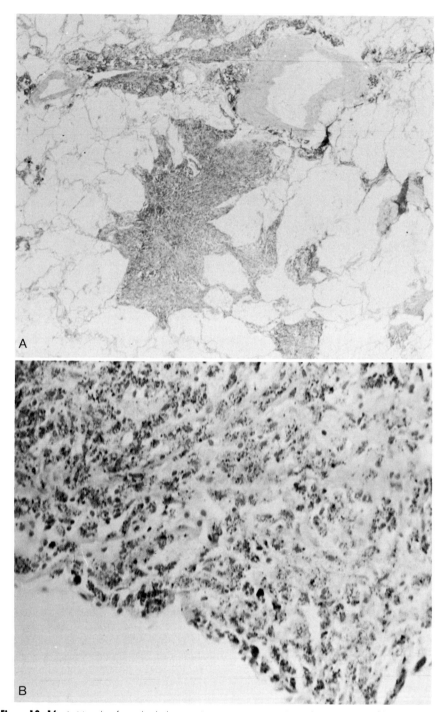

Figure 13–16. *A*, Macule of simple shale miner's pneumoconiosis. *B*, High-power view of lower part of same lesion showing dust-laden macrophages.

The mineral is resistant to heat and has low electrical conductivity. Thus, it is very valuable in the manufacture of high-grade refractories. It is also used in the manufacture of porcelain for laboratory ware, of spark plugs and thermocouples, and in alumina silica refractory bricks.

The ores are calcined at 1600°C and subsequently crushed and milled. The calcining and crushing processes are dusty. Some of the minerals are converted to

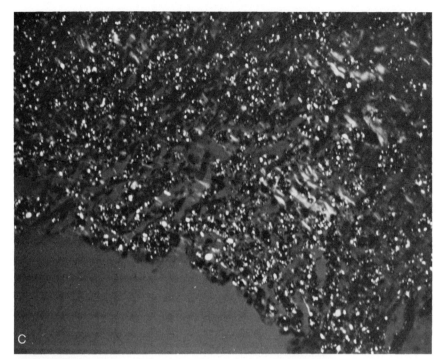

Figure 13–16 *Continued C,* Same area of macule viewed through polarized light showing doubly refractile silicate particles.

mullite, and the latter may occur in leaf-like or needle form. Middleton examined 13 workers in 1936 who had been exposed to sillimanite dust and noted minimal radiographic changes without accompanying symptoms.[48] Whether these changes were significant is not certain. There is some evidence that exposure to sillimanite may cause interstitial pulmonary fibrosis in exposed workers[99] and also in experimental animals,[100] but the possibility that contamination with cristobalite was responsible for the changes in humans must be kept in mind.

Nepheline

Nepheline is a hard rock consisting mainly of the feldspar albite. It is composed of sodium, potassium, and aluminum silicates and is mined in Canada. The rock is milled into a powder for use in glazing pottery. Deposits of nepheline are uncommon, and therefore, few workers are exposed to the dust. Nevertheless, there has been a report of one man who was heavily exposed for 4 years in whom massive fibrosis developed.[101] The dust to which he was exposed apparently contained no free silica, and the disease was attributed to nepheline. The radiographic features of two subjects from Ontario, Canada, with nepheline-induced pneumoconiosis are shown in Figure 13–17.

Mullite

Mullite is a crystalline aluminum silicate that may be found widely in nature or may be formed in various processes, such as the calcining of kaolin. A report was published of granulomatous pulmonary fibrosis in workers exposed to mullite in Australia, where alunite clays had previously been calcined to produce potash.[102] The residue was being reclaimed, because of its highly absorbent properties, as a cat litter. Three men working in very dusty conditions had radiologic evidence of interstitial lung disease, and a biopsy specimen in one showed a fibrosing granulomatous pneumonitis.

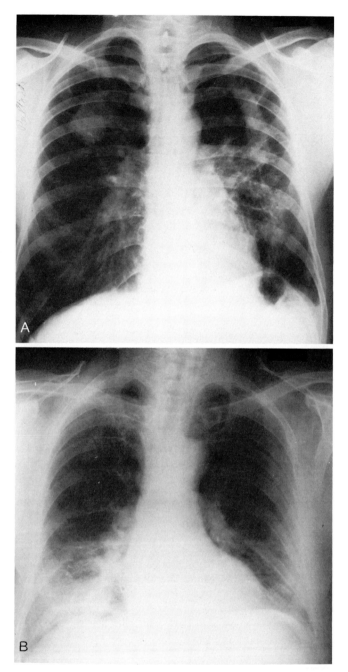

Figure 13–17
Two subjects with nepheline-induced pneumoconiosis, one showing typical complicated disease (A) and the other process appearing more like subacute silicosis (B). (Courtesy of Dr. D. L. Holness.)

Cummingtonite-Grunerite

Cummingtonite-grunerite is the nonasbestiform variant of amosite. The crystals cleave into fragments but have a different shape and properties from those of amosite fibers. The taconite deposits of iron ore situated around Lake Superior and those found in Norway are significantly contaminated by cummingtonite-grunerite, as also are the gold deposits found in the Homestake Mine in South Dakota. Taconite tailings that were produced by the Reserve Mining Company, which is situated in Minnesota near Duluth, used to be dumped into Lake Superior. Examination of the Duluth water supply revealed a fairly large number of these fibers were present. Initially, such fibers were regarded as asbestos, and the media made much of the fact that asbestos fibers were present in the Duluth water supply. Initial fears, engendered by irresponsible reporting of cummingtonite-grunerite not only in the water supply of Duluth but also in various beers and other commonly consumed beverages, eventually proved groundless.[103]

A number of morbidity and mortality studies of the Reserve mining workers have been carried out. None has shown any significant impairment or increased risk of respiratory cancer.[36, 104, 105] In addition, the Homestake miners have been studied on a number of occasions.[34, 35] The first complete study was carried out by McDonald et al. who showed that, although there was an increased SMR from tuberculosis and silicosis, there was no excessive risk of any form of respiratory cancer.[34] Other less well-designed studies purported to show an increased rate of lung cancer,[35] but as indicated, the methodology was inadequate. Some of these studies are discussed earlier in this chapter in the section devoted to talc.[16]

Animal studies have indicated cummingtonite-grunerite displays mild cytotoxic effects *in vitro*, but when fed to rats, no harm ensued.[106] No silicosis or increased rate of lung malignancy occurred, despite a high concentration of free silica present in the iron ore.

Wollastonite

Wollastonite consists of needle-like particles or fibers which are sufficiently long and thin to cause concern as to its possible carcinogenic effect. It also is an acicular chain silicate, with calcium as the predominant cation and is used in ceramics and insulating materials and as an abrasive. The mining and milling of the mineral is done in such a way as to limit the production of long fibers. However, wollastonite has also been used as a substitute for asbestos, and this has led to the use of ore deposits which often contain longer fibers.

Only a few epidemiological studies have been carried out in humans. One study done in Finland was reported to show small irregular opacities in 30% of their subjects and bilateral pleural thickening in 28%.[107] The reliability of the radiographic interpretations is open to question, and much of the so-called pleural thickening may turn out to have been pleural fat deposits. Moreover, in the Finnish study, magnified films were used for the detection of pneumoconiosis, and this is likely to lead to over-reading.

One hundred eight wollastonite workers employed at an open pit in New York State who mined relatively pure wollastonite were studied. No respiratory abnormalities were found, but a limited number of subjects had scanty rounded opacities on their radiographs.[108] The same workers were restudied in 1984.[109] There was the suggestion that the $FEV_1/FVC\%$ and peak flow declined slightly with cumulative exposure, but this may have been a nonspecific effect of dust. Some subjects who showed simple pneumoconiosis at the time of the first radiographic examination in 1976 had a repeat examination in 1982, and no progression was noted. In general, workers in the United States had less exposure than did the Finnish workers. No abnormalities were observed in the study group, no increased risk of lung cancer was found, and mesothelioma was not described.[110]

Pott et al. carried out experiments showing that the long-fiber wollastonite does not cause mesothelioma by injection or lung cancer by inhalation.[111] This may be related to the fact that wollastonite does not persist in the tissues, although no evidence for this is yet available. It would seem that, at this juncture, wollastonite is probably relatively innocuous, although in view of the fact that the mining methods have changed, studies of subjects using the newer methods of extraction are desirable.

Erionite

Erionite is a zeolite and has a fibrous configuration. It is a hydrated alumina silicate and, like perlite, has a common origin from volcanic activity. The zeolites are formed by hydrothermal degradation of volcanic glass. Their crystalline lattice structure makes them useful as molecular sieves, catalyst carriers, and ion-exchange media.

Zeolites can be synthesized to yield cubic crystals that are believed to be relatively innocuous. Natural deposits of zeolite often contain long or fibrous crystalline forms, which are coarse but likewise thought to be relatively harmless. In contrast, erionite often occurs in a relatively pure state and may present a hazard.

Erionite occurs in Oregon and Cappadocia, Asia Minor. Most of the fibers are more than 5 μm long and less than 0.1 μm in diameter. Macrophage culture tests suggest that these fibers have a penchant for inducing lung fibrosis. By the same token, intraperitoneal and intrapleural injection of erionite fibers lead to a high proportion of mesotheliomata in rats and other animals.[112]

Baris et al. described a number of villages in Cappadocia where there was a high incidence of mesothelioma.[113] In many subjects, the mesothelioma had been preceded by pleurisy and the development of circumscribed pleural thickening. It was first thought that asbestos might be responsible, but subsequent investigations showed that the subjects had no significant asbestos exposure. There was strong epidemiological evidence to incriminate erionite, and furthermore, the pathological findings suggested that erionite exposure was responsible. Many families use local rock in the building of houses. Erionite fibers were also present in the soil. In certain villages, neither pleural plaques nor pleurisy was reported. In these, it was found that the zeolites consisted of fibers which were coarser and thicker.[114]

The zeolite deposits found in Oregon have not been shown to induce either lung fibrosis or mesothelioma in humans, but they are located in an extremely sparsely populated area. Deposits of erionite are also found in New Zealand.

A few preliminary studies of the pathology of erionite suggests that the fibers survive almost indefinitely in lung tissue (Fig. 13–18). Malignant lymphoma has also been observed in mice following intraperitoneal injection of fibrous erionite. One study has shown that the number of helper/inducive T cells was significantly decreased among those with pleural fibrosis and acute pleurisy but not among those with pleural plaques only.[115] The significance of these findings is rather dubious.

Perlite

Perlite originates from volcanic eruptions and is a precursor of the zeolites. Its physical structure resembles small beads. The latter are composed of concentric onion-like layers of glass separated by water. When the glass beads are heated, they increase in volume but decrease in density, forming softer compressible pellets which are used as fillers in the construction industry and also to improve the quality of heavy soil. Prolonged exposure to perlite is not thought to be associated with radiographic changes. Some deposits of perlite are contaminated by fibrous zeolite, and the possibility must be considered that such exposures could lead to pleural plaques and, in addition, mesothelioma.[116]

MANMADE MINERAL FIBERS

Synthetic fibers have been produced and used commercially since the middle of the last century. The manner in which manmade mineral fibers (MMMF) are produced varies according to the required characteristics and properties of the fibers. MMMF can be classified according to their function and physical properties. They include insulation wool, continuous filaments, and fibers synthesized for a specific purpose. Insulating wool is produced from metal slag, igneous rock, and glass. The fibers are first melted and then spun down by rapid rotation which is induced by steam jets under high pressure. They are then interwoven and interspersed into fibrous mats. The fibers are then bound to the mat or other insulating material by the introduction of a resin. Insulation wool is used mainly for limiting

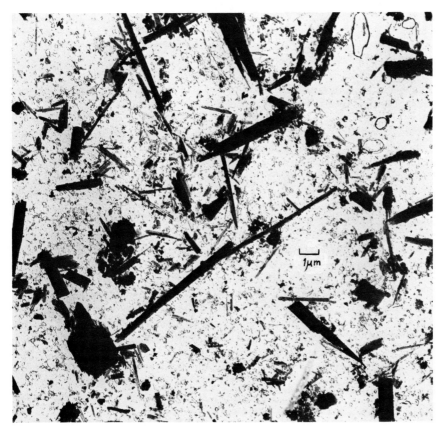

Figure 13–18. Electron microscopic view (× 9257) of erionite from Nevada, showing many fine fibrous particles.

thermal or acoustic stimuli. The fibers used in the manufacture of insulating wool vary in size, but some fibers are relatively thin with a diameter of less than 3 microns. Continuous-filament fiber is incorporated in fabrics and in insulation materials and as a means of rendering plastics and cements more durable and heat resistant. Special-purpose fibers are often made by applying intense heat to kaolin, aluminum, or silica to render them molten. Alumina fibers are often referred to as "whiskers." Flame-attenuated glass and ceramic fibers are also included in the special-purpose category. Most fibers are coated with a binder, which is a biologically inert, polymerized resin.

As mentioned earlier in this chapter, the potential carcinogenicity of a fiber is related to its aspect ratio and its propensity for persistence in the body.[28–31] MMMF tend to divide transversely rather than along the vertical axis. They are also broken down more rapidly into smaller fragments.[117, 118] For the most part, the manufacture of MMMF is associated with the generation of less respirable fibers than occurs in an asbestos textile mill.[119] Nonetheless, it must be borne in mind that glass and other MMMF, such as alumina whiskers, provided their aspect ratios and their penchant for persistence are sufficient, when introduced into the pleura of animals, can lead to the development of mesothelioma-like tumors.[31, 120] This property has generated some concern. As a result, there have been a fair number of studies carried out in humans to ascertain whether there is an increased risk of lung cancer and mesothelioma in those who manufacture or use MMMF.

Over the past several years, the results of two large epidemiological studies have been published.[121, 122] These studies involved more than 40,000 production and maintenance workers. The studies were designed specifically for the purpose of ascertaining whether MMMF could cause the same diseases and health effects as asbestos. The findings of the two studies have many similarities. Those workers concerned with the manufacture of fibrous wool from rock and slag had an increased rate of lung cancer, which only became apparent 20 years or more after the first exposure. The excess risk was slightly higher in European than in American workers, an excess of 40% versus 30%. Workers manufacturing fibrous wool from glass had a 10% excess, both in Europe and in the United States. Those workers involved in the production of glass filaments had no excess risks.

After reviewing these findings, Doll concluded that there may be an excess risk of lung cancer in the rock/slag workers and also among those workers producing glass wool.[123] Enterline, however, pointed out that one of the difficulties in attributing a causal relationship between respiratory cancer and MMMF is that the estimated fiber concentrations to which workers were purportedly exposed were relatively low.[124] This had been previously alluded to by McDonald at a meeting in Copenhagen when he reviewed the epidemiological findings and expressed the opinion that, given the low exposure levels, a greater excess of lung cancer would not be observed, even when dealing with asbestos.[125] Somewhat later, Doll made a similar comment and expressed the opinion that the low fiber counts were difficult to associate with any risk that could be equated with the effects of chrysotile and that the observed risk would suggest that MMMF were more carcinogenic than was chrysotile asbestos.[123] He went on to express the opinion that, even had the studies dealt with workers exposed to chrysotile asbestos, excesses of the magnitude that were observed would not have been expected. Furthermore, he proffered an alternative explanation, suggesting that the exposure estimates were probably too low.

When we consider the fact that animal studies have shown that fiber for fiber, MMMF are much less carcinogenic than asbestos, the anomalies noted earlier become difficult to explain.[28–31] Exposure estimates between the two large studies referred to here resulted from a concerted effort, and there was a remarkable measure of agreement between the two.

After reviewing the data, Enterline suggested that prior exposures to other agents may have played a role in the excess risk noted, and he pointed out that some of the workers had worked in a mineral wool production plant where the estimated exposure to respirable fibers was 1.5 f/cc.[124] Similar findings were noted in the European study. He further concluded that, in the rock slag workers where exposure was greatest, no more than a 10% excess in lung cancer should have been observed. He went on to express the opinion that the 30% to 40% excesses noted in the two studies were difficult to explain and implied that there may be other factors involved, including the fact that many of the workers may have been exposed to asbestos in the past. This hypothesis was subsequently confirmed, at least in four of the six plants in the study in the United States. However, in the four plants in which asbestos was used, the excess of respiratory cancer did not differ from that of two plants where asbestos was not used.

Other possible explanations are related to the fact that MMMF workers are exposed to a wide variety of agents, in addition to the fibers themselves. These include furnace fumes, often containing polycyclic aromatic hydrocarbons, and contaminants were often present in the feed stock. It was further noted that the excess of cancer in the rock slag workers was mainly due to the use of slag rather than rock.[124] The possibility of contamination of the slag from arsenic was suggested.[121]

Enterline goes on to point out that the epidemiological data on MMMF workers suggest that it is the slag workers who have the most impressive excess of respiratory cancer.[124] He doubts whether the smaller excesses among glass workers and others have any significance and believes that they may be explained by differing habits. He further goes on to suggest that carcinogenic contaminants in the slag may be responsible for the excess risk and wonders whether these contaminants are incorporated in the fibers themselves. As a result, the United States Environmental Protection Agency proposed classifying rock slag wool as a probable animal carcinogen and a possible human carcinogen. This proposal, however, was based on inadequate evidence and could greatly affect the rock and slag wool industry, besides misleading the general public. Moreover, this conclusion is not supported by animal experiments.

It has also been suggested that the inhalation of MMMF may lead to the development of pulmonary fibrosis.[126] Most of the early work conducted in this area had suggested that this was not the case,[127] although there have been a few reports purporting to show an effect.[119] A follow-up of workers employed in seven MMMF production plants has recently been published.[128] A suitable group of blue collar workers was selected as referents. A low prevalence of small opacities, all at the 1/0 or 1/1 profusion levels, was found. For MMMF workers, 1.6% of 1435 were shown to have small opacities present in the lungs. In the reference population, the figure was 0.7%. Ventilatory capacity was similar in both populations and, for the most part, suggested that both were healthy and did not differ from other blue collar workers. An initial analysis suggested a dust-induced, dose-related radiographic response, but this was shown to be absent following a better controlled reanalysis. The authors concluded that there were no adverse clinical, functional, or radiographic signs or effects of exposure to MMMF in workers in the production plants.

Other fibers, besides MMMF, are occasionally used commercially. These include carbon and alumina fibers, neither of which has been noted to induce any disease in humans.

REFERENCES

1. Occupational Safety and Health Administration, Definition of asbestos, asbestos fibers, and fibers. Federal Register 1910, 93a, June 7, 1972.
2. Ross, M., Kuntze, R. A., and Clifton, R. A., Definitions for asbestos and other health related silicates. *In* Levadie, B., ed., ASTM STP 8344. Philadelphia, American Society for Testing and Materials, 1984, pp. 139–147.
3. Langer, A. M., Nolan, R. P., and Addison, J., On talc, tremolite and tergiversation. Correspondence. Br. J. Ind. Med. 48, 339, 1991.
4. Langer, A. M., Nolan, R. P., and Pooley, F. D., Phyllosilicates: associated fibrous minerals. *In* Bignon, J., ed., Health Related Effects of Phyllosilicates. NATO/ASI Series, Vol. G.21. Berlin, Springer Verlag, 1990, pp. 59–61.
5. Pooley, F. D., Asbestos mineralogy. *In* Antman, K., and Aisner, J. E., eds., Asbestos Related Malignancy. Orlando, Grune and Stratton, 1987, pp. 3–30.
6. Merewether, E. R. A., Annual Report of the Chief Inspector of Factories and Workshops for England and Wales. London, His Majesty's Stationery Office, 63, 1933, and, 64, 1934.
7. Porro, F. W., Patten, J. R., and Hobbs, A. A., Jr., Pneumoconiosis in the talc industry. AJR Am. J. Roentgenol., 47, 507, 1942.
8. Dreesen, W. C., and Dalla Valle, J. M., Effects of exposure to dust in two Georgia talc mills and mines. Public Health Rep., 50, 131, 1935.
9. Gardner, L. U., Quoted by Porro et al. AJR Am. J. Roentgenol., 47, 507, 1942.
10. Siegal, W., Smith, A. R., and Greenburg, L., The dust hazard in tremolite talc mining. Including roentgenological findings in talc workers. AJR Am. J. Roentgenol., 49, 11, 1943.
11. Kleinfeld, M., Messite, J., and Tabershaw, I. R., Talc pneumoconiosis. Arch. Ind. Health, 12, 66, 1955.
12. Kleinfeld, M., Messite, J., Shapiro, J., et al., Lung function in talc workers: a comparative physiologic study of workers exposed to fibrous and granular talc dust. Arch. Environ. Health, 9, 559, 1964.
13. Kleinfeld, M., Messite, J., Shapiro, J., and Swencicki, R., Effect of talc dust inhalation on lung function. Arch. Environ. Health, 10, 431, 1965.
14. Kleinfeld, M., Messite, J., Kooyman, O., and Zaki, M., Mortality among talc miners and millers in New York State. Arch. Environ. Health, 14, 663, 1967.
15. Kleinfeld, M., Giel, C. P., Majeranowski, J. F., and Messite, J., Talc pneumoconiosis. A report of six patients with postmortem findings. Arch. Environ. Health, 7, 101, 1963.
15a. Kleinfeld, M., Messite, J., and Langer, A. M., A study of workers exposed to asbestiform minerals in commercial talc manufacture. Environ. Res., 6, 132, 1973.
16. Reger, R., and Morgan, W. K. C., On talc, tremolite and tergiversation. Br. J. Ind. Med., 47, 505, 1990.
17. McCormick, W. E., Talc pneumoconiosis. Correspondence. JAMA, 149, 778, 1952.
18. Leophonte, P., and Didier, A., French talc pneumoconiosis. *In* Bignon, J., ed., Health Related

Effects of Phyllosilicates. NATO/ASI Series, Vol. G.21. Berlin, Springer Verlag, 1990, pp. 203–209.

19. Fine, L. J., and Peters, J. M., Respiratory morbidity in rubber workers. II. Pulmonary function in curing workers. Arch. Environ. Health, 31, 6, 1976.

20. Fine, L. J., Peters, J. M., Burgess, W. A., and Di Beradinis, L. G., Studies of respiratory morbidity in rubber workers. Part IV. Respiratory morbidity in talc workers. Arch. Environ. Health, 31, 195, 1976.

21. Delzell, E., and Monson, R. E., Mortality among rubber workers. III. Cause specific mortality 1940–1975. J. Occup. Med., 23, 677, 1978.

22. Delzell, E., and Monson, R. E., Mortality among rubber workers. VIII. Industrial products workers. Am. J. Ind. Med., 6, 273, 1984.

23. Wegman, D. H., Peters, J. M., Boundy, M. G., and Smith, T. J., Evaluation of respiratory effects in miners and millers to talc free asbestos and silica. Br. J. Ind. Med., 39, 233, 1982.

24. Fletcher, C. M., Peto, R., Tinker, C., and Speizer, F. E., The Natural History of Chronic Bronchitis. Oxford, Oxford University Press, 1976, pp. 233–253.

25. Gamble, J. F., Fellner, W., and DiMeo, M. J., An epidemiologic study of talc workers. Am. Rev. Respir. Dis., 119, 741, 1979.

26. Gamble, J., Greife, A., and Hancock, J., An epidemiological industrial hygiene study of talc workers. Ann. Occup. Hyg., 26, 841, 1982.

27. Kleinfeld, M., Messite, J., and Zaki, M. H., Mortality experiences among talc workers: a follow up study. J. Occup. Med., 16, 345, 1974.

28. Wagner, J. C., Experimental production of mesothelial tumours of the pleura by implantation of dusts in laboratory animals. Nature, 196, 180, 1962.

29. Wagner, J. C., Berry, G. L., and Timbrell, V., Mesothelioma in rats after inoculation with asbestos and other materials. Br. J. Cancer, 28, 173, 1973.

30. Stanton, M. F., and Wrench, C., Mechanisms of mesothelioma induction with asbestos and fibrous glass. J. Natl. Cancer. Inst., 48, 797, 1972.

31. Stanton, M. F., Layard, M., Tegeris, A., et al., Carcinogenicity of fibrous glass: pleural response in relation to fiber size. J. Natl. Cancer. Inst., 58, 587, 1977.

32. Smith, W. E., Hubert, D. D., Sober, H. J., et al., eds., Proceedings of the Conference on Occupational Exposures to Fibrous and Particulate Dusts and Their Extension into the Environment. Dust and Disease Pathotoxicology. Park Forest, IL, Pathotox Publishers, 1979, p. 335.

33. McConnell, E. E., Toxicology and Carcinogenesis. Studies of Tremolite. NTP technical report 277. NIH publication no. 90, 2531. Washington, D.C., U.S. Department of Health and Human Services, 1990.

34. McDonald, J. C., Gibbs, G. W., Liddell, F. D. K., and McDonald, A. D., Mortality after long exposure to cummingtonite-grunerite. Am. Rev. Respir. Dis., 118, 271, 1978.

35. Brown, D., Kaplan, S. D., Zumwalde, M., et al., Retrospective cohort mortality study of underground gold mine workers. In Goldsmith, D. F., Winn, D. M., Shy, C. M., eds., Silica, Silicosis, and Lung Cancer: Controversy in Occupational Medicine. New York, Praeger, 1984, pp. 335–350.

36. Cooper, W. C., Wong, O., and Graebner, R., Mortality of workers in two Minnesota taconite mining and milling operations. J. Occup. Med., 30, 506, 1988.

37. Brown, D. P., Dement, J. M., and Wagner, J. L., Mortality patterns among miners and millers occupationally exposed to asbestiform talc. In Lemen, R., Dement, J. M., eds., Proceedings of the Conference on Occupational Exposure to Fibrous and Particulate Dusts and Their Extension into the Environment. Dust and Disease. Pathotoxicology. Peak Forest South, IL, Paradox Publishers, 1979, pp. 317–324.

38. Gamble, J., A nested case control study of lung cancer among New York talc workers. Int. Arch. Occup. Environ. Health, 64, 449, 1993.

39. American Thoracic Society Official Statement, Health effects of tremolite. Am. Rev. Respir. Dis., 142, 1453, 1990.

40. Case, B. W., On talc, tremolite and tergiversation. Correspondence. Br. J. Ind. Med., 48, 357, 1991.

41. Reger, R. B., and Morgan, W. K. C., On talc, tremolite and tergiversation. Correspondence. Br. J. Ind. Med., 48, 358, 1991.

42. British Thoracic Society and Medical Research Council of Great Britain, A survey of the long term effects of talc and kaolin pleurodesis. Br. J. Dis. Chest., 73, 285, 1979.

43. Meunier, A., Thomassin, J. H., and Decarreau, A., Geological occurrence of phyllosilicates: application to kaolinite, talc, sepiolite, and palygorskite deposits. In Bignon, J., ed., Health Related Effects of Phyllosilicates. NATO/ASI Series, Vol. G.21. Berlin, Springer Verlag, 1990, pp. 15–29.

44. Morgan, W. K. C., Donner, A., Higgins, I. T. T., et al., The effects of kaolin on the lung. Am. Rev. Respir. Dis., 138, 813, 1988.

45. Hale, L. W., Gough, J., King, E. J., and Nagelschmidt, G., Pneumoconiosis of kaolin workers. Br. J. Ind. Med., 13, 251, 1956.

46. Gibbs, A. R., Human pathology of kaolin and mica pneumoconiosis. In Bignon, J., ed., Health Related Effects of Phyllosilicates. NATO/ASI Series, Vol. G.21. Berlin, Springer Verlag, 1990, pp. 217–226.

47. Clarke, G. M., Phyllosilicates as industrial minerals. In Bignon, J., ed., Health Related Effects of Phyllosilicates. NATO/ASI Series, Vol. G.21. Berlin, Springer Verlag, 1990, pp. 31–45.

48. Middleton, E. L., Industrial pulmonary disease due to the inhalation of dust. Lancet, 1, 59, 1936.
49. Lynch, K. M., and McIver, F. A., Pneumoconiosis from exposure to kaolin dust: kaolinosis. Am. J. Pathol., 30, 1117, 1954.
50. Edenfield, R. W., A clinical and roentgenological study of kaolin workers. Arch. Environ. Health, 5, 28, 1960.
51. Warraki, S., and Herrant, Y., Pneumoconiosis in china clay workers. Br. J. Ind. Med., 20, 226, 1963.
52. Sheers, G., Prevalence of pneumoconiosis in Cornish kaolin workers. Br. J. Ind. Med., 21, 218, 1983.
53. Kennedy, T., Rawlings, W., Baser, M., and Tockman, M., Pneumoconiosis in Georgia kaolin workers. Am. Rev. Respir. Dis., 127, 215, 1983.
54. Oldham, P. D., Pneumoconiosis in Cornish clay workers. Br. J. Ind. Med., 40, 131, 1983.
55. Altekruse, E. D., Chaudhary, B. A., Pearson, M. G., and Morgan, W. K. C., Kaolin dust concentrations and pneumoconiosis at a kaolin mine. Thorax, 39, 436, 1984.
56. Lapenas, D., Gale, P., Kennedy, T., et al., Kaolin pneumoconiosis: radiologic, pathologic and mineralogic findings. Am. Rev. Respir. Dis., 130, 282, 1984.
57. Wagner, J. C., Pooley, F. D., Gibbs, A., et al., Inhalation of china stone and china clay dusts: relationship between the mineralogy of dust retained in the lungs and pathological changes. Thorax, 41, 190, 1986.
58. Ogle, C. G., Rundle, E. M., and Sugar, E. T., China clay workers in the southwest of England: analysis of the radiograph readings, ventilatory capacity, and respiratory symptoms in relation to type and duration of exposure. Br. J. Ind. Med., 46, 261, 1989.
59. Dick, J. A., Morgan, W. K. C., Muir, D. C. F., and Reger, R. B., Significance of irregular opacities in the chest roentgenogram. Chest, 102, 251, 1992.
60. Sepulveda, M. J., Vallyathan, V., Attfield, M. D., et al., Pneumoconiosis and lung function in a group of kaolin workers. Am. Rev. Respir. Dis., 127, 231, 1983.
61. Morgan, W. K. C., Kaolin and the lung. Am. Rev. Respir. Dis., 127, 141, 1983.
62. Baser, M. E., Kennedy, T. P., Dodson, R., et al., Differences in lung function and prevalence of pneumoconiosis between two kaolin plants. Br. J. Ind. Med., 46, 773, 1989.
63. Davies, R., Griffiths, D. M., Johnson, N. F., et al., The cytotoxicity of kaolin towards macrophages in vitro. Br. J. Exp. Pathol., 65, 453, 1984.
64. Middleton, E. L., Proceedings of the International Conference on Silicates, Geneva, 1938. Published by ILO, Studies and Reports, Series F. J. Ind. Hyg., No. 17, pp. 25 and 134. D. S. King and Sons, London, 1940.
65. McNally, W. D., and Trostler, I. S., Severe pneumoconiosis caused by inhalation of fuller's earth. J. Ind. Hyg., 23, 118, 1941.
66. Gartner, H., Die Bleicherde-Lunge. Arch. Gewerbepath. Gewerbehyg., 13, 508, 1955.
67. Campbell, A. H., and Gloyne, S. R., A case of pneumoconiosis due to the inhalation of fuller's earth. J. Pathol., 54, 75, 1942.
68. Tonning, H. O., Pneumoconiosis from fuller's earth. Report of a case with autopsy findings. J. Ind. Hyg., 31, 41, 1949.
69. Sakula, A., Pneumoconiosis due to fuller's earth. Thorax, 16, 176, 1961.
70. Skulberg, K. R., Gylseth, B., Skaug, V., and Hanoa, R., Mica pneumoconiosis: a literature review. Scand. J. Work. Environ. Health, 11, 65, 1985.
71. Pimentel, J. C., and Menezes, A. P., Pulmonary and hepatic granulomatous disorders due to the inhalation of cement and mica dusts. Thorax, 33, 219, 1978.
72. Davies, D., and Cotton, R., Mica pneumoconiosis. Br. J. Ind. Med., 40, 22, 1983.
73. Dreesen, W. C., Dalla vale, J. M., Edwards, T., et al., Pneumoconiosis among mica and pegmatite workers. Washington, D.C., U.S. Public Health Service Bulletin, no. 250, 1940.
74. Vestal, T., Winstead, J. A., and Joliet, P. V., Pneumoconiosis among mica and pegmatite workers. Ind. Med., 12, 11, 1943.
75. Heimann, H., Markowitz, S., Iyer, C., et al., Silicosis in mica mining in Bihar, India. Arch. Ind. Hyg. Occup. Med., 8, 420, 1953.
76. Li Weizu, A., A preliminary report on the conditions of the mica mine dusts causing lung disease. Chest. J. Prev. Med., 14, 177, 1980.
77. Landas, S. K., and Schwartz, D. A., Mica associated pulmonary interstitial fibrosis. Am. Rev. Respir. Dis., 144, 718, 1991.
78. Smith, A. R., Pleural calcification resulting from exposure to certain dusts. AJR Am. J. Roentgenol., 67, 375, 1952.
79. Chahinian, P., Pajak, T. F., Holland, J. F., et al., Diffuse malignant mesothelioma: prospective evaluation of 69 patients. Ann. Intern. Med., 96, 746, 1982.
80. Amandus, H. E., Althouse, R., Morgan, W. K. C., et al., The morbidity and mortality of vermiculite miners and millers exposed to asbestiform tremolite/actinolite. Part III. Radiographic findings. Am. J. Ind. Med., 11, 27, 1987.
81. McDonald, J. C., Sébastien, P., and Armstrong, B., Radiological survey of past and present vermiculite miners exposed to tremolite. Br. J. Ind. Med., 43, 445, 1986.
82. Lockey, J. E., Brooks, S. M., Jarobek, A. M., et al., Pulmonary changes after exposure to a vermiculite contaminated fibrous tremolite. Am. Rev. Respir. Dis., 129, 952, 1984.
83. McDonald, J. C., McDonald, A. D., Sébastien, P., and Moy, K., Health of vermiculite miners exposed to trace amounts of fibrous tremolite. Br. J. Ind. Med., 45, 630, 1988.

84. Sluis-Cremer, G. K., and Hessel, G. A., Palabora vermiculite. *In* Bignon, J., ed., Health Related Effects of Phyllosilicates. NATO/ASI Series, Vol. G.21. Berlin, Springer Verlag, 1990, pp. 227–234.

85. Amandus, H. E., and Wheeler, R., The morbidity and mortality of vermiculite miners and millers exposed to tremolite-actinolite. Part II. Mortality. Am. J. Ind. Med., 11, 15, 1987.

86. McDonald, J. C., McDonald, A. D., Armstrong, B., and Sébastien, P., Cohort study of vermiculite miners exposed to tremolite. Br. J. Ind. Med., 43, 436, 1986.

87. Wagner, J. C., Griffiths, D. M., and Munday, D. E., Experimental studies with palygorskite dusts. Br. J. Ind. Med., 44, 749, 1987.

88. Pairon, J. C., Jaurand, M. C., Gaudichet, A., et al., Therapeutic and domestic uses of attapulgite and sepiolite. *In* Bignon, J., ed., Health Related Effects of Phyllosilicates. NATO/ASI Series, Vol. G.21. Berlin, Springer Verlag, 1990, pp. 249–263.

89. Sors, H., Gaudichet, A., Sébastien, P., et al., Lung fibrosis after inhalation of fibrous attapulgite. Thorax, 34, 695, 1979.

90. Gamble, J., Sieber, W. K., and Wheeler, R. W., A cross sectional study of U.S. attapulgite workers. Ann. Occup. Hyg., 32(Suppl.), 475, 1988.

91. Waxweiler, R. J., Zumwalde, R. D., Ness, G. O., and Brown, D. P., A retrospective cohort mortality study of males mining and milling attapulgite clay. Am. J. Ind. Med., 13, 305, 1988.

92. Begin, R., Masse, S., and Sébastien, P., Assessment of fibrogenicity of attapulgite. *In* Bignon, J., ed., Health Related Effects of Phyllosilicates. NATO/ASI Series, Vol. G.21. Berlin, Springer Verlag, 1990, pp. 395–403.

93. Pott, F., Bellman, R., Mukle, H., et al., Intraperitoneal injection studies for the evaluation of the carcinogenicity of fibrous phyllosilicates. *In* Bignon, J., ed., Health Related Effects of Phyllosilicates. NATO/ASI Series, Vol. G.21. Berlin, Springer Verlag, 1990, pp. 319–329.

94. McConnochie, K., Lyons, J. P., Bevan, C., and Wagner, J. C., A study of Spanish sepiolite workers. *In* Proceedings of VIIth International Conference on Pneumoconiosis, Part I. US Dept of Health and Human Services, Pittsburgh, PA, Aug. 1988, p. 96.

94a. McConnochie, K., Bevan, C., Newcombe, R. G., et al., A study of Spanish sepiolite workers. Thorax, 48, 370, 1993.

95. Seaton, A., Lamb, D., Rhind Brown, W., et al., Pneumoconiosis of shale miners. Thorax, 36, 412, 1981.

96. Phibbs, B. P., Sundin, R. E., and Mitchell, R. S., Silicosis in Wyoming bentonite workers. Am. Rev. Respir. Dis., 103, 1, 1971.

97. Timár, M., Kendrey, G., and Juhasz, Z., Experimental observations concerning the effects of mineral dust on pulmonary tissue. Med. Lav., 57, 1, 1966.

98. Amadis, Z., and Timár, M., Studies on the effects of quartz, bentonite and coal dust mixtures on macrophages in vitro. Br. J. Exp. Pathol., 59, 411, 1978.

99. Gartner, H., and van Marwych, C., Lungenfibrose durch Sillimanit. Dtsch Med Wochenschr., 72, 708, 1947.

100. Jotten, K. W., and Eickhoff, F. W., Lung changes from sillimanite dust. Arch. Gewerbepath., 12, 223, 1954.

101. Barrie, H. J., and Hosselin, L., Massive pneumoconiosis from a rock dust containing no free silica. Nepheline lung. Arch. Environ. Health, 1, 109, 1960.

102. Musk, A. W., Greville, H. W., and Tribe, A. E., Pulmonary disease from occupational exposure to an artificial aluminium silicate used for cat litter. Br. J. Ind. Med., 37, 367, 1980.

103. Round the World. Asbestos in water. Lancet, 2, 1256, 1972.

104. Clark, T. C., Harrington, V. A., Asta, J., et al., Respiratory effects of exposure to dust in taconite mining and processing. Am. Rev. Respir. Dis., 121, 956, 1980.

105. Higgins, I. T. T., Glassman, J. H., Oh, M. S., and Cornell, R. G., Mortality of reserve mining company employees in relation to taconite dust exposure. Am. J. Epidemiol., 118, 710, 1983.

106. Hilding, A. C., Hilding, D. A., Larson, D. M., and Aufderheide, A. C., Biological effects of ingested amosite, asbestos taconite tailings diatomaceous earth and Lake Superior water in rats. Arch. Environ. Health, 36, 298, 1981.

107. Huuskonen, M. S., Tossavainen, A., Koskinen, H., et al., Wollastonite exposure and lung fibrosis. Environ. Res., 30, 29, 1983.

108. Shasby, D. M., Peterson, M. R., Hodous, T. K., et al., Respiratory morbidity of workers exposed to wollastonite through mining and milling. *In* Lemen, P., Dement, J. M., eds., Dust and Disease. Park Forest, IL, Pathotox Publishers, 1979, pp. 251–256.

109. Hanke, W., Sepulveda, M. J., Watson, A., and Jankovic, J., Respiratory morbidity in wollastonite workers. Br. J. Ind. Med., 41, 474, 1984.

110. Huskonen, M. S., Jarvisalo, J., Koskinen, H., et al., Preliminary results from a cohort of workers exposed to wollastonite in a Finnish limestone quarry. Scand. J. Work. Environ. Health., 9, 169, 1983.

111. Pott, F., Roller, M., Zeim, U., et al., Carcinogenicity studies of natural and manmade fibres with the intraperitoneal test in rats. *In* Bignon, J., Peto, J., and Saracci, eds., IARC Sci. Publ. No. 90, Lyon, France, 1989, p. 173.

112. Wagner, J. C., Skidmore, J., Hill, R. J., and Griffiths, D. M., Erionite exposure and mesothelioma in rats. Br. J. Cancer, 51, 727, 1985.

113. Baris, Y. I., Sahim, A. A., Ozesmi, M., et al., An outbreak of pleural mesothelioma and chronic fibrosing pleurisy in the village of Karain/Ürgüp in Anatolia. Thorax, 33, 181, 1978.

114. Baris, Y. I., Simonato, L., Artvinli, M., et al., Epidemiological and environmental evidence of the health effects of exposure to erionite fibres. Int. J. Cancer., 39, 10, 1987.
115. Ozesmi, M., Patiroglu, T. S., Hillerdal, G., and Ozesmi, C., Peritoneal mesothelioma and malignant lymphoma in mice caused by fibrous zeolite. Br. J. Ind. Med., 42, 746, 1985.
116. Elmes, P. C., Perlite and other nuisance dusts. J. R. Soc. Med., 80, 403, 1988.
117. Wright, G. W., and Kuschner, M., The influence of varying lengths of glass and asbestos fibres on tissue response in guinea pigs. In Walton, W. H., ed., Inhaled Particles 4, Part 1. Oxford, Pergamon Press, 1977, pp. 455–476.
118. Klingholz, R., Technology and production of manmade mineral fibres. Ann. Occup. Hyg., 20, 153, 1977.
119. Hill, J. W., Health aspects of manmade mineral fibres: a review. Ann. Occup. Hyg., 20, 161, 1977.
120. Piggott, G. H., Gaskell, B. A., and Ishmael, J., Effects of long term inhalation of alumina fibres. Br. J. Exp. Pathol., 62, 323, 1981.
121. Enterline, P., Marsh, G. M., Henderson, V., and Callahan, C., Mortality update of a cohort of U.S. manmade mineral fibre workers. Ann. Occup. Hyg., 31, 625, 1987.
122. Simonato, L., Fletcher, A. C., and Cherrie, J. W., The International Agency for Research in Cancer historical cohort study of MMMF production workers in seven European countries. Ann. Occup. Hyg., 31, 603, 1987.
123. Doll, R., Symposium on MMMF Copenhagen October 1986. Overview and conclusions. Ann. Occup. Hyg., 31, 805, 1987.
124. Enterline, P. E., Role of manmade mineral fibres in the causation of cancer. Editorial. Br. J. Ind. Med., 47, 145, 1990.
125. McDonald, J. C., Peer review. Mortality of workers to MMMF: current evidence and future research. In Biological Effects of Man-Made Mineral Fibres; Proceedings of WHO/IARC Conference. Copenhagen, 1982. Copenhagen, World Health Organization, 1982, p. 369.
126. Enterline, P. E., March, G., and Esmen, N. A., Respiratory diseases among workers exposed to man-made mineral fibers. Am. Rev. Respir. Dis., 128, 1, 1983.
127. Weill, H., Hughes, J. M., Hammad, Y., et al., Respiratory health in workers exposed to man made vitreous fibers. Am. Rev. Respir. Dis., 128, 104, 1983.
128. Hughes, J. M., Jones, R. N., Glindmeyer, H. W., et al., Follow up study of workers exposed to man made mineral fibres. Br. J. Ind. Med., 50, 658, 1993.

14

Asbestos-Related Diseases

W. Keith C. Morgan

J. Bernard L. Gee

Asbestos is a generic term applied to a number of metamorphic fibrous mineral silicates. Most governmental agencies and learned societies include six minerals as asbestos, namely, chrysotile, crocidolite, amosite, anthophyllite, actinolite, and tremolite. Of the six, the first three, and to a lesser extent anthophyllite, either are or have been in the past, used extensively commercially. In contrast, tremolite and actinolite have rarely been used for commercial purposes. At present, more than 90% of the asbestos mined is chrysotile, a fact of importance when contemporary asbestos-related hazards are under consideration.

All forms of asbestos belong to one of two distinct groups of minerals, i.e., the serpentine or the amphibole group (Fig. 14–1).[1] The former consists of serpentiform fibers, while the latter consists of needle-like or rod-shaped fibers. Chrysotile is the only member of the serpentine group; the remainder are amphiboles, which have common biological and mineralogical qualities that are not shared by chrysotile. The crystalline structure of the amphiboles is similar, and they can often only be distinguished on the basis of their chemical composition (Table 14–1). In the divided state, the amphibole fibers often lie in parallel formations. In contrast, chrysotile appears as extremely fine, uniform fibers that often can be seen only with an electron microscope. Chrysotile fibers combine in a number of ways to produce varying shaped fibril bundles. Asbestos has certain unique physical, chemical, and heat-resistant properties that allow it to be woven into heat-resistant products that are of great industrial value.

It is important to bear in mind that various minerals with the same chemical composition can exist either as asbestiform or as nonasbestiform forms.[2] Thus, the nonasbestiform variants of chrysotile, crocidolite, and amosite are respectively known as antigorite, riebeckite, and cummingtonite-grunerite. Similar variants occur with anthophyllite, tremolite, and actinolite, but their nonasbestiform variants have no specific names and are referred to as nonasbestiform anthophyllite, tremolite, and so forth. Further discussion of the distinction between the asbestiform and nonasbestiform forms of these minerals is to be found in Chapter 13.

HISTORY AND GEOLOGICAL OCCURRENCE

The fireproof properties of asbestos were noted some 2000 years ago. According to Pooley,[1] the Romans used small amounts of asbestos to weave cremation cloths, and both the Chinese and Egyptians wove asbestos fibers into mats. The Romans termed asbestos *amianthus,* which according to Hunter means "without miasma, undefiled or incorruptible."[3] Pooley pointed out that there is some doubt about the origin of the meaning of the term asbestos.[1]

Asbestos was discovered in the Ural Mountains in Russia early in the 18th

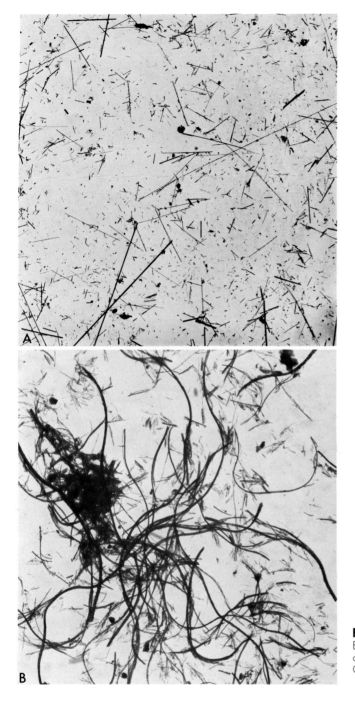

Figure 14-1
Electron micrographs of U.I.C.C. standard samples of asbestos. ×3750. A, Crocidolite. B, Chrysotile.

Illustration continued on following page

century. Subsequently, a factory was set up for the manufacture of asbestos products during the rule of Peter the Great. It was used in the manufacture of women's gloves and handbags for about half a century. In the early 19th century, commercial asbestos mining commenced in Italy, and in 1860, asbestos was discovered in Quebec, Canada. This was a chrysotile deposit, and mining started in 1878. The fiber became popular, and over the years, the amount of asbestos mined greatly increased. Some deposits of chrysotile are contaminated by small amounts of tremolite. Blue asbestos, or crocidolite, was discovered on the Orange River of South Africa in 1815, and amosite was discovered in Central Transvaal at the turn

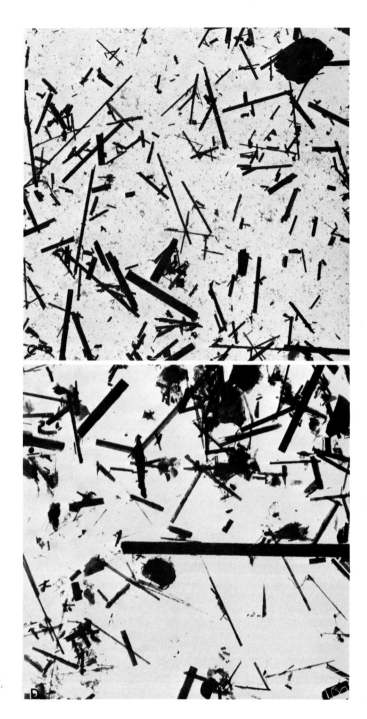

Figure 14–1 *Continued*
C, Amosite. D, Anthophyllite. (Courtesy of Dr. V.
Timbrell and Mr. M. Griffiths.)

of the century. Subsequently, deposits of chrysotile were discovered in other countries, including Russia and Zimbabwe. Crocidolite was also mined for a limited time in the Wittenoom mine in Western Australia. The major deposits of anthophyllite that were commercially mined are located in Finland, although in the past, some mining of anthophyllite took place in the United States. Tremolite has been mined in Italy, Pakistan, Turkey, and South Korea, but the quantities mined and its uses have been relatively limited.

The major producer of asbestos in the Western world was Quebec, where, in the early 1980s, between 1.5 and 2 million tons were mined annually. The annual

Table 14–1
■
Types of Asbestos

Serpentine	Amphiboles
Chrysotile $Mg_6Si_4O_{10}(OH)_8$	Amosite $(FeMg)_7(Si_8O_{22})(OH)_2$
	Crocidolite $Na_2(Fe_3)_2(Fe_2)_3Si_8O_{22}(OH)_2$
	Anthophyllite $(MgFe)_7(Si_8O_{22})(OH)_2$

production is now around one half of what it was. Russia, or what was the Soviet Union, is a major producer of chrysotile; however, its annual output is unknown but is thought to be around 2 to 3 million tons a year. This was used exclusively in the Eastern Bloc countries.

Until recently, there was a great demand for asbestos in the United States; however, since the new legislation and regulations and the proposed but legally unsustained ban by the Environmental Protection Agency, the demand for this valuable mineral has greatly decreased.

MINING, PRODUCTION, AND USES

Deposits of asbestos are removed either by surface or underground mining. Most of the large deposits in the Eastern townships of Quebec are open cast (surface) mines. The process involves drilling and blasting, processes which are often dusty, but the fact that asbestos deposits are intermingled with the surrounding rock tends to limit the amount of asbestos liberated into the air. Over the last 30 years, industrial hygiene measures have suppressed the formation of dust. The result is that the mining of asbestos has become much less hazardous. Underground mining is used to a limited extent in many countries; however, dust suppression in such mines, while more difficult, can be effected. Exposure to silica is an additional hazard of asbestos mining that is experienced in South Africa and certain other countries, including Zimbabwe.

Once the mineral has been removed, it is crushed and milled, usually at the mine, to release the fibers. Asbestos is then blended in a machine similar to a rotatory concrete mixer. The asbestos residue is then passed through a magnetic separator to remove certain mineral impurities. It is cleaned further on rotatory shaker screens where grit and the larger fiber fragments are eliminated. An additional cleaning process that was formerly known as ''willowing'' is sometimes carried out. The material is then ready for carding, which is now done by a wet dispersion process. Usually, cotton (about 5% to 10% by weight) is added to the asbestos, and both fibers are then mixed in a picking machine. On occasion, the asbestos is fed into the carding machine, with both fibers being fed separately into the breaker card. An excellent description of the British and American asbestos textile industries is found in the reports of Merewether and Dreessen.[4, 5] Their descriptions of the processes relate to practices prevailing 60 or more years ago; however, the principles have remained much the same to the present time. Dust control, however, is now far more effective.

One of the more important uses of asbestos is in the manufacture of asbestos cement products, in particular, tiles, corrugated roofing, gutters, water and drain pipes, and chimneys. The fibers are milled to an appropriate size and then mixed with cement to form a slurry, which is then passed on a conveyor to be made into sheeting or into molds for pipes and so forth. Water is then removed, and the product is air cured for about 1 month. Many of the pipes that are used to convey natural gas and oil contain a significant amount of amosite asbestos. Asbestos, particularly chrysotile, has been also extensively used in the manufacture of floor tiles, as a reinforcing agent, and as a filler in asphalt floorings, and it used to be incorporated in vinyl tiles. Asbestos has been extensively used for insulation and in fireproofing, and it was frequently sprayed onto girders in buildings to prevent the girder from buckling when exposed to extreme heat in a fire. Without such insulation, the building would usually collapse. Asbestos has also been extensively used in passenger, cargo, and warships for fire proofing and insulation.

Asbestos textiles nowadays contain only chrysotile. Asbestos fibers are mixed with cotton, hemp, or manmade fibers, which are then carded, spun, and woven prior to being plaited. Chrysotile is used in the manufacture of brake linings and in the bases of clutches where it is combined with graphite, phenolic resins, polymers, and various other metals, including beryllium. Crocidolite and chrysotile were used in cigarette filters for a limited time.[6] Crocidolite was used in the manufacture of gas masks during the Second World War and caused a number of deaths from mesothelioma in Britain, the United States, and Canada.[7, 8] Anthophyllite, as mentioned earlier, has more limited uses but has been used as a filler in rubber and castings, in ceiling tiles, and in the chemical and oil industries.

Finally, it must be remembered that not only miners and millers but also those using end products may develop asbestos-induced disease. Other workers who carry out their tasks near to those working directly with asbestos likewise may have certain asbestos-related conditions.[9–11] Asbestos-related diseases, at one time, occurred commonly in welders working in shipyards and even, occasionally, in those more remote from its use, for example, in bystanders in the vicinity of a site where asbestos was being installed or removed. In such bystanders, the disease was seldom as severe as it was in those who were in direct contact, e.g., insulators. In a few instances, asbestos-related diseases have occurred in the immediate vicinity of asbestos mills and factories that used mainly crocidolite. The wives of asbestos workers have developed mesothelioma or pleural plaques from repeated handling of their husband's work clothes.[12, 13]

HISTORICAL ASPECTS AND EFFECTS OF EXPOSURE TO ASBESTOS

The inhalation and deposition of asbestos in the respiratory tract leads to the following conditions:

1. Asbestosis, i.e., a diffuse fibrotic condition of the lung.
2. Carcinoma of the lung in subjects who have established asbestosis.
3. Malignant mesothelioma of the pleura and peritoneum.
4. Asbestos-induced effusion, which often leads to diffuse pleural thickening.
5. Pleural plaques or circumscribed pleural thickening, which may proceed to calcification.

In the past, it has also been claimed that asbestos exposure caused gastrointestinal cancer and carcinoma of the larynx. The evidence for this is far from convincing, and indeed, most authorities now believe that there is no increased incidence of either of these forms of malignancy in subjects who have either been exposed to asbestos or have asbestosis.[14, 15] Asbestosis was first described by Montague Murray at the turn of the century.[16] Subsequently, a series of articles was published that described the clinical and radiographic features of the condition.[17–20] The initial reports described a fibrotic condition of the lungs that occurred in those who were employed in the mining and weaving of asbestos. His Majesty's Inspector of Factories noted that, in the 1920s, a large number of subjects who were employed in asbestos mills were becoming disabled and dying prematurely of lung disease. They therefore recommended a study of asbestos mills of Britain, and this was carried out by Merewether and Price.[4] Their report gave an excellent description of the disease and its incidence and prevalence. In addition, it made it clear that there was a dose-response relationship, i.e., the more the exposure, the greater the risk of developing asbestosis. In those days, when the levels of asbestos in the air were around 100 million particles per cubic foot (mppcf), the average latency period for the onset of disease was between 7 and 10 years. In exceptional circumstances, as little as 2 years of exposure was sufficient to induce the disease. Merewether recommended that a major effort should be made to improve industrial hygiene in the mills and predicted correctly that, with better ventilation and improved industrial hygiene, the disease would become less frequent.[4, 21] Subsequently, Dreessen et al., in a well-designed study, came to similar conclusions.[5] In this study, they surveyed three North Carolina cotton mills in the mid 1930s. Unfortunately, a large number of the employees at the mills had been let go shortly before the study commenced, and there was a paucity of subjects with prolonged exposures. Dreessen and coworkers realized the deficiencies in their study and called attention to the main defects. Moreover, an attempt was made to trace and examine the 150 or so subjects who had ceased to be employed in the immediate period prior to the study. They concluded that, provided the worker was exposed to less than 5 mppcf, it was unlikely that asbestosis would develop, but in doing so, they recognized the need for dust control. In retrospect, this was an error; however, the investigators were well aware of the problems associated with the short observation period.

The risk to end-product users was not recognized until the late 1950s and early 1960s.[9–11] Prior to that, there had been sporadic case reports of asbestosis occurring in pipefitters, welders, and others.[22–24] Most such reports suggested the condition developed as the result of exceptional or unusual exposure. In this regard, the introduction to the Merewether report specifically noted that the contents of the report applied to textile workers only.[19]

Fleischer et al., in a well-designed study, investigated the likelihood of asbestosis developing in pipefitters and insulators in the United States Navy Shipyards.[25] These investigators again had a limited number of subjects with long exposure, but their findings tended to confirm the validity of Dreessen's recommended standard, i.e., 5 mppcf. They also pointed out that, although insulators and others in the shipbuilding industry were exposed to short-term high concentrations of asbestos, textile millers had continued exposure to a relatively constant amount most of the working day.[25] Subsequently, the reports of Selikoff et al.[10] and Balzer and Cooper[11] demonstrated that a significant risk existed in users of the finished product, e.g., insulators, laggers, and those who were involved in cutting asbestos sheeting. This was confirmed by Marr.[26] It also became clear that the 5-mppcf standard did not prevent asbestosis and that, after 15 or 20 years, many subjects had progressive and disabling asbestosis.[10, 11]

Throughout the 1930s and 1940s, there were a number of case reports in which asbestosis and lung cancer occurred in the same subject.[23, 27–29] A few investigators tentatively suggested there might be a cause-and-effect relationship. However, analyses of mortality data suggested that no such risk was apparent.[30] It was Doll's classic 1955 report that provided the necessary epidemiological evidence to indicate that what had formerly been an impression, namely, that there was an increased incidence of lung cancer in subjects with asbestosis, became almost certain.[31] Doll specifically limited the increased risk of lung cancer to subjects with asbestosis and did not regard asbestos exposure in the absence of fibrosis as a cause of an increased risk of lung cancer. These observations have subsequently been confirmed on many occasions.[32–37]

The shrewd observations of a surgeon and chest physician in South Africa provided the first suspicion that exposure to certain types of asbestos might lead to the development of a malignant tumor of the pleura, known as mesothelioma.[38] Dr. Sleggs, who was a superintendent of a tuberculosis sanitorium, had noted that a minority of subjects who were initially diagnosed as having tuberculous pleurisy went on to develop an intractable fibrothorax and a fatal invasive tumor that extended into the mediastinum.[39] Subsequently, Marchand, a surgeon who had operated on several such patients, asked Wagner, who was a pathologist, to examine the tissues of those subjects who developed the rather distinctive and persistent pleural effusion. They concluded that the tumors were mesotheliomata and showed that nearly all their subjects originated from the region around the Asbestos Mountains, which stretched from Cape Province some 400 miles north, and that most of them had been exposed to crocidolite in the Kimberley area of the Orange Free State. The discovery of the association between asbestos exposure and mesothelioma has recently been described by Wagner.[39] Before the observations of Sleggs and colleagues, the cause of mesothelioma had been unknown and unsuspected, despite an unreferenced and unsubstantiated statement that indicates otherwise.[40]

It is now clear that asbestosis, lung cancer, and mesothelioma are all dose related[41] and that not all asbestos fibers are equally dangerous as far as the induction of lung cancer and mesothelioma are concerned.[42]

INHALATION, DEPOSITION, AND MEASUREMENT OF ASBESTOS IN THE AIR

Asbestos fibers are generally deposited as a result of interception (see also Chapters 7 and 9). This process occurs when longer fibers are carried into the smaller conducting airways, respiratory bronchioles, and alveoli. When a fiber encounters a bifurcation, it straddles the bifurcation and is deposited. Most longer fibers (>5 μm) are deposited in the respiratory and terminal bronchioles, although the alveoli are not entirely spared. Short fibers are often carried to the alveoli. If they are shorter than 4 to 5 μm in length, most will be removed by the lungs' clearance mechanisms. The animal studies of Gardner called attention to the mechanical injury that asbestos induces.[43] Subsequently, it became evident that the longer and thinner fibers are the most hazardous and show the greatest carcinogenic effects.[44] Fibers up to 40 to 60 μm in length may be found in the lung parenchyma and the distal air passages.[45] These are much too large to be removed by macrophages and, once deposited, are unlikely to be cleared unless they disintegrate as a result of leaching or are fractured, phenomena that occur often with chrysotile and fiberglass but only to a very limited extent with the amphiboles.[42, 46–48]

Historically, the standard method of measuring airborne asbestos levels used a membrane filter and optical microscopy.[49] Samples were collected on cellulose filters; the size and number of fibers was counted by phase-contrast microscopy. Only fibers with a 3:1 aspect ratio and 5 μm or greater were counted. Gravimetric measurements of fibers, although sometimes used, have no relevance as far as biological or pathological activity of fibers is concerned. Phase-contrast microscopy, while counting all fibers of 5 μm in length, does not differentiate asbestos fibers from those of cotton, talc, or cellulose or of vegetable origin. Similarly, fibers less than 0.3 μm in breadth are missed by optical microscopy; moreover, the detection limit of the membrane filter is 0.1 fibers per cubic centimeter (f/cc). The measurement of ambient air levels of asbestos requires transmission electron microscopy (TEM). All fibers can be seen with TEM, and their asbestos type can subsequently be identified by energy dispersive x-ray analysis or with selected area electron diffraction.[50, 51] These techniques are infinitely more expensive.

The conversion of gravimetric measurements to fibers per cubic centimeter is difficult and is discussed at some length in the Report of the Ontario Royal Commission.[50] Although this body recommended a conversion factor of 30 fibers/ng, i.e., 1 f/cc as being equivalent to 33,000 ng/m^3, they added a number of caveats, emphasizing that the risk of such small numbers of fibers, especially those fibers that are extremely small, is entirely unknown and may constitute either no or an undetectable hazard.

The standard for asbestos varies between different countries. The current Occupational Safety and Health Administration (OSHA) standard in the United States is 0.2 f/cc. In Canada, the standard varies according to the type of asbestos and the province. In Ontario, the accepted standard is 1 f/cc for chrysotile, 0.5 f/cc for amosite, and 0.2 f/cc for crocidolite. Cumulative exposure is expressed as fiber-years or as the average annual exposure multiplied by the years worked, e.g., 2 f/cc for 15 years equals 30 fiber-years. Most countries, other than the United States and South Africa, have different standards for chrysotile and the other amphiboles.

SPECIFIC OCCUPATIONAL RISKS

The risk of the development of asbestosis and associated other conditions was first described in millers and miners of asbestos. Subsequently, users of the end product were also found to be at risk. As such, pipefitters, laggers, and those who made asbestos mattresses for insulation were likewise found to be exposed under certain circumstances to sufficient asbestos fibers to induce disease. Shipyard workers and insulators were particularly at risk. Construction workers who used asbestos insulation likewise were subsequently shown to be at risk, as were workers in railroad repair sheds where asbestos was used to insulate the boilers and the engines of steam trains. Other risks were also encountered in those workers working in power stations. The evidence that maintenance work with brake linings is hazardous is tenuous, and the chrysotile that is used in brake lining is converted by heat to nonfibrous forsterite.[52, 53] Crocidolite was used for a short time during the Second World War in Great Britain for the manufacture of brake linings, and it is probable that, in some subjects, mesothelioma developed as a result of such exposure. Nonetheless, the overall risk in those who manufacture brake linings and other friction materials is now extremely low.[54]

It is impossible to catalogue the various uses of asbestos completely since they differ from country to country, but asbestos has been used for insulating welding rods, in the manufacture of ropes, and as a binder for bricks used in furnaces and kilns. Those workers involved in the demolition of buildings that contain asbestos may be repeatedly exposed, albeit for relatively short periods, to high concentrations. Most of the *in situ* asbestos-containing products in buildings are harmless unless they are cut with hand saws, drilled, or abraded with high-speed tools. The inclusion of chrysotile in fireproof garments, for the most part, has not been associated with the release of a significant number of fibers. Asbestos has also been included in many domestic appliances, such as electric toasters, iron rests, and hair dryers, and there is limited evidence that, as these appliances become older and disintegrate, there may be liberation of asbestos fibers.

Contamination of the water supply by asbestos and nonasbestiform fibers is not uncommon. There is, however, no evidence to suggest that ingested asbestos fibers constitute a risk.[55] In addition, it has been known for some time that asbestos filters were used for the filtration of various beers, wines, and soft drinks, but again, there is no evidence that the ingestion of such fibers is associated with any risk. The belief that the water supply of Duluth, Minnesota, was contaminated by asbestos has been shown to be fallacious. Fibers were found in the water supply, but these turned out to be the nonasbestiform form of amosite, namely, cummingtonite-grunerite. It has not been possible to trace any ill effects from the dumping of taconite tailings in Lake Superior from whence the Duluth water supply is drawn.[56]

Asbestosis

The term *asbestosis* should be reserved for the fibrotic condition of the parenchyma. It is not entirely appropriate to refer to pleural plaques or pleural thickening induced by asbestos as pleural asbestosis. During the 1920s and 1930s, asbestosis was exceedingly common, and it often took as little as 7 to 8 years for the manifestations of the disease to become obvious.[4] With the introduction of better ventilation and, in the United States, the development of the threshold limit value (TLV), the latency period increased to 15 to 25 years.[5, 10, 11, 25] Nevertheless, severe asbestosis still developed in workers in certain industries, especially after prolonged exposure. With the gradual tightening up of the regulations, it is now reasonably certain that no new cases of asbestosis or asbestos-related lung cancer are developing when the standard of 1 f/cc is followed. Moreover, the 2-f/cc standard of the early 1970s probably prevented the development of asbestosis during a normal working lifetime. For the past several years, a series of articles have been published indicating that, if asbestos in the air is kept to 1 f/cc or less for the usual working lifetime of 35 to 40 years, there is no increase in the rate of either lung cancer or asbestosis.[32–37] These conclusions are based mainly on exposure to chrysotile, and they may not necessarily apply to those subjects who are exposed to between 1 and 2 f/cm^3 of crocidolite or amosite.

Symptoms

The most common presenting symptoms of asbestosis are a dry cough (unless the subject also happens to be a cigarette smoker, in which case, the cough may be productive) and shortness of breath. The onset of such symptoms is insidious, and the affected worker usually does not seek advice until the condition is well established. The shortness of breath gradually worsens, especially with continuing exposure. As time goes by, the severely affected asbestotic subject gradually loses weight, and this is directly related to the severity of the disease. The evidence suggests that separation from further exposure when the disease is detected early in its course, that is to say, when the radiological category is either category 1/0 or 1/1, is seldom followed by significant progression.[57]

Signs

The earliest physical signs of the development of asbestosis are the presence of persistent crackles at both bases. As the disease progresses, the crackles become more profuse and extend from the bases to the middle and upper zones. They are heard during inspiration only and are medium or coarse in character.[58] At the time subjects become short of breath, they are almost invariably tachypneic at rest. The latter is often overlooked in that the affected subject is not obviously short of breath, except on exertion. Clubbing of the fingers occurs in around 15% to 20% of subjects and tends to be found in those subjects with a relatively poor prognosis.[59] Central cyanosis with warm extremities may be found, and later on, cor pulmonale develops. The latter is manifested by ''a'' waves in the jugular pulse, right ventricular hypertrophy, and a right ventricular gallop.

Radiographic Features

Asbestosis is characterized by the development of irregular small opacities on the chest radiograph.[60] The lower zones are first affected, but as the disease progresses, the middle and upper zones become involved, although usually to a lesser extent. Small irregular opacities are divided into s, t, and u types, according to their size.[61] The standard films representing the s, t, and u types are available from the International Labour Office (Geneva, Switzerland). In around 20% to 30% of subjects, the parenchymal changes are accompanied by pleural thickening, with or without calcification. If diffuse *en face* pleural thickening is present in the lower zones, it is extremely difficult, if not impossible, to assess accurately whether any parenchymal changes are present. The *en face* pleural changes closely mimic those seen in parenchymal disease and are often attributed to pulmonary fibrosis.

The early changes seen in a subject in whom parenchymal asbestosis develops are related to the vascular markings, which seem to extend more peripherally toward the pleura than in a normal film (Fig. 14–2). Such appearances, however,

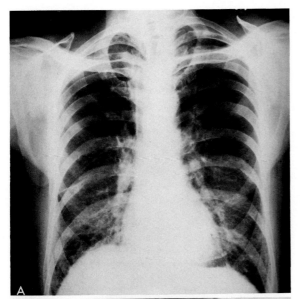

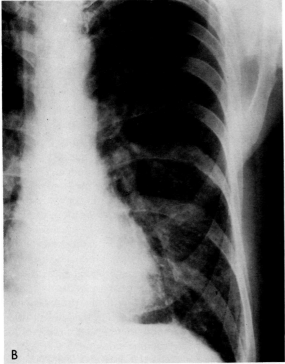

Figure 14–2
A, Chest radiograph of dock worker engaged for 20 years in repair work in ships' engine rooms, showing early changes of basal asbestosis and loss of volume, shown by depressed horizontal fissure, in right lower lobe. B, Close-up view of left base of A, showing fine linear opacities of type s. Some of these shadows may be pleural. (Courtesy of the late Dr. J. Lyons.)

can be mimicked by a high kV chest radiograph.[60] As the fibrosis progresses, the small vessels appear to undergo interruption or disruption from the superimposition of small nodules (Fig. 14–3). Occasionally, fine peripheral shadows that rather resemble Kerley B lines may develop.[62] It is important to stress that these early changes are not specific and may be seen in elderly patients, in subjects who have incipient left ventricular failure, in early cryptogenic fibrosing alveolitis, in other causes of pulmonary fibrosis (such as scleroderma), and in persons who are heavy smokers.[63, 64] With progression of the disease, the changes become more obvious, the opacities become denser and more pronounced, and as mentioned earlier, they gradually spread to involve the remainder of the lung. Occasionally, there is a

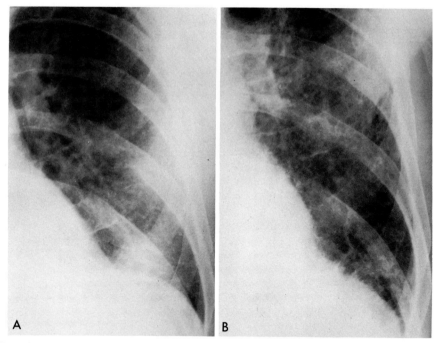

Figure 14–3. Development of asbestotic fibrosis in a shipyard demolition worker. *A,* Radiograph taken in 1967, showing only minimal linear and nodular changes at the bases. *B,* Radiograph taken in 1973, showing extensive basal fibrosis and honeycomb change. (Courtesy of the late Dr. J. Lyons.)

"ground-glass veiling" in which the disease process is composed mainly of s-type opacities and creates an initial erroneous impression of an acinus-filling process. An asbestos-induced pleural effusion that results in a fibrothorax can also create a ground-glass opacity in one hemithorax, but usually there is the telltale involvement and obliteration of the costophrenic angle. Rounded opacities are rarely seen in the chest radiograph of a patient with asbestosis unless there has also been exposure to silica, such as occurs in the manufacture of asbestos cement[60, 65, 66] or when Caplan's syndrome is present[24] (Fig. 14–4).

Large opacities are not seen in patients with asbestosis unless there has been a combined exposure to both asbestos and silica.[67] The pattern produced in typical asbestosis is often referred to as reticulonodulation, i.e., an interlacing network with the superimposition of scattered nodules. In advanced pulmonary asbestosis, honeycombing may appear in the lower zones[60] (Fig. 14–5). With the progression of asbestosis to category 3 and the development of honeycombing, the subject often has some degree of pulmonary hypertension. In addition, there is a shrinkage of the lungs, unless there is coincident emphysema from cigarette smoking.

The presence of irregular opacities in those exposed to asbestos may be due to early asbestosis but can also result from cigarette smoking.[63, 64] Significant radiographic interstitial changes are much more frequent in asbestos workers who are cigarette smokers than they are in nonsmokers.[63, 64, 68] It is, however, important to remember that such changes may occur with other dusts and even in the absence of any exposure to dusts.[64]

Progression of asbestosis is becoming increasingly uncommon. Although Selikoff et al. reported frequent and marked progression from category 0 and category 1 to higher categories over a period of 10 to 28 years, it needs to be borne in mind that most of their workers continued to be exposed to asbestos and, in addition, continued to smoke.[69] Although this information did not appear in their abstract, it was apparent that this was so from the verbal presentation. The belief that the progression of asbestosis is either inevitable or probable, whether the subject is

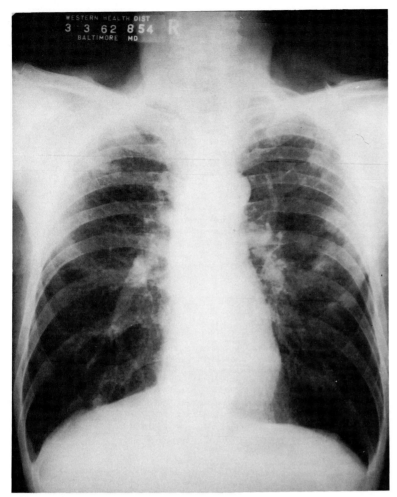

Figure 14–4. Caplan's syndrome in a shipyard welder. Multiple rounded nodules are evident in both lungs. The subject later developed rheumatoid arthritis. (From Morgan, W.K.C., Rheumatoid pneumoconiosis in association with asbestos. Thorax, 19, 433, 1964.)

removed from further exposure or not, was held for many years,[70] but it is now clear that this view is incorrect. Recently, there have been a number of studies indicating that progression is by no means invariable.[57, 71, 72] Among the factors that influence whether progression is likely to occur is the type of asbestos inhaled. Progression is much less frequent in those exposed to chrysotile than it is in those exposed to the amphiboles, and of the amphiboles, crocidolite-induced asbestosis appears more likely to progress and at a faster rate than does asbestosis induced by other types of asbestos.[42] A recent study by Gaensler et al. showed that disease progressed in only 13% to 15% of subjects exposed to asbestos.[57] Included in the study were 522 subjects who had been followed for 6 or more years. It was also clear from this study that asbestosis is a disappearing disease in the United States and Canada, and the authors make the point that, in 1950, 47.6% of subjects first seen already had asbestosis. This decreased to around 18% among those first exposed from 1950 to 1959, and among those first exposed after 1959, only 2% had the condition. Again, it was evident that, in smokers, there was a significantly higher proportion of subjects whose disease progressed, and progression was far more likely to occur in those who had a short latency period than in those in whom fibrosis did not develop until after 20 years. When progression is assessed, it is difficult to take into account the effects of asbestos that has already been deposited

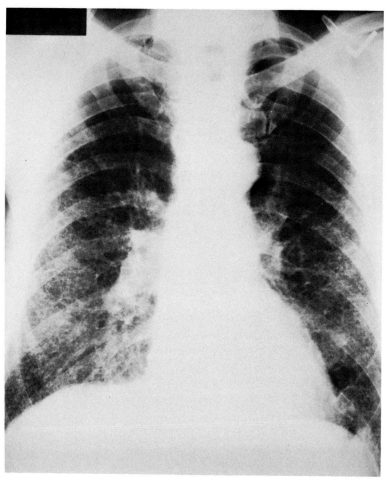

Figure 14–5. Category 2/3 asbestosis showing predominantly basal involvement with honeycombing. The subject was a former insulator.

in the lungs since it is likely that the effects of asbestos present in the lungs persist for several years in those in whom the prior exposure has been heavy.[73] In those in whom further exposure ceased, there may be progression for 4 or 5 years, but there is then a decline in the rate of progression unless the disease, when initially diagnosed, was severe and disabling. There is much evidence to suggest that, once the disease has remained unchanged for 10 years, providing no further exposure occurs, it is likely to remain unchanged for the rest of the subject's life.[57]

The International Labour Office classification has been used to predict life expectancy.[74] Subjects with category 1/2 or above have an increased death rate not only from respiratory failure and asbestosis but, more importantly, from lung cancer and, to a limited extent, mesothelioma. If the subject has only minor changes, i.e., 1/1 or below, it is difficult to detect any excess death rate from lung or any other cancer, with the exception of mesothelioma.

Computed tomography (CT) is more sensitive than is the chest radiograph for demonstrating underlying parenchymal changes in early asbestosis.[75–77] The CT scan is particularly useful in making a diagnosis of parenchymal fibrosis when there are multiple *en face* pleural plaques since, on a posteroanterior (PA) film, such plaques can mimic parenchymal change. Lobar fissures are not well seen in the CT scan, and those publications purporting to show the presence and thickening on the interlobar fissures as evidence of asbestos-related disease are unconvincing since these changes are entirely nonspecific. High-resolution CT scans are sensitive and should be used to complement pulmonary function tests and standard radiologic procedures rather than to replace them.[76, 78] Some of the changes may be masked by gravity-dependent densities. Interstitial lung disease is manifested by thickened septal and interlobular lines and nongravity-dependent lines or dense lines not related to the vessels. Honeycombing is seen in more advanced disease and is well seen in the CT scan (Fig. 14–6). When a patient is examined supine, changes may be observed in the posterior basal segment of the lower lobe caused by pooling of blood from gravity. These changes may resemble infiltrates, and if so, the patient should be rescanned in the prone position. It should, however, be remembered that other fibrotic conditions of the lung, including fibrosing alveolitis, scleroderma, and bronchiolitis obliterans with organizing pneumonia, may closely mimic the changes of asbestosis and are sometimes indistinguishable. Furthermore, the relationship between the images of the high-resolution CT scan in persons with abnormal chest radiographs and changes in lung function has not yet been documented.

Lung Function

Symptomatic asbestosis is virtually always associated with an increase in the stiffness of the lungs and impaired gas exchange.[79–81] As the lungs become stiffer, all lung volumes decrease, except in those subjects who also have emphysema from cigarette smoking.[82] In the latter, the residual volume (RV) and total lung capacity (TLC) may be normal or even somewhat increased, depending on the relative severity of the asbestosis compared with the extent of any emphysema present. The measurement of lung volumes by helium mixing is frequently unreliable under such circumstances. The diffusing capacity (DL_{CO}) is likewise reduced and, in general, becomes abnormal before there is a change in blood gases or before there is a

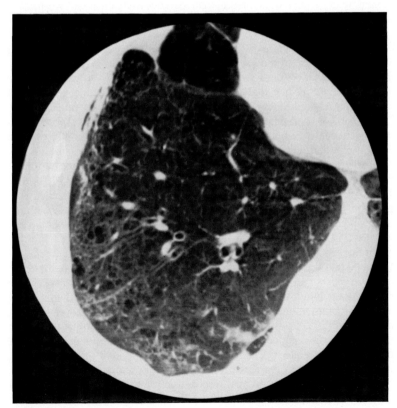

Figure 14–6. High-resolution CT scan of subject with asbestosis. Note thickened septa and moderately advanced interstitial fibrosis. Note honeycombing. (Courtesy of Dr. Linda Hutton.)

significant fall in lung volumes.[79, 81, 83, 84] The DL_{CO} is sensitive but lacks specificity[85] and may be decreased by up to 30% in unexposed smokers. The severity of the abnormalities of lung function are related to the radiographic category.[82] With progression of disease, the tidal volume (V_T) increases, and there is an absolute increase in the minute volume. The static compliance falls, and there is an increase in elastic recoil at TLC. Hypoxemia is frequent in the higher categories, and there is sometimes a further fall in the partial oxygen pressure with exercise.[79, 84] The type of impairment found in asbestosis is similar to that found in all types of interstitial pulmonary fibrosis, whether of industrial or nonindustrial origin.

The DL_{CO} is one of the more sensitive tests for detecting early asbestosis, and the reduction is often present before there are changes in lung volumes.[79, 83, 85] Nonetheless, serial measurements of lung volumes provide a means of following a population exposed to asbestos.[82] An increase in exercise ventilation is often present, but here again, there is a lack of specificity.

A number of attempts have been made to detect asbestosis at a presymptomatic stage when lung volumes and most other tests, including the chest radiograph, are normal.[86, 87] Most have depended on the use of sophisticated tests of lung mechanics. Comparison of asymptomatic asbestos miners with a reference group suggests the possibility of lower maximal expiratory flows for a given transpulmonary pressure.[86] Unfortunately, such tests tend to be nonspecific and overly sensitive, have a wide range for the predicted values, and are not readily reproducible. Such studies involve swallowing an esophageal balloon, and few workers, particularly if asymptomatic, are willing to undergo regular testing of this type.

Exercise testing can provide useful information in asbestos-exposed workers. Agostoni et al. studied 120 asbestos workers who complained of dyspnea with a mean exposure of 34 years; 63% were smokers.[88] Only 4% of their subjects had normal radiographs; 35% had pleural changes, 5% had parenchymal disease only, and the remaining 56% had both pleural and parenchymal changes. Restrictive impairment was present in 25% of the workers, and obstructive impairment was present in 27%. Only 26% of the workers had ventilatory limitation, and this was 3.5 times as common in the smokers as in the nonsmokers. Cardiac limitation on exercise was present in 37% of the subjects and was more common than ventilatory limitation, suggesting that dyspnea was more likely to be related to cardiac rather than to lung disease. A further study of 348 asbestos-exposed subjects who had been referred by the United States Department of Labor resulted in rather similar findings.[89] Sue et al. showed that the FEF_{25-75} did not identify airways obstruction that had not been detected by the $FEV_1/FVC\%$. The $A-a(O_2)$ was more often abnormal in smokers than in nonsmokers. The authors concluded that smoking was the main cause of airways obstruction and also made a major contribution to limitation of exercise in this group of 348 men.

Much has recently been made of small airways dysfunction in asbestos-exposed populations since such changes are evident pathologically.[90] According to Rodriguez-Roisin et al., maximal expiratory flow volume curves may be abnormal despite a normal TLC and FVC; however, this study included only three lifelong nonsmokers in the group of 40.[91] It might be argued that persons who had smoked for some time and had then given the habit up some years previously should not be regarded as nonsmokers and that it could not be guaranteed that their former habit had no effect on their lung mechanics. Other studies purported to show that small airways disease is common and is associated with symptoms and a lower FEF_{25-75} and occasionally with a reduced FEV_1.[92, 93] However, many of the subjects in these latter two studies were seeking compensation and, as such, are not comparable to a general population of asbestos workers. Moreover, it is apparent that the FEF_{25-75} is an unsatisfactory test unless corrected for lung volumes and is no longer recommended as an accurate measure of airways obstruction.[94] The problem of small airways disease has been admirably put into perspective by Bègin et al.[95] These investigators used complete and sophisticated tests of lung mechanics and went on to calculate upstream airways resistance and isoflow volumes. They showed that lifelong nonsmoking asbestos workers had small airways obstruction develop which was associated with an increased upstream resistance. The airflow limitation was seen mainly in those with pulmonary restrictive impairment. In those who had no real restrictive impairment, the effects on small airways function were minimal and unlikely to be associated with symptoms.

Studies of regional lung function have shown that there is impaired ventilation in the lower zones of subjects who have asbestosis, but in subjects with circumscribed pleural plaques, basal ventilation is not impaired.[96]

The physiological determination of pulmonary impairment in asbestos-exposed populations may be imprecise and inaccurate, especially in those seeking compensation.[97] This may result from submaximal efforts during the performance of spirometry and during the measurement in of the DL_{CO}, from the effects of smoking, and from other naturally occurring disease. Moreover, some subjects either misrepresent or downplay their cigarette smoking histories.[98] The determination of a carboxyhemoglobin level should be an important component of disability determination in such subjects. The emphasis that is placed on certain sophisticated tests, such as the FEF_{25-75}, flows at low lung volumes, and tests of small airways function, e.g., closing volume, are inappropriate since these tests, while interesting physiologically, play no role in the determination of disability.

Finally, it is imperative to use appropriate reference values and predictive equations for the subjects being tested.[94] These need to take into account racial differences and also the avoidance of predicted values based on a population from one region of a country which may bear little relationship to a normal population from a different region or country. Similarly, the pseudorestrictive effects of obesity on lung function often go unrecognized.

Diagnosis of Asbestosis

The diagnosis of asbestosis usually has to be made without a histological examination of lung tissue since it is rarely justifiable to carry out an open biopsy of the lung to establish a diagnosis for compensation purposes only. The diagnosis of asbestosis must be based on a careful consideration of all relevant clinical findings but ultimately depends on clinical judgment. The essential criteria for a diagnosis of asbestosis are as follows.[99]

1. **A suitable history of exposure to asbestos.** In this regard, it is necessary to take into account not only the duration of exposure but also the dates and decades during which most of the exposure took place. In the 1940s and 1950s, asbestosis became evident in a significant number of subjects after 10 to 15 years of exposure; however, since the adoption of the 2-f/cc TLV, the likelihood of asbestosis developing in a subject in a comparable period is remote. Thus, the prevalence of asbestosis in one mill in Great Britain fell from 80% to 3% from 1929 to 1957.[100] In this context, there has to be a suitable interval between first exposure and when the disease becomes detectable.
2. **The presence of small irregular opacities of the s, t, and u type in the chest radiograph.** In most instances, a profusion of 1/1 or more provides strong circumstantial evidence that fibrosis is present, although it by no means indicates the cause of such fibrosis. Category 1/0 is regarded by the International Labour Office as the earliest category suggesting asbestosis. It must also be remembered that other conditions, in particular, cigarette smoking, are frequently associated with the development of irregular opacities in the lower zones, although for the most part, the profusion of such opacities is seldom greater than 1/0 or 1/1, a range at which interobserver error in readings of 0/1 to 1/1 is appreciable.[63, 64]
3. **A characteristic pattern of lung impairment with a FVC below the lower limit of normal.** A concomitant and comparable reduction of the FEV_1 and TLC should also be present. An isolated reduction of the FVC in the absence of other criteria for the diagnosis cannot be relied upon, particularly in the presence

of even moderate obesity. Abnormalities of gas transfer, as exemplified by a reduction in the DL_{CO} are common, even in early disease, but are nonspecific.[84, 85]

4. **The presence of bilateral middle to late inspiratory crackles at the lung bases with, in some instances, the crackles being heard elsewhere in the lungs.** Crackles usually manifest themselves first in the posterior basal regions of the lungs.

The most important criteria for a diagnosis of asbestosis are a suitable history of exposure and, in addition, definite radiographic evidence compatible with interstitial fibrosis. Even when both are present, considerable caution is necessary, and it is appropriate to look for other criteria to make the diagnosis more certain. The validity of the diagnosis increases with the increasing number of positive criteria. There are rare occasions when asbestosis may be present in the absence of a radiographic abnormality, but such cases usually need confirmation by biopsy.[101]

In making a diagnosis of asbestosis, it must be remembered that crackles may be heard in 5% to 8% of normal subjects,[102] that the radiographic changes of asbestosis may be mimicked by other interstitial disorders and by the effects of cigarette smoking,[63, 64] and that the same pattern of lung function abnormalities may be seen in all forms of interstitial fibrosis of the lungs. In this context, it is pertinent to bear in mind that cryptogenic fibrosing alveolitis and other causes of interstitial fibrosis can occur in asbestos-exposed workers.[103] In a study of 176 asbestos-exposed persons in whom lung tissue was available, nine were found to have the clinical features of asbestosis, but light microscopic examination of the lung tissue did not demonstrate asbestos bodies. Lung tissue from these nine were compared by analytical electron microscopy with lung tissue from nine persons with idiopathic pulmonary fibrosis and also with tissue from nine persons who met the American Thoracic Society (ATS) criteria for asbestosis.[99] The lung burdens for chrysotile, actinolite, and tremolite in all three groups were similar. In those subjects who had the criteria for asbestosis, the lung burdens for amosite and crocidolite were three to four orders of magnitude greater than that in the others.[103] These results indicate that nonspecific interstitial lung disease among asbestos-exposed persons seems to be higher than expected because of the method of case selection in those who undergo biopsy.

Pathological Findings

The early lesion in animals and humans is located in the alveoli and bronchioles. After the deposition of asbestos fibers, macrophages migrate into the terminal bronchioloalveolar units. With severe exposure, an alveolitis develops, and if the exposure persists, the alveolitis progresses and is accompanied by the deposition of fibrous proteins and in particular collagen.[5, 21] As a result, the lungs become noncompliant and stiffer. Even though the lower regions of the lungs are most affected, autopsy studies show that the whole lung is involved, although there may be regional differences in the degree of alveolitis and fibrosis.[104] Macroscopically, the lungs are of a nondescript gray color, are shriveled, and contracted, with the fibrosis being most marked in the lower lobes (Fig. 14–7). Large conglomerate shadows are rare, as indicated in the section dealing with the radiologic findings of asbestosis; however, Caplan nodules may be found in asbestosis.[24]

Inhaled asbestos is deposited in the lungs as a fiber. With the passage of time, many asbestos fibers in the lung become coated with a proteinaceous iron-staining material, which leads to the formation of asbestos bodies that have a characteristic appearance.[18, 104, 105] The shaft or body tends to be beaded, while the ends appear clubbed. The asbestos body appears as a yellowish intercalated structure varying from 10 to 115 μm in length and develops initially within macrophages. The fibers become coated with ferritin. The iron-containing protein stains with potassium ferricyanide, producing the brilliant Prussian blue hue. It is the deposition of ferritin

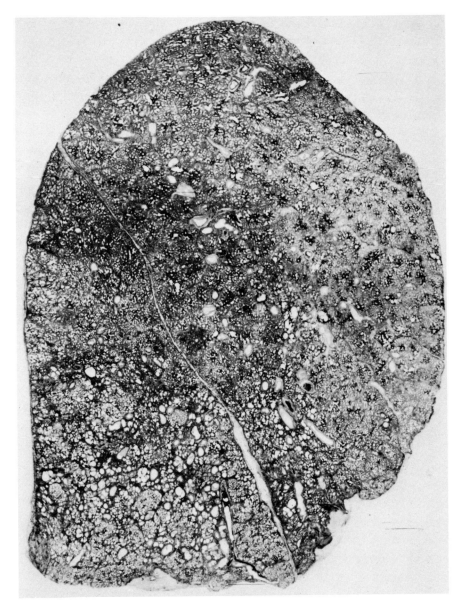

Figure 14–7. Whole-lung (Gough) section from patient with asbestosis, showing fibrotic changes and cyst formation in the lower lobe, with less marked changes in the lingula.

that is responsible for the tuberous appearance of the asbestos body. Similar-appearing bodies may be formed from talc fibers, aluminum whiskers, fiberglass, silicon carbide, and other fibers. Hence, it is preferable to refer to the characteristic iron-coated fiber as a ferruginous body until the core has been identified *(vide infra)*.

The *sine qua non* of asbestosis is the presence of fibrosis in association with numerous asbestos bodies (Fig. 14–8). Fibrosis by itself does not denote asbestosis, and even if there are a few asbestos bodies, this in itself does not make a diagnosis of asbestosis unless such bodies are suitably numerous.

Asbestos is found in the lung as bare or uncoated fibers and as coated fibers or asbestos bodies (Fig. 14–9). The latter are easily seen with a light microscope and are specific markers of asbestos exposure. In contrast, uncoated fibers are mostly invisible in normal histological sections with most being below the resolu-

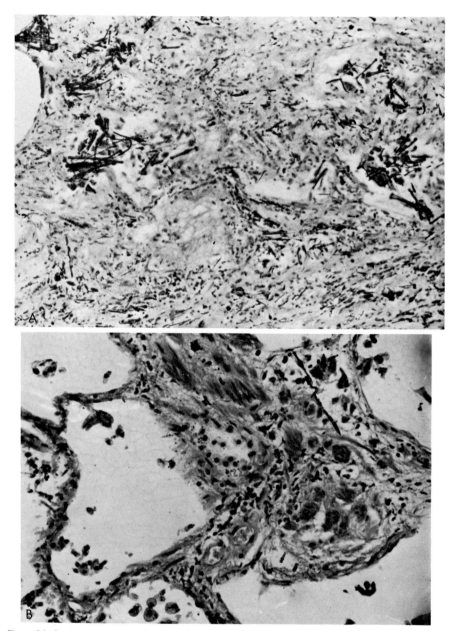

Figure 14–8. *A,* Low-power photomicrograph of lung of patient with severe asbestosis, showing masses of asbestos bodies and fibers situated in air spaces distorted by fibrosis. *B,* Medium-power photomicrograph of lung from an early case of asbestosis, showing relatively few asbestos bodies in a focus of interstitial fibrosis.

tion of the light microscope[106] (see Fig. 14–9*B*). Moreover, should a fiber be detected by optical microscopy, there is no way of demonstrating whether it is an asbestos body or a ferruginous body formed from talc, fiberglass, or other fibers that may be present in the lung. For the most part, asbestos fibers that have been in the body for any length of time lose their birefringence when viewed with polarized light. The available evidence suggests that, at the present time, once the fiber is coated, it can no longer induce fibrosis and, moreover, is not carcinogenic.[106–108]

Asbestos bodies were first described in nonoccupationally exposed urban dwellers by Thomson et al.[109] Subsequently, it was shown that the lungs of normal urban dwellers in North America and Europe contain a limited number of asbestos

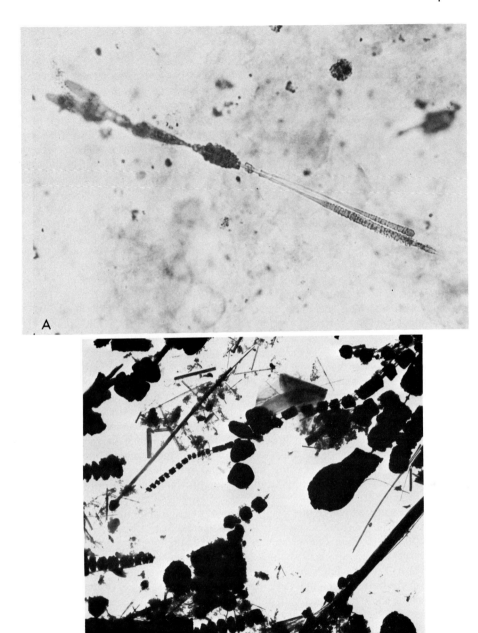

Figure 14–9. *A,* Two asbestos fibers, approximately 100 μm long, coated with iron-protein complex, from sputum of patient exposed to asbestos dust. *B,* Electron micrograph (×5000) showing asbestos bodies and fibers in lung tissue. Note the relative thinness of the fibers compared with the bodies. Many fibers are seen to be uncoated, and their diameters would put them beyond the power of resolution of light microscopy.

bodies.[110, 111] Their presence does not denote disease, and as far as is known at the present time, they are unassociated with any other clinical manifestations of asbestos exposure. It is extremely unlikely that they ever lead to any clinical manifestations of asbestos-related disease. Asbestos bodies are also often found in the sputum of persons exposed to asbestos (see Fig. 14–9A), whether or not they have asbestosis, and they may continue to be expectorated for years after exposure has ceased.

The number of asbestos bodies in the sputum is related, albeit imprecisely, to the extent of prior exposure.[112]

Other bodies with an identical appearance to asbestos bodies may be found in the lungs of nonasbestos-exposed subjects.[105, 106, 110] These likewise are coated or lined with ferritin and appear similar, and for this reason, it is probably preferable to refer to such bodies as ferruginous bodies until it has been proved that their core consists of asbestos. Gross et al. showed that ferruginous bodies may develop from glass wool, talc, fibrous alumina, silicon carbide, and various phyllosilicates but can, however, be differentiated from true asbestos bodies by electron microscopy, which enables identification of the ferruginous body's core.[110] They also inferred, incorrectly, that most of the so-called ferruginous bodies found in the lungs of the general population did not arise from asbestos exposure. This was shown by Langer et al. not to be the case.[113] These workers were able to demonstrate that, with energy dispersive x-ray analysis of the individual cores, nearly all such ferruginous bodies were composed of asbestos. It now seems that, with the exception of erionite, any ferruginous body with a clear, usually straight, and colorless core, as seen with an optical microscope, can be assumed to be an asbestos body.

Quantitative assessment of the number of asbestos bodies present in the lung can be made by counting the number of asbestos bodies in tissue sections. This is relatively inaccurate, and there is a variation in the number of bodies between different lobes and different regions of the lung.[42] It has been shown that the number of asbestos bodies varies between the right and left lungs and between different lobes of lung.[45, 114] In general, the number of asbestos fibers tends to be greater in the upper than in the lower lobes.

Similar observations have been made with uncoated fibers, which tend to be twice as common in the upper lobes as in the lower.[115] Churg studied the concentration of amosite fibers in the periphery of normal human lung tissue.[116] He showed that the concentration is greatest in the apex and least in the periphery of the lower lobe. This distribution is the opposite to what we would expect based on the characteristic findings of the most severe fibrosis being commonly located in the lower lobes. The type of asbestos that is found in the lungs of nonoccupationally exposed persons varies according to the region in which the subject lives. Thus, in Vancouver, Churg found 0.3×10^6 fibers of chrysotile and 0.4×10^6 fibers of tremolite compared with 0.001×10^6 fibers of amosite and crocidolite present per gram of dry lung tissue.[106] The weight of an average pair of dried normal lungs is around 40 g, affording an approximate estimate of the total lung burden. Different proportions of the various types of asbestos, however, have been found by Churg and Warnock in the lungs of the inhabitants of San Francisco[111] compared with those of Vancouver. Although the amphiboles are relatively indestructible and tend to persist in the lungs almost indefinitely, it is now realized that chrysotile leaches out and that the number of chrysotile fibers present in the lungs declines significantly with the passage of time. Even so, studies of miners with established fibrosis in Quebec show that numerous asbestos bodies are present. The number of cores composed of tremolite is about the same or slightly exceeds those of chrysotile. In addition, many uncoated fibers may also be found.[104, 117, 118]

There is a continuum in the number of fibers that may be present in the lungs. Thus, there are relatively few to be found in the lungs of urban dwellers who are not occupationally exposed, but with appropriate methods, at least a few fibers can be demonstrated post mortem in almost 100% of such persons.[106] Subjects with severe established asbestosis show the greatest number of fibers. Those patients with asbestos-induced conditions that are dose related, namely, asbestosis, asbestos-induced lung cancer, and mesothelioma, all have a large number of fibers present in the lungs, and this is particularly true for asbestos-induced lung cancer and asbestosis. As mentioned earlier, an excess risk of lung cancer is seen only in subjects who have overt asbestosis. The number of fibers present in the lungs of subjects with mesothelioma is appreciably less but is still much greater than previously recognized. Table 14–2 shows the range of fibers found in the lungs of

Table 14–2
■
Fiber Content ($\times$ 10^6 gm of Dry Lung)

Urban Dwellers (No Occupational Exposure)	Coated	Uncoated	Both
North America	< 0.001	< 0.025	< 0.05
United Kingdom[41]	—	0.01	—
Australia[119]	—	95% < 0.25	—
Occupational exposure			
No fibrosis: occupational exposure	0.02–0.07	0.10–0.30	0.2–0.4
Plaques	0.1–0.8	0.3–1.0	0.25–2.0
Mesothelioma	0.10–10	0.5–50	0.2–100
Mild fibrosis	0.1–20	1.0–50	1.0–60
Moderate fibrosis	0.5–50	2.0–200	2.5–300
Severe fibrosis	20–150	80–2000	80–2500

various occupationally and nonoccupationally exposed groups. Although the data in the table are based on a variety of studies published by other investigators, it must be realized that comparisons between them are difficult since, after several laboratories have examined the same tissues, the absolute fiber counts were found to vary widely. Such differences are probably a consequence of differing methods and techniques. Nevertheless, all laboratories showed concordance in reporting high, medium, and low numbers of fibers. Thus, there was a consensus among laboratories as far as what constituted high and low fiber counts, and there was usually agreement between the fiber burden and the specific disease diagnosed.

It is essential to express the fiber count as number of fibers per gram of dry lungs. Subjects dying with pulmonary edema or extensive pneumonia have heavy lungs, and if the fiber count is expressed per gram of wet lung, there may be an underestimation. It must also be realized that it is futile to seek asbestos fibers in neoplastic tissue since there are virtually none present in lung cancer itself, and the same is usually true for mesothelioma. In contrast, the lungs in a subject with mesothelioma usually show numerous coated and uncoated fibers.[41, 119] All in all, there is little doubt that fiber counting provides valuable data in relation to the number of asbestos bodies necessary to induce the various manifestations of asbestos exposure.

Mechanisms in Asbestosis with Reference to Bronchoalveolar Lavage

Bronchoalveolar lavage (BAL) has been used to determine asbestos disease mechanisms in humans and provides some assessment of the type of inflammatory process implied by the term *asbestosis*. The features of such lavage include (1) a polymorphonuclear leukocytosis of up to 10% in nonsmokers and a significantly higher response in smokers with asbestosis; (2) on occasion, excess eosinophils; (3) variable reports of lymphocyte patterns with small increases but little change in the helper/suppressor cell ratios (CD4-CD8) (changes in cytotoxic lymphocytes have, however, been described in workers with pleural plaques); (4) asbestos bodies are also in the BAL fluid and, although found in nonoccupationally exposed subjects, in an increased prevalence in persons with asbestosis; and (5) no report of excess basophils, which occur in idiopathic pulmonary fibrosis.

The main features of asbestosis are those of a neutrophilic alveolitis and are similar to those found in fibrosing alveolitis and the pulmonary fibroses that are found in association with collagen vascular disease.[120] The presence of neutrophils implies the chronic production of oxidizing agents, such as hydrogen peroxide, superoxide anion, and so forth, which are consistent with the latter's role in tissue injury (Chapter 11). In addition, free active leukocyte collagenase has been detected in BAL fluid from asbestotic subjects. This enzyme, which degrades certain collagen types, is not inhibited by the major BAL fluid antiprotease, alpha-1-antiprotease, the activity of which is impaired by the oxidants. Thus, two components of the tissue injury mechanisms are identifiable in BAL fluid. The finding of neutrophils in BAL fluid implies the presence of chemotaxins. There are several cytokines with such activities, some of which have been identified in BAL fluid. These are produced by alveolar macrophages exposed to asbestos fibers *in vitro*. Also, interferon-gamma, a lymphokine, is also released from asbestos-exposed macrophages. There is preliminary evidence that an active BAL fluid inflammatory process is associated with epithelial cell dysplasia, a mechanism that may play a role in the airways neoplasia that occurs in asbestosis.[121]

Although clearly not generally necessary in clinical investigation, BAL has shed light on the mechanisms of asbestosis and can be used to detect an alveolitis before radiological or lung function abnormalities become apparent. These features also suggest possible therapeutic applications. Antioxidants, e.g., retinols and vitamin A, may be of benefit, and liposomes that contain superoxide dismutase or catalase ameliorate experimental asbestosis. Further agents that impair neutrophil diapedesis may be useful, e.g., the quinolines (mepacrine), which reduce leukocyte migration into the alveoli and decrease macrophage-derived chemotactic factor in acute silica installation experiments.[122]

Pleural Reactions to Asbestos

The pleural reactions to asbestos can be divided into pleural plaques (circumscribed pleural thickening), pleural effusion, and diffuse pleural thickening. The latter is usually a complication of an asbestos-induced effusion.

Pleural Plaques

The first description of pleural plaques in association with asbestos exposure is probably that of Sparks, who described small irregular calcific deposits on the diaphragmatic pleura and along the lower thoracic walls.[123] Other isolated descriptions of extensive pleural thickening in asbestotic patients are to be found in the publications of Wood and Gloyne[22] and of Dreessen et al.,[5] but the latent period for the development of asbestosis in the 1920s and 1930s was generally too short for plaques to develop. Thus, many subjects had died from the effects of asbestosis before there was time for pleural plaques to become obvious. Moreover, in many instances, pleural plaques and diffuse pleural thickening were attributed to tuberculosis, despite the lack of an ability to demonstrate tubercle bacilli. Pleural calcification similarly usually takes at least 20 years to become obvious radiographically, and then only around 5% of those with plaques show calcification.[124]

The best early descriptions of pleural plaques and calcification can be found in the reports of Porro et al.[125] and of Siegal et al.[126] These were published in the early 1940s and were based on observations made in talc workers. Subsequently, Cartier[127] and Lynch and Cannon[128] in the late 1940s recognized bilateral pleural calcification as an effect of exposure to asbestos.

Pleural plaques were first described as *zuckerguss* or sugar icing.[129] Later, Bohlig et al. coined the term *harmlos-skurriller Schönheitsfehler,* i.e., harmless beauty marks.[130] Presumably, this complimentary term originated because it was thought that pleural plaques were benign and unassociated with either symptoms or impairment.

Over the past 30 years, there have been a number of publications that have studied the effects of asbestos-induced pleural thickening on lung function.[131] Unfortunately, most of these publications did not distinguish or separate pleural plaques (circumscribed thickening) from diffuse pleural thickening. The latter condition might more aptly be termed a fibrothorax. An asbestos-induced effusion which is complicated by the development of a pleural peel, a complication that also occurs in other conditions such as tuberculous pleurisy, hemothorax, and empyema, frequently results in restrictive impairment and breathlessness.

Pleural plaques are most commonly found on the lower lateral chest wall and on the central portion of the diaphragm (Figs. 14–10 and 14–11). Although they seldom become radiographically evident in less than 15 years from first exposure, once they appear, they usually slowly increase in size. Calcification starts about 10 to 15 years after first exposure but does not become evident radiographically until later. The proportion of subjects with radiographic evidence of calcification increases significantly with the further passage of time.[124] Pleural thickening and calcification induced by asbestos-free talc cannot be distinguished radiographically from that produced by asbestos. Calcification of the pericardium may also occur (Fig. 14–12). In general, most plaques start on the lateral wall and tend to extend around the curvature of the chest, either anteriorly or posteriorly, but this is by no means invariable. Plaques may form on the anterior or posterior thoracic walls rather than the lateral chest wall, but this is somewhat unusual. When such *en face* plaques are evident on the chest x-ray film, they appear often as ''crab-like'' outlines with no clear superior margin (Fig. 14–13). In around 80% of asbestos workers who worked during the 1950s and 1960s and who had more than 5 years of exposure, small mushroom-like plaques could be identified post mortem on the diaphragmatic pleura. In most instances, these were not apparent on the plain radiograph.

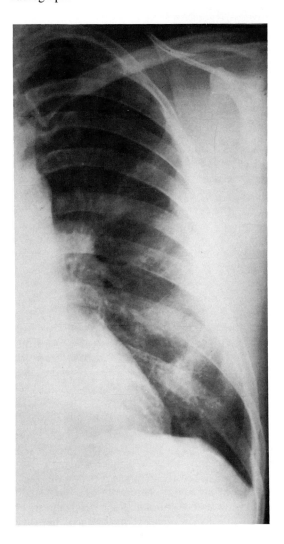

Figure 14–10
Radiograph showing lateral wall and *en face* pleural thickening. A fleck of calcium is present in the left diaphragm.

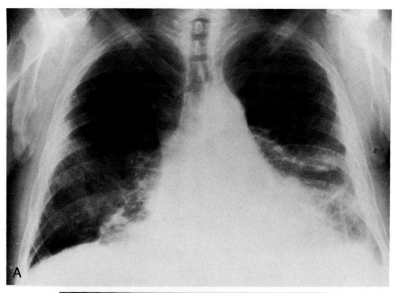

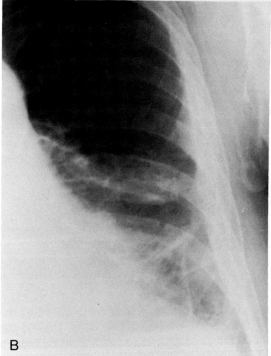

Figure 14–11. *A*, Radiograph showing lateral wall and diffuse thickening on the left side. The right side shows *en face* thickening and early circumscribed thickening on the lateral wall. Note the ill-defined heart shadow. *B*, Magnified view of the left side of the subject shown in *A*. Note the diffuse haziness and opacification in the left lower and middle zones.

Radiographically, the pleural plaque appears on the lower third of the chest wall as a smooth regular linear shadow that bridges the gap between the ribs.[132] The width of the plaque often varies appreciably. *En face* plaques situated on the anterior or posterior chest wall are often mistaken for parenchymal disease. Such plaques, however, seldom can be seen on the lateral chest wall, and this should alert the interpreter that the shadow seen on the PA radiograph probably arises from the pleura. Oblique films often delineate the plaques more clearly, but they

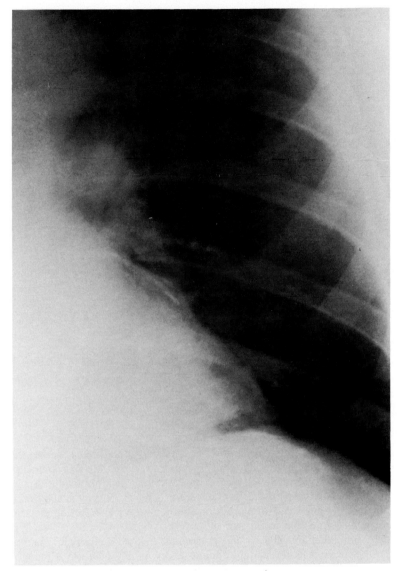

Figure 14–12. Radiograph showing pericardial calcification.

also introduce a number of false-positive readings.[133] CT scanning remains the "gold standard" that provides the ideal way of demonstrating pleural plaques and minor calcifications, but it should be remembered that no standard scans for categorizing pleural thickening or parenchymal fibrosis exist. Pericardial calcification may also be demonstrated by means of CT scans and is often found in association with pleural plaques. Calcification usually begins at the periphery of the pleural plaque, and it is the deposition of calcium that creates the crab-like outline. Under such circumstances, calcification of the *en face* plaque appears as a circinate margin.

The differential diagnosis of pleural plaques, especially in the absence of calcification, is frequently difficult. In the overweight population found in North America, pleural fat pads commonly mimic pleural plaques[134] (Fig. 14–14). Typically, a pleural fat pad starts at the apex, runs down the lateral wall, and may extend to the costodiaphragmatic junction. In some instances, extrathoracic fat can also produce an appearance suggesting extensive pleural thickening. A careful study

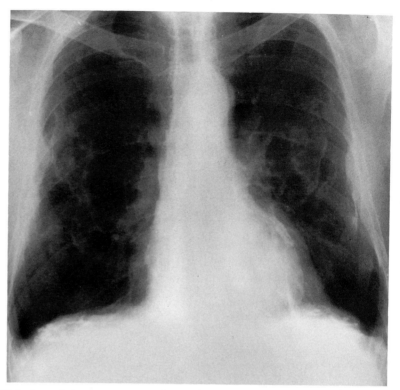

Figure 14–13. Radiograph showing extensive *en face* and diaphragmatic calcification. Note the crab-like contours in the *en face* pleural calcifications.

of the extrathoracic shadows, however, shows how they overlap the thoracic cage. This finding is helpful in distinguishing fat pads from true thickening. Extrathoracic muscles, in particular, the serratus anterior, may also mimic pleural plaques. Such shadows often extend outside the thoracic cage and tend to be saw-shaped and regular. Companion shadows can similarly cause difficulties in interpreting pleural plaques. Tuberculous infection and a hemothorax may lead to calcification, but they are usually unilateral and involve the visceral rather than the parietal pleura. Rib fractures likewise can, under certain circumstances, mimic plaques. Although silicosis can cause pleural calcification, this is less common and is usually associated with eggshell calcification of the hilar glands. The calcification induced by talc is clinically and radiographically indistinguishable from that induced by asbestos; however, it is uncommon to see parenchymal disease associated with talc-induced plaques. In contrast, pleural plaques are found in many subjects who also have definite asbestosis. Rarely, pleural plaques are seen in "bystanders" or family members who have not been occupationally exposed (Fig. 14–15).

It has also been suggested that visceral pleural thickening is a useful indicator of asbestos exposure.[135] Although it is correct to maintain that visceral thickening occurs fairly frequently after prolonged asbestos exposure in the absence of asbestosis and, indeed, may undergo calcification, there are many other causes of visceral pleural thickening, including pneumonia, tuberculosis, pulmonary embolism, and other conditions. Rockoff et al., in their article, compared their asbestos-exposed cohort with a reference population who had no known asbestos exposure and who were selected from a group of 257 patients of whom 157 were then excluded because of either inadequate radiographs or a history of thoracic trauma or pulmonary or heart disease.[135] Clearly, the reference group should have included those with pulmonary and cardiac disease since only by doing so is it possible to determine the sensitivity, specificity, and predictive value of visceral pleural thick-

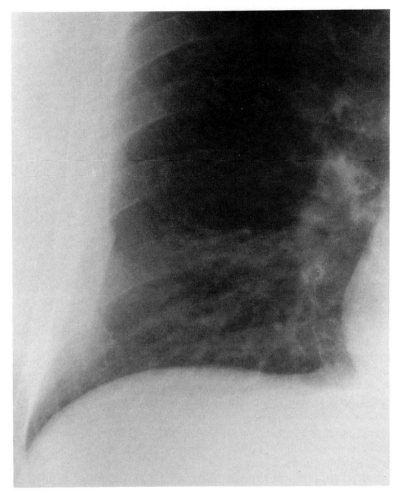

Figure 14-14. Radiograph showing subject with extensive pleural and chest wall fat mimicking pleural thickening. Confirmation obtained by CT scanning.

ening. It is apparent that such pleural changes are relatively nonspecific and are found in a variety of thoracic diseases. As such, little reliance can be placed on them as an index of asbestos exposure. It is probably simpler to take a work history!

Certain investigations have suggested that cigarette smoking increases the prevalence of pleural disease in those exposed to asbestos.[136] Whether this is really so is uncertain, especially in the absence of confirmation by CT scanning. There is no doubt that many smokers, especially those who also consume alcohol, tend to be heavier than nonsmokers and are more likely to have pleural fat pads diagnosed, at least in a plain chest radiograph.

Pleural Plaques and Lung Function

The effects of pleural plaques on lung function have become a source of contention. There are a number of explanations for the disparate findings and divergent opinions as to whether circumscribed plaques induce significant respiratory impairment. First, as mentioned, many investigators have included in their study population all subjects who have pleural thickening, whether circumscribed or diffuse. Thus, it is well accepted that many subjects with diffuse pleural thickening have a significant reduction in lung volumes and evidence of restrictive

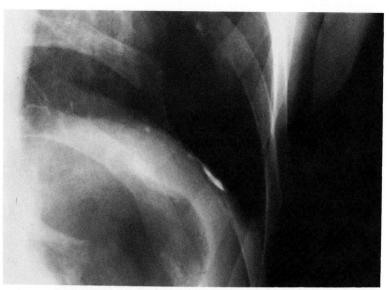

Figure 14–15. Calcified diaphragmatic pleural plaque in a 32-year-old woman whose father was an insulator. She herself had never worked with asbestos. (Courtesy of Dr. D. Ahmad.)

impairment.[137] This type of diffuse thickening is recognized and distinguished from circumscribed pleural thickening by obliteration of the costophrenic angle and evidence of a fibrothorax. Second, in the presence of pleural changes, in particular, in those with extensive *en face* thickening, it is often impossible to exclude parenchymal fibrosis unless a high-resolution CT scan has been carried out.[60, 75–77] Third, in some instances, the investigators have ignored the effects of smoking and obesity on lung function and have chosen either an unrepresentative study population or have not used a suitable reference group.

Oliver et al. claim to have demonstrated restrictive impairment in subjects with asbestos-related pleural plaques.[138] Their exposed subjects were 8 years older and, in addition, significantly heavier smokers than was their control group. No data for mean weight were available, and it appears that the evidence for pleural plaques was based on the interpretation of one reader, although three readers were involved. Fridriksson et al., in a study of Swedish workers exposed to asbestos, found that those with pleural plaques had significantly reduced lung volumes and also stiffer lungs.[139] They concluded, however, that the lung function changes were a consequence of parenchymal asbestosis rather than pleural plaques. In a recent article, Bourbeau et al. claimed that "the complaint of dyspnea with strenuous activities was also significantly related to the width and extent of chest wall thickening independent of parenchymal disease."[140] These authors went on to assert that, in asbestos-exposed subjects, "isolated pleural plaques were associated with a significant reduction in the FEV_1 and FVC which cannot be attributed to the presence of radiographic or subradiographic pulmonary fibrosis." The group of subjects who were selected with pleural thickening were then subdivided into those with diffuse and circumscribed thickening. As controls, they used a group of asbestos workers without evidence of pleural thickening. Unfortunately, those with pleural changes were older, appreciably fatter, shorter, and smoked more than did the controls. It became evident that the severity of any breathlessness that was noted in those with circumscribed pleural thickening did not differ significantly from the reference population, once smoking had been taken into account. Although the FEV_1 and FVC were slightly lower in those with isolated pleural plaques than in the controls, only the FVC achieved statistical significance, and the mean difference was 70 ml. In true restrictive impairment, one would expect both the FEV_1

and the FVC to be reduced to the same extent, along with a similar decrement in the TLC.

Another recent report claimed to have shown that circumscribed pleural plaques had an effect on lung function, but the subject selection and methods are suspect.[141] All active and retired members of a Sheet Metal Workers' Union were offered a union-sponsored medical evaluation. Of those contacted, only 46% (1223 subjects) participated. It is likely that those who did so were more likely to have symptoms and to be interested in compensation, and many went on to seek compensation as a result of the examination. Moreover, spirometry was not carried out according to ATS standards, and nose clips were not used. All subjects who underwent spirometry were included, irrespective of reproducibility. In addition, the radiographs were interpreted by only one physician. CT scans were not done to exclude pleural fat or to ascertain whether there was significant parenchymal disease. The same investigators subsequently selected 24 subjects from this population.[142] Those chosen were all described as nonsmokers; however, the definition of a nonsmoker included both lifelong nonsmokers and those who had stopped smoking at least 5 years previously. In this study, the spirometric values of those with circumscribed pleural plaques did not differ significantly from the predicted values, although a trend was present.

In contrast to these studies, a carefully carried out study of 1764 persons employed in two large shipyards, three mills, and one asbestos plant was recently published by Gaensler et al.[143] One group of control subjects included 100 normal men older than 40 years of age who had no asbestos exposure and no discernible lung disease. These men presented for pre-employment examinations. The second control group consisted of 154 persons who had been exposed to asbestos for 15 or more years but who had normal radiographs. This group was matched for age and years of exposure with a third group who had circumscribed plaques without diffuse thickening or asbestosis. Among the study group of 1764 subjects with circumscribed plaques, 218 had circumscribed plaques without other abnormalities, and 176 had plaques and asbestosis. Two B readers were used for the examination, one of whom was unaware of the nature and type of exposure. There were 218 persons with circumscribed pleural plaques without diffuse thickening or asbestosis. The lung function with respect to volume, flow, and gas exchange was no different from that of the 150 persons matched for age and years since first exposure who had no detectable plaques or from that of the 100 nonexposed normal subjects. Subjects with diffuse pleural thickening had a significant loss of ventilatory function, especially in regard to lung volumes. Those with circumscribed pleural plaques showed no evidence of a reduction in the DL_{CO}, unless asbestosis was present. In contrast, those with diffuse pleural thickening had a reduction of the DL_{CO} commensurate with the degree of pleural thickening and the decrement in lung volumes.

The evidence at the present time suggests that isolated pleural plaques in the absence of asbestosis or diffuse thickening are not associated with clinically detectable restrictive impairment. Studies purporting to show such a decrement usually have flaws in their methods or in their selection of subjects. Even if it is conceded that there may be a reduction in lung volumes in those with isolated circumscribed pleural plaques, such a reduction as that described by Borbeau et al., i.e., 70 ml in the FVC, is minimal and would be most unlikely to be associated with breathlessness.[140]

Pathological Findings

On pleuroscopy, at postmortem examination, or during thoracic surgery, pleural plaques appear as shiny, white, slightly raised areas—the sugar icing already mentioned.[144] They are located on the parietal thoracic wall and the diaphragmatic pleura (Fig. 14–16). Microscopically, they consist of hyaline fibrous tissue, which is almost completely acellular[145] (Fig. 14–17). There are no inflammatory cells

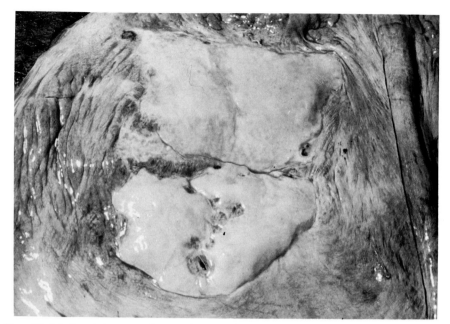

Figure 14–16. Pleural plaques on the central tendon of the diaphragm of a subject who had died of myocardial infarction but who had a history of exposure to asbestos in the building trade.

present in the center of the plaque, but a few low-grade inflammatory changes may be present peripherally. For the most part, plaques are covered by normal mesothelial cells. Asbestos fibers, whether coated or bare, are only very exceptionally found in pleural plaques.[144–147]

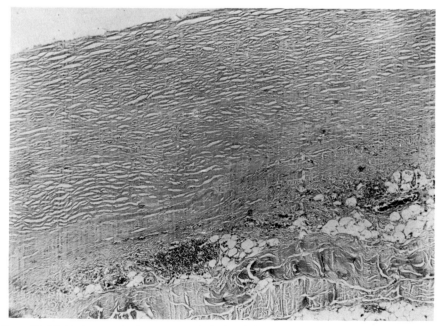

Figure 14–17. Medium-power photomicrograph of pleural plaque showing rows of collagen fibers lying parallel to the surface. The deeper layers contain a few lymphocytes and plasma cells.

Pleural Effusion and Diffuse Pleural Thickening

In 1964, Eisenstadt described an insulator who developed a pleural effusion and suggested that it was related to the inhalation of asbestos.[148] He called the condition "asbestos pleurisy." After his description, a series of additional reports was published.[149-153] Asbestos-induced pleural effusion tends to occur 10 to 15 years after first exposure, but in a few instances, the latent period may be longer. The affected worker usually has few, if any, symptoms, and it is often only later that it is evident from the chest radiograph that the patient has had previous pleurisy with effusion (Fig. 14–18). The effusion tends to persist for several months and often recurs after drainage. Not infrequently, the affected worker may have bilateral effusions. In a few subjects, one side is first affected, and then 1 to 2 years later, an effusion develops on the opposite side.

Shortness of breath and pleuritic pain are the most common symptoms and, initially, may be severe, but they ameliorate with time. However, they may persist for several months. In many instances, pain is absent, and there is a lack of constitutional symptoms. On aspiration, the fluid is usually clear and serous or occasionally fibrinous; not uncommonly, it is hemorrhagic.[153-155] Eosinophils are often present in the fluid and usually indicate prior hemorrhage.[154] The fluid is an exudate with a mixture of cells, including both polymorphonuclear leukocytes and mononuclear cells. Asbestos fibers are not found in the fluid; usually, a needle biopsy specimen of the pleura shows a nonspecific pleuritis. At pleuroscopy, small diaphragmatic plaques may be observed on the parietal chest wall and also on the diaphragmatic pleura.

The development of an unexplained pleural effusion in a middle-aged or elderly man or woman should prompt the patient's physician to ask about exposure to talc or asbestos. In a few instances, the exposure may have occurred while the subject was a bystander or as a result of an avocation. Under such circumstances, the worker was exposed when coworkers were using asbestos, asbestos insulation was installed in the home, or asbestos-containing materials were used for alterations in the home.

Some subjects who have had an asbestos effusion are left with a significant

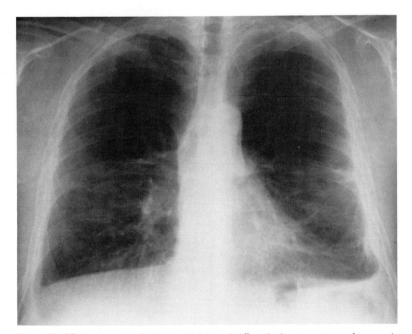

Figure 14–18. Radiograph of subject with bilateral diffuse thickening owing to former asbestos-induced pleural effusions.

fibrothorax.[143, 156] This can be detected on physical examination and is sometimes mistaken on radiological examination for a residual pleural effusion. In general, when there is a significant fibrothorax, the rib spaces are crowded, and the thoracic volume on the affected side is reduced. Radiographically, the costophrenic angle is virtually always obliterated. An asbestos-induced pleural effusion uncommonly leaves a peel, which encases one or the other upper lobe, or occasionally both, causing the formation of a cuirasse on the affected side or sides (Fig. 14–19).[157]

In subjects in whom a significant fibrous peel develops, there is a proclivity to carry out decortication, but this is seldom beneficial. In practice, most fibrothoraces that have followed an effusion tend to improve over a 2- to 3-year period. Moreover, pleurectomy seldom improves function, mainly because the operation itself is usually associated with vigorous bleeding, which in time becomes organized and replaces the original fibrothorax with another.

Epler et al. reported a greater prevalence of idiopathic effusions among asbestos-exposed workers than in workers not exposed to asbestos; in addition, they demonstrated a dose-response relationship between asbestos exposure and the occurrence of pleural effusions.[153]

Pleural Plaques and Lung Cancer

There are a few studies that have suggested that the presence of pleural plaques is associated with an increased incidence of lung cancer. A number of problems exist, not the least of which is the fact that pleural fat is often confused with pleural plaques and that it is often impossible to exclude asbestosis in subjects who have

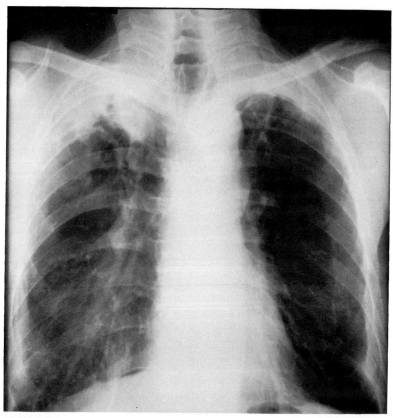

Figure 14–19. Radiograph of an insulator with atelectasis of both upper lobes caused by extensive upper zone pleural thickening. Note retraction of both hila upward. Moderate restrictive impairment was present with a FEV$_1$ and FVC of 52% and 48%, respectively, of the predicted values.

en face plaques without a CT scan. Other confounding factors include smoking, and exposure to radon daughters and other carcinogens. Of 19 studies that have attempted to relate the presence of pleural plaques to an increased incidence of cancer, only four have shown a positive association. The weight of the evidence weighs heavily against this hypothesis.[153a]

Rounded Atelectasis

A peculiar infolding of the pleura, known as rounded atelectasis, occurs in subjects who have had a pleural effusion; nowadays, this is most commonly seen in subjects who have been exposed to asbestos and have developed pleurisy as a result.[158, 159] The peripheral infolding of the lung is the result of associated parietal and visceral pleural thickening and produces an appearance that is often mistaken for a tumor. There are, however, characteristic radiological features which permit differentiation of rounded atelectasis from a true parenchymal tumor.[159, 160]

Rounded atelectasis appears as a spherical or elliptical subpleural opacity with a diameter varying from 2 cm to about 8 to 10 cm at the lung base. The corresponding pulmonary vessels and bronchi follow an arcuate course, and as they converge on the region of atelectasis, they create an impression of a "comet tail."[159, 160] Pleural thickening always accompanies the comet tail; the thickening is greatest adjacent to the rounded atelectasis (Fig. 14–20).

In rounded atelectasis, the interlobar fissure is always thickened, with infolding of the pleural surface. The characteristic features are best demonstrated with a CT scan, which will often reveal an adjacent pleural plaque.[159–161] Once the rounded atelectasis has formed, it tends to persist relatively unchanged. The exact mechanism of the formation of the pseudotumour is uncertain, but it has been suggested that a shrinking fibrous plaque or scar causes intussusception of the inner layers of the pleura into the lung parenchyma, leading to entrapment of a portion of the lung that is caught between the two layers of pleura. The blood vessels and airways that supply the atelectatic area are retracted toward the affected region and pulled closer together. As the pleural thickening increases, so does the atelectasis of the affected lung segment.

Asbestos as a Carcinogen

The inhalation and deposition of asbestos fibers in sufficient quantity can lead to the development of lung cancer and to pleural and peritoneal mesothelioma[31, 38] (Fig. 14–21). All of these conditions are dose related.[41] Although it is often suggested that asbestos-exposed subjects have an increased incidence of laryngeal and gastrointestinal cancer, the evidence in favor of these associations has been repeatedly examined and, for the most part, found wanting.[14, 15, 162]

Lung Cancer

There is no doubt that asbestos is a cocarcinogen and that the presence of asbestosis, at least in smokers, is associated with a significantly increased rate of lung cancer.[163]

It has been estimated that, in the United States, around 430,000 construction workers and 650,000 workers in manufacturing have been significantly exposed to asbestos.[164] Enterline calculated, based on these estimates, that asbestos will play a role in approximately 3% of all lung cancers that occur in the United States.[165] According to his data, there should be approximately 2500 deaths per year; however, it must be remembered that these cannot be attributed to asbestos alone but to asbestos and smoking acting synergistically, with the latter playing a more important role.[163, 164] This assumes an equivalent smoking history, but since smoking has decreased, then the number of deaths that are caused by asbestos will also decline. Elsewhere other projections have estimated higher numbers of exposed workers.[166]

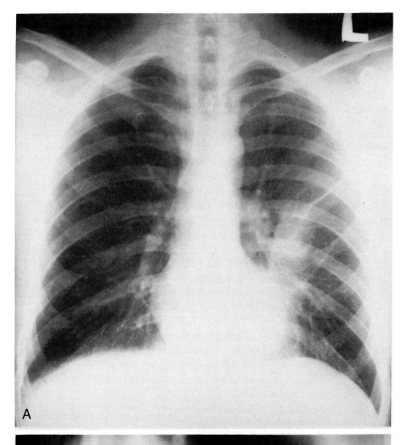

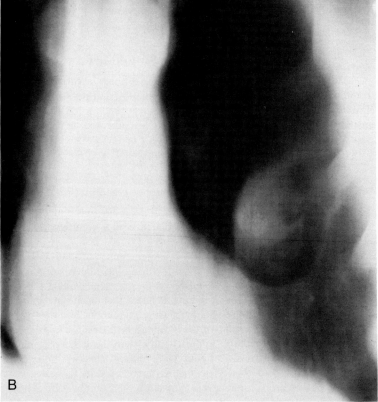

Figure 14–20
Rounded atelectasis. *A*, PA radiograph showing oval opacity with comet tail located in the oblique fissure. *B*, Tomogram showing infolding of the lung with surrounding traction emphysema around the lower margins of the atelectasis. (Courtesy of Dr. Linda Hutton.)

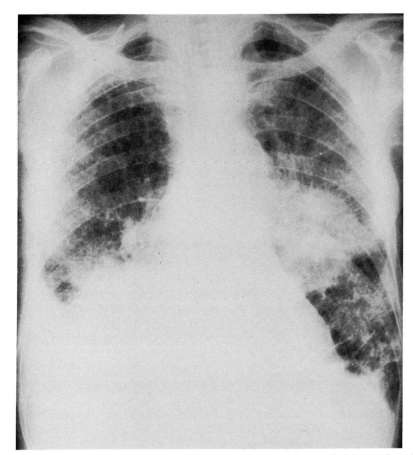

Figure 14–21. Subject with asbestosis, cancer of the left lung, and a mesothelioma on the right.

These latter projections were based on the Selikoff insulation cohort of heavily exposed workers, most of whom were cigarette smokers. The data are not truly representative and exaggerate the hazards of both past and present asbestos exposures. Tendentious pronouncements, such as 18.8 million workers in the United States who have had more than 2 months of exposure in occupations where significant exposure to asbestos may have occurred, are misleading and grossly exaggerate the risk, particularly when no definition of significant exposure data is given.[167] In reality, a 2-month exposure, at least since the days of the 2-f/cc TLV, constitutes an insignificant exposure to chrysotile, and there is no reason to believe that there is any significant risk associated with such a short exposure.[32–37]

That there is a significant excess risk of lung cancer in asbestos workers is clear from Figure 14–22. This graph is derived from the data of Hammond et al. and relates to projections that were made based on the relative risk of cancer associated with different levels of smoking in nonexposed subjects.[168] The predictions for smoking risk are now known to be incorrect,[169] and it is clear that the risk of smoking in the induction of lung cancer has significantly increased mainly because those smokers included in the early surveys are now older and for the most part have continued smoking. As a result, they may have cancer. The relative risk of lung cancer in asbestos workers was said to be increased five to seven times, irrespective of the smoking habit.[168] Nevertheless, only around 30 lifelong nonsmokers with asbestosis have been diagnosed as having lung cancer. If the smoking histories were inaccurate, such as is often the case in those claiming compensation,[98] the excess incidence would disappear completely in nonsmokers.[170] Simi-

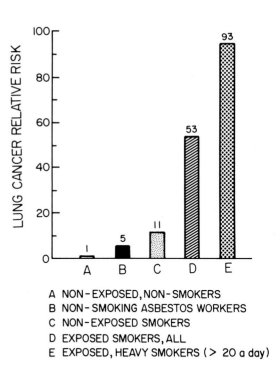

Figure 14–22
Relative risk of lung cancer in those
exposed to asbestos (most had
asbestosis), according to smoking
habit. (Data from Hammond, E.C.,
Selikoff, I.J., and Seidman, H.,
et al. Asbestos exposure, cigarette
smoking and death rates. Ann.
N. Y. Acad. Sci., 330, 473,
1979.)

A NON-EXPOSED, NON-SMOKERS
B NON-SMOKING ASBESTOS WORKERS
C NON-EXPOSED SMOKERS
D EXPOSED SMOKERS, ALL
E EXPOSED, HEAVY SMOKERS (> 20 a day)

larly, in some nonsmoking subjects with asbestosis, secondhand smoke could the-oretically play a significant role in the development of lung cancer.

Wide differences exist between the calculated relative risks of lung cancer according to different statisticians, but such differences are to be expected in the absence of uniform and consistent protocols.[170, 171] Thus, the selection of subjects for studies has differed greatly. Some studies include only those workers with prolonged exposure, i.e., more than 20 years; others include all workers who had been exposed for 6 months or more. Similarly, the smoking histories of the various cohorts included varied greatly, and in a much studied cohort, no attempt was made to include data relating to smoking habits.[172] The latter cohort has shown a decline in the incidence of asbestos-related disease, including lung cancer, with the decline being attributed to decreased asbestos exposure. No attention, however, was given to changes in smoking habits.[173] All these above variables will influence the inci-dence of lung cancer and the relative risk. Moreover, further studies of the surgical, clinical, and autopsy data in the aforementioned cohort were carried out in the asbestos-exposed group in whom lung cancer or mesothelioma developed in order to provide the "best evidence," but no comparable studies took place in the reference population.[14] This adjustment is likely to introduce bias. When all of these caveats are taken into consideration, it is evident that the risk of developing lung cancer is related to the cumulative dose of asbestos, provided the latter is sufficient to induce asbestosis and provided that the worker is also a smoker. The relative risk is greatly increased in heavy smokers, i.e., 40 to 60 times that of nonexposed light smokers. The increased risk of lung cancer is not apparent until there has been an asbestos exposure of at least 15 to 20 years, i.e., a suitable and compatible latent period.[174] Should lung cancer develop in a subject who has only worked for 5 to 8 years prior to the development of the tumor, then it can safely be assumed that the cancer is unrelated to asbestos exposure. There are now a large number of studies indicating that, providing the lifetime cumulative dose is kept below 35 to 45 fiber-years, the risk of lung cancer developing from exposure to chrysotile is no greater than that in the general population.[32–37]

In regard to the development of lung cancer in exposed workers, the assump-tion that there is a linear relationship has received wide but somewhat uncritical acceptance.[171] Such a hypothesis is convenient and simple but is not necessarily valid. Similarly, to infer that the line of identity must pass through the zero point is even less justifiable. Deductions based on observations of the risk of lung cancer in subjects with high exposures cannot be relied on to predict the response to low or trivial exposures. Back extrapolation of the regression line to the zero intercept in many instances is contrived and, although it demonstrates a rather neat and pleasing appearance to the eye, has little statistical justification. It should be borne in mind that there are very few or no excess deaths that occur at the lower exposures and that Liddell and Hanley and others have shown that the intercept varies significantly according to certain mathematical assumptions and to variations in estimates of cumulative exposure.[171, 174] In most instances, there is as much or more mathematical justification for projecting the regression line so that it has either a negative or positive intercept (Fig. 14–23). Moreover, it is assumed that the risk remains constant after exposure has ceased, an assumption that is known to be untrue.[174] To devise a study that would provide the necessary data to confirm the straight line, no threshold hypothesis would require several hundred thousand subjects exposed to very low doses and followed throughout their working lives. Such a cohort is not available nor ever likely to be.

A similar problem prevails in a consideration of the death rate from lung cancer in nonsmoking asbestotic workers. In most studies, there are only one or two excess deaths, and frequently, as Doll and Peto[14] and Berry et al.[98] have pointed out, the risk in nonsmokers appears to be greater than that in smokers. There is no scientific reason to believe that nonsmoking asbestotic subjects are more susceptible to the carcinogenic effects of asbestos than are smokers. This would suggest that smoking histories, at least in many of those claiming compensation, which is almost invariably the case in subjects who have died of lung cancer, cannot be relied on.[98]

The relative risk of developing lung cancer depends on a number of factors, including[175]

1. Dose.
2. Fiber type.
3. The job and type of exposure, whether as a miner, miller, or as an end user, and so forth.
4. Smoking history.
5. Presence of pulmonary fibrosis.

Dose-Response Relationships and Type of Work Exposure

A number of studies have been carried out to estimate the effects of cumulative asbestos exposure on the induction of lung cancer and the level of risk.[14, 163] For the

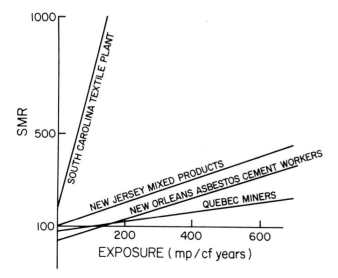

Figure 14–23
SMR for lung cancer according to exposure in several different groups of workers.

most part, an approximately linear trend has been shown with increasing cumulative exposure, providing allowance is made for a latency period of 15 to 20 years. The lung cancer risk is expressed as either a ratio of observed lung cancer cases to that of the expected, or alternatively, the ratio may be multiplied by 100 and expressed as a standardized mortality ratio (SMR). The estimated risk of lung cancer has varied considerably from study to study. A number of reviews in which the estimated slopes and the various factors that might influence the steepness of the slopes have been analyzed.[171, 174] These have been alluded to earlier. To confuse the issue, it seems probable that the risk of lung cancer is also related to fiber type.[175]

One study of amosite factory workers suggested that this amphibole was a greater hazard than crocidolite, but many defects existed in regard to dose estimates in the control population.[176] In addition, even when the type of asbestos used is similar, the risk varies according to the industrial process; miners have the least risk and millers and end users, the greatest.[177, 178] The method of statistical analysis also greatly influences the calculated extent of the risk and the slope of the line. Low risk and gradual regression slopes have been reported in workers manufacturing friction products,[54] in chrysotile miners,[163] and in those producing asbestos cement.[179] In these workers, the main type of asbestos involved was chrysotile, and only rarely was amphibole used.

Recently, a further follow-up study of the 1891 to 1920 birth cohort of chrysotile miners and millers in Quebec was published.[180] This analysis takes into account dust exposure, cigarette smoking, and the presence of asbestosis. The SMR for lung cancer rose nonsignificantly from 1.25 to 1.39, although deaths from mesothelioma increased from 8 to 25. The mortality rates from asbestos and mesothelioma were strongly associated with exposure. The risk of lung cancer in non-smokers was not increased. The risk of mesothelioma was higher at the Thedford mines than at the mines at Asbestos. Not all mesothelioma deaths were in miners, and five occurred in a small asbestos factory that used commercial amphiboles.

Fiber Type

Several studies in which the association between asbestos exposure and the development of mesothelioma was clearly apparent also indicated that those who worked with crocidolite were at most risk.[39, 42, 54] Since the publication of these studies, a growing body of evidence has come to the fore that indicates that crocidolite is also a greater hazard as far as the development of lung cancer is concerned.[14, 42] Hughes recently reviewed 30 or so articles that compared the observed to expected death rates in a number of cohorts where there was information identifying the type or types of asbestos used.[175]

In some extensively studied cohorts, there appears to be confusion or amnesia as to the type of asbestos used.[172] Thus, in a review of the death rates in asbestos insulation workers, Seidman and Selikoff[172] criticize Mossman et al.[181] for stating that crocidolite fibers are the predominant cause of mesothelioma in the United States, asserting that this is not so since "crocidolite was not utilized by the insulation workers studied by us."[172] This pronouncement contradicts a number of statements that appear in volume 132 of the *Annals of the New York Academy of Sciences,* a volume that was edited by the late Dr. Selikoff himself. Thus, Hendry, a Johns Mansville geologist, noted that, in 1963, 17,000 tons of crocidolite were used in the United States for the manufacture of filters, packing, insulation, and certain types of lagging.[182] Selikoff et al. later stated that crocidolite was found in a number of magnesia insulating blocks.[183] Further data in this volume indicate that, by 1954, the amount of blue asbestos imported from South Africa into the United States exceeded the amount of amosite.[184] Thus, it is abundantly apparent that large amounts of crocidolite were used for insulation in the 1940s, 1950s, and early 1960s. These data also rebut Mancuso who stated that railroad machinists were exposed to chrysotile only.[185]

The evidence that chrysotile is less hazardous and less likely to induce lung cancer than is crocidolite has slowly been accumulating. The data that suggest the lesser risk associated with chrysotile come from a limited number of studies in which it has been possible to make a comparison of dose-response relationships. More recently, a number of investigators have compared lung cancer risks in a series of cross-sectional studies to examine the carcinogenicity of the various fibers. These have been reviewed by Hughes.[175] For those workers exposed primarily to chrysotile, regardless of the type of occupational exposure, the lung cancer risk was 25% or less above background rates. The corresponding rates for crocidolite exposed cohorts was 100% higher. The risk for those manufacturing friction products differed, with the higher risk being present in the cohort with the shorter mean employment time and the lowest exposure.[177, 186] This suggests other factors, e.g., prior smoking habits were responsible for the increased risk. If only those workers with long-term exposures were included, then the relative risk of lung cancer was only minimally elevated (1.11) and was similar to that in the other study.[177] In those studies relating to insulation workers, those who had been exposed to chrysotile only had no increased risk, while those who had worked with both chrysotile and amphibole (mainly amosite) did. Much the same applies to those cohorts who worked with asbestos cement. Only in the United States textile industry is the evidence unconvincing that amphibole *vis-à-vis* chrysotile usage is associated with an increased risk of lung cancer. It has been suggested that, in the one study in which only chrysotile exposure occurred and in which the results were out of line, the concomitant inhalation of mineral oil, a carcinogen itself, may have been responsible for the increased risk of lung cancer.[187] This has been disputed.

Although the evidence that chrysotile is less of a risk than the amphiboles in regard to lung cancer is not overwhelmingly convincing, the case for it is fairly persuasive. For the most part, the added risk of exposure to chrysotile is around 20%. For mixed exposures, the comparable figure is 50% and for amphiboles alone, 100% to 380%. The amphiboles also seem more potent in their ability to produce radiographic abnormality, fibrosis, and associated pulmonary function impairment.[42, 175]

Pulmonary Fibrosis

The original description by Doll of the increased occurrence of lung cancer in asbestos mill workers indicated that the increased risk was present only in those workers who had asbestosis.[31] In this context, the fact that the lung cancer occurs more commonly in subjects, particularly in smokers, with various types of nonoccupational pulmonary fibrosis, including pulmonary scleroderma, fibrosing alveolitis, and other collagen vascular diseases, provides an excellent paradigm.[188]

Since Doll's classic article,[31] it has been suggested that asbestos exposure alone in the absence of asbestosis increases the risk of lung cancer; however, the currently available evidence indicates that the increased incidence of lung cancer occurs only in those who both smoke and have asbestosis.[175] A recent study of South African amphibole miners showed that, of those with lung cancer, 69% had evidence of asbestosis and that the latter was statistically significant after taking into account age and smoking.[189] The duration of exposure was an important risk factor. This study was, however, conducted in miners who underwent a postmortem examination, and it is doubtful whether the family of any miner who died with lung cancer that might be related to occupation would forego the chance of compensation by not requesting a necropsy. In addition, a prospective study of the asbestos cement industry studied lung cancer in relation to the radiographic presence of small opacities.[190] No excess was evident in the absence of definite radiographic evidence of 1/0 or more. However, it must be remembered that the radiographic change of category 1/0 may be produced by cigarette smoking in the absence of significant asbestos exposure. A prior study had shown similarly that miners in Quebec had no increased risk of lung cancer unless their radiograph was interpreted as 1/1 or greater.[74] Moreover, in the latter study, in some subjects, there was a long period between the last radiographic examination and death, making it possible for some subjects to have had fibrosis develop after surveillance ceased.

A relatively recent study claimed to have shown that all subjects with lung cancer had evidence of pulmonary fibrosis.[191] Of 450 deaths from confirmed lung cancer, 138 had tissue available for histological examination. Although 82% had definite radiographic evidence of asbestosis, 18% did not. This study is suspect for at least two reasons. First, the specimens were taken from "nonmalignant tissue" adjacent to the tumor, and small areas of fibrosis could have resulted from radiation therapy, chemotherapy, and infection. Second, the definition of minimal fibrosis adopted by these workers differed from the definition used by other investigators.[191] Thus, subpleural connective tissue was considered as part of the investigation by Kipen et al.,[191] whereas most jurisdictions require intra-alveolar and interalveolar fibrosis as the necessary histological criteria for asbestosis.[192] Moreover, it is essential to demonstrate a substantial number of asbestos bodies and fibrosis since it is clear that other nonoccupational parenchymal fibroses can occur in asbestos workers.[103]

Aside from these studies, there is a wealth of statistical data indicating that, in the absence of sufficient exposure to induce asbestosis, it is impossible to demonstrate an increased risk of lung cancer. As far as chrysotile is concerned, the risk of lung cancer does not appear to be increased, provided the dust level is kept below 1 f/cc during a working life of 5 days a week for 35 to 40 years.[32–37] Whether this is true in regard to the other types of asbestos is uncertain, but clearly the risk is small.

Lung Cancer in Shipyard Workers

It is often assumed that shipyard workers were exposed formerly to relatively high levels of asbestos and thus were at risk of asbestosis, lung cancer, and mesothelioma. Although it has been fairly clear since the early 1960s that insulators in the 1940s, 1950s, and 1960s were at an increased risk of asbestosis, lung cancer, and mesothelioma, there has been a facile tendency to assume that all those involved in shipbuilding were likewise at risk. This is not so, and the levels of asbestos to which welders, shipfitters, riggers, mechanics, burners, caulkers, etc. were exposed were significantly less than those to which insulators were exposed. Thus, Nicholson showed that only 3.5% of the fibers generated in the cutting of a calcium silicate block of insulation containing chrysotile were more than 5 μm in length.[193] In a separate study, Nicholson et al. showed that, in asbestos cement, barely 1% of the fibers were longer than 5 μm.[194]

In a survey of indirect occupational exposure during shipboard insulation work, it was found that the average exposure to asbestos in insulators when ventilation was poor was 11.5 f/cc; however, the average exposure for a noninsulator was 2.5 f/cc.[195] It was assumed by Nicholson et al. that a large proportion of the fibers that were in the air surrounding the insulators either settled to the ground or were diluted as they moved away from the center of activity.[194] Only 0.4% of the fibers to which the noninsulators were exposed were shown by electron microscopy to be greater than 5 μm. Thus, indirect exposure to asbestos in noninsulators was appreciably lower than in insulators.

Table 14–3 shows the observed versus expected deaths for lung cancer in most of the studies that have been carried out in the various trades involving shipbuilding.[195–201] For the most part, these studies do not include insulators and it will be seen that the observed/expected ratio is either normal or modestly elevated. As such, it is explicable by differences in smoking habits and so forth.[202] In one study by Puntoni et al. in which the ratio was possibly elevated, the authors suggested that other exposures could account for the slight excess of the ratio.[195] It has moreover been shown that, with the cessation of exposure to asbestos, there is a decline in the incidence of lung cancer and mesothelioma.[173]

Table 14–3
■
Shipyard Workers with Asbestos Exposure

Study Reference and No. of Subjects	Observed	Expected	Observed Expected
Puntoni, et al. (1979)[195] 2190	123	54.9	2.24
Rossiter, et al. (1980)[196] 6292	84	119.7	0.70
Nicholson and Selikoff (1984)[197] 1918	35	25.9	1.35
Kolonel, et al. (1985)[198] 7971	61	56.1	1.09
Newhouse, et al. (1985)[199] 3489	85	73.8	1.15
Sanden and Jarvholm (1987)[200] 3787	11	9.8	1.12
Melkind, et al. (1989)[201] 4778	53	31.3	1.69

Histological Findings and Site of Asbestos-Related Lung Cancer

All histological types of lung cancer occur in asbestos-exposed populations. The early suggestion that an asbestos-associated cancer was more likely to be an adenocarcinoma and peripherally situated is difficult to substantiate for a variety of reasons.[203] Firstly, although the diagnosis of lung cancer can be made relatively easily, histological typing, at least in a substantial minority of subjects, is much more difficult. This is particularly true for undifferentiated nonsmall cell carcinomata. A number of studies have shown that experts often render disparate opinions.[203, 204] Secondly, there are often differences of opinion as to the histological type when the same pathologist looks at surgical, cytological, and autopsy specimens. Thirdly, adenocarcinoma is becoming much more common in Europe and North America, and the increase is mainly related to cigarette smoking.[203, 205] Finally, there is a regrettable but easily understood tendency to attribute all lung cancer that occurs in asbestos-exposed subjects to their occupation when, in reality, the increased risk of this form of cancer is present only in those with parenchymal asbestos-induced fibrosis. The inclusion of subjects with lung cancer but no fibrosis confounds any conclusions that may be drawn as to the relative frequency of occurrence of the various histological types. There is, nevertheless, some indication that adenocarcinomata are more common among subjects with asbestos-induced lung cancer.[206, 207] The evidence that oat cell carcinoma is related to the presence of asbestosis is much more tenuous. The fairest, most objective approach in deciding whether the cancer should be attributed to asbestos is to use the generally accepted criterion that there must be asbestosis present in the lungs. The fiber burden also provides useful circumstantial evidence (*vide supra*).[42]

The lobe of origin of the cancer has also been considered by various investigators.[208, 209] Lung cancer originates most commonly in the upper lobes, and this contrasts with the changes of asbestosis, which are much more apparent and more severe in the lower lobes. Nevertheless, as mentioned earlier in this chapter, there is evidence to indicate that the fiber burden is often greater in the upper lobes.[45, 114, 115] Weiss calculated the relative risk at which the attribution to asbestos equaled its attribution to smoking and other causes.[209] At a relative risk of above 2.81, upper lobe cancers were more likely to be caused by asbestos than other factors; for lower lobe cancers, the relative risk was 1.55. Weiss concluded that these data might be useful in deciding about the cause of cancers that occur in asbestos-exposed subjects, with particular reference to whether or not they have asbestosis.

There are always considerable difficulties in correcting for effects of smoking in lung cancer SMRs. Two suggested ranges of error have been proposed from 2.0 to 1.5. The latter figure, which was suggested by Axelson, is a reasonable lower limit which should be exceeded before definite evidence of lung cancer can be accepted, at least in the earlier asbestos cohorts who were more heavily exposed and who also smoked more.[210]

The mechanisms whereby asbestos induces lung cancer are discussed elsewhere in Chapter 11. Suffice it to say that smoking has been shown to delay the clearance of asbestos fibers from the lungs and increases the penetration of such fibers into the walls of the airways.[211]

MESOTHELIOMA

The term *mesothelioma* is used to describe both a benign pedunculated pleural tumor associated with hypertrophic osteoarthropathy and also a diffuse malignant tumor of the pleura, peritoneum, pericardium, or rarely, the tunica vaginalis. Only diffuse malignant mesothelioma is related to asbestos exposure.

Etiology and Natural History

Epidemiological studies suggest that 75% to 80% of malignant mesotheliomata are associated with prior asbestos exposure.[41, 212, 213] The tumor, however, has also been associated with exposure to fibrous erionite or zeolite, a nonasbestiform fibrous mineral.[214, 215] The relationship between asbestos exposure and the development of mesothelioma was established by Wagner et al.[38, 39] A number of earlier reports of mesothelioma occurring in asbestos workers had been published prior to the Wagner et al.[38] study, but these were case reports in which the authors seldom made a direct association between the subject's former occupation and the development of the tumor. The earliest report was that of Wedler who described two former asbestos workers with mesothelioma.[216] It has been suggested that the association of mesothelioma with asbestos exposure was suspected in the 1940s,[40] but the only reference cited in support of this statement is an individual case report, which is quoted by Parkes in his 1973 review.[217] The reference in the Parkes article makes it apparent that the association was recorded in a doctoral thesis but was never published in a journal. Although there are some who imply that the relationship between asbestos exposure and mesothelioma was known in the 1940s and 1950s, it needs to be borne in mind that many able pathologists denied, even in the late 1940s and 1950s, the existence of mesothelioma and maintained that mesothelial tumors were secondary deposits from a primary adenocarcinoma elsewhere in the body.[218]

The incubation period for malignant mesothelioma varies but is usually from 15 to 40 years. Most mesotheliomata develop 25 to 40 years after the first exposure.[213, 219] The evidence suggests that, once the lungs of the susceptible subject have been primed by a sufficient dose of asbestos, then the development of the tumor is inevitable. Thus, some subjects in whom mesotheliomata develop late in their lives have not been exposed to the mineral for 20 to 35 years.[8] It has also become evident that, contrary to previous teaching, mesothelioma does not develop as a consequence of miniscule or extremely short-lived exposures consisting of 1 week to 10 days. Although it is true that mesothelioma may occur after relatively short exposure, such exposures are usually from 6 months to 2 to 3 years and have been fairly intense. Mesothelioma has also been reported in infants and in subjects with no history of exposure to asbestos.[220] Other causes of mesothelioma have been postulated,[221] including radiation[222, 223] and organic fibers.[224]

There is little doubt that mesothelioma has increased in frequency with the widespread use of asbestos. At the present time, it is likely that the tumor is overdiagnosed, and the risks of contracting it are exaggerated. In 1951, Hochberg noted that, in a series of more than 60,000 autopsies drawn from various American and European cities during the period from 1910 to 1949, malignant pleural tumors were found in 0.07% of subjects.[225] Some of these pleural tumors probably were secondary deposits from nondetected primaries elsewhere. From 1950 to 1970, a rate of 0.24% was observed in 70,000 autopsies drawn from eight similar cities.[226] Although this is a significant increase compared with the prior data, the incidence of mesothelioma remains distinctly uncommon even now. Enterline described 10 reports published before 1961 which described 31 subjects with a mesothelial tumor who had either asbestosis or a history of asbestos exposure.[227]

Incidence and Frequency

Mesothelioma remains a relatively rare tumor, and this is especially so in the general population. The most recent United States data indicate a mesothelioma incidence rate of about 14 to 15 subjects per million population for men.[228] This amounts to about 1750 male cases per year in the United States. In women, the risk is around two subjects per million population per year, i.e., about 250 per year. There is a birth cohort effect, i.e., the incidence of mesothelioma increases with age but diminishes by 70 years of age. Peritoneal mesothelioma remains relatively uncommon, and the rate has not been increasing to the same extent as has that of pleural mesothelioma. In Canada, in the period between 1960 to 1983, there was an increase in male cases from around 0.5 per million to 2 per million.[229] No increase in female cases occurred over the comparable period. A similar pattern has been observed in Great Britain.[230] The fact that the incidence in male patients has been increasing in the United States, Great Britain, and Canada, while that for female patients has remained substantially the same, indicates that occupational exposure is the prime cause of the increase.[229]

Influence of Fiber Type and Other Factors

Occupational exposure is of paramount importance as the cause of mesothelioma, and although it is apparent that asbestos is the major risk, it needs to be borne in mind that, in about 20% to 25% of subjects with mesothelioma, there is no occupational exposure to asbestos.[213, 221] There have been a number of reports of several members in one family with mesothelioma, but not all of these could be explained by a common exposure.[219]

In the early epidemiological studies of the relationship between asbestos exposure, lung cancer, and mesothelioma, little attention was paid to the type of asbestos inhaled. Moreover, the issue was often obscured by the fact that mixed exposures were frequent. Over the past 20 years, much has been done to separate the effects of different types of asbestos.[231] In the past decade, McDonald et al., in a series of articles, compared proportional mortality rates from mesotheliomata and lung cancer with reference not only to the type of industrial exposure, i.e., whether mining, the manufacture of textiles, or of friction products, and so forth, but also to the fiber type[226, 228, 229] (Table 14–4). The few relatively pure exposures that have taken place have provided valuable information. These involved crocidolite,[232] tremolite,[233] chrysotile (sometimes contaminated by tremolite),[234] amosite,[235, 236] and anthophyllite.[237] In nearly every instance, the frequency of mesothelioma was much higher in those exposed to the amphiboles, with crocidolite being associated with the greatest risk. Anthophyllite is an exception and seldom, if ever, causes mesothelioma.[237] A more recent review of the Finnish experience of mesothelioma and lung fiber burden re-examined by TEM shows that all but one of the lungs of their subjects with mesothelioma contained either crocidolite or amosite, suggesting Finnish anthophyllite causes few or if any such tumours (Siesko, A., personal communication, 1993). An excellent and comprehensive review of the role of asbestos and other fibers indicates that chrysotile has a much lower potential for causing asbestos-induced disease, in particular, mesothelioma.[238]

It might be inferred from the high dust concentrations that prevailed in the

Table 14–4

■

Proportional Mortality Rates from Mesothelioma and Excess Lung Cancer in 36 Male Asbestos-Exposed Cohorts

Fiber Type	Deaths			Proportional Mortality Rate/1000	
	All	Mesothelioma*	Excess lung cancer†	Mesothelioma	Excess lung cancer†
Mining					
Chrysotile	3511	11(0)	47	3.1	13.4
Amphiboles	1640	55(9)	98	33.5	59.8
Manufacturing					
Chrysotile	2136	2(1)	61	0.9	28.6
Amphiboles	892	36(15)	112	33.6	125.6
Mixtures	8751	176(54	380	20.1	43.4
Insulation					
Mixtures	2749	238(139)	452	86.6	164.4
Shipyards					
Mixtures	1517	39(2)	− 10	25.7	—

*Figures in parentheses beside mesothelioma cases represent peritoneal cases.
†Lung cancer excess over expected.
Modified from McDonald, J.C., and McDonald, A.D., Epidemiology of mesothelioma from estimated incidence. Prev. Med., 6, 426, 1977; and Connelly, R.R., Spirtas, R., Myers, M.H., et al., Demographic patterns for mesothelioma in the United States. J. Natl. Cancer Inst., 78, 1053, 1987.

Quebec asbestos mines in the 1940s and 1950s, along with the miners' long work histories, that a fair number of mesotheliomata should have occurred. In practice, mesothelioma was, and is, a rarity in miners in Quebec. The fact that chrysotile leaches out of the lungs, and hence is less likely to induce mesothelioma, has been discussed previously. Recent studies have shown that Quebec asbestos often contains some asbestiform tremolite. Thus, Pooley, in an examination of the lungs of 20 miners and millers with parenchymal fibrosis in Quebec, found more tremolite fibers relative to the number of chrysotile fibers,[239] despite asbestiform tremolite being present in only trace amounts in the ore and dust generated by mining and crushing.[240] The concentrations of amosite, crocidolite, and tremolite fibers were determined in a series of lungs taken from autopsied subjects with mesothelioma and were matched with an appropriate reference group. The number of fibers of crocidolite, amosite, and tremolite and of typical asbestos bodies differed significantly in subjects with mesothelioma and the referents.[241] However, concentrations of chrysotile, nonasbestiform anthophyllite, and other identifiable minerals were similar.[242] The relative risk of mesothelioma was proportional to the percentage of amphibole fibers greater than 8 μm in length. Wagner et al. had previously shown that the chrysotile content of the lungs reaches an upper limit and remains at that particular limit despite further exposure.[243] They suggested that further retention of fibers did not occur. Whether this is partly an effect of the fact that many serpentine chrysotile fibers are deposited before reaching the smaller airways[244] or entirely because chrysotile is removed more rapidly from the lungs than are the amphiboles is unknown.

It has also been suggested, but remains unproved, that various organic fibers can induce lung cancer and mesothelioma.[224, 245] Studies have been carried out to ascertain whether the inhalation of manmade mineral fibers is associated with an excessive risk of mesotheliomata. No relationship has been noted,[246] although the latency as yet may be too short for the development of mesothelioma.

A number of cases of domestic exposure have been described, as mentioned earlier.[38, 247, 248] Neighborhood exposure was first described by Wagner et al. in children who played around the blue asbestos mines in South Africa.[38] Some of these children may have also been exposed in the households of asbestos miners. Most studies have shown that, in neighborhood studies, the incidence was either very low or nonexistent.[247, 248]

Mesothelioma of the Peritoneum, Pericardium, and Tunica Vaginalis

Peritoneal and pericardial mesotheliomata occur less frequently than pleural mesothelioma. It is presumed that peritoneal mesotheliomata are caused by asbestos fibers migrating from the lung periphery through the diaphragm into the peritoneum, by ingested fibers making their way through the gut wall into the peritoneum, or by the swallowing of fibers that have been removed from the lungs by the mucociliary escalators. Although the passage of fibers through the gut wall has been shown to occur experimentally in animals that had been fed various types of asbestos fibers,[249] it was not possible to induce an excess number of mesotheliomata or to induce gastric or colonic cancers.[250–252] The effects of various ingested asbestos fibers are well reviewed in a publication of the National Toxicology Program.[253] There seems to be little or no evidence that chrysotile ever causes peritoneal mesothelioma.[254] Primary pericardial mesothelioma is extremely rare and is usually believed to be unrelated to asbestos exposure. Some have suggested that it can result from the asbestos fibers migrating from the lung to the pleura. The rare mesothelioma of the tunica vaginalis testis presents as a mass surrounding the testicle and usually is associated with a hydrocele. Prior exposure to asbestos is common, although it is difficult to imagine how asbestos could be selectively deposited in the tunica vaginalis and yet spare the peritoneum.[255] This rare form of tumor may be the one form of mesothelioma that can be cured by surgery since it is often indolent and slow growing.

Symptoms and Signs

Pleural mesothelioma usually presents as unilateral chest pain, which is often pleuritic. Initially, the pain is transient, but with the passage of time, it becomes persistent, migrates centrally, and is no longer made worse by breathing or coughing. As the disease progresses, the patient starts to lose weight and becomes increasingly breathless. The breathlessness is directly related to the size of the tumor and to compression and collapse of the lung or lungs. The typical signs initially are those of pleural effusion. As the mesothelioma grows, however, the hemithorax flattens, and signs of a fibrothorax often develop. Concomitantly, the mediastinum shifts to the affected side. Occasionally, after the effusion has been aspirated or the patient has undergone open pleural biopsy, seeding of the tract or of the scar occurs (Fig. 14–24). It used to be thought that secondary deposits in other organs were rare, but this is not the case. As the tumor grows, it may compress and invade the great veins of the thorax and the pericardium. Arrhythmias are common and tend to persist in the late stages when pericardial invasion is far advanced. Death usually occurs within 18 months to 2 years as a consequence of terminal bronchopneumonia and involvement of the vessels around the hila. A minority of patients, somewhere around 15%, survive 3 to 4 years. Bilateral mesotheliomata are rare but occur.

Radiographic Findings

Pleural mesothelioma usually presents as a large pleural effusion (Figs. 14–25 to 14–27). In a minority of subjects, several pleural-based solid lesions may also occur. There may be evidence of old pleural plaques or of asbestosis. The latter are present in around 20% of subjects with pleural mesotheliomata. Serial radiographs invariably show a slow extension of the tumor, often with the disappearance of pleural fluid. As the tumor progresses, the fluid becomes loculated. In peritoneal mesothelioma, around one half of the subjects show one or other of the classic radiographic features of prior exposure to asbestos.

CT scans are useful in determining the extent of the mesothelioma and ascertaining whether adjacent organs are involved. They are particularly helpful in delineating the extent of the tumor, which is often irregular and difficult to assess

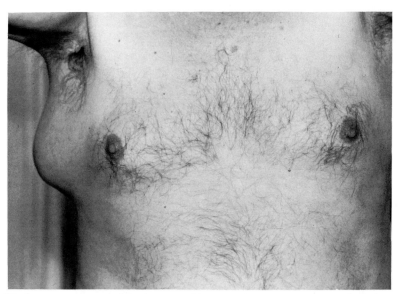

Figure 14–24. Showing involvement of the thoracic wall by a mesothelioma. The subject had undergone a pleuroscopy, and the tract became seeded by the mesothelioma.

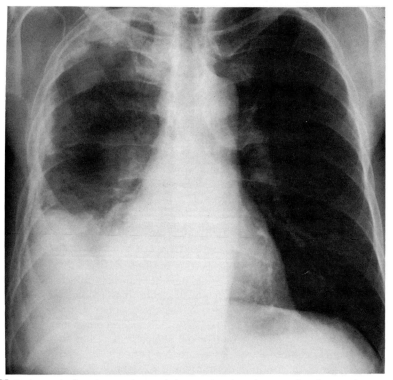

Figure 14–25. Radiograph of a subject with mesothelioma. Note the rather typical scalloping along the lateral thoracic wall.

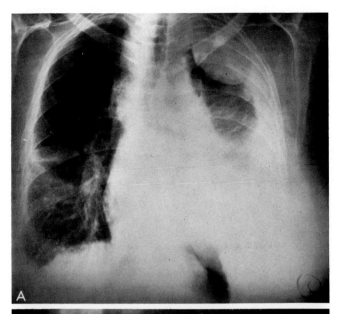

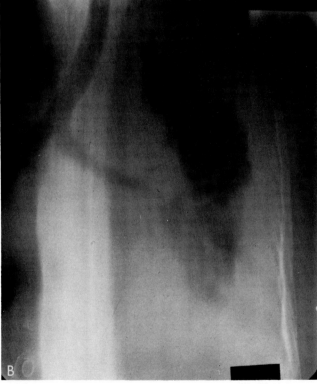

Figure 14–26
A, Radiograph of 60-year-old woman who denied any exposure to asbestos, either occupationally or environmentally. Nevertheless, large numbers of asbestos bodies and typical asbestos-type pleural plaques were found at autopsy, after her death from malignant mesothelioma. *B,* Tomogram showing tumor masses encasing left lung and compressing lobar bronchi.
Illustration continued on following page

from a PA radiograph. The tumor's mushroom-like or crenated margins may encroach on and extend into and through the lung and diaphragm, occasionally leading to esophageal obstruction and invasion of the bowel and mesentery. Satellite lung nodules can occasionally be seen in the lungs and are present in around 5% to 15% of subjects.[256] Later there may be periosteal reaction and rib destruction.

Laboratory Findings

Mesothelioma usually leads to a restrictive ventilatory defect. If an obstruction is present, it is usually related to other factors, such as cigarette smoking. Early in

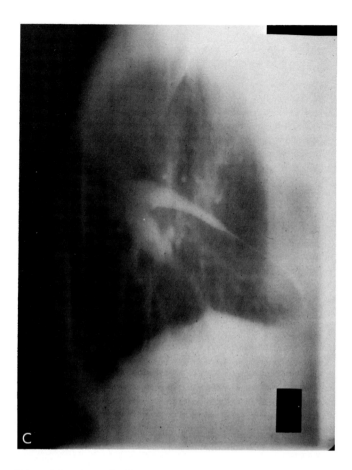

Figure 14–26 *Continued*
C, Lateral tomogram of right lung. This tumor spread across the upper mediastinum, causing superior vena caval obstruction, and infiltrated the fissures in the right lung.

the course of the condition, laboratory findings are not helpful, but as the patient becomes sicker, anemia may occur. A high concentration of hyaluronic acid may be found in the pleural fluid of subjects with mesotheliomata, but this is by no means invariable and is present in only about one third of those affected.

Diagnosis

Mesothelioma should be considered when there is a suitable history of exposure to asbestos and, in addition, a suitable latent period. Thoracentesis and needle biopsy of the pleura usually give negative findings and are seldom helpful. Multiple pleural biopsies obtained blindly with an Abrams or Cope needle may be successful in making the diagnosis. Some of the specimen should be processed in glutaraldehyde for electron microscopy. The most promising diagnostic technique appears to be pleuroscopy. Under these circumstances, the tumor can sometimes be well visualized, and sufficient samples can be taken for a definitive diagnosis. If this is not feasible, then open biopsy can be carried out. In most instances, however, the diagnosis can be made clinically, especially if there is a suitable history of exposure and the presence of radiographic stigmata of prior exposure to asbestos. Open biopsy is often carried out to confirm the diagnosis so that patients and their relatives may claim compensation.

Peritoneal mesothelioma usually presents with ascites, increasing abdominal pain, and a palpable mass.[257] Eventually, the patient may have obstruction and disseminated intravascular coagulation along with thrombophlebitis.

Pathological Findings

The pathological diagnosis of mesothelioma is fraught with difficulty. The symptoms and signs may be closely mimicked by secondary deposits in the pleura

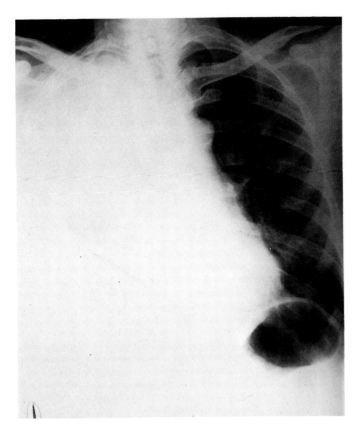

Figure 14–27
Chest radiograph of a man who had worked for 30 years as a marine engineer, with intermittent slight exposure to asbestos lagging in ships' engine rooms, showing massive right pleural effusion.

and lung from a carcinoma situated elsewhere. In many instances, the primary tumor is small and undetectable, despite an extensive search for it. Most commonly, it is an adenocarcinoma in the gut or kidney. In the case of peritoneal mesothelioma, carcinoma of the ovary may present major diagnostic difficulties. Sarcomatous deposits in the pleura or peritoneum can also mimic mesotheliomata, and this applies to both the gross and microscopic appearances. With modern techniques, most mesotheliomata can be distinguished from carcinoma, but in about 5% to 10% of subjects, a definitive opinion as to the origin of the tumor is not possible.

The typical mesothelioma found at autopsy is a firm hard mass of whitish or grayish tissue which envelops the adjacent structures, including the lung and the great vessels (Figs. 14–28 and 14–29). The pleural space is obliterated. Gelatinous material is often present in small cysts that are located inside the tumor. For the most part, the tumor spreads diffusely but, in some instances, appears to have areas where it is relatively circumscribed. The tumor starts on the parietal surface, but nodules are often found on both the visceral and parietal pleura. About 50% of subjects with mesothelioma have distant metastases.[258, 259] The lymph glands are not infrequently involved, and secondary deposits may be found in heart, bone, liver, adrenal glands, and even the retina.

Peritoneal mesotheliomata often entrap loops of bowel and may extend into the liver and other organs and sometimes into and through the diaphragm. It is frequently difficult to separate peritoneal mesothelioma from abdominal adenocarcinoma, in particular, that arising from the ovary.[260]

Mesotheliomata are usually divided into epithelial sarcomatous and mixed types. Peritoneal mesothelioma occurs histologically as epithelial and sarcomatous varieties. In around 30% or so, both epithelial and sarcomatous elements are present. Epithelial tumors are divided into tubopapillary, epithelioid, adenomatoid, and desmoplastic varieties; the sarcomatous variants are either fibrosarcomatous or desmoplastic.

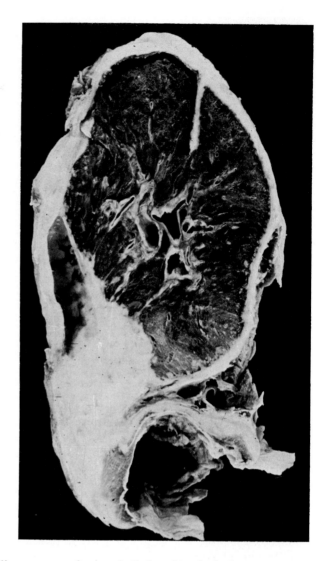

Figure 14–28
Sagittal section of left lung, pleura, and diaphragm showing symphysis of both pleural layers by a malignant mesothelioma. The fissure and diaphragm are also involved.

Epithelial mesotheliomata are of several distinct histological patterns. The tubopapillary type is composed of branching tubules and papillae with a fibrous core that is lined by flattened or cuboidal cells. Mitoses are often few. The cells lining the papillae can be columnar rather than cuboidal (Fig. 14–30). A minority of epithelial mesotheliomata appear to be composed of cells similar to the reactive mesothelial cells seen in pleural fluids. If this is the case, a diagnosis of a small primary carcinoma elsewhere must be excluded. Some epithelial mesotheliomata have smaller cells and are difficult to distinguish from carcinomata. A few have a strong dense collagenous stroma with only scattered tumor cells. This is the desmoplastic variant, which is also seen in sarcomatous mesotheliomata.

The sarcomatous variety is often cellular and morphologically identical to a fibrosarcoma or malignant fibrous histiocytoma (Fig. 14–31). The desmoplastic variety is exceedingly difficult to diagnose and to separate from normal reactive pleura. A more complete description of the histological features is to be found in Chapter 8 of Churg and Green's text, *Pathology of Occupational Lung Disease.*[261]

Histochemical and Immunochemical Aspects

The identification and separation of malignant mesothelioma from secondary deposits caused by carcinoma are rendered more precise by the use of a number of

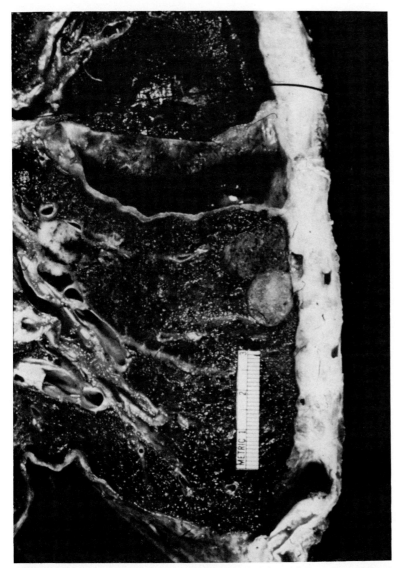

Figure 14–29. Postmortem specimen showing a thick peel of mesothelioma surrounding the lung with secondary deposits in the lung presumably caused by hematogenous or lymphatic dissemination.

immunohistochemical techniques. Pleural mucin is not secreted by mesotheliomata, but hyaluronic acid frequently is. Table 14–5 shows the routine stains that are used to take advantage of these characteristics.

The demonstration of antibodies to carcinoembryonic antigens (CEA), keratin proteins, and milk fat globule (MFG) proteins is frequently helpful in distinguishing mesothelioma from an adenocarcinoma. CEA is a complex glycoprotein that has been noted to be present in adenocarcinomata of the lung and absent in diffuse malignant mesothelioma. Although this is not invariable, CEA is found in around 90% of adenocarcinomata of the lung and in only 10% of malignant mesothelioma.[262] If CEA findings are positive in mesothelioma, the reactivity is usually much less than that found in adenocarcinomata. The argument, however, still persists as to whether diffuse malignant mesothelioma ever contains CEA. Although carcinomata of the breast, ovary, stomach, and colon are usually CEA positive, this rule is not invariable. In contrast, carcinomata of the kidney and prostate are seldom CEA positive. Keratin proteins are widely distributed in normal and neoplastic

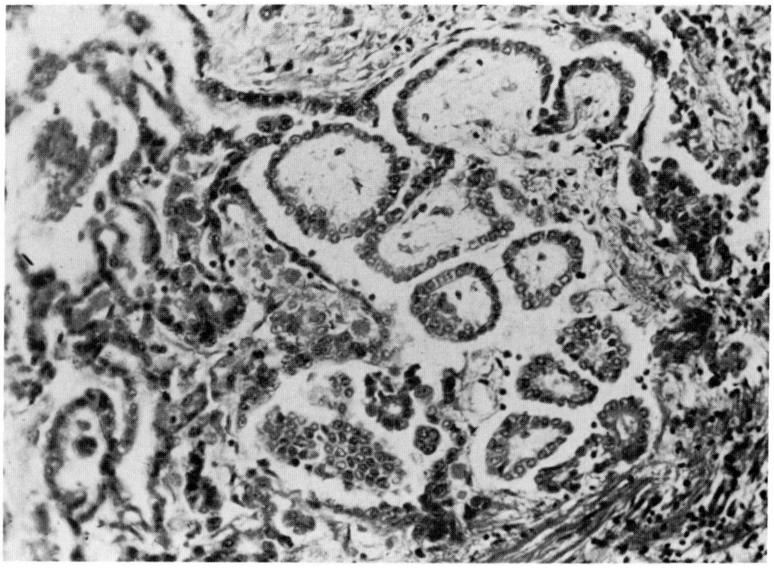

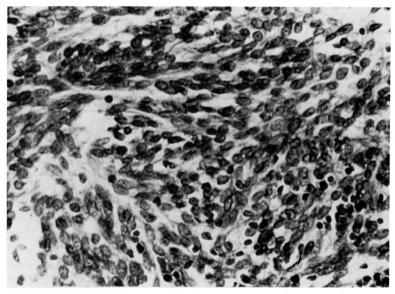

Figure 14–30. Photomicrograph of epithelial type of mesothelioma showing tubopapillary glandular structures.

epithelial cells. They appear as very fine fibers and are visible on electron microscopy after appropriate fixation. They are present in mesotheliomata, and when suitable stains are used, they are easily detectable.[263] In contrast, in adenocarcinomata, they are usually few or absent.[262] Subsequent studies, however, produced variable results, with keratin being absent in a minority of mesotheliomata. They found that adenocarcinoma of the lung also stains with keratin.[264] It has also been suggested that antibodies to MFG proteins stain carcinomata but not mesotheliomata. Here again, there is doubt as to whether this is indeed correct.[265, 266]

Electron Microscopic Findings

Electron microscopy has been increasingly used with the object of demonstrating the ultrastructural features that are specific to mesothelioma.[267] It has been said

Figure 14–31. Photomicrograph of sarcomatous type of mesothelioma.

Table 14–5

■

Histochemical Staining Reactions of Mesothelioma and Adenocarcinoma

Reaction	Mucopolysaccharide	Mesothelioma	Adenocarcinoma
Periodic acid-Schiff	Neutral	Negative	Positive
Hyaluronidase, alcian blue, or colloidal iron	Hyaluronic acid	Positive	Negative
Mucicarmine	Neutral to weakly acidic	Negative	Positive

to be used to characterize the structure of the secretory epithelial cells and fibroblastic cells that are found in sarcomatous mesothelioma,[266] but here again, there is controversy as to the usefulness of electron microscopy.[268]

Perhaps the most useful and neglected investigation is the assessment of the number and type of fibers in the lungs of a subject with suspected mesotheliomata. Should there be a fairly large number of fibers and should they be amphiboles, this provides strong circumstantial evidence as to the cause of the disease. However, it must be remembered that it is the lung in which the fibers are present and not the tumor tissue.

Treatment

No effective treatment is known. Although surgery, including pleural pneumonectomy, has been tried, it usually is followed by a further spread of the tumor, usually to the pericardium and to the opposite pleura and peritoneum. Chemotherapy leads to unpleasant side effects, such as baldness, renal failure, and persistent vomiting, but does nothing to alleviate the symptoms or reduce the size of the tumor. Much the same can be said of radiation therapy. A patient who was treated with fast neutron therapy showed no sign of recurrent disease after 78 months.[269]

ASBESTOS AND OTHER MALIGNANCIES

Laryngeal Cancer

Those malignancies that are definitely associated with exposure to asbestos, namely, lung cancer and mesothelioma, came to light as a result of the observations of shrewd clinicians. In contrast, the hypothesis for asbestos exposure and its purported relationship to an increased incidence of laryngeal cancer came about as a retrospective analysis carried out in a cohort of asbestos workers.[270] Such analyses have been referred to as data dredging. In a cohort of 1100 subjects, one death was due to cancer of the larynx when the total expected deaths from respiratory malignancies other than that of the lung was 0.52. This difference of half a death clearly has no statistical significance, but since asbestos was a known carcinogen, the observation was therefore given undue weight. It was suggested that, since asbestos could induce malignancy in the bronchial epithelium, it was assumed that the laryngeal mucous membrane was equally susceptible.

A number of problems occur in trying to determine a cause-and-effect relationship between asbestos exposure and cancer of the larynx. The most obvious of which is that many subjects with this cancer are apparently cured by radiation or surgery. As a result, death rates are relatively low. Similarly, there are a number of confounding factors. Two of these are of great importance, namely, smoking and alcohol. Thus, cancer of the larynx is virtually never seen in a patient who is not a smoker.

Two early case reference studies[271, 272] indicated that the risk of laryngeal cancer was greatly increased in those exposed to asbestos; however, their methods were subsequently questioned by Doll and Peto.[14] Nevertheless, Doll and Peto concluded that asbestos exposure led to a small increase in the frequency of occurrence of laryngeal carcinoma. A subsequent review published by Chan and Gee came to a different conclusion.[273] The latter authors stressed that most studies have not taken alcohol into account, and when it and smoking are considered no increased incidence can be demonstrated. Liddell concluded, after a detailed analysis of all the studies that were available up to 1990, that there was insufficient evidence to confirm the association.[274] He has expressed the same opinion more recently.[275]

Gastrointestinal Cancer

The assertion that gastrointestinal cancer is associated with exposure to asbestos has received a fair amount of acceptance, despite contradictory and often inadequate studies. Many of the studies that have shown a positive association have been flawed. Here again, there are a number of confounding factors, in particular, ethnic origin and diet, e.g., gastrointestinal cancer is more common in Scandinavians and in those who eat hot, spicy, and smoked foods. It is also more common in blue collar workers and is strongly related to social class. Furthermore, many of the early deaths that were attributed to gastric and colonic cancer in the shipyards of Belfast were probably due to mesothelioma.[276]

The association between gastrointestinal cancer and asbestos exposure was critically reviewed by Doll and Peto in 1985.[14] Firstly, they described the problem of misdiagnosis and pointed out that peritoneal mesothelioma was not generally recognized until 1965. Secondly, they commented on the studies of Selikoff et al.,[166] in which further clinical and pathological evidence of the cause of death and the certified cause of death were sought for all members of the asbestos workers union in North America who were enrolled in their study. Additional information was obtained in 71% of the 2771 deaths, and this enabled the causes of death to be categorized in two ways: by the underlying cause (as stated on the death certificate) and by "the best available evidence" that the investigators had obtained. Doll and Peto point out that the use of different methods can give different results. They refer to an article by Heasman and Lipworth, which showed that 107 of 353 deaths attributed to gastric cancer by the clinicians were not confirmed at autopsy, although 86 gastric cancers found in the same series had not been diagnosed during life.[277] They also criticized Selikoff for using United States national rates to calculate the number of expected deaths. Taking into consideration the fact that insulation workers in the United States and Canada are wholly manual workers and likely to have resided in large towns, this factor would not explain the many excess deaths caused by lung cancer but could have contributed materially to a small excess of death from other causes such as mesothelioma. Finally, asbestos did not produce gastrointestinal cancer when given in large doses by mouth.[278, 279] Edelman more recently reviewed the available data and came to the conclusion that there is no increased risk of gastrointestinal cancer in those exposed to asbestos.[15]

Malignancy to Other Sites

There are occasional reports of an increased incidence of carcinoma of the ovary, carcinoma of the breast, and so forth in those exposed to asbestos. As such, these can be attributed to chance since there is no evidence that they occur consistently and more frequently in asbestos-exposed workers.

Asbestos in Buildings

Societal concern over asbestos in buildings is real but often assumes panic proportions in spite of the publication of the reports of various commissions, symposia, and so forth[49, 55, 280–282] and a report in *Science*.[283] The relevant data are summarized in the Health Effects Institute report[280] and by Corn et al.[284] With electron microscopic techniques, most airborne fiber (greater than 5 μm in length) levels were about 0.0001 f/cc, with the 90th percentile of observations rarely exceeding 0.005 f/cc. Levels were often comparable in buildings and outside air samples. Although transient higher levels undoubtedly can occur, these levels pose no measurable societal risk. As with cigarette smoking, in which the dose is the product of packs a day times years smoked, so asbestos "dose" is expressed as fibers per cubic centimeter times years. Thus, for building dwellers, the present dose estimate is 0.0001 × 1 day × 60 years, i.e., 0.006 f/cc-years. This contrasts with the present United States OSHA standard of 0.2 f/cc times working 8 hours a day 5 days a week for 30 years, which yields a dose of 6 f/years. The OSHA standard is set so as to pose a minimal asbestosis risk over a working life. A comparison of these doses explains why no case of asbestosis has occurred in a building dweller as opposed to asbestos workers or their families. In fact, there is good reason to believe that asbestosis, as a clinical entity, requires well in excess of 30 f/years. This argument in itself is strong enough but is reinforced when two other features are considered. There is little doubt that there is a threshold exposure below which asbestosis does not occur. This threshold level is imprecisely known but is in the order of 1 to 2 f/years. Furthermore, since most buildings contain chrysotile, a biodegradable fiber type, rather than amphiboles, the exposure will not exceed the rate of degradation, implying that the true *in situ* lung exposure to chrysotile is overestimated by the assumption of fiber persistence implicit in the use of fiber-years to define the exposure.

In regard to lung cancer, to the extent that asbestosis is a prerequisite for the ascription of lung cancer to asbestos, the absence of nonoccupational or societal asbestosis risk means there is no lung cancer risk. Certainly, the effect of asbestos on societal lung cancer pales into insignificance in the face of cigarette smoking.

The risk that is most feared is mesothelioma, particularly, in children, since the long latency from first exposure of this tumor poses a greater risk than for adults. However, there are several cogent reasons to rate even this risk as minuscule. First, the use of amphiboles in most buildings in the United States and Canada is rare, whereas chrysotile is at least partly biodegradable and, therefore, will not persist in the lung. Second, chrysotile causes many fewer mesotheliomata than do the amphiboles, particularly, crocidolite. Third, even with crocidolite and also paraoccupational exposure notwithstanding, there is good reason to believe there is a threshold for mesothelioma, probably on the order of 5 f/years for crocidolite.[285] There is currently no evidence that airborne building amphibole levels can ever produce an exposure of 5 f/years, even over the alloted 3 to 7 years spent in school. Among women not generally occupationally exposed to asbestos, the incidence of mesothelioma has not risen in the United States, Canada, and most European countries over the last 20 years.[228, 229, 280, 286, 287] Were societal asbestos risks significant, a rise would be expected since asbestos has been used in the construction of buildings for more than 50 years.

In regard to pleural disorders, asbestos effusions only occur in an occupational setting. Pleural plaques, a disorder occurring with less asbestos exposure than that which causes asbestosis, could serve as a marker of societal asbestos exposure. Indeed, there are geographical variations in plaque prevalence which are not entirely understood.[288–290] However, studies of their prevalence in buildings, with and without *in situ* asbestos, should provide a measure of risk. The only reliable study originates from Paris and did not show any differences in plaque prevalence in those Parisians working in asbestos-containing buildings compared with an appropriate reference group.[291]

In spite of these considerations, societal fears persist, often deliberately fostered by news media and sometimes by ill-considered professional pronouncements. If society is not to return to the dark ages, such unjustified fears need to be counteracted by a sane scholarly account of the asbestos risks in the context of other societal risk.[181, 292] The Ontario Royal Commission report considered the risk of death from driving to work greater than that from working in asbestos-containing buildings.[282]

SUMMARY

Over the past 30 to 40 years, much publicity has been given to the harmful effects of asbestos. Although it is true that there have been a substantial number of deaths associated with the use of this mineral, medical knowledge of the hazards of exposure to asbestos is now sufficient to prevent most of its harmful effects. The hyperbole used by certain lawyers who have a financial interest in asbestos litigation, the illogical attempt by the Environmental Protection Agency to ban asbestos, the distorted propaganda put forth by many of the environmental groups and the lunatic fringe, have done United States and Canadian industry, not to mention the general public, a great disservice. In addition, unnecessary fears have been engendered. No attempt has been made to determine the number of lives saved by the use of asbestos as a fire-resistant agent or its use in the manufacture of asbestos cement pipes to supply drinking water and to effect sewage disposal.

In a somewhat different context, the number of casualties caused by burns in the Royal Navy warships during the Falklands War, and on the USS Stark when the latter was hit by an Exocet missile in the Persian Gulf, was appreciably greater than expected because of the exclusion of asbestos insulation from these ships. One third of all Royal Navy casualties in the Falklands War had burns, and in the overall campaign, burns accounted for 14% of all injuries.[293] The comparable figure in the 1939 to 1945 war was 1.5%. Thus, burn casualties were almost 10 times as common in the recent conflict in which relatively inflammable materials, such as aluminum, were used in the construction of the ships and in which asbestos had not been used for fire control. Nor should it be forgotten that the Challenger disaster was a consequence of substituting a nonasbestos-containing putty used to seal the O rings of the craft.

The total number of deaths in the United States caused by mesothelioma and asbestos-related lung cancer in any 1 year during the 1980s would be around 6700 to 7300.[165, 227] These data, however, reflect asbestos exposure in the 1940s, 1950s, and 1960s. The projected death rate from asbestos exposure during the 1970s and 1980s, when the TLV Federal Standard was 2 f/cc or less and during which chrysotile was the main type of asbestos used commercially, will be far less. New cases of asbestosis are not occurring, and as a result, asbestos-related lung cancer will disappear over the next several years. New cases of mesothelioma will become relatively rare. Forty-five per cent of all male and 21.5% of all female cancer deaths in the United States are due to lung cancer.[294] Thus, cigarette smoking, in the main alone, but also in conjunction with other agents, will cause 157,000 lung cancer deaths in the United States. These figures ignore the role of cigarette smoking as a cause of coronary artery disease, emphysema, and airways obstruction. Clearly, those government agencies whose responsibilities include protection of the environment need to establish their priorities, and instead of recommending the removal of asbestos from all buildings or trying to achieve unattainably low levels of silica in the air, need to concentrate on the control of major hazards.

REFERENCES

1. Pooley, F.D., Asbestos Mineralogy. *In* Antman, K., and Aisner, J., eds., Asbestos Related Malignancy. Orlando, FL, Grune and Stratton, 1987, pp. 3–27.
2. Ross, M., Kuntze, R.A., and Clifton, R.A., Definitions for asbestos and other health related silicates. *In* Levadie, B., ed., ASTM STP. Philadelphia, American Society for Testing and Materials, 1984, pp. 139–147.
3. Hunter, D., The Diseases of the Occupations, 6th ed. London, Hodder and Stoughton, 1978, pp. 990–991.
4. Merewether, E.R.A., and Price, C.W., Report on the Effects of Asbestos Dust on the Lungs and Dust Suppression in the Asbestos Industry. London, His Majesty's Stationery Office, 1930.

5. Dreessen, W.C., Dallavalle, J.M., Edwards, T., et al., A Study of Asbestosis in the Asbestos Textile Industry. Public Health Bulletin 241. Washington, D.C., U.S. Government Printing Office, 1938.

6. Talcott, J., Thurber, W., Gaensler, E., et al., Mesothelioma in manufacturers of asbestos containing cigarette filters. Lancet, 1, 392, 1987.

7. Jones, R.S., Roberts, G.H., Pooley, F.D., et al., The consequences of exposure to asbestos dust in a wartime gas mask factory. *In* Wagner, J.C., ed., Biological Effects of Mineral Fibres 2. IARC publication number 30. Lyon, IARC Publications, 1980, pp. 637–653.

8. McDonald, A.D., and McDonald, J.C., Mesothelioma after crocidolite exposure during gas mask manufacture. Environ. Res., 17, 340, 1978.

9. Frost, J., George, J., and Moller, P.F., Asbestosis with pleural calcification among insulation workers. Dan. Med. Bull., 3, 202, 1956.

10. Selikoff, I.J., Churg, J., and Hammond, E.C., The occurrence of asbestosis among insulation workers in the United States. Ann. N. Y. Acad. Sci., 132, 139, 1965.

11. Baizer, J.L., and Cooper, W.C., The work environment of insulation workers. Am. Ind. Hyg. Assoc. J., 29, 222, 1968.

12. Newhouse, M.L., and Thompson, H., Mesothelioma of pleura and peritoneum following exposure to asbestos in the London area. Br. J. Ind. Med., 22, 261, 1965.

13 Epler, G.R., Fitzgerald, M., Gaensler, E.A., and Carrington, C.B., Asbestos related disease from household exposure. Respiration, 39, 229, 1980.

14. Doll, R., and Peto, J., Asbestos: Effects on Health of Exposure to Asbestos. Health and Safety Commission. London, Her Majesty's Stationery Office, 1985.

15. Edelman, D.A., Exposure to asbestos and the risk of gastrointestinal cancer: a reassessment. Br. J. Ind. Med., 45, 75, 1988.

16. Murray, M., Departmental Committee for Compensation for Industrial Diseases. Cd 3495 and 3496. London, His Majesty's Stationery Office, 1907, p. 127.

17. Cooke, W.E., Pulmonary asbestosis. B.M.J., 2, 1024, 1927.

18. McDonald, S., Histology of pulmonary asbestosis. B.M.J., 2, 1025, 1927.

19. Oliver, T., Clinical aspects of pulmonary asbestosis. B.M.J., 2, 1026, 1927.

20. Pancoast, K.K., Miller, G., and Landis, H.R.M., A roentgenologic study of the effects of dust inhalation on the lung. Trans. Soc. Am. Phys., 32, 97, 1917.

21. Merewether, E.R.A., The occurrence of pulmonary fibrosis and other pulmonary affections in asbestos workers. J. Ind. Hyg., 12, 198, 1930.

22. Wood, W.B., and Gloyne, S.R., Pulmonary asbestosis. Lancet, 2, 1383, 1934.

23. Holleb, H.B., and Angrist, A., Bronchiogenic carcinoma in association with pulmonary asbestosis. Am. J. Pathol., 18, 123, 1942.

24. Morgan, W.K.C., Rheumatoid pneumoconiosis in association with asbestos. Thorax, 19, 433, 1964.

25. Fleischer, W.E., Viles, F.J., Gade, R.L., and Drinker, P., A health survey of pipe-covering operations in constructing naval vessels. J. Ind. Hyg. Toxicol., 28, 9, 1946.

26. Marr, W.T., Asbestos exposure during naval vessel overhaul. Am. Ind. Hyg. Assoc. J., 25, 264, 1964.

27. Gloyne, S.R., A case of oat cell carcinoma of the lung occurring in asbestosis. Tubercle, 18, 100, 1936.

28. Gloyne, S.R., Two cases of squamous carcinoma of the lung occurring in asbestosis. Tubercle, 17, 5, 1935.

29. Lynch, K.M., and Smith, W.A., Pulmonary asbestosis: III. Carcinoma of the lung in asbestos silicosis. Am. J. Cancer, 14, 56, 1935.

30. Kennaway, E.L., and Kennaway, N.M., A further study of the incidence of cancer of the lung and larynx. Br. J. Cancer, 1, 260, 1947.

31. Doll, R., Mortality from lung cancer in asbestos workers. Br. J. Ind. Med., 12, 81, 1955.

32. Thomas, H.F., Benjamin, I.T., Elwood, P.C., and Sweetnam, P.M., Further follow up of workers from an asbestos cement factor. Br. J. Ind. Med., 39, 273, 1982.

33. Ohlson, C.-G., and Hogstedt, C., Lung cancer among asbestos cement workers: a Swedish cohort study and a review. Br. J. Ind. Med., 42, 397, 1985.

34. Hodgson, J.T., and Jones, R.D., Mortality of asbestos workers in England and Wales. 1971–81. Br. J. Ind. Med., 43, 158, 1986.

35. Gardner, M.J., Winter, P.D., Pannett, B., and Powell, C.A., Follow up study of workers manufacturing chrysotile asbestos cement products. Br. J. Ind. Med., 43, 726, 1986.

36. Sluis-Cremer, G.K., and Bezuidenhout, B.N., Relation between asbestosis and bronchial cancer in amphibole asbestos miners. Br. J. Ind. Med., 46, 537, 1989.

37. Neuberger, M., and Kundi, M.I., Individual asbestos exposure: smoking and mortality—a cohort study in the asbestos cement industry. Br. J. Ind. Med., 47, 615, 1990.

38. Wagner, J.C., Sleggs, C.A., and Marchand, P., Diffuse pleural mesothelioma and asbestos exposure in the North Western Cape Province. Br. J. Ind. Med., 17, 260, 1960.

39. Wagner, J.C., The discovery of the association between blue asbestos and mesotheliomas and the aftermath. Br. J. Ind. Med., 48, 399, 1991.

40. Becklake, M., Asbestos-related disease of the lungs and other organs. Am. Rev. Respir. Dis., 114, 187, 1976.

41. Whitwell, F., Scott, J., and Grimshaw, M., Relationship between occupations and asbestos fibre

content of the lungs in patients with pleural mesothelioma, lung cancer, and other diseases. Thorax, 32, 377, 1977.

42. Churg, A., Analysis of lung asbestos content. Br. J. Ind. Med., 48, 649, 1991.

43. Gardner, L.U., Chrysotile asbestos as an indication of subtle differences in animal tissue. Am. Rev. Respir. Dis., 45, 762, 1941.

44. Stanton, M.F., Layard, M., Tergeris, A., et al., Relation of particle dimensions to carcinogenicity in amphibole asbestos and other fibrous minerals. J. Natl. Cancer Inst., 67, 965, 1981.

45. Gylseth, B., and Baunan, R., Topographic and size distribution of asbestos bodies in exposed human lungs. Scand. J. Work. Environ. Health, 7, 190, 1981.

46. Morgan, A., Holmes, A., and Davison, W., Clearance of sized glass fibres from the rat lung and their solubility in vivo. Ann. Occup. Hyg., 25, 317, 1982.

47. Bellman, B., Muhle, H., Pott, F., et al., Persistence of man made fibres (MMMF) and asbestos in rat lungs. Ann. Occup. Hyg., 31, 693, 1987.

48. Churg, A., Wright, J.L., Gilks, B., et al., Rapid short-term clearance of chrysotile compared with amosite asbestos in the guinea pig. Am. Rev. Respir. Dis., 139, 885, 1989.

49. Measurement of asbestos fibres in the workplace (B). In Report of the Royal Commission on Matters of Health and Safety Arising from the Use of Asbestos in Ontario, Vol. II. Toronto, Ontario Ministry of Attorney General, Queen's Printer for Ontario, 1984, pp. 371–374.

50. Asbestos in Buildings. In Report of the Royal Commission on Matters of Health and Safety Arising from the Use of Asbestos in Ontario. Toronto, Ontario Ministry of Attorney General, Queen's Printer for Ontario, 1984, pp. 561–574.

51. Burdett, G.J., and Rood, A.P., Membrane filter dust transfer technique for the analysis of asbestos fibres or other inorganic particles by transmission electron microscopy. Environ. Sci. Technol., 17, 643, 1983.

52. Hickish, D.E., and Knight, K.L., Exposure to asbestos during brake maintenance. Ann. Occup. Hyg., 13, 17, 1970.

53. Williams, R.L., and Muhlbaier, J.L., Asbestos brake emissions. Environ. Res., 29, 70, 1982.

54. Berry, G., and Newhouse, M.L., Mortality of workers manufacturing friction material using asbestos. Br. J. Ind. Med., 40, 1, 1983.

55. What is the health risk from the ingestion of asbestos fibres? In Report of the Royal Commission on Matters of Health and Safety Arising from the Use of Asbestos in Ontario. Toronto, Ontario Ministry of Attorney General, Queen's Printer for Ontario, 1984, pp. 310–313.

56. Round the World Column. Asbestos in water. Lancet, 2, 1256, 1973.

57. Gaensler, E.A., Jederlinic, P.J., and McLoud, T.C., Radiographic progression of asbestosis with and without continued exposure. Proceedings of the VIIth International Pneumoconiosis Conference, Part I. Publication no. 90–108. Washington, D.C., Department of Health and Human Services, 1990, pp. 386–392.

58. Murphy, R.L.H., Gaensler, E.A., Holford, S.K., et al., Crackles in the early detection of asbestosis. Am. Rev. Respir. Dis., 129, 375, 1984.

59. Coutts, I.I., Gilson, J.C., Kerr, I.H., et al., Significance of finger clubbing in asbestosis. Thorax, 42, 117, 1987.

60. Solomon, A., and Sluis-Cremer, G.K., Radiological features of asbestosis. In Solomon, A., and Kreel, L., eds., Radiology of Occupational Chest Disease. New York, Springer-Verlag, 1989, pp. 47–85.

61. International Labour Office, Guidelines for the Use of the ILO International Classification of Radiographs of Pneumoconiosis. No. 23, revised, Occupational Safety & Health Series. Geneva, International Labour Office, 1980.

62. Fletcher, D.E., and Edge, J.R., The early radiological changes in pulmonary and pleural asbestosis. Clin. Radiol., 21, 355, 1970.

63. Weiss, W., Cigarette smoke, asbestos and small irregular opacities. Am. Rev. Respir. Dis., 130, 293, 1984.

64. Dick, J., Morgan, W.K.C., Muir, D.C., and Reger, R.B., The significance of small irregular opacities in the chest radiograph. Chest, 102, 251, 1992.

65. Solomon, A., The radiology of asbestosis. Environ. Res., 3, 320, 1970.

66. Weil, H., Waggenspack, C., and Bailey, W., Radiographic and physiologic patterns amongst workers engaged in the manufacture of asbestos cement products. J. Occup. Med., 15, 248, 1973.

67. Solomon, A., Goldstein, B., Webster, I., et al., Massive fibrosis in asbestosis. Environ. Res., 4, 430, 1971.

68. Hnizdo, E., and Sluis-Cremer, G.K., Effect of tobacco smoking on the presence of asbestosis at postmortem and on the reading of irregular opacities on roentgenograms in asbestos-exposed workers. Am. Rev. Respir. Dis., 138, 1207, 1988.

69. Selikoff, I.J., Seidman, H., Lilis, R., and Herman, Y., Predictive significance of lesser degrees of parenchymal and pleural fibrosis. Prospective study of 1,117 asbestos insulation workers. Jan 1, 1963–Jan 1, 1988. Morbidity experience (Abstract). Proceedings of the VIIth International Pneumoconiosis Conference, Part 1. Publication no. 90–108. Washington, D.C., U.S. Government Printing Office, 1990, p. 703.

70. Wagner, J.C., Susceptibility to asbestos related disease. In Glen, H.R., ed., Proceedings of Asbestos Symposium, Johannesburg, 1977. Handburg, S.A., National Institute of Metallurgy, 1978, pp. 109–113.

71. Rubino, G.F., Newhouse, M., Murray, G., et al., Radiological changes after cessation of exposure among chrysotile workers in Italy. Ann. N. Y. Acad. Sci., 530, 157, 1979.

72. Jones, R.V., Diem, J.E., Hughes, J.M., et al., Progression of asbestos effects: a prospective longitudinal study of chest radiographs and lung function. Br. J. Ind. Med., 46, 97, 1989.

73. Becklake, M.R., Liddell, F.D.K., Manfred, J., and McDonald, J.C., Radiological changes after withdrawal from asbestos exposure. Br. J. Ind. Med., 36, 23, 1979.

74. Liddell, F.D.K., and McDonald, J.C., Radiological findings as predictors of mortality in Quebec asbestos miners. Br. J. Ind. Med., 37, 257, 1980.

75. Katz, D., and Kreel, L., Computed tomography in pulmonary asbestosis. Clin. Radiol., 30, 207, 1979.

76. Begin, R., Boctor, M., and Bergeron, D., et al., Radiographic assessment of pleuropulmonary disease in asbestos workers. Br. J. Ind. Med., 41, 373, 1984.

77. Muller, N.L., and Miller, R.R., Computed tomography of chronic diffuse infiltrative lung disease. Part 1. State of the Art. Am. Rev. Respir. Dis., 142, 1206, 1990.

78. Aberle, D.R., Gamsu, G., and Ray, C.S., High resolution CT of benign asbestos-related diseases. Clinical and radiographic correlation. Am. J. Roentgenol., 151, 883, 1988.

79. Wilson, R., and Hugh-Jones, P., The significance of lung function changes in asbestosis. Thorax, 15, 109, 1960.

80. Muldoon, B.C., and Turner-Warwick, M., Lung function studies in asbestos workers. Br. J. Dis. Chest., 66, 121, 1972.

81. Murphy, R.L.H., Gaensler, E.A., Ferris, B.G., et al., Diagnosis of asbestosis. Observations from a longitudinal survey of shipyard pipe coverers. Am. J. Med., 65, 488, 1978.

82. Becklake, M.R., Fournier-Massey, G., McDonald, J.C., et al., Lung function in relation to chest radiographic changes in Quebec asbestos workers. Bull. Physio-Pathol. Resp., 6, 637, 1970.

83. Murphy, R.L.H., Gaensler, E.A., Redding, R.A., et al., Low exposure to asbestos. Gas exchange in ship pipe coverers and controls. Arch. Environ. Health, 25, 253, 1972.

84. Bader, M.E., Bader, R.A., and Selikoff, I.J., Pulmonary function in asbestosis of the lung: an alveolar-capillary block syndrome. Am. J. Med., 30, 235, 1961.

85. Ferris, B.G., Epidemiology Standardization Project. Recommended standardized procedures for pulmonary function testimony: III C. Am. Rev. Respir. Dis., 118 (Suppl.), 67, 1978.

86. Jodoin, G., Gibbs, G.W., Macklem, P.T., et al., Early effects of asbestos exposure on lung function. Am. Rev. Respir. Dis., 104, 525, 1971.

87. Peress, L., Hoag, H., White, F., and Becklake, M.R., The relationship between closing volume, smoking, and asbestos dust exposure (Abstract). Clin. Res., 23, 647a, 1975.

88. Agostoni, P., Smith, D.D., Schoene, R.B., et al., Evaluation of breathlessness in asbestos workers: results of exercise testing. Am. Rev. Respir. Dis., 135, 812, 1987.

89. Sue, D.Y., Oren, A., Hansen, J.E., and Wasserman, K., Lung function and exercise performance in smoking and nonsmoking asbestos exposed workers. Am. Rev. Respir. Dis., 132, 612, 1985.

90. Wright, J.L., and Churg, A., Severe diffuse small airways abnormalities in long term chrysotile asbestos miners. Br. J. Ind. Med., 42, 556, 1985.

91. Rodriguez-Roisin, R., Merchant, J.M., Cochrane, G.M., et al., Maximal expiratory flow volume curves in workers exposed to asbestos. Respiration, 39, 158, 1980.

92. Kilburn, K.H., Warshaw, R., and Thornton, J.C., Signs of asbestosis and impaired function in women who worked in shipyards. Am. J. Ind. Med., 8, 545, 1983.

93. Kilburn, K.H., Warshaw, R.H., Einstein, K., and Bernstein, J., Airways disease in non-smoking asbestos workers. Arch. Environ. Health, 40, 293, 1985.

94. American Thoracic Society, Lung function testing: selection of reference values and interpretative strategies. Am. Rev. Respir. Dis., 144, 1202, 1991.

95. Bègin, R., Cantin, A., Berthiaume, Y., et al., Airway function in life time nonsmoking older asbestos workers. Am. J. Med., 75, 631, 1983.

96. Seaton, D., Regional lung function in asbestos workers. Thorax, 32, 40, 1977.

97. Harber, P., Tashkin, D.P., Lew, M., and Simmons, M., Physiologic categorization of asbestos exposed workers. Chest, 92, 494, 1987.

98. Berry, G., Newhouse, M.L., and Antonis, P., Combined effects of asbestos and smoking on mortality from lung cancer and mesothelioma in factory workers. Br. J. Ind. Med., 42, 12, 1985.

99. American Thoracic Society. The diagnosis of nonmalignant diseases related to asbestos [statement]. Am. Rev. Respir. Dis., 134, 363, 1986.

100. Gilson, J.C., Problems and perspectives: the changing hazards of exposure to asbestos. Ann. N. Y. Acad. Sci., 132, 696, 1965.

101. Epler, G.T., McLoud, T.C., Gaensler, E.A., et al., Normal chest roentgenograms in chronic diffuse infiltrative lung disease. N. Engl. J. Med., 298, 934, 1978.

102. Murphy, R.L.H., Ferris, B.G., Burgess, W.A., et al., Effects of low concentrations of asbestos. Clinical, environmental, radiologic and epidemiologic observations in shipyard pipe coverers and controls. N. Engl. J. Med., 285, 1271, 1971.

103. Gaensler, E.A., Jederlinic, P.J., and Churg, A., Idiopathic pulmonary fibrosis in asbestos exposed workers. Am. Rev. Respir. Dis., 144, 689, 1991.

104. Craighead, J.E., Abraham, J.L., Churg, A., et al., The pathology of asbestos associated diseases: diagnostic criteria and a proposed gradient scheme. (Report of Pneumoconioses Committee of the College of American Pathologists and NIOSH.) Arch. Pathol. Lab. Med., 106, 544, 1982.

105. Gaensler, E.A., and Addington, W., Asbestos or ferruginous bodies. N. Engl. J. Med., 280, 488, 1969.
106. Churg, A., Nonneoplastic diseases caused by asbestos. *In* Churg, A., and Green, F.H.Y., eds., Pathology of Occupational Lung Diseases. New York, Igaku-Shoin, 1988, pp. 224–234.
107. Gough, J., and Heppleston, A.G., The pathology of the pneumoconioses. *In* King, E.J., and Fletcher, C.M., eds., Industrial Pulmonary Diseases. Boston, Little Brown, 1960, pp. 23–35.
108. Vorwald, A.J., Durkan, T.M., and Pratt, P.C., Experimental studies of asbestosis. Arch. Ind. Hyg. Occup. Med., 3, 1, 1951.
109. Thomson, J.G., Kaschula, R.O.C., and MacDonald, R.R., Asbestos: a modern day urban hazard. S. Afr. Med. J., 37, 77, 1963.
110. Gross, P., deTreville, R.T.D., and Haller, M.N., Pulmonary ferruginous bodies in city dwellers. Arch. Environ. Health., 19, 186, 1969.
111. Churg, A., and Warnock, M.L., Analysis of the cores of asbestos bodies from members of the general population. Patients with probable low-degree exposure to asbestos. Am. Rev. Respir. Dis., 120, 781, 1979.
112. Roggli, V.L., Greenberg, S.D., McLarty, J.W., et al., Comparison of sputum and lung asbestos body counts in former asbestos workers. Am. Rev. Respir. Dis., 122, 941, 1980.
113. Langer, A.M., Rubin, I.B., and Selikoff, I.J., Chemical characterization of asbestos body cores by electron microprobe analysis. J. Histochem. Cytochem., 20, 723, 1972.
114. Gylseth, B., and Skaug, V., Relation between pathological grading and lung fibre concentration in a patient with asbestosis. Br. J. Ind. Med., 43, 756, 1986.
115. Morgan, A., and Holmes, A., Distribution and characteristics of amphibole asbestos fibres, measured with a light microscope, in the left lung of an insulation worker. Br. J. Ind. Med., 40, 45, 1983.
116. Churg, A., The distribution of amosite asbestos in the periphery of the normal human lung. Br. J. Ind. Med., 47, 677, 1990.
117. Rowlands, N., Gibbs, G.W., and McDonald, J.C., Asbestos fibres in the lungs of asbestos miners and millers. Ann. Occup. Hyg., 29, 305, 1982.
118. Holden, J., and Churg, A., Asbestos bodies and the diagnosis of asbestosis in chrysotile miners. Environ. Res., 39, 232, 1986.
119. Roger, A.J., Determination of mineral fibre in human lung tissue by microscopy. Ann. Occup. Hyg., 28, 1, 1984.
120. Hayes, A.A., Rose, A.H., Musk, A.W., et al., Neutrophil chemotactic factor release and neutrophil alveolitis in asbestos exposed individuals. Chest, 94, 521, 1988.
121. Merrill, W., Carter, D., and Cullen, M.R., The relationship between large airway inflammation and airway metaplasia. Chest, 100, 131, 1991.
122. Mikes, P.S., Polomski, L.L., and Gee, J.B.L., Mepacrine impairs neutrophil response after acute lung injury in rats: effects on neutrophil migration. Am. Rev. Respir. Dis., 138, 1464, 1988.
123. Sparks, J.V., Pulmonary asbestosis. Radiology, 17, 1249, 1931.
124. Selikoff, I.J., The occurrence of pleural calcification among asbestos insulation workers. Ann. N. Y. Acad. Sci., 132, 351, 1965.
125. Porro, F.W., Patton, J.R., and Hobbs, A.A., Pneumoconiosis in the talc industry. Am. J. Roentgenol., 47, 507, 1942.
126. Siegal, W., Smith, A.R., and Greenburg, L., The dust hazard in tremolite talc mining, including roentgenologic findings in talc workers. Am. J. Roentgenol., 49, 11, 1943.
127. Cartier, P., Contribution à l'étude de l'amiantose. Arch. Mal. Prof. Med., 10, 589, 1949.
128. Lynch, K.M., and Cannon, W.M., Asbestosis VI. Analysis of forty necropsied cases. Dis. Chest, 14, 874, 1948.
129. Brosig, W., Zuckergrass der Pleura. Allg. Path. Anat., 71, 52, 1939.
130. Bohlig, H., Dalquen, P., and Hain, E., Epidemiologie asbestbedingter Gesundheitsschäden. Internist (Berl.), 13, 318, 1972.
131. Leathhart, G., Pulmonary function tests in asbestos workers. Trans. Soc. Occup. Med., 18, 46, 1968.
132. Sargent, E.N., Jacobsen, G., and Gordonson, J.S., Pleural plaques: a signpost of asbestos inhalation. Semin. Roentgenol., 12, 287, 1977.
133. Reger, R.B., Ames, R.G., Merchant, J.A., et al., The detection of thoracic abnormalities using posterior-anterior (PA) vs PA and oblique roentgenograms. Chest, 81, 290, 1982.
134. Sargent, E.N., Boswell, W.D., Jr., Rolls, P.W., and Markovitz, A., Subpleural fat pads in workers exposed to asbestos: distinction from non-calcified pleural plaques. Radiology, 152, 273, 1984.
135. Rockoff, S.D., Kagan, E., Schwartz, A., et al., Visceral pleural thickening in asbestos exposure: the occurrence and implications of thickened interlobar fissures. J. Thorac. Imaging, 2, 58, 1987.
136. McMillan, G.H.G., Pethybridge, R.J., and Sheers, G., Effect of smoking on attack rates of pulmonary and pleural lesions related to asbestos dust. Br. J. Ind. Med., 37, 268, 1980.
137. Wright, P.H., Hanson, A., Kneel, L., et al., Respiratory function changes after asbestos pleurisy. Thorax, 35, 31, 1980.
138. Oliver, L.C., Eisen, E.A., Greene, R., and Sprince, N., Asbestos-related pleural plaques and lung function. Am. J. Ind. Med., 14, 649, 1988.
139. Fridriksson, H., Hedenstrom, H., Hillerdal, G., et al., Lung parenchymal changes in persons with pleural plaques. Work III. *In* Hillerdal, G., ed., Pleural Plaques, Occurrence, Exposure, and Clinical

Importance. Uppsala, Sweden, Acta Universitatis Upsaliensis Abstracts of Uppsala Dissertations from Faculty of Medicine, no. 363, 1980, p. 157.

140. Bourbeau, J., Ernst, P., Chrome, J., et al., The relationship between respiratory impairment and asbestos related pleural abnormality in an active work force. Am. Rev. Respir. Dis., 142, 837, 1990.

141. Schwartz, D.A., Fuortes, L.J., Galvin, J.R., et al., Asbestos induced pleural fibrosis and impaired lung function. Am. Rev. Respir. Dis., 141, 321, 1990.

142. Schwartz, D.A., Galvin, J.R., Dayton, C.S., et al., Determinants of restrictive lung function in asbestos-induced pleural fibrosis. J. Appl. Physiol., 68, 1932, 1990.

143. Gaensler, E.A., Jederlinic, P.J., and McLoud, T.C., Lung function with asbestos-related pleural plaques. In Proceedings of the VIIth International Pneumoconiosis Conference, Part 1. Publication no. 90–108. Washington, D.C., Department of Health and Human Services, 1990, pp. 696–702.

144. Hertzog, P., Toty, L., Personne, C., and Roujeau, J., Plaques pleurales, pariétales, fibrohyalines. J. Fr. Med. Chir. Thor., 26, 59, 1972.

145. Roberts, W.C., and Ferrans, V.J., Pure collagen plaques on the diaphragm and pleura. Gross, histologic and electron microscopic observations. Chest, 61, 357, 1972.

146. Meurman, L.O., Asbestos bodies and pleural plaques in a Finnish series of autopsy cases. Acta Pathol. Microbiol. Scand. Suppl. No. 181, 1966.

147. Herbert, A., Pathogenesis of pleurisy, pleural fibrosis and mesothelial proliferation. Thorax, 41, 176, 1986.

148. Eisenstadt, H.B., Asbestos pleurisy. Dis. Chest, 46, 78, 1964.

149. Gaensler, E.A., and Kaplan, A.I., Asbestos pleural effusion. Ann. Intern. Med., 74, 178, 1971.

150. Sluis-Cremer, G.K., and Webster, I., Acute pleurisy in asbestos exposed persons. Environ. Res., 5, 380, 1972.

151. Chahinian, P.H., Hirsch, A., Bignon, J., et al., Les pleurisies asbestosiques non-tumorales. Rev. Fr. Mal. Respir., 1, 5, 1973.

152. Hillerdal, G., Nonmalignant asbestos pleural disease. Thorax, 36, 669, 1981.

153. Epler, G.R., McLoud, T.C., and Gaensler, E.A., Prevalence and incidence of benign asbestos pleural effusion in a working population. JAMA, 247, 617, 1982.

153a. Smith, D.O., Plaques, cancer and confusion. Chest, 105, 8, 1994.

154. Mårtennsson, G., Hagberg, S., Pettersson, K., and Thiringer, G., Asbestos pleural effusion: a clinical entity. Thorax, 42, 646, 1987.

155. Boutin, C., Viallat, J., Farisse, P., and Chous, R., Pleurisies asbestosiques benignes. Poumon Coeur, 31, 111, 1975.

156. Wright, P.H., Hanson, A., Kreel, L., and Capel, L.H., Respiratory function changes after asbestos pleurisy. Thorax, 35, 31, 1980.

157. Hillerdal, G., Pleural and parenchymal fibrosis mainly affecting the upper lung lobes in persons exposed to asbestos. Respir. Med., 84, 129, 1990.

158. Dernevik, L., Gatzinsky, P., Hultman, E., et al., Shrinking pleuritis with atelectasis. Thorax, 37, 252, 1982.

159. Hillerdal, G., and Hemmingson, A., Pulmonary pseudotumors and asbestosis. Acta Radiol. (Stockh.), 21, 615, 1980.

160. Mintzer, R.A., Gore, R.M., Vogelzang, L., et al., Rounded atelectasis and its association with asbestos-induced pleural disease. Radiology, 139, 567, 1987.

161. Case records of the Massachusetts General Hospital. N. Engl. J. Med., 308, 1466, 1983.

162. Liddell, F.D.K., Other aspects of asbestos related malignancies. In Liddell, F.D.K., and Miller, K., eds., Mineral Fibers and Health. Boca Raton, FL, CRC Press, 1991, pp. 188–190.

163. Mossman, B.T., and Craighead, J.E., Mechanisms of asbestos associated bronchogenic cancer. In Antman, K., and Aisner, J., eds., Asbestos Related Malignancy. Orlando, FL, Grune and Stratton, 1987, pp. 132–150.

164. National Institute of Occupational Safety and Health. Hazard Surveys. Rockville, MD, National Institute of Occupational Safety and Health, 1973.

165. Enterline, P.E., Proportion of cancer due to exposure to asbestos. In Peto, R., and Schneiderman, M., eds., Quantification of Occupational Cancer (Banbury report no. 9). Cold Spring Harbor, NY, Cold Spring Harbor Laboratory, 1981, pp. 19–34.

166. Nicholson, W.J., Perkel, G., Selikoff, I.J., et al., Cancer from occupational asbestos exposure: projections 1980–2000. In Peto, R., and Schneiderman, M., eds., Quantification of Occupational Cancer (Banbury report no. 9). Cold Spring Harbor, NY, Cold Spring Harbor Laboratory, 1981, pp. 87–107.

167. Nicholson, W.J., Perkel, G., and Selikoff, I.J., Occupational exposure to asbestos: population at risk and projected mortality. Am. J. Ind. Med., 3, 259, 1982.

168. Hammond, E.C., Selikoff, I.J., and Seidman, H., Asbestos exposure, cigarette smoking and death rates. Ann. N. Y. Acad. Sci., 330, 473, 1979.

169. Surgeon General, Report of 1989. Reducing the Health Consequences of Smoking: 25 Years of Progress. Rockville, MD, Centers for Disease Control, Office on Smoking and Health, 1989, pp. 121–162.

170. Enterline, P.E., Estimating health risks in studies of the health effects of asbestos. Am. Rev. Respir. Dis., 113, 175, 1976.

171. Liddell, F.D.K., and Hanley, J.A., Relations between asbestos exposure and lung cancer SMRs in occupational cohort studies. Br. J. Ind. Med., 42, 389, 1985.

172. Seidman, H., and Selikoff, I.J., Decline in death rates among asbestos insulation workers associated with diminution of work exposure to asbestos 1967–1986. Ann. N. Y. Acad. Sci., 601, 300, 1990.

173. Sanden, A., Garoholin, B., Larsson, S., et al., The risk of lung cancer and mesothelioma after cessation of asbestos exposure: a prospective study of shipyard workers. Eur. Respir. J., 5, 281, 1992.

174. Acheson, A.D., and Gardner, M.J., Health and Safety Executive (U.K.), Asbestos: the control limit for asbestos. In Health and Safety Commission, An Update of the Relevant Sections of the Ill Effects of Asbestos Upon Health. London, Her Majesty's Stationery Office, 1983.

175. Hughes, J.M., Epidemiology of lung cancer in relation to asbestos exposure. In Liddell, F.D.K., and Miller, K., eds., Mineral Fibres and Health. Boca Raton, FL, CRC Press, 1991, pp. 136–143.

176. Seidman, H., Selikoff, I.J., and Gelb, S.K., Mortality experience of amosite asbestos factory workers: dose response relationships 5 to 40 years after onset of short-term work exposure. Am. J. Ind. Med., 10, 479, 1986.

177. McDonald, A.D., Fry, J.S., Woolley, A.J., and MacDonald, J.C., Dust exposure and mortality in an American chrysotile asbestos friction products plant. Br. J. Ind. Med., 41, 151, 1984.

178. McDonald, J.C., Liddell, F.D.K., Gibbs, G.W., Eyssen, G.E., and McDonald, A.D., Dust exposure and mortality in chrysotile mining, 1910–1975. Br. J. Ind. Med., 37, 11, 1980.

179. Hughes, J.M., Weill, H., and Hammad, Y.Y., Mortality of workers employed in two asbestos cement manufacturing plants. Br. J. Ind. Med., 44, 161, 1987.

180. McDonald, J.C., Liddell, F.D.K., Dufresne, A., and McDonald, A.D., The 1891–1920 birth cohort of Quebec chrysotile miners and millers: Mortality 1970–88. Br. J. Ind. Med., 50, 1073, 1993.

181. Mossman, B.T., Bignon, J., Corn, M., et al., Asbestos: scientific developments and implications for public policy. Science, 247, 294, 1990.

182. Hendry, N.W., The geology, occurrences and major uses of asbestos. Ann. N. Y. Acad. Sci., 132, 31, 1965.

183. Selikoff, I.J., Churg, J., and Hammond, E., The occurrence of asbestosis among insulation workers in the United States. Ann. N. Y. Acad. Sci., 132, 139, 1965.

184. United States Department of the Interior. Tables compiled by industry 1945–1963. Ann. N. Y. Acad. Sci., 162, 762, 1965.

185. Mancuso, T.F., Relative risk of mesothelioma among railroad machinists exposed to chrysotile. Am. J. Ind. Med., 13, 639, 1988.

186. Newhouse, M.L., and Sullivan, K.R., A mortality study of workers manufacturing friction materials 1941–1986. Br. J. Ind. Med., 46, 176, 1989.

187. McDonald, J.C., and McDonald, A.D., Epidemiology of asbestos related lung cancer. In Antman, K., and Aisner, J., eds., Asbestos Related Malignancy. Orlando, FL, Grune and Stratton. 1987, pp. 31–55.

188. Turner-Warwick, M., Lebowitz, M., Burrows, B., et al., Cryptogenic fibrosing alveolitis and lung cancer. Thorax, 35, 496, 1980.

189. Sluis-Cremer, G.K., and Bezuidenhout, B.N., Relation between asbestosis and bronchial cancer in amphibole asbestos miners. Br. J. Ind. Med., 46, 537, 1989.

190. Hughes, J., and Weill, H., Asbestos as a necessary precursor of asbestos related lung cancer: results of a prospective mortality study in asbestos products manufacturing. Br. J. Ind. Med., 48, 229, 1991.

191. Kipen, H.M., Lilis, R., Suzuki, Y., et al., Pulmonary fibrosis in asbestos insulation workers with lung cancer. Br. J. Ind. Med., 44, 96, 1987.

192. Rudd, R.M., Pulmonary fibrosis in asbestos insulation workers with lung cancer. Correspondence. Br. J. Ind. Med., 44, 428, 1987.

193. Nicholson, W.J., Case study: asbestos. The TLV approach. Ann. N. Y. Acad. Sci., 271, 152, 1976.

194. Nicholson, W.J.C., Holaday, D.A., and Heimann, H., Direct and indirect occupational exposure to insulation dusts in United States shipyards. Occupational Safety and Health Series, Safety and Health in Shipbuilding and Ship Repairing, Vol. 27. Geneva, International Labour Office, 1972, pp 37–47.

195. Puntoni, R., Vercelli, M., Merlo, F., et al., Mortality among shipyard workers in Genoa, Italy. Ann. N. Y. Acad. Sci., 330, 353, 1979.

196. Rossiter, C.E., and Coles, R.M., HM Dockyard, Devonport, 1947 Mortality Study. In Wagner, J.C., ed., Biological Effects of Mineral Fibres, Vol. 2. Lyon, IARC Scientific Publications, 1980, pp. 713–721.

197. Nicholson, W.J., and Selikoff, I.J., Mortality Experience of 1918 Employees of Electric Boat Company, Groton, Connecticut. New York, Environmental Sciences Laboratory, Mount Sinai, School of Medicine, 1984.

198. Kolonel, L.N., Yoshizawa, C.N., Hirohato, T., et al., Cancer occurrence in shipyard workers exposed to asbestos in Hawaii. Cancer Res., 45, 3924, 1985.

199. Newhouse, M.L., Oakes, D., and Wooley, A.J., Mortality of welders and other craftsmen at a shipyard in N.E. England. Br. J. Ind. Med., 42, 406, 1985.

200. Sanden, A., and Jarvholm, B., Cancer morbidity in Swedish shipyard workers. Int. Arch. Occup. Environ. Health, 59, 455, 1987.

201. Melkild, A., Langard, S., Andersen, A., et al., Incidence of cancer among welders and other workers in a Norwegian shipyard. Scand. J. Work Environ. Health, 15, 387, 1989.

202. Editorial. What proportion of lung cancers are occupational? Lancet, 2, 1238, 1978.

203. Ives, J.C., Buffler, P.A., and Greenberg, D., Environmental association and histopathologic patterns of carcinoma of the lung. Am. Rev. Respir. Dis., 128, 195, 1983.

204. Feinstein, A.R., Gelfman, N.A., and Yesner, R.A., Observer variability in the histopatologic diagnosis of lung cancer. Am. Rev. Respir. Dis., 101, 671, 1970.

205. Vincent, R.G., Pickren, J.W., Lane, W.W., et al., The changing histopathology of lung cancer: a review of 1682 cases. Cancer, 39, 1647, 1977.

206. Whitwell, F., Newhouse, M.L., and Bennett, D.R., A study of the histological cell types of lung cancer in workers suffering from asbestosis in the United Kingdom. Br. J. Ind. Med., 31, 298, 1974.

207. Hourihane, D.O., and McCaughey, W.T.E., Pathological aspects of asbestosis. Postgrad. Med. J., 42, 613, 1966.

208. Kannerstein, M., and Churg, J., Pathology of carcinoma of the lung associated with asbestos exposure. Cancer, 30, 14, 1972.

209. Weiss, W., Lobe of origin in the attribution of lung cancer to asbestos. Br. J. Ind. Med., 45, 544, 1988.

210. Axelson, O., Confounding from smoking in occupational epidemiology. Br. J. Ind. Med., 46, 505, 1989.

211. McFadden, D., Wright, J., Wiggs, B., et al., Smoking inhibits asbestos clearance. Am. Rev. Respir. Dis., 133, 372, 1986.

212. Greenberg, M., and Lloyd Davies, T.A., Mesothelioma register, 1967–1968. Br. J. Ind. Med., 31, 91, 1974.

213. Milne, J.E.H., Thirty-two cases of mesothelioma in Victoria, Australia: a retrospective survey related to asbestos exposure. Br. J. Ind. Med., 33, 195, 1976.

214. Baris, Y.I., Sahin, A., and Ozesmi, M., An outbreak of pleural mesothelioma and chronic fibrosing pleurisy in the village of Karain/Urgup in Anatolia. Thorax, 33, 181, 1978.

215. Hillerdal, G., and Baris, Y.I., Radiological study of pleural changes in relation to mesothelioma in Turkey. Thorax, 38, 443, 1983.

216. Wedler, H.W., Ber den Lungenkrebs bei Asbestose (pulmonary cancer in asbestosis). Dtsch. Arch. Klin. Med., 191, 189, 1943.

217. Parkes, W.R., Asbestos-related disorders. Br. J. Dis. Chest, 67, 261, 1973.

218. Willis, R.A., Pathology of Tumors. St. Louis, C.V. Mosby, 1948.

219. Browne, K., The epidemiology of mesothelioma. J. Soc. Occup. Med., 33, 190, 1983.

220. Brenner, J., Sordillo, P.P., and Magill, G.B., Malignant mesothelioma in children. Med. Pediatr. Oncol., 9, 367, 1981.

221. Peterson, J.T., Greenberg, S.D., and Buffler, P.A., Non-asbestos related malignant mesothelioma. A review. Cancer, 54, 951, 1984.

222. Antman, K.H., Corson, J.M., and Frederick, P., Malignant mesothelioma following radiation exposure. J. Clin. Oncol., 1, 695, 1983.

223. Lerman, Y., Learman, Y., Schachter, P., et al., Radiation associated malignant pleural mesothelioma. Thorax, 46, 463, 1991.

224. Das, P.B., Fletcher, A.G., and Deodhare, S.G., Mesothelioma in an agricultural community of India: a clinicopathological study. Aust. N. Z. J. Surg., 46, 218, 1976.

225. Hochberg, L.A., Endothelioma (mesothelioma) of the pleura. Am. Rev. Respir. Dis., 63, 150, 1951.

226. McDonald, J.C., and McDonald, A.D., Epidemiology of mesothelioma from estimated incidence. Prev. Med., 6, 426, 1977.

227. Enterline, P.E., Asbestos and Cancer: The First Thirty Years. Pittsburgh, PA, P.E. Enterline, 1978.

228. Connelly, R.R., Spirtas, R., Myers, M.H., et al., Demographic patterns for mesothelioma in the United States. J. Natl. Cancer Inst., 78, 1053, 1987.

229. McDonald, A.D., and McDonald, J.C., Epidemiology of malignant mesothelioma. In Antman, K., and Aisner, J., eds., Asbestos Related Malignancy. Orlando, FL, Grune & Stratton, 1987, p. 31.

230. Jones, R.D., Smith, D.M., and Thomas, P.G., Mesothelioma in Great Britain in 1968–1983. Br. J. Cancer, 51, 699, 1985.

231. Liddell, D., Epidemiological observations on mesothelioma and their implications for non-occupational exposure to asbestos. In Spengler, J.D., Ozkaynak, H., McCarthy, J.F., and Lee, H., eds., Proceedings of Symposium on Health Effects of Exposure to Asbestos in Buildings, December 14–16, 1988. Cambridge, MA, Harvard University Energy and Environmental Policy Centre, 1989.

232. Armstrong, B.K., DeKlerk, N.H., Musk, A.W., and Hobbs, M.S.T., Mortality in miners and millers of crocidolite in Western Australia. Br. J. Ind. Med., 45, 5, 1988.

233. McDonald, J.C., McDonald, A.D., Armstrong, B., and Sèbastien, P., Cohort study of mortality of vermiculite miners exposed to tremolite. Br. J. Ind. Med., 43, 436, 1986.

234. McDonald, J.C., Liddell, F.D.K., Gibbs, G.W., et al., Dust exposure and mortality in chrysotile mining, 1910–75. Br. J. Ind. Med., 37, 11, 1980.

235. Seidman, H., Selikoff, I.J., and Gelb, S.K., Mortality experience of amosite asbestos asbestos factory workers: dose response relationships 5 to 40 years after onset of short-term work exposure. Am. J. Ind. Med., 10, 479, 1986.

236. Acheson, E.D., Gardner, M.J., Winter, P.D., and Bennett, C., Cancer in a factory using amosite asbestos. Int. J. Epidemiol., 13, 3, 1984.

237. Meurman, L.O., Kiviluoto, R., and Hakama, M., Mortality and morbidity among the working population of anthophyllite asbestos miners in Finland. Br. J. Ind. Med., 31, 105, 1974.

238. Gibbs, A.R., Role of asbestos and other fibers in the development of diffuse malignant mesothelioma. Thorax, 45, 649, 1990.

239. Pooley, F.D., An examination of the fibrous mineral content of asbestos lung tissue from the Canadian chrysotile mining industry. Environ. Res., 12, 281, 1976.

240. Gibbs, G.W., Qualitative aspects of dust exposure in the Quebec asbestos mining and milling industry. In Walton, E.H., ed., Inhaled Particles III. Surrey, England, Unwin Bros. Ltd., 1970, p. 783.

241. Sébastien, P., Bégin, R., Case, B.W., and McDonald, J.C., Inhalation of chrysotile dust. In Wagner, J.C., ed., Biological Effects of Chrysotile. Philadelphia, J.B. Lippincott, 1987, p. 783.

242. McDonald, J.C., Armstrong, B., Doell, D., et al., Mesothelioma and asbestos fiber type—evidence from lung tissue analysis. Cancer, 63, 1544, 1989.

243. Wagner, J.C., Gerry, G., Skidmore, J.W., and Timbrell, V., The effects of the inhalation of asbestos in rats. Br. J. Cancer, 29, 252, 1974.

244. Timbrell, V., Physical factors as aetiological mechanisms. In Bogovski, P., Gilson, J.G., Trimbell, V., and Wagner, J.C., eds., Biological Effects of Asbestos. IARC publication no. 8. Lyon, IARC Scientific Publications, 1973, p. 295.

245. Rothschild, H., and Mulvey, J.J., An increased risk for lung cancer mortality associated with sugar cane farming. J. Natl. Cancer Inst., 68, 755, 1982.

246. Doll, R., Symposium on MMMF, Copenhagen, October 1986: Overview and Conclusions. Ann. Occup. Hyg., 31(4B), 805, 1987.

247. Vianna, N.J., and Polan, A.K., Non-occupational exposure to asbestos and malignant mesothelioma in females. Lancet, 1, 1061, 1978.

248. McDonald, A.D., and McDonald, J.C., Malignant mesothelioma in North America. Cancer, 46, 1650, 1980.

249. Sébastien, P., Masse, R., and Bignon, J., Recovery of ingested asbestos fibers from the gastrointestinal lymph in rats. Environ. Res., 22, 201, 1980.

250. Gross, P., Harley, R.A., Swinberne, L.M., et al., Ingested mineral fibers, do they penetrate tissue or cause cancer? Arch. Environ. Health, 29, 341, 1974.

251. Smith, W.E., Hubert, D.D., Sobel, H.J., et al., Health in experimental animals drinking water with and without amosite and other mineral particles. J. Environ. Pathol., Toxicol., 3, 277, 1980.

252. Donham, K.J., Berg, J.W., Will, L.A., et al., The effects of long term ingestion of asbestos on the colon of 344 rats. Cancer, 45, 1073, 1980.

253. McConnell, E.E., Toxicology and Carcinogenesis Studies: Studies of Tremolite. NTP Technical Report 277. NIH publications no 90–2531. Washington, D.C., U.S. Department of Health and Human Services, 1990.

254. Omenn, G.S., Merchant, J., Boatman, E., et al., Contribution of environmental fibers to respiratory cancer. Environ. Health Perspect., 70, 51, 1986.

255. Antman, K., Cohen, S., Dimitrov, N.V., Malignant mesothelioma of the tunica vaginalis testis. J. Clin. Oncol., 2, 447, 1984.

256. Wechsler, R.J., Rao, V., and Steiner, R.M., The radiology of malignant mesothelioma. Crit. Rev. Diagn. Imaging, 20, 283, 1984.

257. Kannerstein, M., and Churg, J., Peritoneal mesothelioma. Hum. Pathol., 8, 83, 1977.

258. Elmes, P.C., and Simpson, M.J.C., The clinical aspects of mesothelioma. Q. J. Med., 45, 427, 1976.

259. Roberts, G.H., Distant visceral metastases in pleural mesothelioma. Br. J. Dis. Chest., 70, 246, 1976.

260. Kannerstein, M., Churg, J., McCaughey, W.T.E., and Hill, D.P., Papillary tumors of the peritoneum in women: mesothelioma or papillary carcinoma. Am. J. Obstet. Gynecol., 127, 306, 1977.

261. Churg, A., Neoplastic asbestos-induced diseases. In Churg, A., and Green, F.M., eds., Pathology of Occupational Lung Disease. New York, Igaku-Shoin, 1988, pp. 292–297.

262. Corsun, J.M., and Pinkus, G.S., Mesothelioma: profile of keratin protein and carcinoembryonic antigen. Am. J. Pathol., 108, 80, 1982.

263. Schlegel, R., Banks-Schlegel, S., McLeod, J., and Pinkus, G.S., Immunoperoxidase localization of keratin in human neoplasms. A preliminary survey. Am. J. Pathol., 1010, 41, 1980.

264. Loosli, H., and Hurlimann, J., Immunohistologic study of malignant diffuse mesotheliomas of the pleura. Histopathology, 8, 793, 1984.

265. Battifora, H., and Kopinski, M.I., Distinction of mesothelioma from adenocarcinoma. An immunohistochemical approach. Cancer, 55, 1679, 1985.

266. Battifora, H., and Kopinski, M.I., Distinction of mesothelioma and reactive mesothelial cells from adenocarcinoma: an immunohistochemical study. Lab. Invest., 50, 4A, 1984.

267. Wang, N.S., Electron microscopy in the diagnosis of pleural mesotheliomas. Cancer, 31, 1046, 1973.

268. Dardick, I., Al-Jabi, M., McCaughey, W.T.E., et al., Ultrastructure of poorly differentiated diffuse epithelial mesotheliomas. Ultrastruct. Pathol., 7, 151, 1984.

269. Blake, P.R., Catterall, M., and Emerson, P.A., Pleural mesothelioma treated by fast neutron therapy. Thorax, 40, 72, 1985.

270. Mancuso, T.F., and Coulter, E.J., Methodology in industrial health studies: the cohort approach, with special reference to an asbestos company. Arch. Environ. Health, 6, 210, 1963.

271. Stell, P.M., and McGill, T., Asbestos and laryngeal carcinoma. Lancet, 2, 416, 1973.

272. Morgan, R.W., and Shettigara, P.T., Occupational asbestos exposure, smoking, and laryngeal carcinoma. Ann. N. Y. Acad. Sci., 271, 308, 1976.
273. Chan, C.K., and Gee, J.B.L., Asbestos exposure and laryngeal cancer: an analysis of the epidemiologic evidence. J. Occup. Med., 30, 23, 1988.
274. Liddell, F.D.K., Laryngeal cancer and asbestos. Br. J. Ind. Med., 47, 289, 1990.
275. Liddell, F.D.K., Other aspects of asbestos related malignancy. *In* Liddell, D., and Miller, K., eds., Mineral Fibers and Health. Boca Raton, FL, CRC Press, 1991, pp. 180–190.
276. Elmes, P.C., and Wade, O.L., Relationship between exposure to asbestos and pleural malignancy in Belfast. Ann. N. Y. Acad. Sci., 132, 549, 1965.
277. Heasman, M.A., and Lipworth, L., Accuracy of certification of death GRO. Studies on medical and population studies. No. 20. London, Her Majesty's Stationery Office, 1966.
278. Bolton, R.E., Davis, J.M.G., and Lamb, D., The pathological effects of prolonged asbestos ingestion in rats. Environ. Res., 23, 134, 1982.
279. Condie, L.W., Review of published studies of orally administered asbestos. Environ. Health Perspect., 53, 3, 1983.
280. Symposium on Health Aspects of Exposure to Asbestos in Buildings. Presented at Harvard University, Energy and Environmental Policy Center, John F. Kennedy School of Government, Cambridge, MA, December 14–16, 1988.
281. World Health Organization, Report on Occupational Exposure Limit for Asbestos, Oxford, United Kingdom, April 10–11, 1989. Geneva, World Health Organization, 1989.
282. Report of the Royal Commission on Matters of Health and Safety Arising from the Use of Asbestos in Ontario, Part IV, Vol. 2. Toronto, Ontario Ministry of the Attorney General, Queens Printer for Ontario, 1984, pp. 534–634.
283. Zeckhauser, R.J., and Viscusi, W.K., Risk within reason. Science, 248, 559, 1990.
284. Corn, M., Crump, K., Farrar, D.B., et al., Airborne concentrations of asbestos in 71 school buildings. Reg. Toxicol. Pharmacol., 13, 99, 1991.
285. Ilgren, E.B., and Browne, K., Asbestos related mesothelioma: evidence for a threshold in animals and humans. Reg. Toxicol. Pharmacol., 13, 116, 1991.
286. Gardner, M.J., Acheson, E.D., and Winter, P.D., Mortality from mesothelioma of the pleura during 1968–78 in England and Wales. Br. J. Cancer, 46, 81, 1982.
287. Anderson, M., and Olsen, J.H., Trend and distribution of mesothelioma in Denmark. Scand. J. Work Environ. Health, 14, 145, 1988.
288. Bazas, T., Oakes, D., Gilson, J.C., et al., Pleural calcification in northwest Greece. Environ. Res., 38, 239, 1985.
289. Hillerdal, G., Pleural changes and exposures to fibrous minerals. Scand. J. Work Environ. Health, 10, 473, 1984.
290. Hillerdal, G., Pleural plaques in Sweden among immigrants from Finland: with an editorial note. Eur. J. Respir. Dis., 64, 386, 1983.
291. Cordier, S., Lazar, P., Brochard, P., et al., Epidemiologic investigation of respiratory effects related to environmental exposure to asbestos inside insulated buildings. Arch. Environ. Health, 42, 303, 1987.
292. Mossman, B.T., and Gee, J.B.L., Medical progress: asbestos related diseases. N. Engl. J. Med., 320, 1721, 1989.
293. Richards, T., Medical lessons from the Falklands. B.M.J., 286, 790, 1983.
294. Shopland, D.R., Eyre, H.J., and Pechacek, T.F., Smoking attributable cancer in 1991: is lung cancer now the leading cause of death among smokers in the United States? J. Natl. Cancer Inst., 83, 1142, 1991.

15

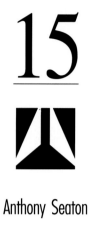

Anthony Seaton

Coal Workers' Pneumoconiosis

■

The history of coal mining is inextricably linked to the history of the industrial development of nations, and the fortunes of coal miners and their risks of disease reflect this linkage.[1-3] Coal has been dug from surface outcroppings since ancient times, and such individual activity can still be found in communities in poor countries and in poor communities in rich countries. However, the European industrial revolution of the late 18th and early 19th century, especially in Great Britain, France, and Germany, brought about a need for large amounts of coal as fuel for the factories and transport systems. The invention of the steam pump in the mid-18th century allowed underground coal mines to be exploited fully by the removal of flood water. By the mid-19th century, the British coal industry was producing 100 million tons a year. The coal not only provided the fuel for factories, iron and steel production, and transport but also became the major source of domestic fuel. This was the era of urban smoke pollution, which was to last 100 years in Great Britain until it was finally controlled after its effects on the epidemic mortality of town dwellers were recognized in the 1950s.[4] Another probable consequence of domestic coal burning was the occurrence of skin and scrotal cancer in chimney sweeps' apprentices, first recorded by Pott in 1775.[5]

Coal mining in the United States followed in the footsteps of the European industry, starting in the early 19th century in Appalachia and rapidly growing into a major industry involving also Illinois, Indiana, Utah, and Colorado. More recently, as other countries have embarked on industrialization, they also have based their development on a rapidly expanding coal industry, and today, the early history of the West's development of coal has been mirrored in nations such as China and India.

As coal has been central to the economic development of nations, so the fortunes of coal miners have risen and fallen as a barometer of economic health. Coal mines characteristically occur in rural areas and, in times of boom, attract workers in search of wages. The imperatives of capitalism have led to real or perceived exploitation of workers in the search for maximizing profit. In times of recession, the same workers find themselves without jobs. Thus, coal mining became, through the 19th and 20th centuries, the main battleground between capitalism and organized labor. Nowhere was this more so than in the United States,[6] where the importation of large numbers of central Europeans into Appalachia to work in nonunion mines led to a series of armed conflicts between miners and the coal companies' private army, the Balwin Felts Agency. Although never quite reaching the same level of violence, this history of industrial conflict was also seen in Great Britain and other developed countries. The power of the miners lay in their ability to organize and in the value of coal to the economy. In the United States, from the 1930s, an uneasy truce has obtained, negotiated between union and employers, allowing increasing mechanization to drive down the cost of coal so that it remains competitive at the cost of a progressive reduction in jobs in the industry. In Great Britain, nationalization of the industry in 1948 was hailed as a new era for the miners. However, the government, as the new owners, soon found that economic factors, often without their direct control, determined the fate of the industry. In particular, competition from cheap oil and gas forced the worldwide coal industry to cut its costs and its labor force. Where coal is easily won, as in the huge strip mines in the United States and Australia, or where labor is cheap, as in South America or China, the costs are low, and bulk transport has allowed such industries to compete with the older coal fields, resulting in the closure of most of the mines in western Europe.

The history of coal miners' diseases has been no less turbulent than that of the industry itself. Coal workers' pneumoconiosis was first described in Scottish miners in the 1830s,[7, 8] but Laennec, in his classic textbook on auscultation published in 1819, had recognized the black pigmentation of coal miners' lungs.[9] For many years thereafter, controversy raged about the diseases of miners,[10, 11] in particular, whether coal dust inhalation was harmful. The view promoted by two notable scientists, J. S. Haldane and Leroy Gardner, was that it was not. Was the disease seen in the lungs of coal miners due to quartz? What was the relationship between symptoms and coal dust exposure? The early history of coal miners' lung diseases has been reviewed by Meiklejohn, and the interested reader is referred to these classic articles.[1–3]

There has never been any doubt in the minds of coal miners that inhalation of dust is harmful to their health, a belief fortified over the last 200 years by their experience of the frequency of respiratory disease in their communities. However, more objective observers have always been ready to point to the confounding effects of poor housing and nutrition, overcrowding, and more recently, cigarette smoking. There have apparently also been real fluctuations in the prevalence of disease in mining communities. Lung disease was undoubtedly very common in the 19th century, yet Arlidge, an astute observer, believed that, by the end of that century, it was becoming much less common.[12] Haldane and Gardner both assumed, on the basis of *in vitro* studies of coal dust and of awareness of the low quartz content of most such dust, that it was harmless, and their views gained widespread support at the time. Indeed, the concept that coal workers' pneumoconiosis and silicosis are one and the same persisted in Great Britain until the 1940s, in the United States until the 1960s, and in some countries to this day.

Light began to be shed on the problems of coal miners' disease in the 20th century, when the chest radiograph began to be used in clinical diagnosis. Radiologists and pathologists in South Wales, the most heavily mined region of Britain, became aware of the real frequency of serious lung disease. The work of Collis and Gilchrist[13] and Gough et al.[14] in Cardiff first established that coal dust, independent of quartz, could cause serious and fatal disease. In 1936, the British Medical Research Council (MRC) recognized the seriousness of the then current epidemic of lung disease and established its Pneumoconiosis Unit under the direction of Charles Fletcher in Cardiff in 1945. This coincided with the election of Britain's first postwar Labour government and was followed by nationalization of the mines. In 1950, the National Coal Board's Pneumoconiosis Field Research (PFR) started, an epidemiological program that has answered many of the main questions relating to coal miners' diseases.[15, 16] In the United States, the problem was recognized somewhat later and probably never reached the level of severity that occurred in Great Britain. In 1966, the United States Public Health Service established the Appalachian Laboratory for Occupational Respiratory Diseases (ALFORD) under Keith Morgan in West Virginia, and this unit continues, as the Appalachian Laboratory for Occupational Safety and Health, to lead American research in these diseases.

The very important change in research attitudes that came about with the foundation of the MRC unit in Cardiff was the emphasis on epidemiological rather than experimental studies. The principles of standardization of techniques, including measurement of lung function, of symptoms by questionnaire, and of radiological change by the use of standard radiographs, that form the basis of all respiratory epidemiology were either formulated in this unit or were promoted by its staff under its second director, John Gilson. These techniques were applied and adapted by the PFR in the National Coal Board and its Institute of Occupational Medicine in Edinburgh and by ALFORD in Morgantown, West Virginia.

The early research,[17] together with clinical observations, had shown that coal miners were at risk of simple pneumoconiosis (although there was some doubt as to its harmfulness), complicated pneumoconiosis or progressive massive fibrosis, and chronic cough and sputum production.[18] Risks of tuberculosis and lung cancer probably reflected those of the miners' social milieu rather than being a consequence of mining.[19, 20] Thus, the important practical research questions in 1950, at which time, in some 6000 miners a year, coal workers' pneumoconiosis was developing in Great Britain, were "How much and what kinds of dust cause pneumoconiosis?" and "What dust levels need to be maintained to prevent miners falling ill with respiratory disease?" These were the questions that the British PFR set out to answer. The results of this research have been applied worldwide, including the United States, in setting dust standards in coal mines.[21, 22]

The seriousness of the pneumoconiosis problem in the years during and after the Second World War in Europe and the United States was such that coal industries had to take action, action that was often hastened by widespread public sympathy for the plight of mining communities after awful accidents. One such, the explosion in the Farmington mine in West Virginia, in which 78 miners died, was the final stimulus to the passage of the United States Federal Coal Mine Health and Safety Acts of 1969 and 1977,[23] which, *inter alia,* mandated dust standards for United States coal mines intended to prevent pneumoconiosis. Over this period, important advances were made in understanding the principles of dust control and in devising means of measuring respirable dust.[24] The maintenance of acceptably safe levels of dust in mines became a practical proposition.

In general, it is now true that coal workers' pneumoconiosis has become a relatively uncommon condition in the highly mechanized, well-ventilated mines of the western world. Mechanization, while often generating more dust, means that far fewer people are exposed, and the hours worked are much shorter than they were traditionally. Shot-firing, with its attendant dust and gases, is less used as long-wall mining becomes more prevalent, but the specter of the disease is still present. A relaxation of dust control, an increase in working hours, and the introduction of new, dustier methods can always lead to a resurgence of the problem. Meanwhile, the newer coal industries in China and other poorer countries are now seeing the start of major pneumoconiosis epidemics that can only be prevented by applying the lessons learned the hard way in the West.

THE WORK OF THE COAL MINER

Strip Mining

The most efficient sector of the coal industry is strip or open cast mining. This is possible where the coal seams are close to the surface and can be reached by the removal of the superficial layers of earth and rock known as the overburden. The excavation of overburden is carried out by diggers, the rock being broken up by explosives. Large-scale machinery is used, including drills that are used to place the charges. Once the coal has been uncovered, it is removed by excavators and giant drag lines and transported by truck to the tipple or coal preparation plant. Dust is generated throughout the process, but since it takes place in the open air, the levels rarely approach those of underground mines. However, some workers are at risk of disease, i.e., the drill operators may be exposed to high levels of quartz, while laborers who are not protected by being in enclosed machine cabs may be exposed to high levels of dust at the site of digging or tipping operations (Fig. 15–1).[25] It should be noted that climate would be expected to have an important influence on dust exposure. The damp, cool conditions of Europe encourage less airborne dust than do hot dry subtropical or desert conditions. However, the relatively small work force and the ease with which enclosed cabs and water suppression can be used to control dust exposure mean that well-regulated strip mining should entail little hazard to the work force.[26]

Underground Mining

Most coal occurs too far underground, or in too sensitive an environment, for strip methods to be employed. Deep mining requires access to the seams, either by a shaft or by a horizontal or sloping tunnel, known as a drift. Once the seam is reached, a number of different methods may be used to get the coal. The traditional method, used in relatively shallow mines where seams are thick and the coal is plentiful, is the room-and-pillar method, whereby tunnels are driven in parallel through the coal and connected by lateral communicating tunnels, thus leaving pillars of coal to support the roof. This method obviously causes problems with achieving adequate ventilation to dilute dust and remove mine gases at points of coal cutting, and these are addressed by hanging curtains, or brattices, to channel the air flow in the appropriate direction. Originally, the coal was broken up by explosives, but increasingly, it is removed in modern mines by coal cutting machines (Fig. 15–2).

A more efficient method, widely used in Europe and increasingly in the United States, is long-wall mining. This is suitable also for very deep coal and thin seams where maximum extraction is economically essential. A pair of tunnels, usually about 100 m apart, are driven to the coal seam and joined together through the seam. A coal cutting machine, a continuous miner, traverses the face cutting coal which falls onto a moving conveyor belt for removal. The coal cutter progressively cuts into the seam in transverse runs while other miners take the two lateral tunnels forward. The roof above the miners' heads on the face is held up by powered roof supports, operated by hydraulic jacks. As the face moves forward, so the miners move the roof supports with it, allowing the roof to fall in behind them. Thus, the long-wall face moves forward into the coal seam, continuously extracting the coal. If the seam becomes very narrow, or if there are intrusions of rock (dirt bands) in

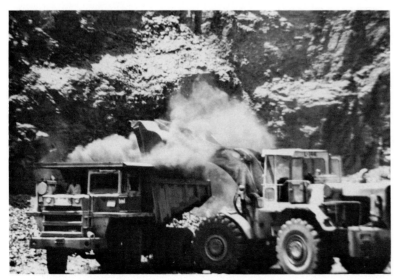

Figure 15–1. Coal loading at the face of a large open pit mine. Note the high levels of dust but relative ease with which workers could be protected by operating in air-conditioned cabs.

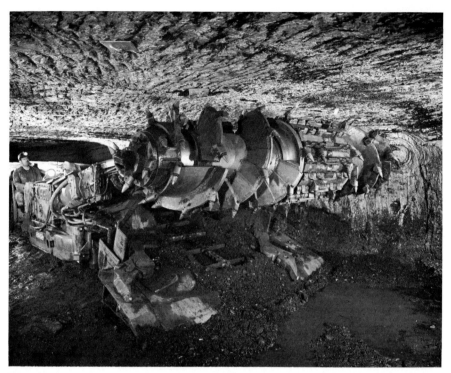

Figure 15–2. Continuous miner. The cutting head of this Joy Continuous Miner is designed to cut automatically an arched roof, thereby making the roof more stable and lessening the chance of roof falls. Coal is ripped from the seam and falls to the floor, where it is collected by gathering arms and a conveyor belt, which are built into the machine. (Courtesy of Joy Manufacturing Co.)

it, the coal cutter will remove minerals other than coal and the composition of the dust may accordingly alter from place to place.

A typical modern mine will have several long-wall faces, often at different levels, operating simultaneously. The mine is ventilated by powerful fans at the surface, which push or draw air through the sequence of tunnels, ensuring that adequate ventilation occurs on the long-wall face. Again, brattices and air locks are used to ensure that ventilation goes where it is needed.

In the search for greater productivity, variations on the long-wall method have been used from time to time. One such is retreat mining, whereby the tunnels are driven to the far end of the seam and the mining takes place in the opposite direction. Another is the single-entry face, which dispenses with the second tunnel and is thus effectively a long tunnel across the seam with a continuous miner operating within it. This obviously causes serious problems with ensuring adequate ventilation because it requires ducted extraction or fresh air delivery.

The underground miner is clearly at greater risk of inhaling significant amounts of dust and gases than a surface counterpart. Face workers, who operate where coal is cut and transferred and where the roof falls in, and shot firers, who drill into the coal to place explosive charges, are at greatest risk from dust exposure. Here, the primary preventive measure is ventilation, but water sprayed at points of dust generation, such as onto the picks of coal cutters, drills, the roof supports when moving forward, and coal transfer points, is an important secondary method. Miners who bore shafts and tunnels, sometimes called headers or hard headers, may be at risk of silicosis rather than coal workers' pneumoconiosis. Other face workers, in traditional mines, may be involved in roof bolting, i.e., drilling upward above the face into hard rock to insert the bolt and plate used to support more friable and looser rock above the miners' heads. These men are exposed to a fine dust that may contain high concentrations of quartz and are thus also at risk of silicosis. Some transport systems underground involve railroads, and brakemen or drivers may use sand on the tracks to improve the grip of the wheels. Again, silicosis has been described in these workers. Other underground workers, who are exposed to less dust than face workers, are maintenance and electrical technicians. Workers on the surface tipple and coal preparation plant are also exposed to dust and may be at risk of pneumoconiosis, as may workers on the quayside or in the holds of ships involved in coal transportation.

The physical work of mining has been much reduced in modern mines compared with the arduous pick and shovel and hand drilling methods still used in traditional parts of the industry. Nevertheless, moments of severe exertion are required, especially in handling heavy machinery, tunnel arches, and cables, and sometimes in getting to and from the face. Although these activities, in what is generally a less fit work force than heretofore, result in a high incidence of musculoskeletal problems, they do not place the same ventilatory demands on miners at times of coal cutting and thus reduce, to some extent, dust intake.

THE COMPOSITION OF COAL

Coal is not a mineral of fixed composition. Formed from dead vegetation over the past 250 to 300 million years, it exists on a spectrum from very hard, brittle black anthracite at one extreme to crumbly brown lignite at the other. Less formed matter, peat, also serves as a source of fuel in many parts of the world. Coal is graded by rank; the rank reflects its carbon content and thus combustibility. Anthracite is the highest ranked coal, with a carbon content around 98%. Lower ranked coals, known as bituminous and sub-bituminous, have contents around 90% to 95% carbon.

When coal is burned, a residue of ash remains. This nonorganic matter is in the original coal and in dust derived from it as kaolinite, mica, various complex clay minerals, and quartz. The composition of the ash, and importantly its quartz content, varies very much from mine to mine and from area to area. As will be discussed later, this compositional variety influences the risks of lung disease of men exposed to the dust. Similarly, the rank of coal has an important influence on the risk of disease.

EPIDEMIOLOGY OF COAL MINING DISEASES

Most studies have shown that coal mining does not have an effect on overall life expectancy,[19, 27–29] as is the case with most heavy industries since only relatively healthy, fit people are recruited into the industry. However, increased rates of mortality have been consistently shown for accidents and respiratory diseases,[19] partly balanced by reduced rates for heart disease and lung cancer.[30–32] The most comprehensive mortality study carried out,[29] involving some 25,000 miners over 22 years and including detailed estimates of lifetime dust exposure, showed that cumulative dust exposure is related to the risk of dying from chronic airways disease and that the mortality rate is increased in miners with both complicated pneumoconiosis (progressive massive fibrosis [PMF]) and also, to a lesser extent, simple pneumoconiosis. There was a reduced risk of death from lung cancer, but in this and also in American and Dutch studies, there is a slightly increased risk of stomach cancer, which appears to relate to dust exposure.[33, 34]

The British PFR was designed to answer the two questions posed earlier, i.e., how much and what types of dust cause pneumoconiosis and what dust levels need to be maintained to prevent miners from having respiratory disease? To this end, some 50,000 miners were studied by questionnaire, spirometry, and chest radiography every 5 years over a 25-year period. Crucially, careful estimates of past dust exposure, based on a detailed occupational history and knowledge of dust conditions in their mines, together with prospective measurements of respirable dust exposure by occupational groups, were made. Therefore, it was possible to calculate individual cumulative dust exposures of all men participating in the study. In addition to this detailed information, mortality data were collected, and as far as possible, the lungs of deceased miners were obtained postmortem and examined pathologically and mineralogically. Attempts were also made to obtain information on the health status of those men who left the industry between surveys. This vast epidemiological undertaking was funded by the British National Coal Board, later the British Coal Corporation, and the European Community.

Analyses of the data gathered in this research provided answers that may be used worldwide in the prevention of disease in coal miners, the objective of the exercise. The results may be summarized as follows:

1. The risk of simple pneumoconiosis is related to the worker's cumulative exposure to coal mine dust.[35]
2. The risk of PMF is related to the cumulative exposure to coal mine dust.[36]
3. These risks differ with coal rank, high-rank (high carbon, more highly combustible) coals being more dangerous than lower-rank ones.[35–37]
4. Simple coal workers' pneumoconiosis does not progress or regress significantly after dust exposure ceases, unless there is an important silicotic element.[38, 39]
5. PMF frequently progresses, and often appears for the first time, after dust exposure ceases.[38]
6. Low-rank coals, containing high concentrations of quartz, may cause a rapidly progressive pneumoconiosis resembling silicosis.[39, 40]
7. Chronic cough and sputum, decrement in ventilatory capacity, and the presence of pathological centriacinar emphysema are all associated with cumulative exposure to coal mine dust.[18, 41–44]

Risks of Simple Pneumoconiosis

The risks of category 1 and combined categories 2 and 3 simple pneumoconiosis are illustrated in Figures 15–3 and 15–4. In both cases, the influence of coal

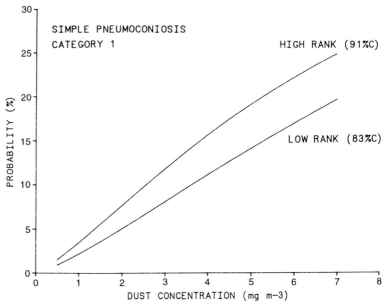

Figure 15–3. Calculated risks of simple pneumoconiosis category 1 developing from exposure to given average or respirable dust concentrations for a working lifetime in miners in the United Kingdom. The two curves represent risks from exposure to coal of different combustibilities or carbon content.

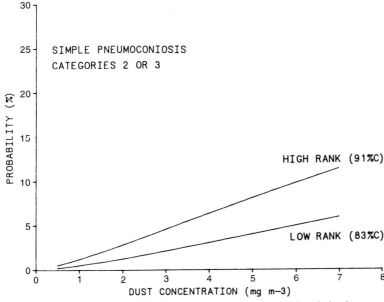

Figure 15–4. Calculated risks of simple pneumoconiosis categories 2 or 3 developing over a working lifetime (see Fig. 15–3).

rank can be seen; higher-rank coals entail higher risk than do lower-rank ones. These risk estimates relate to a working lifetime exposure (35 years) to a given level of dust of known rank. Although they have been made on a population of working miners, in studies of ex-miners, it has been shown that they hold good in these men also.[38] They provide a useful basis for debate about coal mine dust standard setting and have been widely used for this purpose.

These risk estimates refer to conventional simple coal workers' pneumoconiosis, with small rounded opacities. It is now recognized that coal miners also develop small irregular opacities.[45–47] These also occur in relation to dust exposure but seem not to progress beyond the category 1 stage on the International Labour Office (ILO) scale. They are associated epidemiologically with impaired ventilatory capacity, even when age and smoking habits are taken into account.

Studies of coal miners in countries other than Great Britain have also shown similar results. In Germany[48–50] and the United States,[51] exposure-response relationships, varying with coal rank, have been found, and the German studies have pointed to an additional influence of the length of time the dust has been in the lung on the risk of disease. The results of the American studies, which are based on estimates of dust exposure, are illustrated in Figure 15–5.

Risks of Complicated Pneumoconiosis

Similar analyses have shown the risk of PMF in British and other coal miners (Fig. 15–6).[36, 51] Although dust exposure and composition are the most important factors, the presence and category of simple pneumoconiosis on earlier films are also very relevant. Studies of ex-miners have measured the risks of having PMF develop after leaving the industry.[52] These again relate to prior cumulative dust exposure, but they are also strongly influenced by the category of simple pneumoconiosis at the time of leaving. Over an 11-year period after leaving the industry, the risks of PMF range from 37 per 1000 in men with no simple pneumoconiosis to 471 per 1000 in men leaving with category 3 radiological change. Similarly, the risks increase from 9 per 1000 in men with dust exposure less than 50 gh/m³(grams per cubic meter times hours of working life) to 183 per 1000 in men with more than 400 gh/m³. These studies showed that calculations of risks of PMF

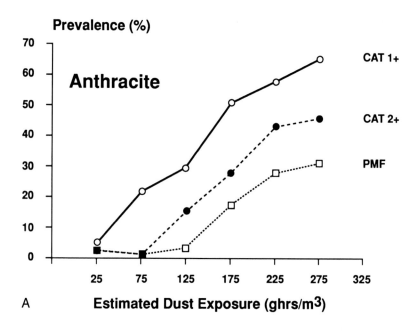

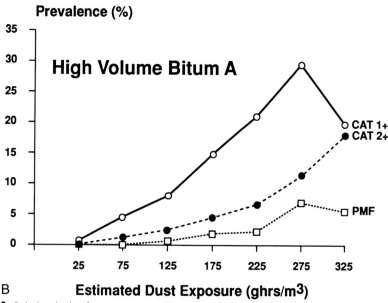

Figure 15–5. Calculated risks of pneumoconiosis in United States Public Health Service studies of coal miners. (Courtesy of Dr. Mike Attfield.)

derived from earlier studies of working miners[53–55] led to substantial underestimates, especially in respect of the risks associated with category 1 simple pneumoconiosis. Once this early stage of radiological disease has been reached, dust exposure has been such that a high risk of PMF is present and persists through the remainder of the worker's life. Thus, preventive strategies should aim at reducing the risks of category 1 simple disease and not rely on excluding workers with this radiological appearance from further dust exposure.

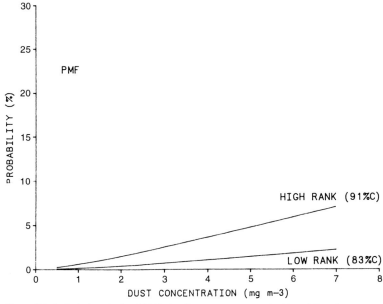

Figure 15-6. Calculated risks of PMF developing in miners in the United Kingdom over a working lifetime (see Fig. 15-3).

Influence of Dust Composition

The influence of coal rank has been mentioned before, and the greater harmfulness of high-rank coals has been noted wherever it was studied, although the explanation remains elusive. However, exposures to coal dust with a quartz concentration greater than about 15% are associated with a high risk of a rapidly progressive form of pneumoconiosis developing that clinically and pathologically has the characteristics of silicosis.[39, 40] This relationship is not straightforward since men exposed to similar concentrations of quartz in different mines may have very different risks of radiological disease, and it is likely that the other ash minerals present in the dust modify the toxicity of the quartz. This is discussed further in the section on pathogenesis.

Coal Dust and Other Respiratory Diseases

Clear relationships have been demonstrated between cumulative coal dust exposure and chronic productive cough after allowing for the effects of smoking.[18, 56, 57] Lung function, measured as the forced expiratory volume in 1 second (FEV_1), has been shown both in cross-sectional and longitudinal studies to decline in relation to increasing underground dust exposure[41–43, 56–60] but not in relation to estimates of exposure to oxides of nitrogen. This decline occurs at a similar rate in smokers and nonsmokers, although the loss of lung function overall is greater in smokers, the two effects being additive.[43, 61] Estimates of the risk of the loss of lung function in relation to dust exposure are shown in Figure 15-7. Expressed in terms of the risk of having a FEV_1 less than 65% predicted at age 47 years, a nonsmoker with no dust exposure has a 3% chance compared with 5% in a smoker. With high dust exposure (approximately 350 gh/m³), the corresponding risks are about 8% and 14%.

These results described earlier come not only from the British PFR but also from other studies in the United States and Australia. Similar results have been reported from Germany,[62] and no studies have failed to show this general relationship. All reports point in the same direction, i.e., that coal dust and cigarette smoke both impair ventilatory capacity. On average, in a population, the loss of lung

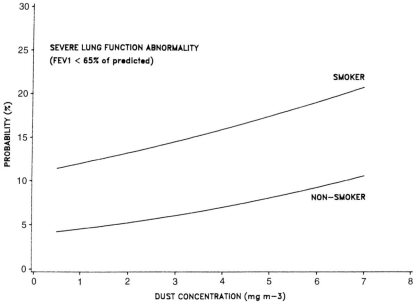

Figure 15–7. Calculated risks of having a FEV$_1$ less than 65% predicted in miners in the United Kingdom over a working lifetime in relation to average exposure to respirable dust, in smokers and lifetime nonsmokers. (Data from Marine, W.M., Gurr, D., and Jacobsen, M., Clinically important respiratory effects of dust exposure and smoking in British coal miners. Am. Rev. Respir. Dis., 137, 106, 1988.)

function is small, but with both cigarettes and coal dust, the variation between individuals is such that some show a greater response that can result in clinical impairment. This is discussed further later. A further point of interest has arisen from studies of young miners. It seems likely that, over the first year or two of exposure to coal dust, there may be an accelerated loss of lung function, which subsequently slows down.[63] It has been speculated that this may mark the initial inflammatory response that can lead to the formation of the coal macule or even to the initiation of the emphysematous process (see Pathogenesis).

Investigations have been carried out to determine the likely explanation of this effect of dust on lung function, and they have pointed to a relationship between dust exposure and pathological centriacinar emphysema after allowing for the influence of smoking.[44] This holds true only if there is evidence in the lungs also of at least simple pneumoconiosis. The relationship concerns the presence rather than the amount of emphysema. Moreover, it is modified by quartz exposure, in that, for a given level of coal dust exposure, the risk of having centriacinar emphysema is less in those who have had a relatively high concomitant quartz exposure. Further studies have shown the relationship between the presence of centriacinar emphysema and dust exposure to be present in lifelong nonsmoking miners.[64]

CLINICAL FEATURES OF COAL WORKERS' PNEUMOCONIOSIS

Simple coal workers' pneumoconiosis is a radiological or pathological diagnosis; there are no associated symptoms or signs. Finger clubbing and inspiratory crackles are not features of the disease, and if these are present, other explanations should be sought. The most important clinical fact to remember about simple pneumoconiosis is that, if the patient is breathless, even in the presence of category 3 disease, another disease is responsible. Although this may often be emphysema related to the worker's smoking habits and dust exposure, on occasion it may be a disease that is responsive to treatment, such as asthma, allergic alveolitis, or sarcoidosis. A blind belief that a dramatic radiographic change in a coal miner must explain symptoms has led many doctors into the trap of failing to treat the treatable. Indeed, the author has seen patients suffer needlessly because of their doctor's unwillingness to consider other diagnoses, especially in the pursuit of claims in civil litigation.

Complicated pneumoconiosis, or PMF, is similarly not responsible for symptoms or signs at an early stage. Only when extensive, multifocal disease is present does the patient become aware of breathlessness and then usually only when there is associated bullous emphysema. At this stage, some patients complain of cough, perhaps associated with bronchial distortion, but usually a progressive, unvarying exercise dyspnea is the only symptom. Ultimately, cor pulmonale may occur,[65] but more usually, the final course is characterized by hypoxic, nonhypercapnic respiratory failure.

At various times in the past, other diseases have been associated either with coal mining or coal workers' pneumoconiosis. Scleroderma is one such;[66] this does seem to be associated with quartz exposure,[67] but the author has yet to see it in a coal miner. Peptic ulcer is associated with chronic airflow obstruction, almost certainly because of the common etiological factor in smoking, but there is no evidence that it is a specific risk of miners. Gastric carcinoma does seem to occur more frequently in coal miners than in the general population. There is, however, no increased risk of tuberculosis or of lung cancer in coal miners with or without pneumoconiosis. The association of coal workers' pneumoconiosis with rheumatoid arthritis, in which distinctive lesions of PMF occur on the radiograph, is known as Caplan's syndrome.[68, 69] This is not associated with any specific pulmonary symptoms or signs (see next section).

Radiological Appearances

Simple Coal Workers' Pneumoconiosis

The appearances of the chest radiograph are described by reference to the ILO standard films and classification of the pneumoconioses (see Chapter 6). The earliest sign is usually either sparse q or, less commonly, r nodules in upper and middle zones, or a more diffuse and barely discernible p shadowing (Figs. 15–8 to 15–10). Such changes only occur after considerable dust exposure and are usually associated with fine irregular shadows in the periphery of the lower zones.[46, 47] Such irregular shadows have previously been ignored in the films of coal miners and are indistinguishable from shadows associated with age, smoking, and a history of productive cough. Nevertheless, they have been shown to be associated with dust exposure in coal mining and other industries and seem to be a nonspecific response.[70–72] Moreover, their presence is associated epidemiologically with a measurable decrement in ventilatory capacity, even when age and smoking habit are taken into account.[46, 47, 73] Kerley B lines can also usually be seen in heavily dust-exposed miners if looked for and probably indicate dust deposition in interlobular septa (Fig. 15–11). There is considerable variability even between very experienced readers in recording the earliest signs of pneumoconiosis, particularly with respect to the presence of irregular shadows and the size (p, q, or r) of rounded shadows. As the lesions become more profuse, there is greater agreement with respect to rounded shadows and their size. However, it should be noted that, on most films with pneumoconiosis, there are nodules of different sizes, and it is often difficult to be confident which is predominant.

The rounded shadows increase in profusion with increasing dust exposure, but there is no evidence that the irregular shadows do so beyond category 1. In addition, the larger r shadows individually increase in size in keeping with the concept that they are usually fibrotic nodules caused by the quartz component of the inhaled dust.[39] In general, r shadows are less profuse than q and tend to occur more in the upper zones originally; p shadows most commonly are first noticed in the middle

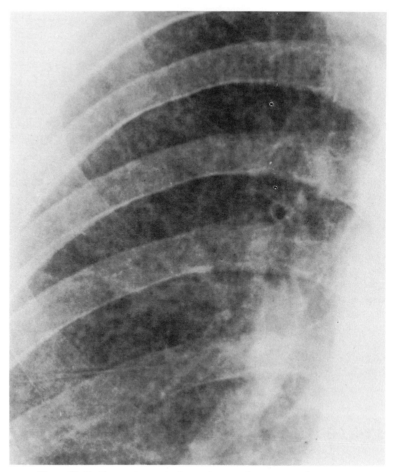

Figure 15–8. Chest radiograph of a coal miner, showing typical q opacities.

zones where the depth of the lung is greatest. After dust exposure has ceased, a change in the profusion of p or q shadows is very unusual.[38] Occasionally, the lesions may disappear when masked by progressive emphysema, but usually when regression or progression is recorded, it can be attributed to a variation in the radiographic or reading technique. In contrast, it is not uncommon for the rarer r shadows to increase not only in size but also in profusion after dust exposure has ceased, in keeping with their silicotic nature.[39]

Progressive Massive Fibrosis

PMF is defined radiologically as a lesion of 1 cm or greater in longest diameter. Studies of serial radiographs of coal miners in the PFR have shown that the radiological appearances of early PMF may differ very strikingly.[74] The most frequent appearances are ghost-like opacities of homogeneous density, sometimes multiple, and usually in the upper zones (Fig. 15–12). These lesions become progressively more dense, and their edges are more clearly defined over the course, usually, of several years. Somewhat less commonly, the lesion appears first as a condensation of irregular streaky shadows (Fig. 15–13). Least commonly, two other types have been described. One, which seems to be associated with a silicotic pathological origin, consists of an aggregation of r-type nodules, and the other includes an initially hazy peripheral condensation of p or small q lesions. As time passes, all these lesions may develop in much the same way, becoming more dense

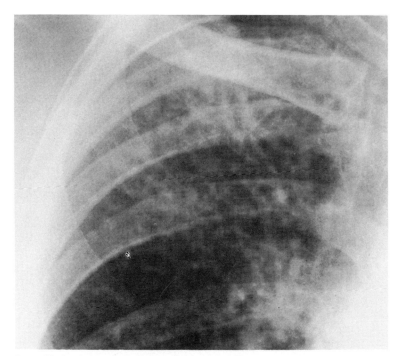

Figure 15–9. Chest radiograph of a coal miner, showing r opacities suggestive of quartz exposure. The upper-zone distribution is typical.

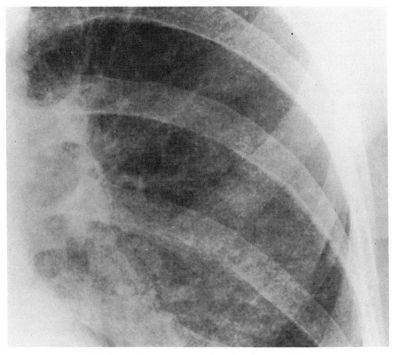

Figure 15–10. The fine p opacities of coal worker's pneumoconiosis.

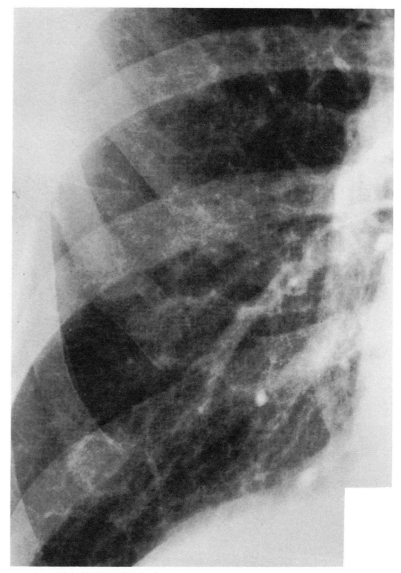

Figure 15–11. Kerley B lines in a healthy coal miner. (Courtesy of Dr. Colin Soutar.)

and better defined, growing progressively, and frequently becoming surrounded by bullous emphysema. Very characteristically, the emphysema separates the lesions from the chest wall (Fig. 15–14). In the later stages, some PMF lesions may be seen to contract and become more dense. However, the pattern and rate of change in size of PMF is very variable and unpredictable.[64] Some lesions may grow while others remain static, and not infrequently, the progression in size of lesions becomes arrested. The only factor so far identified that influences the rate of progression is quartz exposure (and the quartz content of the lung), i.e., the higher the quartz exposure, the more rapid the progression.

The early appearances of PMF described previously are not classifiable by the ILO system and are unfamiliar to most film readers. There is thus much scope for disagreement between readers on whether an early A lesion is present on a coal miner's film. As the lesion increases in size, disagreement is likely to be less, although readers who *record* appearances strictly in terms of the ILO protocol will find more PMF than those who *interpret* the shadows and who are likely to attribute

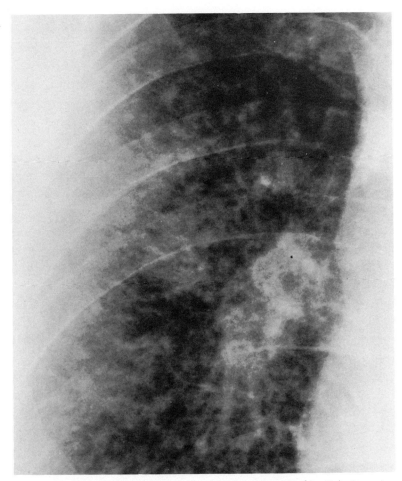

Figure 15–12. Type of PMF. Peripheral consolidation. (Courtesy of Dr. Colin Soutar.)

causation to things other than dust exposure in some cases. Particular problems occur in countries where there is a high prevalence of tuberculosis or pulmonary eosinophilia, when many large irregularly shaped or diffuse shadows may have these etiological factors. The problem is solved by consideration of whether the reading is for clinical or epidemiological purposes. If the former, the possibility of a treatable condition must be borne in mind, and other clinical features and investigations must be taken into account before reaching a diagnosis. If the reading is epidemiological, the appearance of a large shadow should be recorded as A, B, or C if it could reasonably be thought to be due to pneumoconiosis. Bearing in mind the variety of appearances of PMF described earlier, this means that cases of tuberculosis and other conditions will be categorized as PMF, and it is appropriate for the reader to record a clinical comment on the form, so that the possibility of a nondust-related cause can be allowed for in subsequent analyses.

Although PMF usually starts in one lung (most commonly the right), it is usual for further lesions to develop in other parts of both that and the other lung. Most PMF occurs on a background of simple pneumoconiosis, and the risk of PMF developing relates to the category of simple disease, as described in the epidemiology section. PMF may occur after dust exposure has ceased, even when the miner has left the industry with no apparent simple pneumoconiosis, although this will only occur if the worker has had substantial prior dust exposure. Such late-onset PMF can give rise to diagnostic difficulties, and these lesions may be removed by thoracic surgeons who suspect they are carcinomata.

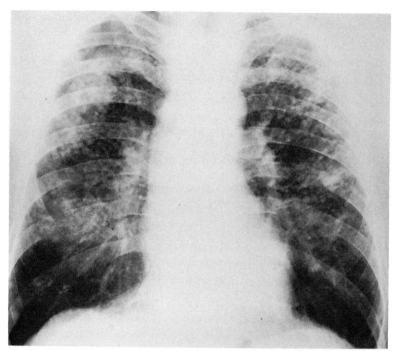

Figure 15–13. Type of PMF. Irregular streaky shadows. (Courtesy of Dr. Colin Soutar.)

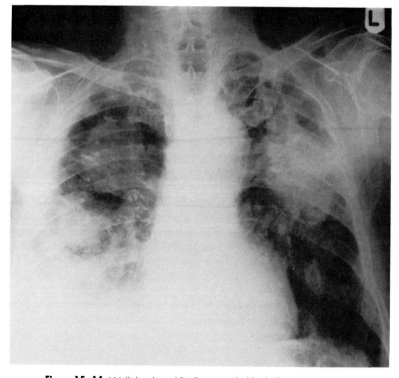

Figure 15–14. Well-developed PMF surrounded by bullous emphysema.

Pulmonary Function

Simple Pneumoconiosis

When reading the literature on lung function in coal miners, which has been described in detail in earlier editions of this book, it is important to appreciate the distinction between the functional deficits attributable to coal mine dust exposure and those attributable to the presence of pneumoconiosis. In studies of ventilatory capacity, it has consistently been shown that there is a decline both in FEV_1 and forced vital capacity (FVC) in relation to indices of dust exposure.[75–77] This impairment is distinct from the fall in FEV_1 and relatively normal FVC associated epidemiologically with smoking. However, studies which have looked for an effect of simple pneumoconiosis itself on FEV_1 and FVC have usually not found one, except in occasional subgroups of the populations studied.[78, 79] Such findings suggest, since pneumoconiosis occurs almost exclusively in people who have high dust exposure, a selection bias in that those workers who survive and in whom pneumoconiosis develops are those who have been most resistant to the effects of dust on lung function; those with impaired lung function have left the industry before pneumoconiosis developed. In general, it can be stated that simple pneumoconiosis *per se* has no important effect on spirometric measures of lung function when prior dust exposure is taken into account.

More subtle changes in lung function, probably of little clinical significance, have been found in simple pneumoconiosis. Several studies have shown that subjects with higher categories of p shadows have lower diffusing capacities than do those with q or r shadows, which suggests a loss of alveolar surface area consistent with pathological studies (see next section).[80–82] A progressive rise in residual volume with the category of simple pneumoconiosis, unaccounted for by smoking habit or airflow obstruction, has also been shown; again, this is consistent with the concept that emphysema or small airways obstruction may be a feature of pneumoconiosis.[83–85] In keeping with this, some studies have also shown evidence of small airways disease (or patchy emphysema) in workers with high categories of simple pneumoconiosis.[86, 87] Similarly, minor abnormalities of gas distribution and of gas exchange have been shown in coal miners with simple pneumoconiosis but without airflow obstruction.[88, 89] Consistent with this evidence of only minor or no abnormality of lung function in association with simple pneumoconiosis, studies of pulmonary hemodynamics have shown elevated pulmonary artery pressures to occur almost exclusively in association with airflow obstruction or PMF. In the rare cases in which it occurs without these factors, the elevation has been slight, and other causes, such as silicosis or obesity, may have been present.[90]

In general, for clinical purposes, in a patient with abnormal lung function and radiological signs of simple pneumoconiosis, it is wise to regard the two as being unassociated and to seek another cause of the functional deficit. Although both may be separate consequences of the same dust exposure, this attitude of mind will prevent treatable conditions from being missed.

Attribution of Functional Abnormalities to Dust Exposure

In medicolegal practice, it may be necessary to give an opinion, on the balance of the probabilities, as to whether breathlessness and abnormal lung function in a patient has been caused by exposure to coal mine dust. There is abundant evidence that reductions in FEV_1 and FVC occur in relation to dust exposure and this deficit may on occasions be severe.[42, 91] However, most coal miners have smoked, and in such cases, the relative contributions of the two harmful substances are a matter for individual judgment, depending on the numbers of cigarettes smoked and an assessment of likely cumulative exposure to dust underground. Occasionally, a lifelong nonsmoker with emphysema and heavy past dust exposure may be seen. In such cases, it is appropriate to rule out asthma by tests of reversibility with bronchodilators and corticosteroids and to assess individual susceptibility by the alpha-1-antitrypsin phenotype. These cases are rare; most patients have had both exposures. It is then a matter for the lawyers to argue questions of liability on the basis of negligence in the light of knowledge at the time the dust exposure occurred. In most instances, evidence that the employer adhered to the national coal mine dust standards at the time of employment should constitute a reasonable defense.

Progressive Massive Fibrosis

As might be expected from a consideration of the pathological findings, the lung function in a patient with PMF depends on the extent of the lesions and of associated emphysema. Two forms of emphysema complicate PMF, i.e., bullous disease, which forms around the PMF lesions, and centriacinar emphysema elsewhere in the lungs. The presence of this latter lesion is strongly associated with prior dust exposure.[44] Thus, studies of lung function in the more advanced stages of PMF have shown evidence both of airflow obstruction and of restriction.[79, 87, 88, 92-94] FEV_1 and FVC are reduced, residual volume is somewhat raised (but usually less so than in simple pneumoconiosis), and diffusing capacity and total lung capacity are usually reduced. Increased alveolar-arterial oxygen differences, wasted ventilation, and increased pulmonary arterial pressure may be found.[90] Compliance depends on the relative proportions of PMF and emphysema but is usually somewhat decreased.[87] Ultimately, hypoxemic respiratory failure and pulmonary hypertension may occur.[90, 95] All of these changes, of course, may be influenced by the additional presence of smoking-related disease.

Caplan's syndrome describes the association of rheumatoid disease and coal workers' pneumoconiosis, in which distinctly rounded lesions appear, often in crops over a short period, on the chest radiograph (Fig. 15–15).[96, 97] The lesions may

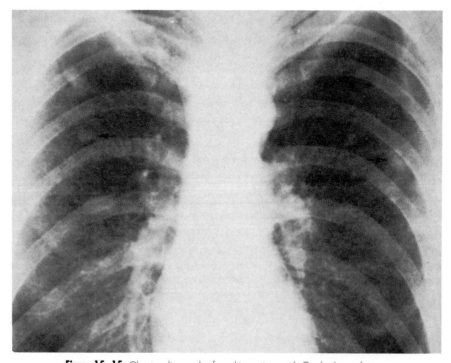

Figure 15–15. Chest radiograph of working miner with Caplan's syndrome.

grow rapidly and often cavitate, after which they may occasionally disappear. They may also calcify. The lesions are usually less than 5 cm in diameter but may be larger. They are not surrounded by emphysema and have no important effect on pulmonary function.[98] The pleura may also be involved, and pleural effusion sometimes occurs. The lung lesions may predate the onset of rheumatoid arthritis, even by several years, but more commonly occur in seropositive patients with subcutaneous rheumatoid nodules. Studies in South Wales suggested that a form of Caplan's syndrome might be a frequent cause of PMF,[99, 100] but this has not been borne out by later studies in United States and the PFR,[101–105] which have shown no link between immunological parameters and PMF. In particular, rheumatoid factors increase in prevalence in coal mining populations with age.

Pathological Findings

Simple Pneumoconiosis

The macroscopic appearance of a coal miner's lung is distinctive, in that it shows black staining of hilar and pulmonary nodes, of centriacinar nodules, and of interlobular septa (Fig. 15–16). In the case of PMF, large masses of black amorphous tissue, often surrounded by bullous emphysema, can be seen (Fig. 15–17). The characteristic microscopic lesion is the coal macule,[106–108] a usually centrilobular accumulation of dust-laden macrophages that originates at the division of the respiratory bronchioles and spreads out into surrounding peribronchiolar tissue and adjacent alveoli. It is commonly surrounded by enlarged air spaces, usually referred to as focal emphysema. The macule contains some reticulin and sometimes includes collagen.

This description of the typical macule covers a wide range of appearances which have been shown to correlate approximately with the different radiographic appearances described previously and which show relationships with both the miner's prior dust exposure and also the dust content of the lung.[109–113] When the following description is read, however, it should be borne in mind that there is considerable variation not only between miners' lungs but also within the lung of any one individual. It is not uncommon to find several of the described lesions in one lung. Nevertheless, patterns emerge, and experienced pathologists who have seen miners' lungs from many different areas are often able to guess the worker's geographical location from a macroscopic sight of the lung.

Some lungs are very markedly dust stained and have very many small pinhead macules, often surrounded by prominent emphysema. The macules contain little or no collagen (Fig. 15–18). Such lungs are likely to have been classified as showing predominantly p opacities on the radiograph in life.[111, 114] The radiographic appearance is probably due to overlap of many very small lesions to give the typical stippled effect. In these cases, which occur especially in miners who have been exposed to high-rank coal, there is a good correlation between dust exposure, lung dust content, and radiological category. In other words, the chest film is a good index of prior dust exposure and dust retention.

At what is perhaps the other end of the spectrum of pathological response to coal dust comes the larger nodule with a clearly silicotic cause central whorled fibrosis, and a surrounding rim of dust and macrophages (Fig. 15–19). However, many coal miners' lungs show an intermediate nodule, with patchy fibrosis and dust deposition and a rather more cellular appearance (Fig. 15–20). Both these and the more silicotic nodules correlate most closely with the r appearances on the radiograph.[111, 114] They do not show a good correlation with dust exposure, but they do relate to higher proportions of retained ash (including quartz) in the lungs. Between the extremes lies a range of appearances of macules, from 1 mm to 1 cm and from mainly cellular to heavily dusted. Lungs from miners with predominantly q opacities on the radiograph, the most common type in most coal fields, usually show a range of pathological appearances within this spectrum.[111, 114] Such lungs

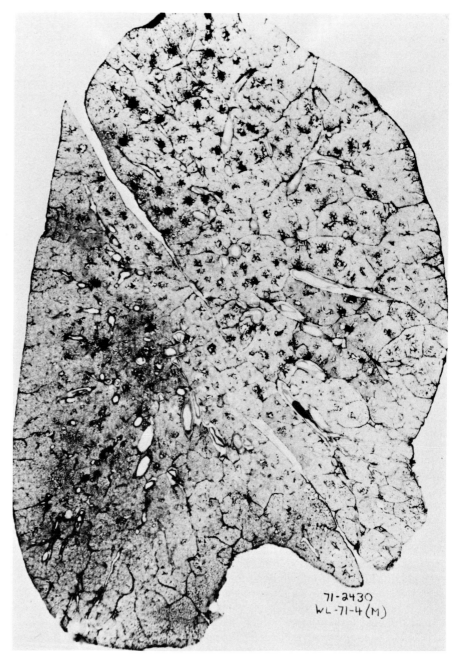

Figure 15–16. Large lung slice of coal miner's lung showing pigmented dust macules and interlobular septa.

show less dust in relation to radiological category than do those with q opacities, and the profusion of macules relates better to lung ash content than to total dust content.

To summarize these studies, lungs which show p opacities on the chest radiograph usually have a high lung dust content and the miner has had a high exposure to high-rank coal. Those with r opacities have usually had less exposure, but it was to dust containing relatively high proportions of ash and quartz. Most miners with pneumoconiosis have intermediate nodules, which reflect a complex cellular reaction to coal and quartz, probably modified by the other components of the ash. This is discussed further in the section on pathogenesis.

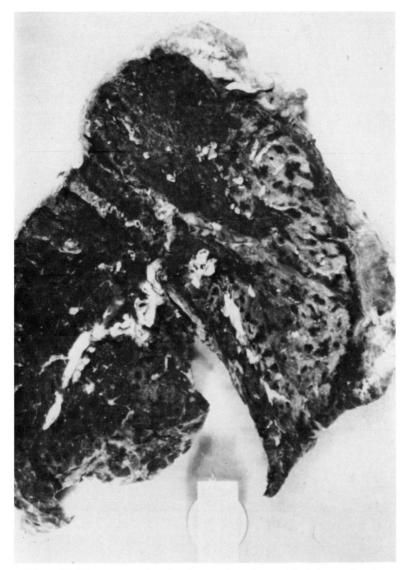

Figure 15–17. Large lung slice of coal miner's lung showing black density of PMF.

Progressive Massive Fibrosis

Macroscopically, PMF is seen as irregularly shaped black masses of tissue, most frequently in apical and posterior segments of upper and lower lobes (Fig. 15–17). Cavitation, usually caused by ischemic necrosis, may be present.[115] The lesions commonly appear to have retracted toward the hilum, where they may cause distortion of bronchi and pulmonary vessels. They are usually surrounded by bullous emphysema, and the uninvolved lung invariably shows simple coal macules, although these may be insufficiently profuse to have been visible radiologically. It is conventional to define pathological PMF as being present when the lesions are greater than 1 cm (or 2 cm on the advice of the American College of Pathologists[108]). However, such criteria are artificial, and it may well be possible to recognize characteristic features in smaller lesions.[100, 116]

As with simple coal macules, in PMF, different pathological patterns have been recognized.[113] Almost all PMF arises in lungs that already show some palpable fibrotic nodules, and in about one third of cases (corresponding generally to those

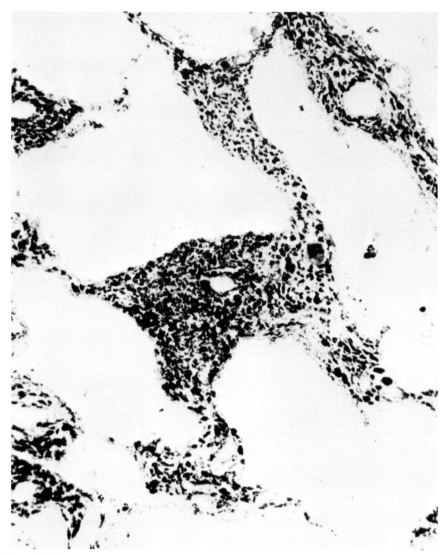

Figure 15–18. Coal macule surrounding distal airway and showing early extension into the pulmonary interstitium.

in which the same process is visible radiologically), the PMF lesion results from coalescence of such predominantly collagenous nodules (Fig. 15–21). In these lesions, the periphery clearly shows aggregating nodules with cellular and dusted edges and fibrotic centers, and bands of granulation tissue and dust within the deeper parts of the mass are often present, indicating earlier aggregations of fibrotic nodules. As with other types of PMF, the center of these lesions may become necrotic, but cavitation is relatively uncommon. It has been shown that the original fibrotic nodules do not occur randomly throughout the lung but tend to be grouped together, most commonly in upper zones, perhaps in the distribution of the pathways of lymphatic drainage.

A rather higher proportion of cases show no defined internal architecture, with a peripheral band of dust-laden cells surrounding a largely amorphous lesion with a necrotic center (Fig. 15–22). Chemical studies of such lesions have shown the collagen to be predominantly in the outer rim; the center consists of mainly fibronectin.[117, 118] The center may show ischemic necrosis and cavitation. Other intermediate types of lesion may also be observed. In some, there is a clearly

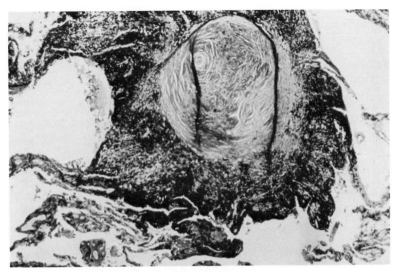

Figure 15–19. Coal macule showing central fibrosis and suggesting silicotic cause.

nodular component but with large irregular intervening areas of dust accumulation; in others, there appears to be a collapse of dust-laden acini intersected with bands of fibrous tissue.

Studies of the dust content of the lungs of miners with PMF have shown them to contain more dust than those with simple pneumoconiosis or no pneumoconiosis. When these results have been compared with calculated dust exposures during the workers' lifetimes, it has become apparent that PMF has occurred in miners who have *retained* a relatively high proportion of the inhaled dust.[113] This, together with the observation that pulmonary and hilar lymph nodes are fibrosed and destroyed in workers with PMF, suggests that interference with the lymphatic drainage of the lung by the products of cells damaged by dust may be an important etiological factor in PMF.

In PMF, the blood vessels in the affected region are obliterated, and changes of pulmonary hypertension may be present in the pulmonary arterial tree elsewhere. The adventitia and media of muscular arteries may be seen to be infiltrated with dust-laden cells, and endarteritis obliterans may be present, especially in proximity to the large lesions.[119] In advanced disease, especially when emphysema is present, right ventricular hypertrophy may be present.[65, 120, 121]

It has become apparent that Caplan's syndrome is an uncommon occurrence in coal miners. Caplan's lesions have a characteristic histological appearance, with peripheral features of the rheumatoid nodule, palisading and necrobiosis, a smoothly rounded shape, and concentric internal rings containing less dust than is usual in other forms of PMF.[122] Ischemic necrosis and cavitation are common features.

Pathogenesis

Studies of the pathogenesis of coal miners' disease have been complicated by the ranges of pathological appearances of simple pneumoconiosis and PMF, by the coincidence in most cases of both fibrosis and emphysema, and by the variability of coal dust from place to place and from time to time. Moreover, since the essential epidemiological relationships between dust exposure and disease have now been well described (and thus the information on which preventative measures can be based is available to the industry), it can be argued that such studies are of academic and scientific interest, as models of disease, rather than of practical value to the health of workers.

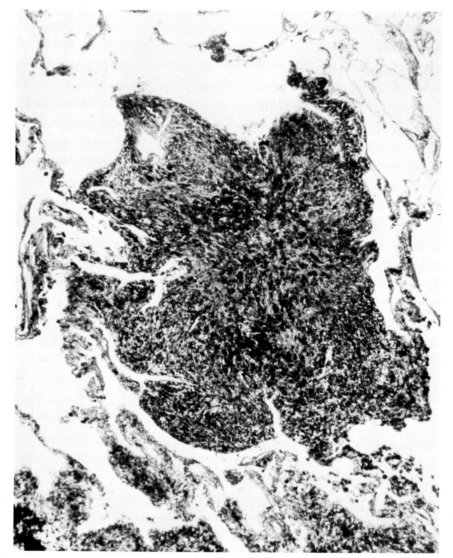

Figure 15–20. Larger coal macule showing coal dust, dust-laden macrophages, reticulin fibers, and minimal collagenous fibrosis.

The questions of perhaps greatest interest are the following:

1. How does coal mine dust cause PMF?
2. Why are there such marked and consistent differences in the risk of pneumoconiosis from one mine to another?
3. What is the relationship between fibrosis and emphysema?

Certain aspects of the pathogenesis are clear. The particles that cause pneumoconiosis are those aerodynamically small enough to reach the acinus and be deposited there. Although this generally means spherical particles between 0.5 and 7 μm, it should not be forgotten that the shape of the particle may be important. Anthracite, for example, has plate-like particles that may have a larger diameter in one dimension and yet still be aerodynamically respirable.[123] Once in the acinus, the foreign particles are engulfed by macrophages, which then attempt to remove them either by the mucociliary mechanism or lymphatic vessels, eventually to the hilar nodes.[124] Any pathological changes that occur are the consequences of the interaction of macrophages, other attracted defensive cells, especially polymorpho-

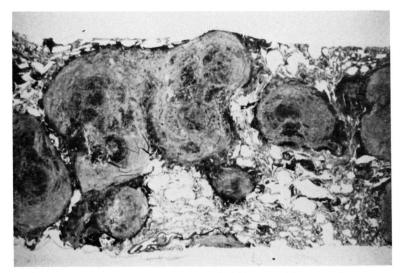

Figure 15–21. Low-power view of PMF in which fibrotic nodules are coalescing.

nuclear leukocytes,[125] and the dust. They are therefore dependent on the toxic effects of the dust particles on the lung cells. In theory, the dust may have a number of effects on cells, i.e., it may immobilize them, kill them, or interfere with their metabolism in such a way that they emit signals to other cells. It seems likely that all three mechanisms play a part in the genesis of dust-related coal miners' diseases.

In vitro studies have shown coal dust to be far less toxic to macrophages than quartz.[126] Free oxygen radicals have been suggested as a cause of lung damage in a variety of circumstances,[127] and it has been suggested that the toxicity of coal dust may depend on its ability to generate free radicals on cleavage planes when crushed.[128, 129] *In vitro* experiments in rats have shown low-rank coal dust to produce a transient macrophage-neutrophil alveolitis after intratracheal instillation and a more prolonged and persistent alveolitis during inhalation experiments, even at doses as low as 10 mg/m³.[130] Macrophages and leukocytes lavaged from the lungs of rats exposed to coal dust have been shown to have markedly reduced chemotaxis,

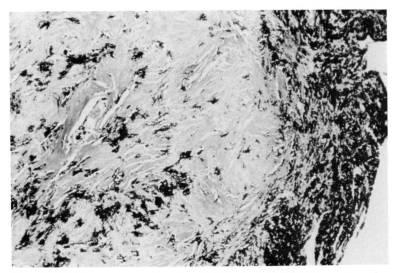

Figure 15–22. Low-power view of periphery of PMF showing cellular outer region and amorphous center.

a finding that may well partially explain their accumulation in the macule and their failure to remove dust from sites of deposition within the lung.[131] Moreover, the inflammatory cells in the lungs of rats exposed to coal dust have an enhanced ability to produce proteases and degrade fibronectin.[132] In these circumstances, alveolar macrophages have been shown to produce the inflammatory mediator interleukin-1.[133] Taken together with the evidence that the lungs of miners with PMF contain more dust per unit lifetime dust exposure, these experimental results suggest that an effect of dust on the motility of macrophages, together with stimulation of the release of mediators of inflammation and tissue breakdown, are central to the pathogenesis of pneumoconiosis and the accompanying inflammation, fibrosis, and emphysema. Differences in the microscopic appearances, including the amounts of cellular infiltration, dust accumulation, and surrounding emphysema, may then hypothetically be related to the type of dust inhaled, including potentially protective effects of some of its components. To date, however, experimental studies have not shown clear correlations between the *in vivo* animal toxicity of coal mine dusts and their recorded epidemiological effects in populations of miners.

It can be seen that the aforementioned hypothesis may explain the pathogenesis of the most common type of PMF, if (perhaps because also of lymphatic blockage) there is accumulation of dust and cells diffusely through part of the lung. Three observed facts in the cause of PMF (namely, its relationship to heavy dust exposure and lung dust content, its propensity to develop in upper zones (especially on the right), and its relative frequency in taller workers) suggest a partly mechanical explanation in terms of dust clearance. Such an explanation fits the observed radiological features of the genesis of PMF, i.e., aggregation of lesions grouped together and sometimes a diffuse haziness of the relevant part of the radiograph prior to the appearance of a clear-cut PMF lesion. In some cases, as stated before, the cause of PMF is very clearly the growth and aggregation of r lesions, which is related to high quartz exposures.

Although the differences in the incidence of pneumoconiosis in different mines are largely explicable on the basis of different dust exposures and different ranks of coal, anomalies remain between mines in which dust exposures and compositions have been similar yet the incidence of disease differs. Attempts to explain this, based on the proportion of minerals, such as clays, with the potential to inhibit surface activity of more toxic components of the dust, have so far been unsuccessful. It remains true that the best guides to future risks of disease in a mine are the current dust levels, the coal's rank and its quartz content, and the past pneumoconiosis record.

The relationship between fibrosis and emphysema, which was commented on by Osler and by pathologists in the 1930s,[134, 135] is intriguing. The work of Cummins is of especial interest, in that he commented on the frequency of emphysema in the lungs of miners with pneumoconiosis, at a time when emphysema was much less common than it was to become, and he was able to show the disruption of the elastic network of the lung.[135] This he thought unlikely to be a compensatory consequence of fibrosis since it occurred also in heavily dusted lungs without much fibrosis. It is a matter of common observation that most diseases that cause pulmonary fibrosis may also be associated with airflow obstruction and pathological emphysema; tuberculosis, sarcoidosis, and farmers' lung are three such conditions. Conversely, fibrosis has been noted in smokers' emphysema. PMF lesions are frequently surrounded by bullae and coal macules by foci of emphysema. It seems logical, in view of the experimental results mentioned earlier, that dust lesions involving the attraction of neutrophils and release of (*inter alia*) proteolytic enzymes are responsible for emphysema and fibrosis, and experimental studies have given some support to this hypothesis.[136] Recent studies of collagen and elastin in human lungs with emphysema also support the concept that inflammation and repair, features of the pneumoconiotic process, are responsible for the development of centriacinar emphysema.[137] The increased risk of centriacinar emphysema in PMF cases away from the lesion and, in simple pneumoconisosis, in relation to dust exposure[44, 64, 138, 139] supports the hypothesis that coal dust exposure sufficient to cause alveolar inflammation and fibrosis also initiates centriacinar emphysema. This seems a likely explanation for the consistent epidemiological finding of decrements in FEV_1 and FVC and a rise in residual volume in relation to the indices of dust exposure in coal miners.

It has been suggested that emphysema in coal miners might be a consequence of exposure to oxides of nitrogen or other products of explosives used underground.[140] Although it is not possible to deny this possibility in individual cases of heavily exposed, nonsmoking miners, epidemiological study of exposures to nitrogen oxides has not shown an effect on ventilatory capacity when age, smoking habit, and coal dust exposure have been allowed for.[141] It seems likely that any such effect must be unusual, perhaps resulting from accidental high exposure of individuals, rather than a general one in the mining population.

PREVENTION AND MANAGEMENT OF LUNG DISEASE IN COAL MINERS

The prevention of pneumoconiosis is based on reductions in the levels of dust to which workers are exposed and the duration of exposure, together with regular surveillance of the exposed work force for early signs of radiological disease. Dust control is effected primarily by ventilation and, thus, dilution of the dust and, secondarily, by the use of water sprayed at points of dust generation. The effectiveness of such measures should be monitored by regular measurement of dust concentrations. In a long-wall face, this is done most conveniently in the return roadway by a static sampler, but in other mining situations, personal samplers on workers, chosen according to a statistically designed strategy, are probably the most useful method. In most countries, statutory standards apply, and failure to comply with these may result in the regulatory authority taking sanctions against the mine operator.

In some mining situations, it may be difficult to achieve adequate dust control. In such circumstances, the use of approved respirators and a limitation of the miners' hours of exposure are additional measures that may be used. These are not, of course, substitutes for good dust control but additional measures that may have to be taken.

If the dust levels currently found in United States and British mines are maintained, it is unlikely that chronic airflow obstruction will be as much a problem in the future as it has been in the past. All the studies have shown the effects of dust to be additional to those of cigarettes, but they have been based, necessarily, on studies of miners with relatively high exposures in the past. Future studies are likely to show a lower excess of airflow obstruction in Western miners, relating more to their cigarette consumption than to their dust exposure. Studies of nonsmoking miners who have worked in the industry since the 1970s will be of particular interest.

Coal mining is one industry wherein regular worker surveillance is worthwhile since early pneumoconiosis can be detected radiologically and, if caught at that stage, is unlikely to progress if future dust exposure is controlled. Radiological examination should be carried out at a frequency dependent on the efficacy of dust control. In Western mines, it need not be more frequent than every 5 years. Where there is a risk of silicosis, especially in tuberculosis-endemic areas, more frequent films may be advisable.

When pneumoconiosis is detected in a miner, the most important aspect of management is good medical advice. The diagnosis conjures up a fearful picture in the mind of the miner, who is often well aware of relatives or friends who have died of the disease. The matter is further complicated in the United States by personal injury litigation. It is the duty of the doctor to put the facts fairly before the patient. The important ones in any individual case relate to the severity of the disease, its prognosis, and the absence of any curative treatment. Fortunately, with early detection, the physician is usually able to reassure the patient about adverse effects on exercise tolerance and prognosis and to encourage the patient to lead a normal life, with one important exception, i.e., that further dust exposure should be controlled. This does not necessarily mean complete exclusion from mining and, therefore, earning a livelihood. An older miner, close to retirement age, might reasonably be allowed to continue in the same job in the belief that the small additional increment in dust exposure is unlikely to make a substantial difference to the outcome. A younger man should properly be advised either to quit dusty work or to transfer to a substantially less dusty part of the operation, although it will usually involve a reduction in income. Of course, in all cases, advice should be given on the dangers of smoking, and if necessary, help should be given to stop the habit. Where PMF is suspected, further dusty work should generally be prevented. Since this condition is nevertheless likely to progress after leaving the industry, follow-up should be arranged so that the progress of the condition can be monitored and the patient advised accordingly. The variability of progression should be stressed, i.e., the condition does not always progress relentlessly and may arrest before the patient becomes disabled. Patients should be informed of this possibility and encouraged to make the most of their lung function by taking part in a physical fitness program.[142] This should always, where relevant, include advice and support in smoking cessation, but the benefits of physical exercise in the rehabilitation of patients with pneumoconiosis are often forgotten, especially where litigation becomes an issue.

REFERENCES

1. Meiklejohn, A., History of lung disease of coal miners in Great Britain, Part I, 1800–1875. Br. J. Ind. Med., 8, 127, 1951.
2. Meiklejohn, A., History of lung disease of coal miners in Great Britain, Part II, 1875–1920. Br. J. Ind. Med., 9, 93, 1952.
3. Meiklejohn, A., History of lung disease of coal miners in Great Britain, Part III, 1920–1952. Br. J. Ind. Med., 9, 208, 1952.
4. Stocks, P., Cancer and bronchitis mortality in relation to atmospheric deposit and smoke. B.M.J., 1, 74, 1959.
5. Pott, P., Chirurgical Works, Vol. 3. London, Hawes, Clark and Collins, 1775, p. 177.
6. Lee, H.B., Bloodletting in Appalachia. Morgantown, West Virginia University Press, 1969.
7. Gregory, J.C., Case of peculiar black infiltration of the whole lungs, resembling melanosis. Edinb. Med. Surg. J., 36, 389, 1831.
8. Marshall, W., Cases of spurious melanosis of the lungs, or of phthisis melanotica. Lancet, 2, 271, 1834.
9. Laennec, R.T.H., Traité de l'Auscultation Médiate. Paris, Brosson et Chaudé, 1819.
10. Fletcher, C.M., Pneumoconiosis of coal-miners. B.M.J., 1, 1015, 1948.
11. Fletcher, C.M., Pneumoconiosis of coal-miners. B.M.J., 1, 1065, 1948.
12. Arlidge, J.J., The Hygiene, Diseases and Mortality of Occupations. London, Percival, 1882.
13. Collis, E.L., and Gilchrist, J.C., Effects of dust upon coal trimmers. J. Ind. Hyg., 10, 101, 1928.
14. Gough, J., Pneumoconiosis of coal trimmers. J. Pathol., 51, 277, 1940.
15. Fay, J.W.J., The National Coal Board's Pneumoconiosis Field Research. Nature, 180, 309, 1957.
16. Seaton, A., Coalmining, emphysema and compensation. Br. J. Ind. Med., 47, 433, 1990.
17. Hart, P.d'A., and Aslett, A.E., Medical Research Council Special Report Series, No. 243. London, H.M. Stationery Office, 1943.
18. Rae, S., Walker, D.D., and Attfield, M., Chronic bronchitis and dust exposure in British coal miners. In Walton, W.H., ed., Inhaled Particles III. Old Woking, UK, Unwin Bros, 1971, p. 883.
19. Enterline, P.E., Mortality rates among coal miners. Am. J. Public Health, 54, 758, 1964.
20. Liddell, F.D.K., Mortality of British coal miners in 1961. Br. J. Ind. Med., 30, 15, 1973.
21. Jacobsen, M., Rae, S., Walton, W.H., and Rogan, J.M., New dust standards for British coal mines. Nature, 227, 445, 1970.
22. Jacobsen, M., New data on the relationship between simple pneumoconiosis and exposure to coal mine dust. Chest, 78, 408s, 1980.
23. Federal Mine Safety and Health Act of 1977. Pub. L No. 91,173. Amended by Pub. L No. 95,164: 101.
24. Hamilton, R.J., and Walton, W.H., The selective sampling of respirable dust. In Davies, C.N., ed., Inhaled Particles and Vapours. Oxford, Pergamon Press, 1961, p. 465.
25. Banks, D.E., Bauer, M.A., Castellan, R.M., and Lapp, N.L., Silicosis in surface coal mine drillers. Thorax, 38, 275, 1983.

26. Fairman, R.P., O'Brien, R.J., Swecker, S., et al., Respiratory status of surface coal miners in the United States. Arch. Environ. Health, 32, 211, 1977.
27. Cochrane, A.L., and Moore, F., A 20-year follow-up of a population sample (aged 25–34) including coal miners and foundry workers in Staveley, Derbyshire. Br. J. Ind. Med., 37, 230, 1980.
28. Ortmeyer, C.E., Costello, J., Morgan, W.K.C., et al., The mortality of Appalachian coal miners, 1963–1971. Arch. Environ. Health, 29, 67, 1974.
29. Miller, B.G., and Jacobsen, M., Dust exposure, pneumoconiosis and mortality of coal miners. Br. J. Ind. Med., 42, 723, 1985.
30. Costello, J., Ortmeyer, C.E., and Morgan, W.K.C., Mortality from heart disease in coal miners. Chest, 67, 417, 1975.
31. Costello, J., Ortmeyer, C.E., and Morgan, W.K.C., Mortality from lung cancer in U.S. coal miners. Am. J. Public Health, 64, 222, 1974.
32. Rockette, H., Mortality Among Coal Miners Covered by the UMWA Health and Retirement Funds. NIOSH Research Report. Publication no. 77–155. Rockville, MD, Department of Health, Education and Welfare, 1977.
33. Matolo, N.M., Gorishek, W.M., Moslander, V., and Dixon, J.A., Coalmining and cancer of the stomach. Rocky Mt. Med. J., 69, 44, 1972.
34. Miejers, J.M.M., Swaen, G.M.H., Slangen, J.J.M., et al., Long term mortality in miners with coal workers' pneumoconiosis in the Netherlands. Am. J. Ind. Med., 19, 43, 1991.
35. Hurley, J.F., Burns, J., Copland, L., et al., Coalworkers' simple pneumoconiosis and exposure to dust at 10 British coalmines. Br. J. Ind. Med., 39, 120, 1982.
36. Hurley, J.F., Alexander, W.P., Hazledine, D.J., et al., Exposure to respirable coalmine dust and incidence of progressive massive fibrosis. Br. J. Ind. Med., 44, 661, 1987.
37. Bennett, J.G., Dick, J.A., Kaplan, Y.S., et al., The relationship between coal rank and the prevalence of pneumoconiosis. Br. J. Ind. Med., 36, 206, 1979.
38. Soutar, C.A., Maclaren, W.M., Annis, R., and Melville, A.W.T., Quantitative relations between exposure to respirable dust and coalmine dust and coalworkers' simple pneumoconiosis in men who have worked as miners but who have left the coal industry. Br. J. Ind. Med., 43, 29, 1986.
39. Seaton, A., Dick, J.A., Dodgson, J., and Jacobsen, M., Quartz and pneumoconiosis in coal miners. Lancet, 2, 1272, 1981.
40. Jacobsen, M., and Maclaren, W., Unusual pulmonary observations and exposure to coalmine dust: a case-control study. Inhaled particles V. Ann. Occup. Hyg., 26, 753, 1982.
41. Rogan, J.M., Attfield, M.D., Jacobsen, M., et al., Role of dust in the working environment in development of chronic bronchitis in British coal miners. Br. J. Ind. Med., 30, 217, 1973.
42. Marine, W.M., Gurr, D., and Jacobsen, M., Clinically important respiratory effects of dust exposure and smoking in British coal miners. Am. Rev. Respir. Dis., 137, 106, 1988.
43. Love, R., and Miller, B.G., Longitudinal study of lung function in coalminers. Thorax, 37, 193, 1982.
44. Ruckley, V.A., Gauld, S.J., Chapman, J.S., et al., Emphysema and dust exposure in a group of coal workers. Am. Rev. Respir. Dis., 129, 528, 1984.
45. Cockcroft, A., Berry, G., Cotes, J.E., and Lyons, J.P., Shape of small opacities and lung function in coalworkers. Thorax, 37, 765, 1982.
46. Cockcroft, A., Lyons, J.P., Andersson, N., and Saunders, M.J., Prevalence and relation to underground exposure of radiological irregular opacities in South Wales coal workers with pneumoconiosis. Br. J. Ind. Med., 40, 169, 1983.
47. Collins, H.P.R., Dick, J.A., Bennett, J.G., et al., Irregularly shaped small shadows on chest radiographs, dust exposure, and lung function in coalworkers' pneumoconiosis. Br. J. Ind. Med., 45, 43, 1988.
48. Reisner, M.T.R., Results of epidemiologic studies of the progression of coal workers' pneumoconiosis. Chest, 78, 406s, 1980.
49. Reisner, M.T.R., Results of epidemiological studies of pneumoconiosis in West German coal miners. In Walton, W.H., ed., Inhaled Particles III. Old Woking, UK, Unwin Bros., 1971, p. 921.
50. Breuer, H., and Reisner, M.T.R., Criteria for long-term dust standards on the basis of personal dust exposure records. Ann. Occup. Hyg., 32(suppl. 1), 523, 1988.
51. Attfield, M.D., and Morring, K., An investigation into the relationship between coal workers' pneumoconiosis and dust exposure in US coal miners. Am. Ind. Hyg. Assoc. J., 53, 486, 1992.
52. Soutar, C.A., and Maclaren, W.M., Progressive massive fibrosis and simple pneumoconiosis in ex-miners. Br. J. Ind. Med., 42, 734, 1985.
53. Cochrane, A.L., The attack rate of progressive massive fibrosis. Br. J. Ind. Med., 19, 52, 1962.
54. McLintock, J.S., Rae, S., and Jacobsen, M., The attack rate of progressive massive fibrosis in British coalminers. In Walton, W.H., ed., Inhaled Particles III. Old Woking, UK, Unwin Bros., 1971, p. 933.
55. Shennan, D.H., Washington, J.S., Thomas, D.J., et al., Factors predisposing to the development of progressive massive fibrosis in coal miners. Br. J. Ind. Med., 38, 321, 1981.
56. Kibelstis, J.A., Morgan, E.J., Reger, R.B., et al., Prevalence of bronchitis and airway obstruction in American bituminous coal miners. Am. Rev. Respir. Dis., 108, 886, 1973.
57. Leigh, J., Wiles, A.N., and Glick, M., Total population study of factors affecting chronic bronchitis prevalence in the coalmining industry of New South Wales, Australia. Br. J. Ind. Med., 43, 263, 1986.

58. Attfield, M.D., and Hodous, T.K., Pulmonary function of US coal miners related to dust exposure estimates. Am. Rev. Respir. Dis., 145, 605, 1992.

59. Leigh, J., and Wiles, A.N., Factors affecting prevalences of mucus hypersecretion and airflow obstruction in the coal industry of New South Wales, Australia. Ann. Occup. Hyg., 32(suppl. 1), 1186, 1986.

60. Seixas, N.S., Robins, T.G., Attfield, M.D., and Moulton, L.H., Exposure-response relationships for coal mine dust and obstructive lung disease following enactment of the Federal Coal Mine Health and Safety Act of 1969. Am. J. Ind. Med., 21, 715, 1991.

61. Attfield, M.D., Longitudinal decline in FEV_1 in United States coal miners. Thorax, 40, 132, 1985.

62. Schmidt, U., Dust and non-specific respiratory disorders in foundry workers and coal miners in the Rhine-Ruhr area. Rev. Inst. Hyg. Mines, 34, 70, 1979.

63. Seixas, N.S., Robins, T.G., Attfield, M.D., and Moulton, L.H., Longitudinal and cross sectional analyses of exposure to coal mine dust and pulmonary function in new miners. Br. J. Ind. Med., 50, 929, 1993.

64. Ruckley, V.A., Fernie, J.M., Campbell, S.J., and Cowie, H.A., Causes of Disability in Coalminers: A Clinico-Pathological Study of Emphysema, Airways Obstruction and Massive Fibrosis. TM 89/05. Edinburgh, Institute of Occupational Medicine, 1989.

65. Fernie, J.M., Douglas, N.A., Lamb, D., and Ruckley, V.A., Right ventricular hypertrophy in a group of coal miners. Thorax, 38, 436, 1983.

66. Rodnan, G.P., Benedek, T.G., Medgser, T.A., and Cammarata, R.J., The association of progressive systemic sclerosis (scleroderma) with coal miners' pneumoconiosis and other forms of silicosis. Ann. Intern. Med., 66, 323, 1967.

67. Sluis-Cremer, G.K., Hessel, P.A., Nizdo, E.H., et al., Silica, silicosis and progressive systemic sclerosis. Br. J. Ind. Med., 42, 838, 1985.

68. Caplan, A., Certain unusual radiological appearances in the chest of coal-miners suffering from rheumatoid arthritis. Thorax, 8, 29, 1953.

69. Caplan, A., Payne, R.B., and Withey, J.L., A broader concept of Caplan's syndrome related to rheumatoid factors. Thorax, 17, 205, 1962.

70. Dick, J.A., Morgan, W.K.C., Muir, D.C.F., et al., The significance of irregular opacities on the chest roentgenogram. Chest 102, 251, 1992.

71. Weiss, W., Cigarette smoking and small irregular opacities. Br. J. Ind. Med., 48, 841, 1991.

72. Seaton, A., Cigarette smoking and small irregular opacities. Br. J. Ind. Med., 49, 453, 1992.

73. Amandus, H.E., Lapp, N.L., Jacobson, G., and Reger, R.B., Significance of irregular small opacities in radiographs of coalminers in the USA. Br. J. Ind. Med., 33, 13, 1976.

74. Soutar, C.A., and Collins, H.P.R., Classification of progressive massive fibrosis of coalminers by type of radiographic appearance. Br. J. Ind. Med., 41, 334, 1984.

75. Soutar, C.A., and Hurley, J.F., Relation between dust exposure and lung function in miners and ex-miners. Br. J. Ind. Med., 43, 307, 1986.

76. Soutar, C.A., Update on lung disease in coalminers. Br. J. Ind. Med., 44, 145, 1987.

77. Hankinson, J., Reger, R.B., and Morgan, W.K.C., Maximal expiratory flows in coalminers. Am. Rev. Respir. Dis., 116, 175, 1977.

78. Cochrane, A.L., and Higgins, I.T.T., Pulmonary ventilatory function of coal miners in various areas in relation to the x-ray category of pneumoconiosis. Br. J. Prev. Soc. Med., 15, 1, 1961.

79. Morgan, W.K.C., Handelsman, L., Kibelstis, J., et al., Ventilatory capacity and lung volumes of U.S. coal miners. Arch. Environ. Health, 28, 182, 1974.

80. Cotes, J.E., and Field, G.B., Lung gas exchange in simple pneumoconiosis of coal workers. Br. J. Ind. Med., 29, 268, 1972.

81. Seaton, A., Lapp, N.L., and Morgan, W.K.C., The relationship of pulmonary impairment in simple coal workers' pneumoconiosis to type of radiographic opacity. Br. J. Ind. Med., 29, 50, 1972.

82. Frans, A., Veriter, C., and Brasseur, L., Pulmonary diffusing capacity for carbon monoxide in simple CWP. Bull. Physiopathol. Respir., 11, 479, 1975.

83. Morgan, W.K.C., Burgess, D.P., Lapp, N.L., et al., Hyperinflation of the lungs in coal miners. Thorax, 26, 585, 1971.

84. Morgan, W.K.C., Seaton, A., Burgess, D.B., et al., Lung volumes in working coal miners. Ann. N. Y. Acad. Sci., 200, 478, 1972.

85. Morgan, W.K.C., Handelsman, L., Kibelstis, J., et al., Ventilatory capacity and lung volumes of U.S. coal miners. Arch. Environ. Health, 28, 182, 1974.

86. Lapp, N.L., and Seaton, A., Lung mechanics in coal workers' pneumoconiosis. Ann. N. Y. Acad. Sci., 200, 433, 1972.

87. Seaton, A., Lapp, N.L., and Morgan, W.K.C., Lung mechanics and frequency dependence of compliance in coal miners. J. Clin. Invest., 51, 1203, 1972.

88. Lapp, N.L., and Seaton, A., Pulmonary function. In Key, M.M., Kerr, I.E., and Bundy, M., eds., Pulmonary Reactions to Coal Dust. New York, Academic Press, 1971, p. 153.

89. Frans, A., Veriter, N., Gerin-Portier, N., and Brasseur, L., Blood gases in simple coal workers' pneumoconiosis. Bull. Physiopathol. Respir., 11, 503, 1975.

90. Lapp, N.L., Seaton, A., Kaplan, K.C., et al., Pulmonary hemodynamics in symptomatic coal miners. Am. Rev. Respir. Dis., 104, 418, 1971.

91. Hurley, J.F., and Soutar, C.A., Can exposure to coalmine dust cause a severe impairment of pulmonary function? Br. J. Ind. Med., 43, 150, 1986.

92. Morgan, W.K.C., and Lapp, N.L., Respiratory disease in coal miners. State of the art. Am. Rev. Respir. Dis., 113, 531, 1976.

93. Gilson, J.C., and Hugh-Jones, P., Lung function in coalworkers' pneumoconiosis. Medical Research Council, Special Report Series no. 290. London, H.M. Stationery Office, 1955.

94. Ulmer, W.T., and Reichel, G., Functional impairment in coal workers' pneumoconiosis. Ann. N. Y. Acad. Sci., 200, 405, 1972.

95. Kremer, R., and Lavenne, F., La circulation pulmonaire dans les pneumoconioses. Poumon Coeur, 22, 767, 1966.

96. Morgan, W.K.C., Caplan's syndrome. Ann. Intern. Med., 55, 667, 1961.

97. Miall, W.E., Caplan, A., Cochrane, A.L., et al., An epidemiological study of rheumatoid arthritis associated with characteristic chest x-ray appearances in coal workers. B.M.J., 2, 1231, 1953.

98. Constantinidis, K., Musk, A.W., Jenkins, J.P.R., and Berry, G., Pulmonary function in coalworkers with Caplan's syndrome and non-rheumatoid complicated pneumoconiosis. Thorax, 33, 764, 1978.

99. Wagner, J.C., and McCormick, J.N., Immunological investigations of coal-workers' disease. J. R. Coll. Phys., 2, 49, 1967.

100. Wagner, J.C., Etiological factors in complicated coal workers' pneumoconiosis. Ann. N. Y. Acad. Sci., 200, 401, 1972.

101. Lippman, M., Eckert, H.L., Hahon, N., and Morgan, W.K.C., The prevalence of circulating antinuclear and rheumatoid factors in United States coal miners. Ann. Intern. Med., 79, 807, 1973.

102. Benedek, T.G., Zawadzki, Z.A., and Medsger, T.A., Serum immunoglobulins, rheumatoid factor and pneumoconiosis in coal miners with rheumatoid arthritis. Arthritis Rheum., 19, 731, 1976.

103. Robertson, M.D., Boyd, J.E., Fernie, J.M., and Davis, J.M.G., Some immunological studies on coalworkers with and without pneumoconiosis. Am. J. Ind. Med., 4, 467, 1983.

104. Soutar, C.A., Coutts, I., Parkes, W.R., et al., Histocompatibility antigens in coal miners with pneumoconiosis. Br. J. Ind. Med., 40, 34, 1983.

105. Boyd, J.E., Robertson, M.D., and Davis, J.M.G., Autoantibodies in coalminers: their relationship to the development of progressive massive fibrosis. Am. J. Ind. Med., 3, 201, 1982.

106. Heppleston, A.G., The essential lesion of pneumokoniosis in Welsh coal workers. J. Pathol., 59, 453, 1947.

107. Heppleston, A.G., The pathogenesis of simple pneumokoniosis in coal workers. J. Pathol., 67, 51, 1954.

108. Kleinerman, J., Pathology standards for coal workers' pneumoconiosis. Report of Pneumoconiosis Committee of the College of American Pathologists. Arch. Pathol. Lab. Med., 103, 375, 1979.

109. Rivers, D., Wise, M.E., King, E.J., and Nagelschmidt, G., Dust content, radiology and pathology in simple pneumoconiosis of coal workers. Br. J. Ind. Med., 17, 87, 1960.

110. Rossiter, C.M., Relation of lung dust content to radiological changes in coal workers. Ann. N. Y. Acad. Sci., 200, 465, 1972.

111. Ruckley, V.A., Fernie, J.M., Chapman, J.S., et al., Comparison of radiographic appearances with associated pathology and lung dust content in a group of coalworkers. Br. J. Ind. Med., 41, 459, 1984.

112. Douglas, A.N., Robertson, A., Chapman, J.S., and Ruckley, V.A., Dust exposure, dust recovered from the lung, and associated pathology in a group of British coalminers. Br. J. Ind. Med., 43, 795, 1986.

113. Davis, J.M.G., Chapman, J., Collings, P., et al., Variations in the histological pattern of the lesions of coal workers' pneumoconiosis in Britain and their relationship to lung dust content. Am. Rev. Respir. Dis., 128, 118, 1983.

114. Fernie, J.M., and Ruckley, V.A., Coalworkers' pneumoconiosis: correlation between opacity profusion and number and type of dust lesions with special reference to opacity type. Br. J. Ind. Med., 44, 273, 1987.

115. Kilpatrick, G.S., Heppleston, A.G., and Fletcher, C.M., Cavitation in the massive fibrosis of coal workers' pneumoconiosis. Thorax, 3, 260, 1954.

116. Wagner, J.C., Immunological factors in coalworkers' pneumoconiosis. In Walton, W.H., ed., Inhaled Particles III. Old Woking, UK, Unwin Bros., 1971, p. 573.

117. Wagner, J.C., Wusterman, F.S., Edwards, J.H., and Hill, R.J., The composition of massive lesions in coal miners. Thorax, 30, 382, 1975.

118. Wagner, J.C., Burns, J., Munday, D.E., and McGee, J., Presence of fibronectin in pneumoconiotic lesions. Thorax, 37, 54, 1982.

119. Wells, A.L., Pulmonary vascular changes in coal-workers' pneumoconiosis. J. Pathol., 68, 573, 1954.

120. Thomas, A.J., Right ventricular hypertrophy in the pneumoconiosis of coal miners. Br. Heart J., 13, 1, 1951.

121. James, W.R.L., and Thomas, A.J., Cardiac hypertrophy in coalworkers' pneumoconiosis. Br. J. Ind. Med., 13, 24, 1956.

122. Gough, J., Rivers, D., and Seal, R.M.E., Pathologic studies of modified pneumoconiosis in coalminers with rheumatoid arthritis (Caplan's syndrome). Thorax, 10, 9, 1955.

123. Addison, J., and Dodgson, J., The influence of the size, shape and composition of individual dust particles on the harmfulness of coalmine dusts: development of methods of analysis. In Proceedings of the 7th International Pneumoconiosis Conference, 1988. Pittsburgh, U.S. Department of Health and Human Services, 1990, p. 287.

124. Vincent, J., and Donaldson, K., A dosimetric model for relating the biological response of the lung to the accumulation of inhaled mineral dust. Br. J. Ind. Med., 47, 302, 1990.

125. Begin, R., Bisson, G., Boilleau, R., and Masse, S., Assessment of disease activity by gallium[67] scanning and lung lavage in pneumoconiosis. Semin. Respir. Med., 7, 275, 1986.

126. Vallyathan, V., Schwegler, D., Reasor, M., et al., Comparative in vitro cytotoxicity and relative pathogenicity of mineral dusts. Ann. Occup. Hyg., 32(suppl. 1), 279, 1988.

127. Brighan, K.L., Role of free radicals in lung injury. Chest, 89, 859, 1986.

128. Dalal, N.S., Suryan, M.M., Vallyathan, V., et al., Detection of reactive free radicals in fresh coal mine dust and their implication for lung injury. Ann. Occup. Hyg., 33, 79, 1989.

129. Castranova, V., Bowman, L., Reasor, M.J., et al., The response of rat alveolar macrophages to chronic inhalation of coal dust and/or diesel exhaust. Environ. Res., 36, 405, 1985.

130. Donaldson, K., Brown, G.M., Brown, D.M., et al., Impaired chemotactic responses of bronchoalveolar leukocytes in experimental pneumoconiosis. J. Pathol., 160, 63, 1990.

131. Brown, G.M., Brown, D.M., and Donaldson, K., Persistent inflammation and impaired chemotaxis of alveolar macrophages on cessation of dust exposure. Environ. Health Perspect., 97, 91, 1992.

132. Brown, G.M., and Donaldson, K., Inflammatory responses in lungs of rats inhaling coalmine dust: enhanced proteolysis of fibronectin by bronchoalveolar leukocytes. Thorax, 46, 866, 1989.

133. Kusaka, Y., Brown, G.M., and Donaldson, K., Alveolitis caused by exposure to coal mine dusts: production of interleukin-1 and immunomodulation by bronchoalveolar leukocytes. Environ. Res., 53, 76, 1990.

134. Osler, W., The Principles and Practice of Medicine, 2nd ed. Edinburgh, Young J. Pentland, 1895, p. 588.

135. Cummins, S.L., The pneumoconioses in South Wales. J. Hyg., 36, 547, 1936.

136. Niewoehner, D.E., and Hoidal, J.R., Lung fibrosis and emphysema: divergent responses to a common injury. Science, 217, 359, 1982.

137. Cardoso, W.V., Sekhan, H.S., Hyde, D.M., and Thurlbeck, W.M., Collagen and elastin in human pulmonary emphysema. Am. Rev. Respir. Dis., 147, 975, 1993.

138. Cockcroft, A., Seal, R.M.E., Wagner, J.C., et al., Post-mortem study of emphysema in coalworkers and non-coalworkers. Lancet, 2, 600, 1982.

139. Green, F.H.Y., Emphysema in coalworkers' pneumoconiosis: contribution by coal and cigarette smoking. Am. Rev. Respir. Dis., 145(suppl.), 321a, 1992.

140. Kennedy, M.C.S., Nitrous fumes and coal miners with emphysema. Ann. Occup. Hyg., 15, 285, 1972.

141. Robertson, A., Dodgson, J., Collings, P., and Seaton, A., Exposure to oxides of nitrogen: respiratory symptoms and lung function in British coalminers. Br. J. Ind. Med., 41, 214, 1984.

142. Cockcroft, A.E., Saunders, M.J., and Berry, G., Randomised controlled trial of rehabilitation in chronic respiratory disability. Thorax, 36, 200, 1981.

16

Other Pneumoconioses

W. Keith C. Morgan

■

ALUMINUM AND THE LUNGS

The term *bauxite* is used to describe those sedimentary rocks that contain the aluminum minerals gibbsite, boehmite, and diaspore. These ores consist for the most part of aluminum oxide, hydroxide, oxyhydroxide, iron oxide, titanium oxide, and aluminosilicates. Most of the world's bauxite deposits are located in the savannah regions of the world extending from 20° north and south of the tropical rain forest belt. The largest bauxite deposits are found in Australia, Guyana, France, Jamaica, and Brazil. There are smaller deposits in Hungary and Surinam.

The mineral is located close to the surface and can usually be readily recovered by open cast mining. From the mine sites, the ore is transported to large rock crushers and subsequently taken to refining installations. Because most of the mining takes place on the surface, occupational dust exposure is relatively limited and less than it would be in an underground mine. There is little, if any, risk of silicosis in the mining of bauxite, mainly because those ores contaminated by silica are not economically worthwhile and thus are seldom mined.

Calcined bauxite is used in corundum production, in which it is mixed with coke and iron and fused in an electric arc furnace at a temperature of around 2000°C. This process involves the emission of fumes of aluminum oxide containing 15% to 55% free silica in the form of cristobalite. Such exposures have been associated with Shaver's disease (see later discussion).[1]

The aluminas are refined from bauxite utilizing the specific temperature-dependent solubility of the minerals boehmite, gibbsite, and diaspore.[2] Purification is carried out in hot caustic solutions so that respiratory exposure to the minerals is negligible. Subsequently the purified aluminas, i.e., aluminum trihydroxide ($Al(OH)_3$)), oxyhydroxides ($AlOOH$), and aluminum oxide (Al_2O_3), are heated to varying temperatures to obtain the properties desired for subsequent commercial use. Aluminum trihydroxide and the oxyhydroxides are heated from 300°C to 850°C, thereby driving off water with the formation of transitional forms of alumina. This leads to an increased surface area, especially in those transitional aluminas that are formed between 400°C and 600°C. The thermodynamic instability of these transitional aluminas has led to the suggestion that they may be biologically active in certain circumstances.[3] With continued heating above 800°C, new transitional aluminas are produced and the surface area decreases. At 1150°C, alpha alumina (corundum) is formed, and this has a significantly decreased surface area.

Until the 1970s, the highly calcined aluminas, particularly alpha alumina oxide, were primarily used in aluminum reduction. For technical reasons, there has been a trend toward the use of the less highly heated and more biologically active aluminas for smelting purposes. Smelting grade aluminas now contain less alpha aluminum and more kappa, delta, theta, and also small amounts of gamma alumina. In the past, the lower temperature transitional patterns, namely, chi and eta, were erroneously referred to as gamma alumina.

The reduction of Al_2O_3 to metallic aluminum involves electrolytic decomposition, whereby the Al_2O_3 is first rendered liquid to permit a direct current to flow through it. This is called the Hall-Heroult process and involves dissolving Al_2O_3 with cryolite (Na_3AlF_6) in a large pot into which dip carbon electrodes. This process leads to the generation of fluoride-containing effluents. The consumable carbon electrodes originally used in the Hall-Heroult process were baked prior to use, and as a consequence, there was a production of large volumes of CO_2 and CO. Exposures at such sites where reduction cells are located involved aluminum oxide and fluorides. Carbon monoxide, sulfur dioxide, and vanadium exposures were minimal and well below present threshold limit values. Alumina has adsorbent properties, and as a result, a fair amount of fluoride used to be carried into the lungs on particles of Al_2O_3, thereby producing an effect on the lungs and skeleton. The early smelters were extremely dusty, but over the past two or three decades the introduction of more stringent industrial hygiene measures has led to a much cleaner environment.

Smelter Work Force

There are five major jobs in the smelter: potroom workers, carbon plant workers, workers involved in cathode relining, and those workers engaged in the casting and maintenance. Potroom workers are exposed to aluminum, fluoride particles from cryolite, hydrogen fluoride gas, and some CO and coke impurities, while the carbon plant workers are exposed to coke and coal tar pitch volatiles but have little exposure to fluorides. The other jobs have no significant exposure to aluminum.

The National Institute for Occupational Safety and Health (NIOSH) in 1977 estimated that in the United States alone there may be 3 million workers with industrial exposure to aluminum compounds.[4] It cannot, however, be inferred that the majority of those exposed are at risk. It will become evident later in the chapter that aluminum for the most part is relatively innocuous.

Pathogenicity of the Alumina

At present there is little or no evidence to suggest that exposure to aluminum oxide in the workplace presents a significant risk to the lungs. The substitution of aluminum oxide for silica-containing abrasives in the Staffordshire pottery industry in Britain is a paradigm of the replacement of a harmful substance by one that is less so.[5] In the early 1900s to around 1935, it was the custom in the Staffordshire pottery industry to embed china articles in ground flint composed of nearly pure silica. The incidence and prevalence of silicosis in pottery workers in the first three decades of the century were a source of governmental concern, and as a result, calcined aluminum was substituted, with a resulting decline in the prevalence of silicosis.[6, 7] Subsequently, the report of Shaver and Riddell dealing with the entity that came to be known as Shaver's disease raised doubts as to the innocuous nature of aluminum oxide.[1]

Early studies in humans suggested that aluminum oxide was harmless and did not induce radiographic evidence of pneumoconiosis or lead to the development of any other chest condition.[5, 8] Subsequent studies of aluminum smelters seemed to confirm the innocuousness of the various forms of alumina.[9]

The early experiences of Gardner et al. in 1944 had shown that amorphous aluminum hydroxide (i.e., gelatinous boehmite), when administered to guinea pigs by inhalation, was nonfibrogenic.[10] It was also noted that the inhalation of an alumina known to have been thermally changed from gibbsite to the chi transition form failed to induce fibrosis. Later, King et al. administered gelatinous boehmite by the intratracheal route and produced fibronodular infiltrates and collagenous fibrosis.[11] They pointed out the disparities that might arise from differing routes of administration, but nevertheless noted that the lesions they had induced bore some resemblance to those reported in the lungs of workers with Shaver's disease.

The results obtained by Gardner et al. in 1944[10] in early inhalation experiments using guinea pigs exposed to the catalytically active transitional alumina, chi, differed completely from those obtained by King et al. when the latter used intratracheal injection.[11] Klosterkotter subsequently exposed rats to massive concentrations of inhaled specific transitional gamma Al_2O_3 (33 mg/m³) but failed to induce pulmonary fibrosis,[12] whereas Stacy et al. in 1959 had succeeded by using the intratracheal route.[13] Klosterkotter, however, had induced pulmonary alveolar proteinosis, from which it would be reasonable to infer that the clearing mechanisms of the lungs had been completely overwhelmed by the magnitude of the dust insult. The weight of the evidence suggests that both catalytically active eta transitional alumina and the large surface area aluminas can induce lung fibrosis in experimental animals, but only when given intratracheally. The pertinence of the intratracheal experiments in relation to workplace exposure to alumina is extremely doubtful, especially since it has been demonstrated that the most reactive of the aluminas, i.e., the chi and gamma forms, when given by inhalation, are nonfibrogenic in experimental animals.

Most studies of occupational exposure have concerned themselves with exposure to aluminum oxide and have not attempted to differentiate the various types of alumina. In doing so, the possibility of different responses being induced by different forms of aluminum oxide is not given consideration. A fairly recent study of 1109 exposed workers in an aluminum smelter that prepared a variety of chemical aluminas has been carried out.[14] Exposure to the more active transitional forms of alumina occurred intermittently from 1958 to 1982, with around 3% of the production consisting of catalytically active chi, eta, and gamma transitional forms. No pneumoconiosis was found, but there was an excess of subjects with an abnormal forced expiratory volume in 1 second (FEV_1); however, the effect of dust was far less than that of smoking.[14] There was also an increased prevalence of small irregular opacities in the chest x-ray films of the most exposed workers, to which both smoking, and to a much lesser extent dust, contributed.[15] A very low prevalence of rounded opacities was noted in this group of workers. Similar findings have been described in other occupations exposed to nonfibrogenic dusts.[16] There is no indication that increased frequency of irregular opacities is specific to alumina exposure. Furthermore, the reduction in ventilatory capacity is probably a consequence of industrial bronchitis which in itself is a nonspecific response.[17]

A more recent study describes nine workers exposed to aluminum oxide from the production of abrasives from Alundum ore.[18] Most had long-term exposure, and all had abnormal chest radiographs (category 1/0 or greater). In three subjects, respiratory symptoms of pulmonary impairment and the radiographic appearance were more severe than in the others, and as a result, an open lung biopsy was carried out. In all three, interstitial fibrosis and honeycombing were found. The lungs were found to contain a variety of metals and silica; and in one, an increased number of asbestos fibers and silica particles were found. As might be expected, the three subjects who underwent a biopsy had an increased aluminum burden in their lungs; however, the burden as measured by the number of aluminum particulates varied greatly. Of the remaining six subjects who had radiographs which showed changes of either category 1/0 or 1/1, all were smokers, and their radiographic changes were likely due to smoking.[15, 16] The finding of a high concentration of aluminum in the lungs is to be expected with long exposure and cannot be construed as indicating that aluminum causes fibrosis. There is nothing to suggest that aluminum workers are not as susceptible to fibrosing alveolitis and other types of interstitial fibrosis as is the general population. Moreover, this subject has been reviewed in detail by Morgan and Dinman[2, 3] and by Abramson et al.,[19] and the evidence for aluminum oxide producing fibrosis appears tenuous and unconvincing.

Pulmonary Aluminosis and the Manufacture of Pyrotechnics

Metallic aluminum does not occur naturally because of the metal's propensity for combining with oxygen to form aluminum oxide. Metallic aluminum on exposure to air is coated immediately with a fine layer of the oxide. The latter is relatively inert, and most workers are exposed to alumina rather than the metal itself, with the result that there are few, if any, occupational hazards.[2] Nevertheless, under exceptional circumstances, exposure to respirable particles of finely divided aluminum flake can occur and in the past has lead to the development of significant pulmonary fibrosis.[20, 21] This is a distinct entity and is not to be confused with Shaver's disease.[1]

Aluminum powder is produced in two forms, flake and granular. The former is produced by stamping cold metal in a ball mill, whereas the granular form is prepared directly from molten metal. Aluminum particles are often inadvertently generated by grinding metal with a corundum wheel; however, the size of such particles is relatively large, with most of them being greater than 100 μm. When smaller particles are produced commercially, this is effected by spraying molten metal through a high velocity jet or atomizer. These particles are smooth, small, spherical or elliptical and are referred to as granular or atomized particles. Flake aluminum is produced by ball milling atomized particles so that they are flattened and leaf-like with an irregular wave and trough-like contour. They have, in addition, a large surface area. Stearin, which is a mixture of hydrolyzed fats, is added in the milling process as a lubricant in order to keep separate the particles and to prevent impact welding. The fatty acids contained in stearin react with aluminum to form a film of aluminum stearate, which greatly slows down the rate of oxygenation of the metal to aluminum oxide. When aluminum powder is used in the preparation of paints, fairly large quantities of stearin are added.

An unusual form of flake powder known as pyro consists of very small particles (less than 1 μm in size) to which lesser amounts of stearin have been added. Pyro was, and is still, used for the manufacture of fireworks. This necessitates the mixing of pyro and carbon into a fine black powder. The stamping machines that were formerly used in this process generated large quantities of respirable dust, and values up to 0.5 mg/m^3 have been recorded.[22]

Pulmonary Hazards of Exposure to Aluminum Dust

At the turn of the century, aluminum flakes were used in Europe as a pigment, and the possible hazards from the use of powdered aluminum were investigated by Koelsch et al.[23] and by Doese.[24] For the most part such investigations were negative. In the 1940s, Goralewski was the first to describe the harmful effects of metallic aluminum powder.[20, 21] He became aware that German workers who manufactured pyro (aluminum powder) developed an acute respiratory illness often within a relatively short time of their starting work. The metal they were producing was used in the manufacture of explosives but was not coated with stearin, which had been the rule prior to 1939. Those who developed aluminosis of the lung had cough, fever, shortness of breath, lethargy, and anorexia. The chest radiograph showed pulmonary shadows, and often pneumothoraces developed. The lungs were later shown to have fibrotic changes. Ten of the original 18 of Goralewski's patients died from the disease.[25] Subsequently, Hunter et al.[26] examined the records of Goralewski and confirmed his findings.[20, 21] As a result, epidemiological studies were carried out on British workers employed in the manufacture of incendiary bombs and aluminum airplane propellers, but no significant hazards came to light. No explanation was apparent for the disparity in the British and German findings, at least at that time; but in retrospect, the aluminum particles generated in Britain were much larger and nonrespirable.[2] Subsequently, Mitchell et al.,[27, 28] Jordan,[29] and McLaughlin et al.[22] described additional subjects with aluminosis.

Clinical Features

The symptoms of aluminosis are similar to those of Shaver's disease. The fibrosis usually develops gradually, often over a period of years. The first complaints are a dry, nonproductive cough and breathlessness. Chest pain is not usual unless there is a spontaneous pneumothorax. A low-grade fever and chest tightness supervene later. On physical examination there is tachypnea and cyanosis in advanced cases, crackles, and sometimes clubbing. The pulmonary function tests show restrictive impairment, often with an abnormal diffusing capacity.[22, 28]

Pathology

The pathological features of aluminosis, both macroscopically and microscopically, are those of nonspecific interstitial pulmonary fibrosis. In this regard it must be remembered that the lungs have a limited way of responding and in doing so produce fibrosis without any specific features. The lungs tend to be smaller than normal, indurated, and grayish-black. The upper lobes are most affected, although the lower lobes are often involved to some extent. Emphysematous blebs, especially at the apices, are often present, but whether they are related to aluminum exposure is uncertain. On sectioning, the lungs show multiple areas of grayish-black fibrous tissue present, mainly in the upper and middle zones, with radiating bands of dense fibrosis. The typical features of silicosis are absent. Microscopically, there is interstitial fibrosis and epithelization of the alveoli. Giant cells may be present. The histological features are for the most part indistinguishable from those of fibrosing alveolitis. Honeycombing appears late in the disease and obliterative endarteritis and perivascular fibrosis may be present. Examination of the lungs reveals a grossly increased aluminum content. The aluminum content of the lungs of subjects with and without aluminosis have not been compared, but it is presumed that those with aluminosis contain more aluminum.

Pathogenesis

Anomalies in the development of parenchymal fibrosis in workers exposed to aluminum remained unexplained until recently. The disease apparently does not occur in plants where aluminum reduction is taking place,[15, 19] nor has it been reported in those industries where alumina has been used for many years.[6, 7] For many years metallic aluminum was administered to metal miners in Canada in the hope of preventing silicosis. As far as is known, none has developed any harmful effects from this procedure.[30, 31] The powder used for the prophylaxis of silicosis was composed of metallic granules and had been prepared by milling nonlubricated pellets of aluminum metal. Presumably the aluminum particles to which the Canadian miners were exposed were covered by a thin layer of oxide, and the metal itself did not come in contact with the lungs.

Goralewski's general observations and description of aluminum lung were made as a result of a series of subjects who developed this condition from 1939 to 1949.[20, 21] He observed that prior studies of German aluminum workers had failed to detect any respiratory hazard and that all of the subjects with aluminum lung had worked in the production of pyrotechnic powders. With remarkable prescience, he concluded that the advent in 1938 of aluminosis may have been related to the change in the lubricant used, and noted that it was about that time mineral oil lubricants started to be used.

In the early 1950s, there were sporadic cases of aluminosis occurring in Britain with similar features to those described by Goralewski.[22, 27–29] All British workers who developed the condition were working with pyro, and this was also true of the early cases described in Sweden by Swensson et al.[32] These observations stimulated King et al. to conduct a series of animal experiments.[11] In the early experiments, he used intratracheal injection of large doses of a metallic aluminum, and with this method he and his workers were able to produce marked fibrosis. Later Corrin in a series of experiments demonstrated that stamped aluminum coated with mineral oil reacts vigorously with water, whereas the granular powder was unreactive.[33] He concluded that the granular particles were inert because they were coated with aluminum oxide. The sudden appearance of aluminum pneumoconiosis in Britain suggested to Corrin that it was substitution of mineral oil for stearin that was responsible.[33, 34] He noted that the mineral oil permits the aluminum flake to react with water. He did a further series of experiments in rats administering up to 100 mg of pyro powder intratracheally and managed to produce extensive fibrosis.[34] He was successful at inducing fibrosis, no matter whether the pyro powder had been coated with stearin or mineral oil, and suggested that the stearin-treated pyro could therefore not be regarded as innocuous. Subsequently, McLaughlin described a subject with aluminosis who had been working with stearin-coated pyro powder. This seemed to confirm that pyro flakes were dangerous regardless of the form in which they were inhaled or given to animals and seemed to refute Corrin's thesis. Despite these later observations, up to 1938 there had been no convincing report of aluminosis occurring in Europe, Britain, or the United States, and it was the introduction of mineral oil–based lubricants in Germany that was responsible for the outbreak observed by Goralewski.[20, 21] In the United States, where mineral oil was never used, no convincing case of aluminosis has ever been described. It became clear with the passage of time that McLaughlin's subject,[22] who was initially said to have worked only with stearin-coated pyro, had worked with flake powder from 1946 to 1949,[2] that is to say, at a time when spindle oil was still used as a lubricant. The same goes for the case reported by Ueda et al.[35]

The weight of the evidence indicates that aluminosis does not occur unless the worker is exposed to high concentrations of flake powder that has been treated with stearin. Corrin's data indicated that the coating of mineral oil could be easily washed free from the flaked surface, so that the water could and did react vigorously with the free metal sites, resulting in the formation of oxygen and aluminum hydroxide and aluminum oxide. In contrast, stearin binds very tightly with aluminum and cannot be washed free from metallic aluminum flakes.[34] This has been discussed in detail by Morgan and Dinman.[2]

Other Respiratory Effects

Potroom Asthma

This asthma-like condition has been described in potworkers regularly exposed to the fumes generated by aluminum smelting.[36] There are around 70 different papers from 20 countries describing potroom asthma; nevertheless, the characteristics of the condition are ill defined, and in some instances investigators have failed to identify that the problem indeed exists.[2, 36] While some studies have suggested that the symptoms of wheezing and shortness of breath are work related and develop following exposure to potroom pollutants, in others there is no obvious relationship to work. The studies that have been carried out suggest that the morbidity and significant impairment, if they occur, are distinctly uncommon. Discher and Breitenstein found that up to 36% of potroom workers had left the job within 1 year of employment, and that fewer than 5% of these workers were under the age of 36.[37] The incubation period for occupational asthma is usually between 6 months and 3 to 4 years. Thus, the early departure of recently hired workers is unexpected and suggests that perhaps the working conditions were responsible for their egress.

The Health Committee of the International Primary Aluminum Institute (IPAI) attempted to assess the features of potroom asthma and its worldwide prevalence.[36]

They conducted an inquiry of 51 smelters in 31 countries and showed, in a population of over 17,000 men, that an acute type of asthmatic response was rare. More recently, airways obstruction that could be either immediate or delayed or of the dual type has been described; however, no specific agent was incriminated as responsible.[38] Chan-Yeung et al. conducted a large epidemiological study in British Columbia; she and her coworkers were unable to find any evidence of asthma in the potroom workers.[39] It was noted that the potroom workers had a higher prevalence of cough and sputum and a lower ventilatory capacity than the control group, but this might well be a nonspecific effect produced by industrial bronchitis. In studies of airways function in an aluminum smelter in Tasmania, Field and Owen claimed to have shown that most of their potroom workers had loss of lung elasticity and a somewhat dubious reduction of the diffusing capacity, along with increased bronchial hyper-reactivity, and an impaired ventilatory capacity.[40] The changes were relatively minor, and their significance remained uncertain.[41] In contrast, Smith has described a group of subjects who showed an increase in respiratory symptoms that was related to work and a waning of the symptoms when off work.[42] A recent study was conducted of 1301 employees in Norwegian aluminum smelters who were examined on at least two occasions.[43] The investigators found that 105 subjects developed some dyspnea and wheezing, and many of these showed an improvement or an absence of symptoms when off work. A dose-response relationship was shown between the development of symptoms and fluoride exposure.[43] A similar increase in symptoms was noted with cigarette smoking. The presence of an allergic diathesis appeared to be unrelated to the development of such symptoms.

In summary, there is some limited evidence to suggest that a specific type of reversible airways obstruction occurs in a small percentage of potroom workers. However, no specific agent has been identified as the cause, and the likelihood of Al_2O_3 playing a role, except as a nuisance dust, is remote. The incidence and prevalence of potroom asthma vary from country to country and from smelter to smelter. Doubt exists as to the specific entity, and it may well be that certain of the subjects who complain of symptoms have idiopathic asthma that is worsened by the inhalation of nonspecific irritants. It is also clear that a nonspecific airways response may occur in nonasthmatic potroom workers, especially those mostly exposed to irritant fumes.[36] The decrement in FEV_1 appears to be nonspecific but sometimes is associated with an increased rate of decline of ventilatory capacity.[2]

Aluminum Exposure and Malignancy

There have been a few studies suggesting that in certain groups of aluminum workers there may be an increased incidence of lung cancer. Unfortunately, most such studies lack smoking histories, and any increase in the standardized mortality ratio (SMR) or relative risk could easily be accounted for by differing smoking habits.[2] Gibbs, in his study, showed no overall excess of malignant neoplasms.[44] There was some suggestion that tar-years of exposure is associated with an increased mortality in those who are exposed to coal tar pitch derivatives given off by the Sodeberg cells.

Aluminum Welding and Fume Exposure

Because of the frequent mixing of aluminum with copper, manganese, zinc, silica, or mixtures of these to produce various alloys, welding is sometimes associated with exposure to multiple metallic oxide fumes.[2] In order to prevent such oxidization, a tungsten or metal inert gas welding process is often used. The volatilization of these metals and their subsequent oxidization outside the inert gas shield are followed immediately by cooling and condensation. This results in the formation of multiple small globules of around 0.01 μm. Since the globules are so small, they are frequently carried to the alveoli; but most tend to remain airborne, apart from those which are deposited as a result of diffusion. It might be expected that such particles would lead to an increased incidence of metal fume fever; however, this is not the case, in that zinc and copper, the usual culprits in this condition, are seldom used in aluminum alloys.[2]

Aluminum Exposure and Alveolar Proteinosis

Several experiments conducted by Gross et al. have shown that when rats were made to inhale fine metallic aluminum in high concentrations, pneumonitis and alveolar proteinosis developed.[45] This condition is characterized by the development of extensive alveolar deposition of an eosinophilic material derived from surfactant. The condition usually arises from the inhalation of free silica, but other mineral dusts may be responsible. Alveolar proteinosis has been noted to occur in hamsters and guinea pigs that have been exposed to metallic aluminum by inhalation, but no such case has been described in humans until recently. When endotracheal injection of aluminum dust was substituted for inhalation, metallic powdered aluminum led to the development of focal fibrosis.[45]

The experiments of Gross et al. are particularly relevant to a case report of Miller et al., who described a 44-year-old man who presented with shortness of breath and a cough.[46] He had worked for 6 years as an aluminum rail grinder, and his chest x-ray film showed diffuse air space disease. At open lung biopsy, the diagnosis of pulmonary alveolar proteinosis was made. Mineralogical analysis of the lungs showed numerous spherical aluminum particles (see Figure 4 of their paper) plus a small amount of iron, kaolinite, and mica. The authors attributed the development of the pulmonary alveolar proteinosis to aluminum dust exposure and indicated that his job as a rail grinder was responsible. This seems unlikely, since grinding rails leads to the formation of small fragments of aluminum, which for the most part are nonrespirable. Furthermore, they have sharp edges and do not have the configuration of heterodispersed spheres. The presence of the latter indicates that the aluminum was present in the air as a liquid aerosol, and subsequently as cooling took place, the spherical particles were formed. This is also likely to be the case in the welder described by Herbert et al.[47] These reports and the observations of Gross et al.[45] make it likely that when high concentrations of extremely small aluminum particles are inhaled over a prolonged period in the form of fumes, pulmonary alveolar proteinosis but not fibrosis develops.

Pulmonary Granulomatosis

There are two reports of chronic granulomatous involvement of the lungs that have been attributed to the inhalation of aluminum.[48, 49] Neither case is fully convincing, and the possibility of other granulomatous conditions has not been excluded. In one subject, the only exposure to aluminum was welding metals in an aircraft industry for 5 years. At the time he left the industry, his chest radiograph was reported as normal, and it was not until 6 years later that he developed the symptoms. In the De Vuyst et al. study, the subject had reportedly been exposed as a chemist to powdered aluminum and alumina. He had multiple other exposures, including cobalt and titanium.[49] Epidemiological tests were carried out, but no relationship between exposure to aluminum and the granulomatous condition was ever demonstrated. Because it was felt that aluminum was responsible, extensive animal experiments were carried out, in none of which were granulomata induced. Furthermore, the fact that in numerous epidemiological surveys of exposure to metallic aluminum and alumina no comparable condition has been identified weighs heavily against the hypothesis that aluminum was responsible in the these two cases. Both papers put forward the hypothesis that the mere presence of large amounts of aluminum in the lungs is of significance, but in neither instance could the pathological changes necessarily be attributed to aluminum. Moreover, any worker who is exposed to aluminum dust for long periods will be bound to retain some in his lungs and have an increased aluminum content.

Shaver's Disease

The condition commonly referred to as Shaver's disease was first described in 1947.[1] More complete descriptions of the condition were published later.[50, 51] It occurs in workers who manufacture alumina abrasives and, in particular, corundum. The latter is composed of bauxite (aluminum oxide) and is extremely hard. It is manufactured in special electrical furnaces. The process involves grinding up bauxite into a powder that is then mixed with iron and coke. The mixture is placed into large iron pots into which carbon electrodes are lowered and is then fused at over 2000°C. During the process, dense white fumes are given off that contain both aluminum oxide and silica. The fumes contaminate the atmosphere in the furnace room, although most escape through openings in the roof.

The fumes generated in the manufacture of corundum were found by Jephcott to consist of between 35% and 65% alumina and 15% and 56% silica, usually in the amorphous form, but often with significant concentrations of cristobalite or tridymite.[52] The silica that was noted in these fumes originated as an impurity in the bauxite. Those who worked with the storage bins and on the cranes in the vicinity of the storage room were at particular risk of developing Shaver's disease.[1, 50]

Shaver's disease was not described until after World War II, despite the fact that during the war years production of corundum was greatly expanded. The disease has been attributed to combined exposure to amorphous silica and mullite.[53] In retrospect, there seems little doubt that the original cases were a result of exposure to free silica, and in particular to cristobalite, which has a greater fibrogenicity than does quartz. Although much discussion of this disorder is provided in reference texts, no new cases have been reported since 1950, and furthermore, there has been an unfortunate tendency on the part of some authors to confuse aluminosis with Shaver's disease. The decline in the incidence of Shaver's disease can be attributed to the reduced exposure of corundum workers to free silica.

CLINICAL FEATURES

The symptoms of affected subjects are related to the degree of radiographic lung involvement.[50, 51] Shortness of breath is the most common complaint. Paroxysms of shortness of breath occur along with chest pain. Sputum production and cough are common; however, the sputum is usually mucoid. Tightness in the chest is frequent, as are weakness and fatigue. Pleuritic pain and acute shortness of breath, when they occur together, suggest the presence of pneumothorax. An acute form of the condition occurs when exposure has been intense, and is characterized by cough, low-grade fever, and chest tightness. In many subjects the acute condition progresses to the chronic disease.

RADIOLOGY

The findings vary according to the severity of involvement, and the less severely affected subject may show little in the way of abnormality.[1, 51] Widening of the mediastinum and elevation of the diaphragm are frequent. Both lungs are usually affected by a diffuse reticulonodular process. As time goes by, numerous blebs appear and regional honeycombing develops. The upper lobes are most affected.

The acute form of the disease is characterized by an acinous filling pattern; however, this would often partially resolve, leaving a reticulonodular pattern. Pneumothoraces were common and often chronic.

PATHOLOGY

At postmortem examination, the lungs were found to be gray-black with pleural thickening and frequent adhesions.[54] Bullae were present on the pleural surface, and fibrotic masses were often present in the upper lobes in those subjects who had the complicated form of the disease.

Microscopically in the acute form the alveolar septa were thickened and the alveoli were suffused with what was often labeled as edema fluid, but more probably was alveolar proteinosis. Interstitial fibrosis was present, but classical silicotic nodules were scanty or more often absent. In chronic Shaver's disease, large conglomerate masses were sometimes present, and, although formed of collagen, they lacked the classical characteristics of complicated silicosis. Obliterative endarteritis and perivascular fibrosis were often present.[1, 50] Subsequent analysis of the lungs of subjects with Shaver's disease showed an increase in both alumina and free silica.[52]

Death, when it occurred, was usually due to progressive respiratory failure; however, no increased risk of tuberculosis was found.

The Effects of Abrasives Containing Aluminum

The two main synthetic abrasives in use are alumina and silicon carbide. The latter is a widely used artificial abrasive with a hardness not much less than that of diamonds. It goes by the usual trade name of Carborundum and is used in the production of abrasive wheels and in the manufacture of boilers and foundry furnaces. Silicon carbide is produced from high-grade sand that has been ground to a fine powder, sodium chloride, and wood dust. These materials are fused in an electric arc furnace at a temperature of about 2400°C, and the resulting fully formed silicon carbide is ground and crushed in mills. Silicon carbide does not contain Al_2O_3, but is often bonded with alumina in grinding wheels.

Aluminum oxide is frequently used in the manufacture of abrasives. The grains of aluminum are compacted and then bonded together prior to being made into grinding wheels or emery cloth. Most grinding wheels are composed of a bonded combination of alumina and silicon carbide.

Carborundum has been thought for the most part to be harmless; however, occasional cases of pneumoconiosis alleged to be related to long, continued exposure to silicon carbide have been described.[55, 56] As such, such subjects showed slight restrictive impairment, with an x-ray film which showed bilateral reticulonodular infiltrates mainly in the upper lobes. In some subjects, ferruginous bodies were noted, the core of which was felt to be composed of silicon carbide.[56]

Natural emery is composed of 50% to 70% Al_2O_3, some hematite, occasionally some magnetite, and usually a little free silica. While there have been a few reports of radiographic abnormalities in emery workers, it is uncertain whether radiographic changes are a consequence of inhaled Al_2O_3 or the other constituents, such as hematite or the other iron ores.[57]

ANTIMONY PNEUMOCONIOSIS

Antimony is closely related to arsenic and readily forms alloys with lead, tin, zinc, and iron. It occurs normally in several forms: stibnite (SbS_3), valentinite (Sb_2O_3), kermesite (Sb_2S_2O), and senarmontite (Sb_2O_3). It is mined in China, South Africa, Russia, Mexico, and Bolivia.

Antimony has been used in the manufacture and plating of vases since the times of the great Egyptian civilizations. Stibnite has also been used as a cosmetic. At present, the metal is used as a constituent of alloys, in the compounding of rubber, in flame proofing, in safety matches, and in paints and lacquers. Antimony is also used in electronic, semiconductive, and thermoelectric devices because of its low electrical resistance, and in medicine as an emetic (tartar emetic) and in the treatment of schistosomiasis. NIOSH has estimated that 1.4 million workers in the United States are potentially exposed to antimony in their occupational environment. Such *ex cathedra* pronouncements, although impressive, for the most part appear to be based on extremely tenuous data and give no indication of the true number of subjects at risk.

The dust that is produced during the mining of antimony often contains some free silica, and the term *silicoantimoniosis* has been coined to refer to the condition of lungs containing both silica and antimony. The antimony ore, when it is processed, is pulverized into a fine dust. High dust concentrations are thus present during the operations of reduction and scaling. Crushing of the ore generates coarse particles that are not retained by the lungs, and most of the other processes are wet and relatively dust-free. However, furnacemen who refine the metal prior to its being alloyed with other metals are exposed to appreciable concentrations of antimony dust.

Antimony pneumoconiosis has been described in individuals working with stibnite.[58] The latter is usually emptied from bags through a grill onto a rotating kiln. The metal is volatilized by the heat and forms a fine white powder at the top of the kiln which escapes into the surrounding atmosphere.

Antimony enters the body through the lungs and skin. The metal is absorbed from the lung parenchyma, taken up by the blood and tissues, and excreted in the feces. Some remains in the red blood cells. The inhalation of antimony may produce rhinitis, bronchitis, and nasal septal perforation. Conjunctivitis and dermatitis occur.

Although antimony may produce radiographic changes in the lung (Fig. 16–1), pulmonary function does not appear to be affected.[59] Histological examination of the lungs of workers exposed to antimony has shown alveolar macrophages laden with dust and congregating in and around the alveolar walls and around small vessels.[60, 61] No fibrosis or significant inflammatory action has been observed, and the characteristic radiographic features are small rounded opacities similar to those seen in siderosis or stannosis. Massive fibrosis has not been reported.

BARITOSIS

Baritosis was first described by Arrigoni among barite miners in Italy.[62, 63] Barite occurs in combination with other minerals such as calcite, fluorite, quartz, and chert. It is found in Mississippi, Nevada, and Georgia, as well as in Italy. Barite is used in the production of lithopone, a white pigment used in paints; in vulcanization; for x-ray studies; and in glass-making. During mining, high concentrations of dust are produced. Baritosis has also been described in a few workers in a lithopone plant in Pennsylvania.[64] Those who were affected had markedly abnormal chest radiographs, and it was noted that one of them had features that closely resembled those previously described by Arrigoni in barytes workers. Further inquiries showed that the men in the lithopone plant were exposed to finely dissolved barium sulfate powder. Doig also reported eight subjects with baritosis in a small factory in which barytes was crushed.[65]

Baritosis is not associated with respiratory symptoms or impairment as far as is known. The radiographic appearances are quite striking (Fig. 16–2). The deposits of barium appear as multiple, extremely dense, small rounded opacities. Some radiographic clearing may occur after exposure ceases. Kerley B lines are sometimes in evidence when silica is present in the inhaled dust, and under such circumstances a mixed-dust pneumoconiosis results. Fibrosis is not a feature of the condition unless inhaled dust has been contaminated by silica or other agents.[66]

BERYLLIOSIS

Beryllium is a rare element that was discovered by Vauquelin in 1798. About 50 different minerals contain beryllium, but of these beryl is of prime importance. Beryl is beryllium aluminum silicate and yields about 12% of the oxide and around 4% of the metal. Most of the ore comes from South America, and the cost, although

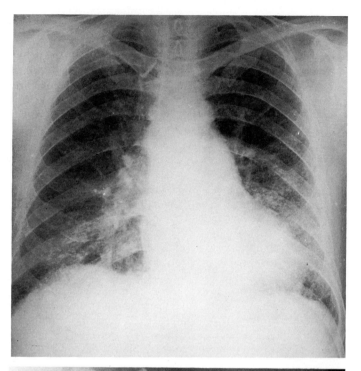

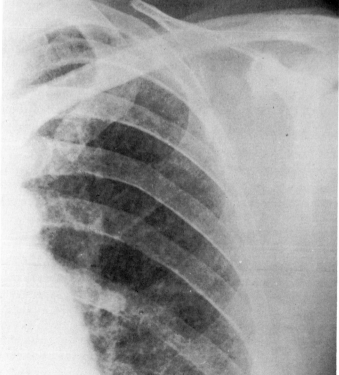

Figure 16–1. Chest radiographs of subject with antimony pneumoconiosis. (Courtesy of the late Dr. E. P. Pendergrass.)

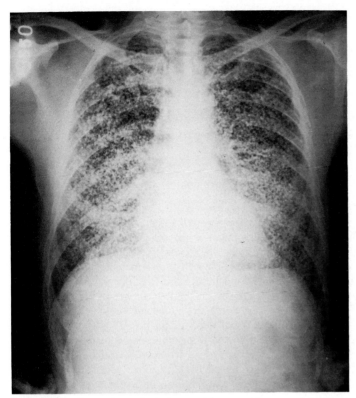

Figure 16–2. Chest radiograph of subject with baritosis. (Courtesy of the late Dr. E. P. Pendergrass.)

fluctuating, is well over $150 per pound. Beryl deposits are found in Argentina, Brazil, India, Zimbabwe, and South Africa. In the United States there are deposits in Colorado, New Mexico, and Utah. Bertrandite is a low-grade ore found in Utah and which is currently being mined.

Beryllium is in demand as a metal because of its lightness and tensile strength. Since it is nonmagnetic and transmits x-rays easily, beryllium is extensively used in x-ray tube manufacture as an alloy in combination with steel, aluminum, and copper. It was also used in the manufacture of fluorescent lighting tubes; however, the recognition of berylliosis led to its replacement in this capacity by other, less toxic substances. Its main uses at the present time are in nuclear physics, since it reduces the speed of fission reactions, in the space program, in the production of fatigue-resistant alloys and heat-resistant ceramics, and as a ''window'' in x-ray tubes.

Production of Beryllium

Two processes are used to extract beryllium from the ore. These are known as the sulfate and the fluoride extractions. In the former, crushed beryl is melted in an arc furnace at 1650°C and poured through a high-velocity water jet to form ''frit.'' Following heat treatment, the frit is pulverized in a ball mill and then mixed with concentrated sulfuric acid. This mixture, known as slurry, is then sprayed onto a revolving sulfating mill. The beryllium is now in water-soluble form and can be separated or leached from the sludge. Ammonia is added to the leached liquid, which is then transferred to a crystallizer in which ammonium alum is crystallized out. The liquor is next treated with chelating agents to hold iron, nickel, and other metals in solution. Sodium hydroxide is added, and this forms sodium beryllate. The latter is hydrolyzed so that beryllium hydroxide is precipitated. Beryllium hydroxide can be easily converted to metallic beryllium or to beryllium salts.

The fluoride process involves sintering in a rotating furnace a mixture of beryl, sodium, silicofluoride, and soda ash. The sintered residue is pulverized, melted, and separated by leaching. Sodium hydroxide is added to the solution of beryllium fluoride that has been formed by leaching. This leads to the precipitation of beryllium hydroxide, which can then be treated as described in the sulfate process.

Several beryllium salts are used industrially: (1) beryllium fluoride (BeF_2), (2) beryllium chloride ($BeCl_2$), (3) beryllium nitrate ($Be(NO_3)_23H_2O$), and (4) beryllium sulfate hydrate ($BeSO_44H_2O$).

Aside from health hazards, beryllium is inflammable, and its degree of inflammability is related to its particle size.

Effects of Beryllium

Beryllium is highly toxic, and exposure can lead to a condition known as berylliosis. The metal may be absorbed through either the lungs or the skin, especially if the latter is not intact. The metal is not absorbed to any extent by the gastrointestinal canal. Although the metal has local effects, these are relatively unimportant compared with the systemic changes that also may occur. Some beryllium combines with a protein and is deposited in the liver, spleen, and bones. A small residue remains in the lungs. In rats, the half-life clearance of beryllium from the lungs exceeds 63 days; however, no comparable data are available in humans.[67] The rate of urinary excretion of the metal depends on how rapidly and in what form the metal has been absorbed. Beryllium persists in bone and liver after it has been almost entirely excreted by the lung. This observation is difficult to reconcile with the fact that berylliosis is said to appear from 15 to 35 years after exposure has ceased and at a time when virtually no beryllium is likely to remain in the lungs.[68, 69]

Cutaneous Effects

It is important to bear in mind that aside from the pulmonary effects of beryllium, the skin is also often affected.[70, 71] Erythematous papular or vesicular rashes occur on the exposed parts of the body after an incubation period of about 2 weeks. They are usually itchy. Accidental implantation of the metal in the skin may produce a "beryllium ulcer" or granuloma. Such ulcers are often chronic. Chronic pulmonary berylliosis may undergo an acute exacerbation when the afflicted subject's skin comes into contact with the metal or its salts. Conjunctivitis is also seen and may occur in association with the pulmonary and cutaneous effects. There is some evidence suggesting that the cutaneous manifestations of beryllium exposure are related to hypersensitivity and that sensitization has to occur first. The more soluble the salts are, the more likely is sensitization to occur. The metal itself is thought not to produce sensitization if the skin is intact. Beryllium fluoride is the most potent sensitizing agent, followed by beryllium chloride and sulfate.

Acute Berylliosis

The acute syndrome affects the nasopharynx, trachea, bronchi, and lung parenchyma.[71, 72] It occurs only when the concentration of respirable beryllium particles in the air is in excess of 100 $\mu m/m^3$.[73] The mucous membranes of the nose become hyperemic and swollen. Ulceration may be present and nasal septal perforation occurs. Tracheitis and bronchitis lead to a dry irritative cough. Substernal pain is common. If the exposure to beryllium is severe and intense, a chemical pneumonia develops. The patient complains of the sudden onset of shortness of breath. He rapidly becomes ill, and death is not uncommon. Physical examination reveals cyanosis, tachycardia, and tachypnea. Fever is unusual unless secondary infection occurs. Crackles are often present, especially in the mid and lower regions of the lungs. The chest film may show an appearance that suggests pulmonary edema. In some instances, the radiographic picture resembles that of an acute miliary process, while in others a patchy acinous filling process is present. If the process develops more slowly, weight loss and anorexia are common.

During the acute process, the patient may be severely hypoxic, and the lungs are stiff and have a low diffusing capacity. The blood count is usually normal.

Treatment consists of giving supplementary oxygen, preferably by mask or nasal catheter. Only if the arterial oxygen level cannot be maintained above 50 mm should mechanical ventilation be considered. Antibiotics are useful in preventing secondary infection, and a combination of penicillin and streptomycin is probably the most effective. Steroids should be given in high doses, although there is no conclusive evidence that they are effective. Most of the changes found in acute beryllium pneumonitis resolve completely within 1 to 4 weeks, but in around 10% of affected subjects chronic berylliosis develops. In the subjects who have died of acute berylliosis, the lungs resemble those seen in acute pulmonary edema. The alveoli are filled with fibrin and red cells, while the alveolar walls are infiltrated with lymphocytes and plasma cells. The trachea and bronchi may show acute tracheitis and bronchitis. Epithelialization of the alveolar walls and organization of the exudate may be seen.

Subacute or Reversible Berylliosis

Sprince and colleagues have advanced the concept of a reversible form of berylliosis.[74] Their conclusions were derived from the results of medical and environmental surveys conducted in a beryllium extraction and processing plant. In 1971 they carried out a cross-sectional study, and in 1974 they conducted a follow-up study. High concentrations of beryllium were found in the ambient air in 1971, sometimes as much as 50 times the recommended level. They reported that 31 workers showed radiographic evidence of interstitial disease and that a further 20 workers had hypoxemia and an increase in $(A-a)O_2$, with 11 showing both radiographic abnormalities and hypoxemia. The follow-up study indicated that the concentrations of beryllium in the air had declined significantly, and concomitantly that a lesser number of subjects showed hypoxemia and radiographic evidence of berylliosis. The authors attributed the amelioration of the hypoxemia and the improvement in the radiographic changes to the lower levels of beryllium in the air, but the evidence they adduced is less than completely convincing. Thus, on the second occasion, although the mean PaO_2 had increased, the $PaCO_2$ had fallen, indicating that the subjects were hyperventilating more, although the hyperventilation may not have accounted entirely for the changes in the PaO_2. In addition, they made no effort to exclude the bias that is introduced by a knowledge of the chronological sequence of the chest x-rays. Similarly, resting $(A-a)O_2$ is a variable test which is not reproducible, and it is unwise to place too much emphasis on it, especially in the presence of hyperventilation. The improvement in PaO_2 was not accompanied by changes in lung volumes, and the possibility exists that a number of workers had an acute process leading to a physiological shunt and ventilation perfusion mismatching and that as time went by the shunt improved, despite the fact that the mechanical properties of the lung and the diffusing capacity remained unchanged. Similar changes have been observed in sarcoidosis. In the latter condition, an improvement in arterial blood gases due to lessening of the $\dot{V}/\dot{Q}$ mismatching with the passage of time and in the absence of treatment is usual, but is seldom accompanied by an improvement in the DL_{co} or in the mechanical properties of the lung unless the subject has been treated with steroids. Nevertheless, the authors' recommendation that the concentrations of beryllium in the ambient air should be rigidly controlled carries weight.[74]

Chronic Pulmonary Berylliosis

This is a systemic disease which produces granulomata throughout the body but particularly affects the lung. The disease was described by Hardy and Tabershaw in 1946.[75] Most of the early case reports were of workers engaged in the manufacture of fluorescent strip lighting; however, in some instances contact was much less close, and wives of beryllium workers have been reported to incur the disease by inhaling beryllium dust from their husbands' clothes. The ambient air around beryllium refineries may contain enough beryllium to lead to the development of chronic berylliosis.[76, 77] Women seem to be more affected than men. In many instances there is a latent period of 10 to 15 years following exposure before the disease appears.[68, 69, 78, 79] Although beryllium is no longer used in the manufacture of fluorescent tubes, there are still two large beryllium refineries in the United States, and sporadic cases of berylliosis are still occurring and are likely to continue to do so.

Clinical Features. Needless to say, a history of exposure to berylliosis is necessary, but as previously noted, it is important to remember that berylliosis is not limited to workers in beryllium refineries. The onset of symptoms is reputed to occur long after exposure has ceased, and it is therefore important to take a complete occupational history.[68, 69, 78, 79] Symptoms of the chronic condition often develop at a time of stress, e.g., during pregnancy or following surgery. At first minimal, dyspnea tends to become progressive and unremitting. A dry unproductive cough is common, and skin lesions may also be present. There may also be a history of previous acute beryllium pneumonitis. In the established cases of chronic berylliosis, there is tachypnea, a small tidal volume, and the typical physical signs found in diffuse fibrosis. Crackles are not common initially. Weight loss and fatigue are also frequent symptoms.

Unfortunately, almost all of the clinical features of berylliosis are also found in sarcoidosis.[78–80] Thus, lymphadenopathy, especially hilar, occurs in both conditions, although both hilar and generalized lymphadenopathy are less common in berylliosis. Hilar adenopathy in the absence of pulmonary changes is rare in berylliosis but common in sarcoidosis. Granulomatous skin lesions are likewise common to berylliosis and sarcoidosis. Hepatic and splenic involvement occur in both diseases, and the spleen may be palpable in both. Salivary gland enlargement and cystic bone changes are felt by some to be peculiar to sarcoidosis. Nephrocalcinosis and hypercalcemia occur in both conditions, and their presence offers no help in distinguishing them. Meningitis, peripheral neuropathy, and involvement of the myocardium have not been reported in berylliosis, but since they are such rare complications of sarcoidosis, they are usually little help in the differential diagnosis. Ocular involvement such as uveitis is peculiar to sarcoid. Uveoparotid fever is not seen in berylliosis, nor is there a change in tuberculin reactivity. Remission is also much more common in sarcoidosis.

Chronic berylliosis is often accompanied by abnormalities of the serum proteins and in this, too, resembles sarcoidosis. Gamma globulin production is predominantly affected; however, in chronic berylliosis, unlike sarcoidosis, the IgG fraction is primarily involved and is elevated in most subjects.[81] Unfortunately, it is also elevated in beryllium workers who have no clinical evidence of acute or chronic berylliosis. Nor are there blood changes specific to either sarcoidosis or berylliosis.

As the disease progresses, the patient becomes increasingly dyspneic. Respiratory rate climbs, arterial oxygen partial pressure falls, and the patient becomes cyanosed. Clubbing may develop. As pulmonary scarring and bleb formation develop, the likelihood of pneumothorax increases. A few scattered wheezes may be heard, and there may be some scattered basal crackles. Gradually, cor pulmonale develops, and right ventricular hypertrophy becomes evident clinically and electrocardiographically. Progression of the disease is slow, however, and a survival time of 15 to 20 years is relatively frequent.

Radiographic Features. The radiographic features of berylliosis are nonspecific. In some instances, radiographic changes may precede the development of symptoms by several years. Both lungs are commonly affected and there is usually a miliary mottling throughout. Bilateral hilar adenopathy is a rare accompaniment (Fig. 16–3). Larger, blotchy coalescent infiltrates are also seen and closely resemble

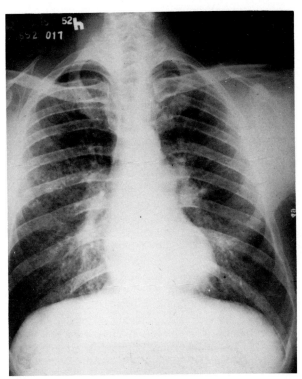

Figure 16–3. Chest film of a 38-year-old man who was exposed to beryllium. There is a fine reticulonodulation present in both lung fields, with bilateral hilar adenopathy. He had no pulmonary function abnormalities other than slight oxygen desaturation on exercise. The question arises as to whether he has berylliosis or has developed sarcoidosis. (Courtesy of the late Dr. Howard Van Ordstrand.)

those seen in sarcoidosis.[82] In long-standing berylliosis, the lungs become small and show widespread reticulonodulation. In some subjects, extensive honeycombing occurs.

Pulmonary Function Abnormalities. These too are entirely nonspecific and are identical to those seen in other diffuse fibroses, including sarcoidosis.[83–85] Typically there is an increased respiratory rate and a reduced tidal volume. The vital capacity, total lung capacity, and residual volume all are decreased, but vital capacity is usually most affected. There is arterial desaturation, a slightly low arterial P_{CO_2}, but a relatively normal pH. The lungs are stiff, and the static compliance is reduced. Elastic recoil pressure at total lung capacity is increased. Late in the course of the disease when cor pulmonale supervenes, minor degrees of airways obstruction may develop. The diffusing capacity is reduced, and serial measurement of this function offers the best means of following the course of berylliosis.

Other Diagnostic Tests. A cutaneous test for berylliosis was first described by Curtis in 1951.[86] The beryllium patch test is often, but by no means invariably, positive in chronic berylliosis. A positive patch test is probably a consequence of delayed hypersensitivity to beryllium. The test is best done with a piece of gauze or filter paper soaked in 1% or 2% beryllium fluoride, sulfate, or nitrate. Metallic beryllium cannot be used for patch testing. A positive reaction is recognized by the development of an erythematous papule in 2 to 3 days. Sneddon biopsied the site of the reaction and showed sarcoid granulomata to be present.[87] There is some evidence that patch testing may lead to an exacerbation of the pulmonary symptoms and to a decrement in pulmonary function.[87, 88] The test is negative in sarcoidosis; and although often positive in chronic berylliosis, it may be negative. In contrast, the Kveim test, which is negative in berylliosis, may be helpful in differentiating the conditions.[89]

Tissue biopsy and spectrographic analysis of the biopsy specimens for beryllium have been singularly unhelpful.[90] The introduction of more refined techniques has made it possible to detect beryllium in patients with granulomata, although this does not necessarily mean that its presence in the granuloma caused the disease.[91] Most workers who have been exposed to beryllium for any appreciable period have beryllium present in their bodies. If the exposure is recent, it may be present in the lungs and urine. However, beryllium persists in the bones and liver for many years, and there may be an increased beryllium content in these organs even though the worker has not been exposed for many years. Spectrographic analysis cannot confirm the presence of the disease, since an excess of beryllium in the tissues is found in most subjects who have at some time in their life worked in a beryllium refinery. Moreover, the severity of chronic berylliosis is unrelated to the beryllium content of the tissues. Similarly, a lung biopsy specimen may have a normal beryllium content when there is excellent circumstantial evidence to suggest the presence of berylliosis. The immunological features of the condition are discussed under the section on pathogenesis.

Pathology. Chronic berylliosis is characterized by the presence of noncaseating granulomata[92] that are indistinguishable from those seen in sarcoidosis. Round cell infiltration is common, but necrosis is relatively rare (Fig. 16–4). Asteroid and Schaumann's bodies may be present. Blebs form late in the disease and may rupture, leading to a pneumothorax. Pleural thickening is usual. Right heart hypertrophy occurs late in the course of the disease, as do pulmonary vascular changes. It has also been suggested that beryllium is a carcinogen. In this regard, the results of studies have been conflicting, and certainly some of those originating from NIOSH have been both poorly controlled and lacking in credibility.[93, 94] At the present time there is little convincing evidence that beryllium is an occupational carcinogen (see Chapter 24).

Treatment. Steroids are felt by some to improve the clinical condition of the patient, although there is no evidence that they have ever produced a cure. When starting treatment of a subject with berylliosis, it is probably best to use a large dose for about a week (75 mg prednisone daily). This should be gradually tapered until the subject is taking the smallest possible dose to control the symptoms, i.e., around 10 to 20 mg daily. There is no indication for megadose steroids. The effects of steroids on the patient's condition are difficult to assess, mainly because of the euphoria they induce. Thus, the patient is best followed by serial and objective pulmonary function tests, e.g., diffusing capacity measurements.

Pathogenesis. A number of cellular responses have been described following experimental exposure to beryllium. Thus, alveolar macrophages take up beryllium particles by phagocytosis and in doing so suffer damage and release lysosomal enzymes. Any beryllium deposited in the alveoli is cleared relatively slowly, probably over a period of months. Initially, macrophage activity is decreased, but there is a subsequent rebound and increase in activity. There is also evidence that macrophages sequester beryllium in the lungs, and in doing so become more active, with the result that lung damage subsequently occurs.[79] Despite the most sensitive and extensive diagnostic efforts, a differentiation between berylliosis and sarcoidosis is not always possible. Sarcoidosis can occur in subjects employed in a beryllium refinery, and conversely, berylliosis occurs in those who have never set foot in a refinery. Thus, there is little doubt that some patients who were diagnosed as having chronic berylliosis probably had sarcoidosis, and it is equally probable that other cases of so-called sarcoidosis were berylliosis. Studies carried out by Marx and Burrell suggest that differentiation between the two conditions is frequently possible. These workers sensitized guinea pigs by repeated intradermal injection of beryllium sulfate.[95] They were able to produce classical delayed hypersensitivity. They then related the skin hypersensitivity to migration inhibitory factor (MIF) and showed a 74% correlation. The sensitivity to beryllium could be transferred by cells. Lymphocytotoxin was also demonstrated in the cells of the sensitized animals but not in those of the unsensitized animals. Subjects with chronic pulmonary

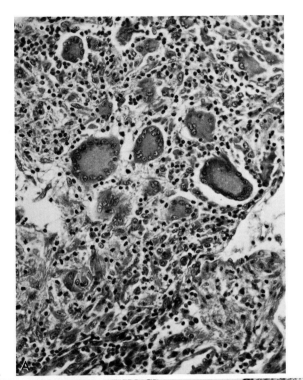

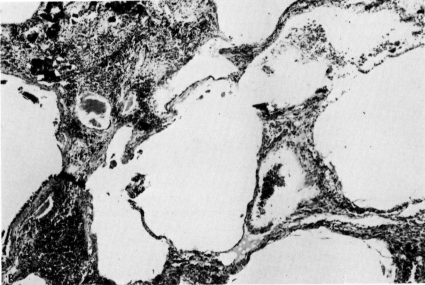

Figure 16–4. *A,* Medium-power photomicrograph of an open lung biopsy specimen. Granulomatous interstitial pneumonitis is present, with obvious giant cells. The beryllium content of the lung was 1.3 μg/100 g of tissue. (Courtesy of the late Dr. Howard Van Ordstrand.) *B,* Chronic beryllium disease with interstitial fibrosis, lymphocytic infiltration, an occasional giant cell, and several Schaumann's bodies (top left). The patient died of pulmonary fibrosis in 1972, having worked at manufacturing fluorescent lights from 1942 to 1949. This is not the same patient as in *A.*

berylliosis were assessed for sensitivity by *in vitro* inhibition of peripheral blood leukocyte migration and showed MIF production when exposed to beryllium sulfate *in vitro.*

Cellular and immune mechanisms of berylliosis have also been studied by Deodhar and coworkers.[96] They studied blast transformation of lymphocytes in subjects with berylliosis, in the presence of beryllium sulfate in tissue cultures. Of their 35 patients, approximately three fifths showed blast transformation. The clinical severity of the disease appeared to be related to the degree of blast transformation. In about half of their subjects, the serum IgA was reported to be significantly elevated. The findings contrast with those of Resnick et al., who found that it was the IgG fraction of the immune globulins that was elevated.[81] Since most of the subjects included in the series of Deodhar and coworkers were taking steroids, and since steroids inhibit blast formation, the authors expressed the opinion that their results provide strong evidence that the etiology of berylliosis is related to immune mechanisms.

Additional support for the hypothesis that the pathogenesis of berylliosis is related to immunological factors came from the studies of Krivanek and Reeves, who demonstrated a delayed type of skin sensitivity in experimental animals.[97] They showed differences in the size of the reactions and in responsiveness according to whether the beryllium was administered to the animal in an ionized or chelated form.

A beryllium lymphocyte transformation test has been developed, and this has been used with some success in the diagnosis of berylliosis.[98] It has been suggested that is possible to identify subclinical berylliosis by screening by lymphocyte transformation tests and bronchoalveolar lavage.[99]

The findings in a subject with chronic berylliosis who underwent bronchoalveolar lavage have been described.[100] The number and proportion of bronchoalveolar T cells were noted to be increased, and the percentage of activated T cells was five times the control value. Both the peripheral blood and the bronchoalveolar lymphocytes proliferated in response to exposure to $BeSO_4$ and BeF_2, but the bronchoalveolar lymphocytes responded more than did the peripheral lymphocytes. The authors suggest that the findings are consistent with berylliosis being a form of hypersensitivity pneumonitis.

The evidence currently available suggests that there is a cell-mediated response to the inhalation of beryllium.[79, 98, 101] This includes:

1. Similar microscopic features in the lungs and lymph nodes to those seen in other cell-mediated reactions.[102]
2. Skin sensitivity reactions.[86]
3. Blast transformation and MIF production from lymphocytes.[95, 96]
4. Selective stimulation of T lymphocytes.[103]
5. The transfer in animal models of cutaneous sensitivity by lymphocytes but not by serum.[79, 104]

Prevention. All unnecessary beryllium exposure must be avoided. Dust control is of paramount importance so that the generation of fumes and dust is kept to a minimum. Wet processes should be used, and the various work areas of the plant should be self-contained as far as possible. Beryllium-containing preparations should be transported as liquids rather than powders. Masks and protective clothing should be worn when concentrations of beryllium in the ambient air are much above the threshold limit value. Nonetheless, it must be realized that even with optimal care, the concentration of beryllium in the air may be sufficient to induce hypersensitivity in some subjects.

The beryllium content of the ambient air should be measured daily. It is recommended that exposure should not exceed 2 mg/m³ of air averaged over an 8-hour period. To protect against the acute form of berylliosis, it has been recommended that a concentration of 25 µg/m³ of beryllium should never be exceeded.[105] Even so, there is good evidence to show that sporadic cases of berylliosis will occur even when exposures remain below the threshold limit value. Such cases are a consequence of the fact that berylliosis is a hypersensitivity disease and that minimal exposures are often sufficient to induce a hypersensitive state.

Pre-employment and periodic medical examinations of all workers in beryllium refineries are recommended, but their value has not been demonstrated. Such examinations should include determination of the vital capacity, the forced expiratory volume, and the flow rates. If possible, the total lung capacity should be measured. Serial chest radiographs at 1-year intervals may conceivably be helpful in controlling the disease.

GRAPHITE AND CARBON PNEUMOCONIOSIS

The term graphite is derived from the Greek word *graphein,* to write. Graphite occurs in three forms: lump, amorphous, and flake. It is also known as plumbago or black lead and is found almost all over the world; however, it is extracted or mined in Austria, Russia, Sri Lanka (Ceylon), Norway, and Korea. Lump graphite is found in veins that traverse igneous rocks. Quartz, feldspar, mica, and other impurities often occur in the veins. Lump graphite is usually removed by underground mining. Amorphous graphite occurs in underground beds often lying between strata of shale, sandstone, or quartz-containing rocks. It is excavated by blasting, and then is hand-loaded into wagons prior to being brought to the surface. Flake graphite more often occurs near the surface as outcrops from sedimentary rock. This form of graphite is removed by the same methods used for open-cast (strip) coal mining. Graphite that is made from petroleum coke is almost pure carbon.

Small traces of free silica are found in most samples of graphite. Certain deposits contain between 3% and 10% of free silica. These higher concentrations are present in some deposits in Sri Lanka, Korea, Namibia, and Italy.[106] After the graphite has been mined, the silica is removed by treating it with hydrofluoric acid and sodium hydroxide. The graphite is then ground, screened, and dried in kilns prior to use. It is used mainly in the manufacture of steel, lubricants, lead pencils, nuclear reactors, and electrodes. Since it conducts electricity, it is often used in generator brushes. Before graphite can be used in any of these processes, it has to be crushed, ground, and milled to a fine powder. It is also used in electrotyping, a method used in the printing industry for duplicating plates. The exact process is described in detail by Gaensler and colleagues.[107]

It has been known for many years that the inhalation of carbon may induce radiographic changes.[108–110] The changes are usually described as a fine basal reticulation or, in some instances, nodulation. The prevalence of carbon pneumoconiosis varies, but Meiklejohn found it in more than half the workers in two carbon plants.[111] While progressive massive fibrosis was first described in German carbon electrode workers,[112] Watson and colleagues have described similar findings in England.[113] They found both simple and complicated pneumoconiosis occurring in carbon-exposed workers. The complicated form was accompanied by massive fibrosis, cavitation, and right ventricular hypertrophy. Similarly, simple pneumoconiosis in carbon workers was pathologically indistinguishable from coal workers' pneumoconiosis, and the condition was characterized by the typical macule and the presence of focal emphysema. Even in subjects with progressive massive fibrosis, the silica content of the lungs was no greater than that found in the lungs of normal subjects. The British and German observations of both simple and complicated pneumoconiosis occurring in non–silica-exposed carbon electrode workers militate strongly against the silica theory of progressive massive fibrosis. Other case reports have emphasized the low silica content found in both forms of carbon pneumoconiosis.[114, 115]

It is felt by some that graphite modifies the fibrogenic action of silica.[116] Thus, while heavy exposure to pure carbon may induce a slight scattered fibrotic reaction, comparable exposures to a mixture of carbon and silica will induce the formation of nodular foci. In the latter instance, it is thought that the large amounts of carbon dust probably overwhelm the clearing mechanisms so that the silica persists in the lung and thereby has an opportunity to induce a fibrogenic response. Adequately controlled studies of the pulmonary function abnormalities that occur in carbon pneumoconiosis are not available. While individual case reports abound, in many instances it is difficult to demonstrate a cause-and-effect relationship between the physiological impairment and the presence of the pneumoconiosis. In some instances, the respiratory impairment is better explained by the presence of concomitant and coincidental chronic bronchitis and emphysema. Nonetheless, a variety of pulmonary function abnormalities have been reported, including alveolocapillary block (diffuse fibrosis), restrictive disease, and obstructive airways disease. One of Gaensler's subjects had massive fibrosis with severe vascular changes and pulmonary hypertension.[107] Analysis of the lungs in three of his subjects revealed no silica in two instances, and 5% cristobalite in the third.

A study of 3086 carbon black workers in 18 plants in seven European countries has been published.[116a] A respiratory questionnaire was administered along with spirometry and chest radiography. Current exposures to respirable dust, sulfur, and carbon monoxide were measured. The levels of gaseous contaminants were too low to permit the generation of exposure indices. A poor response limited the size of the cohort. Thus, 1742 subjects in 15 plants (81%) underwent spirometry and answered the questionnaire, while 1096 subjects from 10 plants (74%) had a chest radiograph taken. Cough, sputum, and the symptoms of bronchitis were found to be associated with increasing exposure to particulate matter. Ventilatory capacity showed a small decrease with increasing dust exposure in both smokers and nonsmokers. Nearly 25% of the radiographs showed small opacities of 0/1 or greater; however, only 10% of the radiographs had a reading of category 1/1 or greater, with only three subjects with category 2/1 or greater. Some of the cohort had other exposures, e.g., to asbestos, welding fumes, and so on. Most of the small opacities were of the irregular type, suggesting that they were related to smoking rather than dust; however, cumulative dust exposure was related to some extent to the radiographic category of 1/0 or greater. In summary, and not unexpectedly, the effects of carbon black seemed very similar to those of coal.

HEMATITE PNEUMOCONIOSIS (SILICOSIDEROSIS) AND OTHER MIXED-DUST FIBROSES

The effects of the inhalation of relatively pure iron are discussed in the section on siderosis; however, many iron miners are exposed not only to iron oxide but also to a fair quantity of free silica. This leads to a condition known as silicosiderosis, or mixed-dust fibrosis. It is seen in the iron miners of Cumbria (England), in the Siegerland miners of Germany, and in the Italian miners of Bergamo. Silicosiderosis seldom occurs without at least 10 years' exposure, and most of the affected subjects have worked in the mines for at least 20 to 30 years.

The first adequate pathological description of the condition was given by Stewart and Faulds.[117] They noted a predominance of diffuse rather than nodular fibrosis, although the latter was present in certain instances. In the diffuse variety of fibrosis, the whole lung is brick red and there is often what appears to be associated focal emphysema. Radiographically, diffuse fibrosis appears as a reticular pattern. The nodular type of silicosiderosis is characterized by the presence of nodules similar to those seen in silicosis; however, in this instance they are red and are located predominantly in the upper lobes. The remainder of the lung appears brick red.

Massive fibrotic lesions may also be seen. Like progressive massive fibrosis of coal workers, the masses are usually situated in the upper lobes. They encroach on the blood and bronchial supply of the affected region and often undergo cavitation. The presence of massive fibrosis in silicosiderosis appears to be closely related to the silica content of the lung, and tuberculosis is a frequent complication. Microscopically the alveolar walls often show aggregated particles of hematite and silica. Other aggregates occur close to the blood vessels and alveolar septa. Peribronchiolar and periarteriolar fibrosis are frequent findings. Many of the silica and hematite particles are picked up by the macrophages and transported in the lymphatics to the regional lymph nodes. Whorled nodules may develop in and along the lymphatic routes. The massive fibrotic areas appear to consist of dense collagenous tissue, heavily impregnated with iron and silica. The adjacent vascular supply is damaged, and endarteritis obliterans is common.

A study of the vasculature of hematite lung showed that the muscular pulmonary arteries between the small fibrotic nodules that characterize the simple form of this condition develop excess longitudinal muscle in the intima, a change that was felt to be a consequence of distortion of these vessels.[118] In some vessels the muscular layer of the intima showed secondary fibrosis. No muscularized pulmonary arteries were observed, and there was an absence of constriction in the terminal region of the pulmonary arterial tree. Vessels adjacent to areas of conglomeration were frequently incorporated into the masses and destroyed by encroachment from fibrous tissue. The occlusive and obliterative changes observed in silicosiderosis were felt to be those of silicosis and not a specific response to hematite. The only peculiar feature of hematite lung is the intense accumulation of iron-containing dust around the pulmonary blood vessels.

There is good evidence that cancer of the lung is found more often in Cumbrian iron miners; however, the cause of the increase is not known.[119] Two theories exist: the first, which seems more probable, relates to the excess radioactivity to which the miners are exposed. In this, it is thought to resemble the radiation-induced lung cancer that occurs in uranium miners. The second theory postulates that the iron ore contains a carcinogenic agent.

The symptoms and signs of silicosiderosis are relatively nonspecific. The miner often complains of shortness of breath, cough, and reddish-brown sputum. The shortness of breath is worse in miners who have massive fibrosis, and many of them develop pulmonary hypertension and cor pulmonale.

Ochre miners also develop silicosiderosis. Ochres are brown-yellow earths that are used in the manufacture of pigments and colors. They are hydrated ferric oxides and are often contaminated with clay, silicates, and a certain amount of free silica. Ochre miners may have reticular and nodular radiographic changes, but massive fibrosis rarely if ever occurs.[120]

Foundry workers are exposed to both iron and silica, but the proportion of free silica to which they are exposed varies greatly according to their job. While it is undoubtedly true that many foundry workers inhale relatively pure iron and hence are not affected by pulmonary fibrosis or respiratory impairment, in a minority appreciable fibrosis occurs owing to the free silica to which they also have been exposed. Mixed-dust fibrosis is commonly seen in foundry welders and burners.[121] The nodule of mixed-dust fibrosis differs macroscopically and microscopically from that seen in classical silicosis. The arrangement of reticulin and collagen fibers is linear or radial rather than concentric, and the outline of the nodule is irregular or stellate.[122] The mixed-dust nodule resembles more closely the coal macule than the typical silicotic nodule. Analysis of the lungs of foundry workers shows that free silica, silicates, and iron are found in varying proportions. The amount of fibrosis is in general related mostly to the free silica content. The radiographic appearances of mixed-dust fibrosis are indistinguishable from those seen in classical silicosis and silicosiderosis. The more dense the radiographic opacities, the greater the amount of iron present in the lungs and the less the likelihood of complicated pneumoconiosis developing. Fettlers and foundry workers show less tendency for their disease to progress radiographically, and there is evidence to indicate that most of the radiologic abnormalities are a reflection of iron deposition rather than silica. Iron itself is nonfibrogenic and attenuates the fibrogenicity of the limited amount of silica that is deposited along with the iron.

A paper described a cluster of three subjects working in a foundry who developed an uncommon type of pneumonia due to *Acinetobacter pneumoniae*.[123] Two of the men died and were noted to have iron particles in their lungs. The latter finding is hardly surprising, despite the fact that the authors try to attribute the pneumonia to the iron and silica that the workers inhaled in the foundry. There is little evidence to corroborate their hypothesis. While the pneumonia may have been a consequence of the organism being present in dust in the foundry, there is little reason to believe that silica or iron in the concentrations to which the workers were exposed predisposed them to this rare form of pneumonia.

Boiler scalers who clean the water tubes and flues of boilers may also develop pneumoconiosis. This is usually a mixed-dust reaction, since the dust to which they are exposed contains free and combined silica, iron, carbon, and various carbonates. The scale of many marine boilers contains a high proportion of silica, i.e., 8% to 10% total silica.[124] Thus, dust exposures in iron and steel workers are usually of the mixed variety and range from pure siderosis at the one extreme to pure silicosis on the other. Most, however, are mixed exposures, and silica, silicates, and numerous other potentially harmful dusts may be inhaled in addition to iron. In some instances, significant exposures to chromium oxide and nickel oxide also occur.[125]

Labrador Lung

An unusual form of mixed-dust pneumoconiosis known as "Labrador lung" has been described in iron miners in West Labrador.[126] The miners were exposed to dust containing iron, silica, and some anthophyllite. Lung biopsies in certain selected subjects have demonstrated large amounts of iron and silica present in the lungs, but in addition some subjects have shown a fair number of ferruginous bodies. A granulomatous reaction was seen in a few biopsies of specimens. These latter findings contrast with the typical silicotic reaction observed in most subjects.

The chest symptoms that occurred in the Labrador miners were nonspecific and appeared to be mainly a consequence of bronchitis. Both simple and complicated pneumoconiosis were observed, although the latter was uncommon. Physiological abnormalities were unimpressive even in the complicated form of the disease. Chest films from affected subjects for the most part showed the presence of typical rounded opacities such as are seen in classical silicosis, but a few radiographs also showed the presence of irregular opacities. The latter in general were relatively sparse (0/1 and 1/0), and most could probably be accounted for by cigarette smoking. In a few instances, however, irregular opacities predominated and were relatively profuse. Pleural thickening was also occasionally observed, as was hilar adenopathy.

Labrador lung is thought to be a mixed pneumoconiosis, with most of the effects being a consequence of silica. Occasionally the presence of anthophyllite produces atypical features and modifies both the radiographic appearances and the pathological features of the lung.

POLYVINYL CHLORIDE (PVC) PNEUMOCONIOSIS

The manufacture of polyvinyl chloride (PVC) is associated with the generation of a varying number of respirable dust particles. Since the administration of PVC dust to animals is known to lead to bronchiolitis, a minor degree of alveolitis, and the formation of granulomata, the possibility that PVC may be a respiratory hazard in humans needs consideration.[127, 128] Over the years there have been isolated case reports of PVC pneumoconiosis, many of them unconvincing, although it is now clear that such a condition exists. A number of epidemiological surveys have also been carried out, but the inferences drawn as a result of such surveys have been suspect, mainly because of a lack of adequate controls and failure to take into account age, cigarette smoking, and other confounding factors.[129, 130]

PVC pneumoconiosis was first described by Szende et al. in 1970.[131] Since then a number of studies have suggested that exposure to PVC dust leads to radiographic changes, respiratory symptoms, and pulmonary impairment. There are few studies of the pathology of PVC pneumoconiosis in humans. Arnaud et al.

describe a subject who had a micronodular infiltrate in his lungs.[132] Histological examination of a drill biopsy specimen revealed infiltration with histiocytes and multinucleated giant cells with some collagenous fibrosis. Macrophage reaction was marked, and the macrophages contained many PVC particles (Fig. 16–5).

A well-designed study of a large group of workers exposed to PVC was published in 1980.[133] In this cross-sectional survey involving 818 workers, PVC exposure was found to be associated with a minimal increase in respiratory symptoms. After taking into account smoking and age, a slight effect was noted on the FVC and FEV$_1$. Smoking and PVC dust appeared to have an additive effect. There were minimal radiographic changes, but these were subtle, and higher grades of simple pneumoconiosis were not noted. PVC pneumoconiosis was characterized by the development of scanty, small, rounded opacities.

Vinyl chloride monomer has effects on other organs, including the liver, where it may produce peripheral fibrosis and lead to the development of angiosarcoma. In addition, a scleroderma-like condition associated with cysts in the fingers and Raynaud's phenomenon has been described.

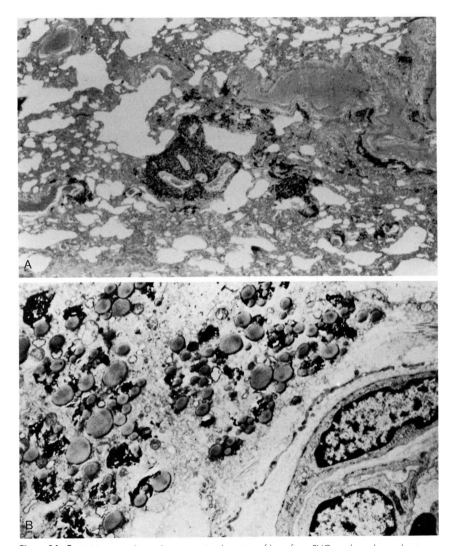

Figure 16–5. *A,* Hematoxylin and eosin–stained section of lung from PVC worker whose chest radiograph showed category 1/1 q opacities. A dust macule containing PVC is present. *B,* Electron microscope photomicrograph of PVC particles in lung macrophage. The subject had undergone resection for a tumor. No pneumoconiosis was visible in radiograph.

SIDEROSIS

The condition of siderosis was described by Zenker in the mid–19th century.[134] The two subjects he reported also had pulmonary tuberculosis, and it can be assumed that the fibrosis which he found in their lungs was more likely the result of tuberculosis than a response to the dust to which they had been exposed. Iron when inhaled in its pure form does not lead to fibrosis; however, it is often inhaled in conjunction with other fibrogenic dusts such as silica.

Siderosis is seen in its purest form in arc welders, oxyacetylene cutters, and silver finishers. During arc welding and oxyacetylene cutting, iron is melted and boiled by the heat of the arc or torch. The iron is emitted as particles of ferrous oxide which are immediately oxidized to ferric oxide and appear as blue-gray fumes. Prolonged inhalation of these fumes can lead to the development of radiographic changes in the lung that are identical to those seen in silicosis.[135, 136]

Silver finishers use what is known as jeweler's rouge to polish their unfinished wares. The rouge is composed of iron oxide and is often applied with a buffer that generates a cloud of small iron and silver particles.[137] The iron miners of Cumbria in Great Britain are subject to silicosiderosis, a condition accompanied by fibrosis and other pathological changes that are not seen in subjects exposed to pure iron. The same is true of the Italian iron miners from Bergamo. Similar changes have been observed in ochre workers.

Welders' Siderosis

Welders' siderosis was described by Doig and McLaughlin in 1936.[135] Since its original description, siderosis has generally been assumed to be benign and unassociated with respiratory symptoms. The bases for this assumption have been, first, the published statistics of mortality and morbidity in the United States and Britain,[138, 139] second, the lack of fibrosis in the lungs of welders,[136, 140] and third, the absence of pulmonary function abnormalities in subjects with marked radiographic abnormalities.[140]

The biological effects of welding have been thoroughly investigated over the past 30 to 40 years. Although the literature on this topic is replete with real and imaginary hazards,[141, 142] a lesser number of carefully carried out studies have indicated that welding, provided adequate precautions are taken, is relatively harmless.[143, 144]

Over the years, welding has evolved from a process that was initially relatively simple, and in which bare iron electrodes were used almost exclusively, into a complex technology in which numerous different electrodes are used.[145, 146] These now consist of a central core and various outer coats that include a variety of different agents. The effluent from welding contains a number of fumes and gases, with some of the latter causing in rare circumstances significant respiratory hazards, including death. The emission and type of fumes vary according to the kind of welding taking place, with manual metal arc and metal inert gas welding having the highest emissions and tungsten inert gas and submerged arc welding the lowest emissions.[145, 146] The volume of fumes and gases emitted during the process depends on the type of electrode used and the shielding gas. The generation of fumes is also influenced by the voltage used, by the welder's or cutter's attention to industrial hygiene, and by the adequacy of ventilation in the workplace. McMillan indicated that 30 different electrodes were being used in the Royal Navy dockyards, and these contained 19 different ferrous and nonferrous alloys.[145]

The likelihood of welding fumes reaching the lung parenchyma depends on their aerodynamic diameter. Manual metal arc welding generates larger particles that tend to agglomerate and hence are seldom deposited in the lungs.[145, 146] Stainless steel workers who use tungsten inert gas welding are usually exposed to lower fume concentrations.[147] The inhalation of fumes depends on several factors, including the concentration of fumes in the breathing zone of the welder, the welder's breathing pattern, and the ventilation present in the workplace. Arc welders, especially when aluminum welding, may be exposed to ozone concentrations of up to 6 to 9 ppm. Such exposures lead to eye and nasal irritation, along with bronchitis.

The potential hazards of welding may be classified as follows:[144]

1. Acute toxic effects, respiratory and systemic
2. Chronic toxic effects
3. Chronic respiratory effects
4. Carcinogenic effects

Acute effects may result from the inadvertent inhalation of cadmium, the oxides of nitrogen, ozone, and phosgene, all of which may be produced under certain circumstances.[144] Metal fume fever is a well-recognized hazard of acute exposure. Among the chronic respiratory effects, siderosis and bronchitis are the most common.[144, 148] Emphysema can develop after a worker has been acutely exposed to cadmium. Asbestosis and silicosis also occur under certain circumstances.[140, 144, 149] Welders may be exposed to a number of carcinogenic materials of which the most common is asbestos. They are also exposed to chromium and nickel during stainless steel welding, but it is unlikely that these metals lead to any excess carcinogenic risk.

Epidemiological Studies

A number of well-controlled studies have been carried out on the chronic effects of welding, especially in regard to the prevalence and effects of bronchitis. In a group of welders from Newport News shipyards, Hunnicutt et al. found that the prevalence of symptoms such as cough and sputum was significantly higher in welders than in nonwelders.[150] There was also an increased prevalence of airways obstruction, but only smoking welders were affected. Similar findings resulted from the study of Boston shipyard welders.[151] Some of the latter, however, had significant exposure to asbestos. In a series of well carried out and detailed studies, McMillan investigated the health of welders employed in the Royal Navy dockyards in Britain.[145, 152–154] He studied morbidity and mortality, lung function, and other indices of ill health.[145] In a general review of the health of welders, he concluded that there was no evidence of a causal relationship between welding and respiratory disease or other ill health, with the exception of injuries, at least among welders in Her Majesty's dockyards.[145, 154] He felt that there may be a small number of welders who are unusually susceptible to the effects of fumes and gases. This included a group of subjects who had previous obstructive airways disease such as asthma or emphysema. Neither of these diseases, however, was related to welding exposure. McMillan and Pethybridge also examined 135 welders aged 45 and over with prolonged exposures. They carried out detailed clinical, radiographic, and lung function studies and concluded that welding did not cause significant clinical abnormalities or impairment of lung function.[153]

Over the last 30 to 40 years, a number of welders have been described in whom symptomatic pulmonary disease has been noted to be present.[144] There has been a tendency to associate the symptoms and any disease present with their occupation. There has usually been no consistency, however, in the type of physiological impairment, and there has been a lack of supportive epidemiological evidence to confirm that the association truly exists. In some instances, analyses of lung tissue have demonstrated numerous elements to be present in the lung parenchyma in excess concentrations, and the assumption was therefore made that their presence had led to fibrosis, when in most instances naturally occurring disease was responsible.[144] The presence of such histological changes has been assumed to be sufficient to implicate the agent that has been deposited in the lungs, despite the fact that in other regions of the lung in which no pathological change has been detected, equal or greater amounts of the foreign agent were present.

A series of reports extending over a number of years have described several welders with respiratory insufficiency, but in most instances smoking histories were not available and the possible role of cigarette smoke was not considered.[155–160] In some subjects emphysema was present, while others had pulmonary fibrosis. It is interesting to note that the majority of the workers described by Charr had worked in the Philadelphia Naval shipyard as welders, and as such they were exposed to asbestos, with several of the cases described as having fibrotic changes and radiographic evidence of reticulonodulation in the lower zones.[156–158] Cyanosis and clubbing of the digits were also often present, findings clearly indicating that the presumptive diagnosis should have been asbestosis. Other reports, including those of Friede and Rachow, are likewise unconvincing in that their subject had obvious heart failure.[159] Some subjects who were reported to have welding-induced disease turned out to have silicotuberculosis.[155, 160]

Elsewhere, Stern et al. reviewed 3600 pathology cases in the Liebow pulmonary pathology collection, and of the total, 29 subjects who were welders were noted to have pulmonary fibrosis.[141] Of the 29 subjects, eight had a history of exposure to talc or asbestos, and a further 10 subjects had no available occupational history, leaving 11 subjects with fibrosis in whom idiopathic pulmonary fibrosis had not been excluded. It was suggested that nitrogen dioxide was the fibrogenic agent in certain of these subjects; however, currently available evidence suggests that nitrogen dioxide induces a subacute bronchiolitis which may be complicated by the development of centrilobular emphysema, in short, the exact antithesis of fibrosis. McMillan, in an extensive study, found that 11 of 328 welders had lung fibrosis, and all were caused by asbestos exposure.[145] Moreover, in a carefully carried out case control study, neither diffusing capacity nor the total lung capacity was significantly different in welders as compared to control subjects.[153] The evidence to indicate that welding fumes induce pulmonary fibrosis is tenuous in the absence of a clear-cut history of exposure to recognized fibrogenic substances such as asbestos, silica, or cadmium.[140, 144, 149] There is little or no evidence to support the contention that nitrogen dioxide, chromium, or any other metal emitted in welding fumes induces pulmonary fibrosis, although the introduction of new technology may lead to new and unrecognized hazards.[144, 153]

As far as chronic findings are concerned, Challen concludes that while iron is nonfibrogenic, welders are often exposed to other dusts, and a mixed-dust pneumoconiosis can occur.[143] Welders tend to smoke more than the general population, and this explains the high prevalence of bronchitis. Some welders who work in confined spaces are exposed to high concentrations of nitrogen dioxide, and Morley and Silk have suggested that pulmonary edema may occur.[161] Aluminum welders may also be exposed to increased concentrations of ozone, and while these may cause acute nasal and respiratory symptoms, there is little evidence to conclude that such exposures have a permanent effect.

Pathology of Welders' Siderosis and Related Conditions

The first descriptions of the pathological effects of iron were recorded by Harding et al.[136] These workers described the pathological findings in four arc welders and an oxyacetylene cutter who came to autopsy. Some of these subjects had been exposed to silica, and in them there was evidence of a mixed-dust fibrosis. The lungs of the cutter showed no fibrosis at all. Harding and his coworkers attributed the fibrosis not to iron oxide but to other constituents of the welding fumes, i.e., silica and possibly some of the gases evolved such as the oxides of nitrogen.

Autopsy studies of silver finishers have shown an absence of fibrosis,[137] and inhalation experiments have similarly shown a lack of fibrosis in animals exposed to iron.[162] Morgan and Kerr described seven subjects with welders' siderosis, four of whom had had lung biopsies.[140] The histological appearances of the biopsied lung showed that while some iron lies free in the alveoli and respiratory bronchioles, most is taken up by the macrophages and can be seen in the lymphatic channels (Fig. 16–6). Fibrosis was not seen except in subjects with mixed-dust

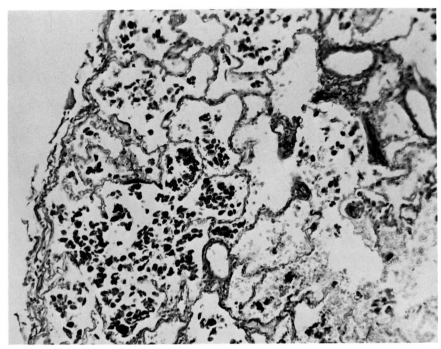

Figure 16–6. Photomicrograph of lung biopsy of subject with welders' siderosis. There is an absence of fibrosis; however, aggregated deposits of iron are much in evidence. Occasional alveolar walls can be seen to be disrupted, but these appearances are due to artifacts introduced in the preparation of the slide. Verhoeff's elastic stain, × 180. (From Morgan, W. K. C., and Kerr, H. D., Pathologic and physiologic studies of welder's siderosis. Ann. Intern. Med., 58, 293, 1963.)

exposures. Analysis of a portion of one subject's lung revealed an iron content of 46 mg of iron per gram of dry lung, which is 15 times greater than the normal level. Despite the greatly increased iron content, no fibrosis was present. Another subject whose lung biopsy showed fibrosis was known to have a mixed-dust exposure, and an excess of silica was found in his lung. While the usual radiographic appearances of arc welder's lung are those of simple silicosis, exceptionally a massive shadow appears (Fig. 16–7).[163, 164] It is felt that when conglomeration is seen in a welder, it can be assumed that the worker has been exposed to dusts other than iron, of which by far the most common is silica. Recent postmortem studies of fume contaminants in the lungs of an arc welder, although providing data as to the lungs' constituents, have added little to our understanding of welders' siderosis.[165]

Radiographic Features of Welders' Siderosis

Siderosis, whatever its occupational origin, has similar appearances to and cannot be distinguished from simple silicosis.[135, 136, 140, 153] Massive shadows are extremely rare. In some instances the small rounded shadows tend to be "harder" and look more circumscribed than those observed in silicosis. They also tend to be more evenly distributed throughout the lung fields, and the predilection for the upper zones is absent.

Pulmonary Function in Welders' Siderosis and in Welders

There seems little doubt that in its pure form siderosis does not lead to pulmonary impairment. In their study of welders, Morgan and Kerr measured all aspects of pulmonary function with the exception of the diffusing capacity.[140]

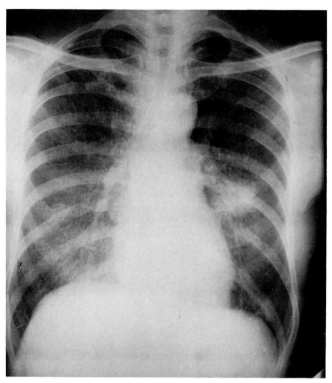

Figure 16–7. Chest radiograph of welder with massive shadow in left lung field. Fine reticulonodulation is present in lower lung fields.

Despite the fact that the subjects had markedly abnormal chest films and despite the fact that the iron content of their lungs was grossly increased, neither the ventilatory capacity, respiratory mechanics, nor the arterial blood gases were abnormal, except in those subjects who had a mixed exposure. At a later date, Stanescu et al. studied the pulmonary mechanics of a group of 16 working welders with abnormal chest films.[166] They compared the welders to a group of 13 unexposed healthy men and showed that arc welders had a statistically significant reduction in the static and functional compliance of the lungs. However, measurement of elastic recoil at total lung capacity did not separate the welders from the control subjects. It is difficult to assess the significance of the results of this investigation, and ideally an additional control group of welders without radiographic abnormalities should have been included. Either way, it is difficult to equate slight changes in static compliance with respiratory symptoms, and the effect, if any, that such changes have on the development of respiratory disability can be assumed to be negligible. Additional studies of lung function, including measurement of the diffusing capacity, have been carried out by Teculescu and Albu.[167] Their results agree with those of Morgan and Kerr, and no functional abnormalities to suggest fibrosis were demonstrated.[140]

Well-controlled epidemiological studies of the respiratory status of welders are few. Hunnicutt et al. studied the ventilatory capacity of 100 welders and an equal number of controls.[150] Although obstructive airways disease was found in both groups, there was no significant difference between them when the effects of smoking were taken into account. Peters et al. studied 61 welders, using a questionnaire, chest film, and more detailed tests of pulmonary function.[151] These workers were unable to show that welders had a significant decrease in pulmonary function when compared to other shipyard workers. Nevertheless, there was some indication that shipyard workers as a whole had a lower ventilatory capacity than did the general population. Like Morgan and Kerr,[140] they concluded that nonsmoking welders do not suffer from a reduction in ventilatory capacity. As mentioned previously, McMillan et al. have studied all aspects of lung function including the diffusing capacity and shown that welding and welders' siderosis are not associated with significant respiratory impairment, with the possible exception of a greater prevalence of airways obstruction among smoking welders.[143, 152–154]

Prevention

Although iron in its pure form appears relatively harmless, some welders and oxyacetylene cutters are exposed to various dusts and fumes other than ferric oxide. In some instances these dusts can lead to fibrosis. Such exposures often include the oxides of nitrogen and ozone and other air pollutants. Siderosis and metal fume fever are seen, and most commonly occur, in welders who work indoors in a poorly ventilated workroom. Both are uncommon when ventilation is adequate and when the welders are working outside.

Silver Polishers' Lung

This differs somewhat from the pure siderosis seen in most welders. The jeweler's rouge that is used for polishing formerly consisted of iron oxide mixed with oil; however, with the widespread use of a buffing wheel, also known as a dolly, the powder is now dampened with water only. The dust generated during the polishing process consists of silver and iron oxide particles. As such, the inhaled iron is picked up by the phagocyte, while the silver combines with the protein of the lung, with the result that the elastic tissue is stained black.

Magnetite and Limonite Pneumoconiosis

Radiological abnormalities have also been observed in workers exposed to magnetite dust[168] (Fig. 16–8). Deposits of magnetite (Fe_3O_4) are found in the northeastern United States. Although radiographic abnormalities have been reported in miners and those who process the ore, respiratory impairment has not been observed.[169] The pulverizing of limonite may also be associated with radiographic abnormality.

STANNOSIS

Tin is an important metal because of its pliability and because it readily forms alloys with other metals. After gold and copper, tin was the earliest metal used by man. According to Hoover and Hoover, the smelting of tin took place in the Neolithic Age, that is to say, about 5000 years ago.[170] Both the Phoenicians and Carthaginians traded with the inhabitants of Cornwall in order to obtain tin.

Deposits of tin are widely distributed throughout the world. Until the industrial revolution, most of the world's tin came from Cornwall, Saxony, and Bohemia. Now most comes from Malaysia, Thailand, Bolivia, Nigeria, and to a lesser extent Zaire and Australia. The most important ore is known as cassiterite (SnO_2); it occurs in veins that are often intimately related to granite and other rocks with a high silica content. Seventy per cent of the world's total production today comes from secondary alluvial deposits that result from the disintegration of primary deposits. In Bolivia, tin is also extracted from various sulfide ores such as stannite (Cu_2FeSnS_2) and tealite ($PbZnSnS_2$).

Lode or underground mining for tin was formerly the main method of extracting the metal. The process involved removing a layer of rock with enough cassiterite in it to make the extraction profitable—that is, at least 1% tin in the rock. However, the concentration of tin in any lode almost never exceeds 10%.[171] A lode

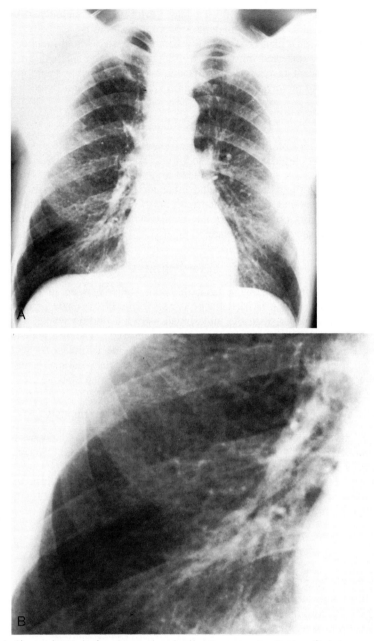

Figure 16–8. *A,* Chest radiograph of worker employed pulverizing magnetite. *B,* Magnified view.

mine is usually started as a tunnel that is bored into the hillside and then often is redirected downward. Some Cornish tin mines went down to a depth of 1000 feet, but elsewhere depths of 3000 feet were not uncommon. The cassiterite-containing rock has to be broken up, and this is mainly done by shot-firing. Compressed air drills are used to bore the holes for the insertion of the explosives. The surrounding strata frequently are composed of rock with a high free silica content, and silicosis used to be common in tin miners. Ventilation and wet drilling have reduced the prevalence of the disease greatly. In Cornish tin mines, hookworm infection also used to be relatively common.

The method of extraction of tin is related to the type of deposit. Cassiterite is usually dredged from the sea or river bed. After it has been dug or excavated, it is washed, and the mud and other superfluous materials are eliminated. In order to achieve this, primary and secondary washing operations are necessary, but even so, the concentrate is usually only about 70% pure.

The inhalation of tin leads to a benign pneumoconiosis known as stannosis. Most of the subjects who develop stannosis are involved in bagging of the concentrate or in smelting operations. During the latter process, hot gases containing minute particles of tin are given off from the molten metal as it leaves the furnace, and it is these particles that are responsible for the development of stannosis.

Stannosis is not associated with symptoms, but there is a relatively distinctive radiographic appearance that resembles welders' siderosis (Fig. 16–9). The small opacities present in the radiograph appear extremely radiopaque. The macroscopic appearances of the lung have been described by Robertson et al.[172] Blackish or gray macules ranging between 2 to 5 mm are present in the lungs (Fig. 16–10). These are relatively evenly distributed, and dust pigmentation of the interlobular septa is often evident. Microscopically the dust foci can be seen to be composed of aggregates of dust-laden macrophages that tend to surround the respiratory bronchioles. Occasionally dust-laden cells may be seen in the alveoli, in the interlobular septa, and in the perivascular lymphatics. Focal emphysema occurs but is not as prominent or as frequent as in coal workers' pneumoconiosis. Fibrosis is absent, and complicated pneumoconiosis (progressive massive fibrosis) does not occur.

There appears to be no evidence of significant pulmonary impairment in stannosis.[172, 173] Analysis of the lungs of subjects dying with, but not because of, stannosis have yielded between 30% and 40% dry weight of tin oxide. There is a reasonably good relationship between the tin content and the radiographic category of subjects with stannosis. Tin oxide is strongly birefringent. It must, however, be realized that very little tin needs to be retained in the lungs before radiographic abnormalities appear, and indeed 10 times as much coal is required to induce the

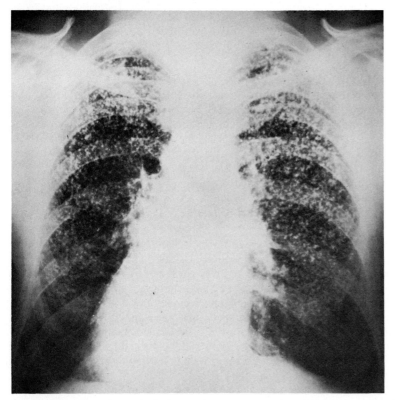

Figure 16–9. Chest radiograph of subject with stannosis. (Courtesy of the late Dr. C. Dundon.)

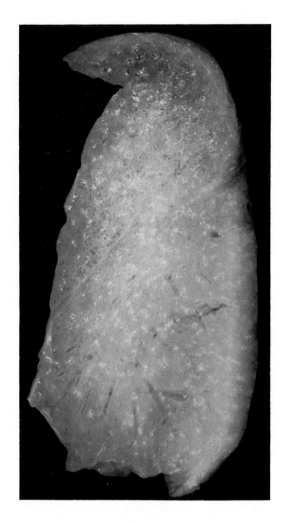

Figure 16–10
Large lung section showing grayish deposits (macules) of tin. The macules range between 2 and 5 mm in size.

same radiographic category. This phenomenon is a consequence of the fact that while tin has an atomic number of 50, carbon has an atomic number of 6.

In conclusion, it appears that although the inhalation of tin produces a benign pneumoconiosis generally known as stannosis, the condition is not associated with either morbidity or a decreased life expectancy, and in this context, one wonders whether it is correct to label the condition a pneumoconiosis.

THESAUROSIS

In 1958, Bergmann et al. described several subjects with a chronic pulmonary disease that they termed thesaurosis or storage disease. The condition occurred in young women exposed to hair spray, and was attributed by them to the inhalation of polyvinylpyrrolidone (PVP), the major constituent of hair sprays.[174] The first two patients described were asymptomatic young women with a history of heavy exposure to hair spray. Both had pulmonary infiltrates and hilar adenopathy. A granulomatous reaction was found in an excised scalene lymph node from one subject. In an attempt to develop an animal model for the condition, Bergmann and colleagues injected hair spray residue into the inguinal region of guinea pigs and produced a granulomatous reaction.

In 1962, Bergmann et al. reported 12 new cases, including three autopsies.[175] They added a more detailed clinical description, claiming that the condition is characterized radiographically by fluffy, hazy infiltrates and hilar adenopathy. They noted that when the use of hair spray was stopped, the disease resolved. Lymph node biopsy revealed findings that varied from reticuloendothelial hyperplasia to frank sarcoid granulomata. The microscopical lesions in the lung resembled those found in interstitial pneumonitis of the Hamman-Rich type; however, in subjects who had the condition for some time, the appearances were more suggestive of fibrosing alveolitis. Granulomata were sometimes seen in the lung. These workers made much of the presence of PAS-positive granules, which they observed in the lung parenchyma, and at first implied that these were a specific finding in thesaurosis. However, since then, the granules have been described in several other conditions. Following Bergmann and colleagues' description, there have been numerous case reports of one or two subjects with so-called thesaurosis.[176-178]

Unfortunately, good evidence that thesaurosis is an entity in its own right is sadly lacking. The name thesaurosis is presumably derived from the Greek *thēsauros,* which in English becomes "thesaurus," and which is best defined as a treasury or repository. Bergmann et al. regarded the condition as a "storage disease"; however, its relative infrequency in persons exposed to hair spray suggests strongly that it is a manifestation of hypersensitivity, if indeed it exists at all.[174, 175] In many reports of so-called thesaurosis, the clinical picture, x-ray findings, and even pathology were almost pathognomonic of sarcoid. Moreover, most subjects with sarcoidosis, in particular those with hilar adenopathy, improve spontaneously. The subjects described by Bergmann et al. could equally well have had sarcoidosis,[174, 175] and the fact that the condition improved when the subjects stopped using the hair spray is likely to have been entirely fortuitous.

A failure to demonstrate PVP in the lungs of several of the subjects who have been reported as having this condition is further circumstantial evidence against the concept of thesaurosis as a distinct disease entity. The fact that PVP has been shown to be retained in the lymph nodes is to be expected, since as an inert substance, once it is deposited in the lungs, it is removed by the macrophage and deposited elsewhere. Animal experiments have likewise failed to give any evidence in favor of the existence of thesaurosis.[179-181] The ultimate acceptance or rejection of thesaurosis must depend on well-controlled epidemiological studies. The study conducted by McLaughlin and Bidstrup best fits this description.[182] These authors were unable to find a single subject with thesaurosis in a survey of 505 hairdressers. A similar study carried out by Sharma and Williams in which the lung volumes and diffusing capacity of 62 exposed cosmetologists were compared to those of 33 control subjects likewise provided no evidence that thesaurosis exists.[183] Larson also failed to find any evidence of ventilatory impairment in users of hair spray.[184] A large study purporting to show that hair sprays are harmful was carried out by Palmer.[185] Using matched pairs, he reported that abnormal radiographs and a reduced vital capacity and single breath diffusing capacity were more common in Utah beauticians. The results, however, are not convincing, and the so-called radiological abnormalities were nonspecific and did not conform to a specific pattern. Moreover, beauticians are notoriously heavy cigarette smokers, appreciably more so than the general population in Utah, who for the most part are Mormons and nonsmokers. In a survey of 227 beauticians, Gowdy and Wagstaff claimed to have identified two types of radiographic abnormality, an airways response and a parenchymal response.[178] They noted increased bronchovascular markings in 11 subjects; however, the significance and indeed the very presence of this nonspecific finding are open to doubt. It is difficult to know whether they are describing nonspecific findings in beauticians, an occasional case of sarcoidosis, or what conceivably might be labeled thesaurosis. In a series of circuitous arguments, they reviewed the evidence for the existence of thesaurosis, and argued that neither clinically, physiologically, pathologically, nor epidemiologically is there anything that differentiates thesaurosis from sarcoidosis. Then by means of *a posteriori* logic they concluded that thesaurosis could conceivably exist. Suffice it to say that in the absence of epidemiological proof, the existence of thesaurosis cannot be accepted.

It is clear that while brief exposure to hair sprays decreases maximal expiratory flows at low lung volumes, the clinical significance of such a finding is doubtful.[186] A response of this type is likely to be nonspecific and of little import and shows only that the agent that has been inhaled has reached the small airways. Nevertheless, it is undoubtedly clear that a small minority of subjects react specifically to the fluorochlorohydrocarbons (Freon) that are used as propellants, and a few develop acute symptomatic bronchoconstriction with the characteristic features of asthma.[187]

TUNGSTEN CARBIDE PNEUMOCONIOSIS (HARD METAL DISEASE) AND RELATED SYNDROMES

The currently available evidence suggests that cobalt rather than tungsten is responsible for hard metal disease. The metal is usually recovered as a by-product of gold and silver mining. Cobalt is especially useful in the manufacture of alloys, and is frequently added to other metals such as aluminum, molybdenum, beryllium, chrome, and tungsten carbide. These alloys find their many uses in the production of hard metal and in the manufacture of certain parts of jet engines and large ferromagnets. Cobalt salts have a characteristic blue tint that is frequently useful in coloring glass and for tinting enamel paints and ceramic glazes.

Hard metal is produced by metallurgical blending of tungsten and carbon, with cobalt being used as a binder. Tungsten carbide is a metal that is extremely hard and resistant to heat and is therefore used in the cutting of metals and in the manufacture of dental drills and bearings. Tools made of hard metal remain sharp at temperatures up to 3000°F.

Tungsten carbide is prepared by mixing extremely fine particles (0.5 to 15 microns) of tungsten and carbon. The majority of such particles are at the lower end of the spectrum and range between 1 and 2 microns. The tungsten carbide is then milled with the addition of between 3% and 25% cobalt. The tiny hard metal crystals are deposited on the cobalt. During this process, nickel, titanium, and other metals may be added according to the desired properties of the hard metal. When the tungsten carbide has been milled, paraffin is added to provide body prior to pressing of the metal into ingots. The mixture of powdered metals is pressed into various shapes and heated to around 1500°C. A variety of coolants and lubricants are used for cutting, grinding, and polishing hard metal parts to precise dimensions. Aerosolization of the coolants creates a mist of metal particles that are readily inhaled.[188] In the coolants, cobalt exists mainly in the dissolved or ionized form in which it is combined with body proteins and can act as a hapten. Metallic cobalt is a lesser hazard, probably because it is non-ionized. In each of these processes fine dust containing both cobalt and tungsten particles is produced. The manufacturing process is described in detail by Bech, Kipling, and Heather.[189]

Respiratory Disease in Tungsten Carbide Workers and Those Exposed to Cobalt

Three main respiratory effects are produced by exposure to hard metal: (1) reversible airways obstruction, (2) hypersensitivity pneumonitis or alveolitis, and (3) pulmonary fibrosis.[190, 191] All of these reactions are relatively uncommon. Those who work with hard metal were once thought to develop either asthma or pulmonary fibrosis, and it was believed that the two conditions were mutually exclusive. In some subjects with hypersensitivity pneumonitis and alveolitis, and in others with early fibrosis, unusual giant alveolar lining cells appear. When these are present, the subject is said to have giant cell interstitial pneumonitis.[192] Airways obstruction and alveolitis may occur in the same subject, and both usually improve spontaneously when the subject is removed from further exposure. Pulmonary fibrosis may gradually develop with continued exposure. It is irreversible and may be associated with few or rarely no radiographic abnormalities.

The manifestations of exposure to cobalt may occur in those who manufacture hard metal parts and also in those who use hard metal tools.[191] Observations in diamond polishers who use high-speed cobalt polishing disks, and in whom exposure to cobalt occurs, have made it clear that the same conditions that occur in those exposed to hard metal are also found in diamond polishers.[193, 194]

In 1940, Jobs and Ballhausen, following examination of a group of 27 German workers, reported that eight of them had an abnormal chest radiograph.[195] A fine reticulonodulation was present. In 1959, Moschinski et al. examined 696 hard metal workers and found a high prevalence of bronchitis.[196] In a substantial percentage of the sample, there also was radiographic evidence of pneumoconiosis. In the United States, Fairhall et al. surveyed almost 2000 tungsten carbide workers. Conjunctivitis, rhinitis, tracheitis, and bronchitis were frequently found. Pruritus and cobalt sensitivity were also common.[197] Some subjects included in this sample had radiographic evidence of a pneumoconiosis.

Much experimental work suggests that cobalt is the responsible agent for both the interstitial and the obstructive syndromes. Harding showed powdered cobalt to be toxic when given intratracheally or by inhalation.[198] He also demonstrated that the metal is much more soluble in plasma than in saline. Moreover, tungsten carbide in the absence of cobalt is inert. Delahant produced chronic bronchiolitis and metaplastic changes in the alveoli with pulverized cobalt but not with tungsten carbide, titanium, or tantalum.[199] In animals, the inhalation of metallic cobalt or cobalt salts leads to pulmonary edema. Repeated inhalations over a fairly long period lead to pulmonary fibrosis. Bronchiolitis obliterans, granulomatous pneumonia, and interstitial fibrosis all may occur following the inhalation of metallic cobalt, with the likelihood of fibrosis developing being related to the dose and duration of inhalation. The administration of cobalt oxide when limited to a few weeks produces a transient pneumonitis.[200] In contrast, continued inhalation of powdered metallic cobalt has been shown to cause permanent changes, stiff lungs, and the laying down of collagen.

Cobalt oxide is less toxic than metallic cobalt. It is felt that the cobalt ions contained in the metal are responsible for most of the deleterious effects. It has been suggested that cobalt impairs oxidative metabolism, and in this regard cysteine has been shown to have an ameliorating influence on lung damage that has been induced by the inhalation of cobalt metal.[201]

Observations of interstitial fibrosis occurring in diamond polishers and referred to earlier provide additional evidence that hypersensitivity pneumonitis and lung fibrosis of hard metal workers are produced by exposure to cobalt and not by other agents in the hard metal.[193, 194]

Hypersensitivity Pneumonitis

This condition is found in hard metal workers and is characterized by acute or subacute episodes of pneumonitis.[188, 191, 192] These occur when a subject is exposed to cobalt while at work. The episodes are characterized by fever, anorexia, and shortness of breath and are often attributed to a viral respiratory tract illness or to bronchitis. The subject is usually compelled to take time off from work. When he or she does so, the symptoms improve but recur when he or she returns to work. Repeated episodes are common, and with the passage of time, usually in about a year, there is a gradual attenuation of the acute episodes. The shortness of breath persists and slowly becomes more severe. In subjects with hypersensitivity pneumonitis, contact dermatitis is not uncommon, and subjects with skin manifestations usually have positive cobalt patch tests.

The chest radiograph may be normal during the acute attack, but more often patchy infiltrates appear. In some instances a fine reticulonodular pattern may be present. Both the bilateral mottling and the patchy infiltration usually disappear gradually after exposure ceases, especially following the initial attack. The characteristic acinus-filling pattern that is seen in certain types of extrinsic allergic alveolitis such as farmer's lung is most uncommon. A return to work is associated with further symptoms and, in addition, recurrence of the radiographic changes.

After some time, lung volumes start to decrease, and this becomes evident on the chest radiograph. Magnetic resonance imaging may show residual parenchymal activity despite a normal chest x-ray.[191] Fibrosis and active inflammation can be distinguished by using T_1- and T_2-weighted magnetic resonance images (MRI) (Fig. 16–11). Concomitantly with the decrease in lung volumes, there is obvious evidence of restrictive impairment, a reduction of the diffusing capacity, and an increased static elastic recoil. The administration of steroids hastens clinical and radiographic improvement, but whether the eventual outcome is influenced is uncertain. Complete resolution usually occurs, but if the patient has been exposed for long periods, restrictive impairment may persist and presumably can be attributed to the laying down of collagenous fibrosis in the lungs.

Many subjects with hypersensitivity pneumonitis show multinucleated giant cells on bronchial lavage or on biopsy (Fig. 16–12). Some subjects show a nongranulomatous reaction characterized by intra-alveolar exudate with some interstitial reaction. The process is initially mild but becomes severe as times goes by. Biopsy specimens usually reveal a type 2 pneumocyte response.

Interstitial Fibrosis

A relatively early and detailed description of hard metal disease is that of Coates and Watson.[202] These workers described 12 subjects with diffuse interstitial lung disease, of whom no fewer than eight died. The early symptoms of hard metal disease are cough and shortness of breath, which progressively worsen.[190, 191, 202] Tachypnea is frequent, and clubbing of the digits and basal crackles are late features of the condition. Pulmonary function measurements reveal reduced lung volumes, arterial desaturation, and a low diffusing capacity. The pattern is that of classical restrictive disease without significant airways obstruction. Death is usually a consequence of pulmonary hypertension and cor pulmonale.

Chest symptoms usually appear before the film becomes abnormal. Disease is seldom seen without at least 10 years of exposure, but longer and shorter periods of exposure have been reported. Radiographically the disease usually presents as a fine reticulonodular pattern in the middle and lower zones, but the upper zones are occasionally predominantly affected. The heart outline is often blurred, as in asbestosis, and a fine honeycombing may develop, as in other pulmonary fibroses.

Although the lungs in hard metal disease usually appear diffusely involved in the chest film, the fibrosis may be distributed in a patchy fashion.[191, 203] The interstitial tissue is infiltrated with histiocytes and plasma cells, and the alveolar septa are thickened by fibrous tissue. The interstitial fibrosis seen in hard metal disease is usually described as a nongranulomatous process characterized by intra-alveolar exudate and some interstitial reaction. Occasionally present is a granulomatous reaction very similar to that seen in berylliosis. Cystic air spaces lined by cuboidal epithelium are found later in the disease. The alveoli contain what are assumed to be desquamated mononuclear cells, probably type II alveolar pneumocytes.

Coates and Watson carried out electron microscopy in several of their subjects. They demonstrated excessive deposition of collagen and elastic tissue in the septa and the presence of multifaceted crystals thought to be tungsten carbide.[203] The alveolar lining cells were markedly affected.

Bronchoalveolar lavage shows a relative increase of lymphocytes and neutrophils in those who have an active alveolitis.[192] It also frequently reveals multinucleated giant cells. The tissue that is obtained with open biopsy from subjects usually shows alveolitis with varying degrees of fibrosis. In those with established fibrosis and severe restrictive impairment, the fibrosis predominates. In six of the seven

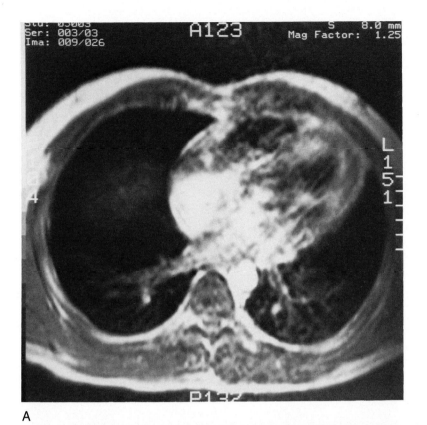

A

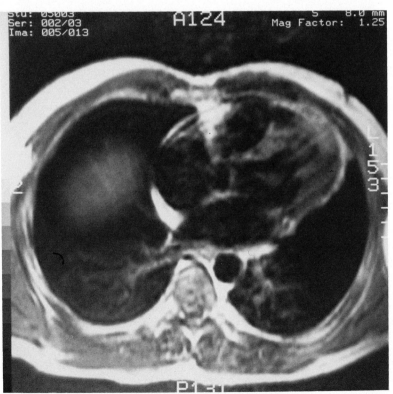

B

Figure 16–11

Magnetic resonance images from a subject with hypersensitivity pneumonitis and mild fibrosis. *A,* T1-weighted image showing both vascular shadows and interstitial fibrosis. The bronchi appear black and the blood vessels white. Note the increased shadowing posteriorly. The differentiation between vascular shadows, alveolitis, and fibrosis is difficult or impossible in T1-weighted images. *B,* T2-weighted image. Arterial blood flow appears black because of high flow rates; venous blood flow appears white because of slowness. Definite early fibrosis is present posteriorly and is adjacent to the bronchovascular markings. The fibrosis is gray, indicating that it is smoldering. Mature nonvascular fibrosis appears black, while active alveolitis is white. (From Cugell, D. W., Morgan, W. K. C., Perkins, D. G., et al., The respiratory effects of cobalt. Arch. Intern. Med., 150, 177, 1990. Copyright 1990, American Medical Association.)

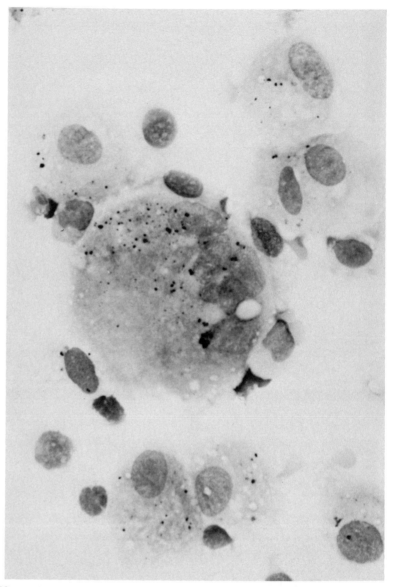

Figure 16–12. Bronchovascular lavage fluid from same patient as in Figure 16–11 showing multinucleated giant cells with cytoplasmic vacuoles. Numerous alveolar macrophages are present containing similar particulate matter. (Giemsa stain × 630)

subjects described by Cugell et al., giant cell pneumonitis was present, and all those who underwent bronchoalveolar lavage had frequent multinucleated giant cells in their lavage fluid.[191]

Sprince et al. surveyed 1039 tungsten carbide workers to determine the prevalence of interstitial lung disease and work-related wheeze.[204] They also studied the extent of cobalt exposure and related it to the prevalence of lung disease, and finally they examined the effects of exposures to the new and old threshold limit values (TLVs), i.e., 50 µg/m^3 and 100 µg/m^3. Nine subjects were found with 1/1 or greater changes in their lungs, however, only one reader interpreted the chest x-rays. Moreover, five of the nine subjects who had x-ray abnormalities had small rounded opacities, an unusual finding in subjects with hard metal disease, especially in the absence of systemic symptoms. No clear differentiation was made between wheeze produced by bronchitis and so-called work-related wheeze. The prevalence of irregular opacities in this group appears similar to that in many other groups exposed to inert dusts in whom cigarette smoking is common.[16] Other studies have shown that interstitial fibrosis is rare or absent in those working with hard metal.[205, 206]

The observation of interstitial fibrosis in diamond workers served to confirm the fact that cobalt alone is responsible for the disease that occurs in hard metal workers and makes it apparent that it is cobalt ions that are responsible.[193] In a more recent survey of 194 diamond polishers, it was suggested that exposure to cobalt below the present TLV of 50 $\mu g/m^3$ may be capable of inducing disease.[194] The diagnosis of hard metal disease in this study, however, was based on symptoms such as cough and shortness of breath, along with exposure to cobalt and their relationship to a reduction in ventilatory capacity as measured by the FVC, FEV_1, $FEV_1/FVC\%$, and FEF_{25-75}. There is some reason to doubt that the effects of the various confounding factors were clearly separated by the statistical methods used.

Obstructed Airways Syndrome

This appears most often to be an allergic response and is characterized by wheezing, cough, and shortness of breath while at work. The symptoms often improve when the subject goes home. In this it resembles, to some extent, byssinosis. There is no evidence that this type of disease progresses to interstitial fibrosis. Bech et al. have shown that in a small proportion of workers who have the obstructive syndrome, the respiratory mechanics deteriorate over the day.[189] Most subjects in whom a severe obstructive response develops leave their job.[188, 205] Coates et al. described this syndrome in more detail.[205] They described nine subjects with the typical syndrome. Itching was present in three of them. The symptoms cleared up after work and on weekends, and recurred when they returned. The syndrome did not develop until the subjects had had between 6 and 18 months' exposure and sensitization had occurred. They showed that cobalt was toxic to the affected subjects' leukocytes, but that tungsten had no effect. Challenge studies with cobalt, but not tungsten, produced an airways response. It is not known whether parenchymal manifestations are related to an allergic predisposition and whether sensitization occurs, but this seems somewhat unlikely, at least from the animal experiments. In contrast, the bronchoconstrictive response is seen in cobalt-induced asthma and airways obstruction and is felt to be an allergic response and has all of the characteristic symptoms of asthma. Although there is no evidence that asthma progresses to interstitial fibrosis, subjects with asthma may also develop hypersensitivity pneumonitis.

The diagnosis of cobalt-induced lung disease is usually based on a history of exposure plus certain other clinical features and laboratory tests. There is evidence to indicate that the disease is more likely to occur when the TLV for cobalt (50 $\mu g/m^3$) is exceeded; however, in many instances no measurements are made of the cobalt levels until after the subject becomes ill, after which a vigorous attempt is made to improve ventilation and other industrial hygiene measurements. Whether the parenchymal manifestations are related to an allergic predisposition and sensitization is unknown, but this seems unlikely, at least from the animal experiments previously described. In contrast, the bronchoconstrictive response may well be related to hypersensitivity and tends to be associated with the cutaneous manifestations of cobalt exposure.

Treatment

No treatment is successful in established interstitial fibrosis, but the alveolitis can be controlled by steroids. There seems, however, to be little doubt that the administration of steroids hastens clinical and radiographic improvement in those subjects who have hypersensitivity pneumonitis. Yet, it must be borne in mind that complete resolution can occur simply by moving the subject from further exposure.

In our experience, steroids not only make the subject feel better but also appear to produce a more rapid improvement in lung function. Nevertheless, a long-term beneficial effect of steroids has not been unequivocally demonstrated.

MISCELLANEOUS PNEUMOCONIOSES

Aside from the well-recognized pneumoconioses, a series of uncommon or esoteric occupationally related conditions have been described.

Bakelite Pneumoconiosis

Two subjects with generalized pulmonary infiltration and exposure to Bakelite have been described.[207] Although Pimentel states that the clinical features of Bakelite pneumoconiosis resemble those of extrinsic allergic alveolitis, his description is less than convincing. According to him, the basic lesion is an epithelial granuloma resembling sarcoid. While Pimentel claims to have developed an animal model, his evidence for the existence of the condition is tenuous, and the existence of Bakelite pneumoconiosis must remain *sub judice.*

Rare Earth Pneumoconioses

A number of elements are referred to as rare earth. These include yttrium, cerium, neodymium, and lanthanum. While intratracheal injection of yttrium and cerium in animals can induce granulomata,[208] there is little evidence that the occupational inhalation of rare earths ever leads to pulmonary fibrosis, although a few reports of radiographic abnormalities induced by cerium have been described. Cerium oxide is used in the optical industry in the manufacture of glassware and in metallurgy. A report from the LaRochelle district of France described two subjects with a miliary process in their lungs which was attributed to the inhalation of cerium oxide.[209]

The subjects had been exposed for 11 and 15 years, respectively. No description of any pulmonary function abnormalities was provided, and there is no evidence that impairment occurs in this condition.

Laundry Workers' Pneumoconiosis

A few subjects who were employed as laundry workers in the pottery district of Britain were reported as developing pneumoconiosis.[210] It is thought that these cases arose from the practice of laundry workers shaking out pottery workers' overalls prior to putting them in the wash. The likelihood is that the radiographic changes were a consequence of exposure to kaolin. No evidence of pulmonary impairment was found in the affected subjects.

Titanium Pneumoconiosis

Titanium oxide is used as a white pigment in the manufacture of paint. The carbide of titanium finds extensive use with tungsten carbide in the manufacture of tools. There is some evidence that titanium oxide may produce radiographic abnormalities similar to those resulting from inhalation of iron and tin; however, there appears to be no associated pulmonary impairment.[211] A paper described a number of symptoms and changes in pulmonary function in a group of 207 titanium workers.[212] Despite description of a multitude of abnormalities, the authors concluded that the clinically significant disease was infrequent.

A more recent study examined the respiratory effects of titanium exposure on 1576 workers who have been exposed for more than 1 year.[213] They were compared to a suitable control group of 901 nonexposed workers. Titanium exposure was not associated with an excess of chronic respiratory disease, pneumoconiosis, or pleural thickening. Furthermore, there appeared to be no excess risk of lung cancer.

Zirconium Pneumoconiosis

Zirconium is a silvery rare metal, and its oxide is used in the manufacture of fused and sintered ceramics and heat-resistant textiles and in the production of furnace bricks. Animal studies for the most part have suggested that zirconium is inert, but it has been shown that the lungs of rats exposed to extremely high concentrations may develop radiographic abnormalities.[214] A slight inflammatory response has been observed.

In humans there is doubt as to whether occupational exposure to zirconium ever leads to pulmonary disease. Reed described a granulomatous pulmonary response in a chemical engineer who was involved in the production of the metal;[215] however, this may well have been fortuitous. McCallum has described small round opacities in eight men working in a zirconium processing plant, but here again the men had a mixed exposure.[216] The weight of the evidence is against the association of zirconium with the development of pneumoconiosis in humans except under rare circumstances.

Pneumoconiosis of Dentists and Dental Workers

Pneumoconiosis has also been described in dental technicians and dental students. Sherson et al. described the development of small opacities in the chest radiographs of dental laboratory technicians.[217] Those with the longest exposures (at least 15 years) had consistently lower lung function as determined by measurement of the ventilatory and diffusing capacities. The differences between those with long and short exposures, however, were not statistically significant. All six subjects who had radiographic evidence of pneumoconiosis were smokers, which could well explain the reduced lung function noted in the group. Of the six affected, one had scleroderma, and the three who were biopsied showed nonspecific interstitial fibrosis. The fact that those who had small opacities in their radiographs were all smokers suggests that they probably had irregular opacities, and the changes may well have been due to smoking.[16] In addition, it is perhaps relevant that the most hazardous job involved the production of chromium cobalt prostheses. Clearly the possibility of cobalt being responsible for certain of the findings, and in particular, the fibrosis, needs to be borne in mind. The significance of the findings described in this study are therefore difficult to assess, especially since other workers have carried out similar surveys with negative findings.[218]

A case report describes a dental student who developed bilateral basal pulmonary infiltrates.[219] An open biopsy revealed interstitial pneumonitis with abundant vacuolated macrophages with electronlucent bodies resembling beads. It was felt that the latter were produced by exposure to an acrylic resin. The infiltrates cleared following cessation of exposure; however, no definite cause-and-effect association between exposure and the development of the disease was demonstrated, and it is preferable to reserve judgement as to the existence of this form of pneumoconiosis until confirmed by others.

Esoteric Pneumoconioses

A number of truly esoteric conditions have recently been described. These include "dung lung," a pneumonitis caused by the inhalation of liquid manure.[220] The inhalation of hydrogen sulfide from liquid manure caused pulmonary edema. Whether this can be regarded as a true pneumoconiosis is a moot point, but it is included under this term.

A case report of "fly ash lung" described a shipyard worker who developed a nonspecific pulmonary interstitial process.[221] The authors suggested that fly ash, an aluminum silicate, may be the responsible agent.

The development of pulmonary fibrosis in a drug-snorting fire-eater seems to be unique.[222] The affected subject was a drummer in a punk rock band who frequently inhaled powdered drugs, including cocaine, barbiturates, and amphetamines, through a rolled up pound-note. His pièce de résistance involved filling his mouth with paraffin (kerosene), which he would then expel through his lips, at the same time igniting the jet. He was observed to have radiographic changes; and after complete investigation, a lung biopsy revealed diffuse pulmonary fibrosis due to the deposition of kerosene and other substances he had been inhaling.

REFERENCES

1. Shaver, C.G., and Riddell, A.R., Lung changes associated with the manufacture of alumina abrasive. J. Ind. Hyg., 29, 145, 1947.
2. Morgan, W.K.C., and Dinman, B.D., Pulmonary Effects of Aluminum. In Gitelman, H.J., ed., Aluminum and Health. New York, Marcel Dekker, 1989, pp. 203–234.
3. Dinman, B.D., Alumina related pulmonary disease. J. Occup. Med., 30, 328, 1988.
4. National Institute of Occupational Safety and Health. U.S. Public Health Service. National Occupational Hazard Survey, Vol. III, Survey Analysis and Supplemental Tables. Washington, D.C., U.S. Government Printing Office, 1977.
5. Meiklejohn, A., The successful prevention of silicosis among china biscuit workers in the North Staffordshire potteries. Br. J. Ind. Med., 20, 255, 1963.
6. Meiklejohn, A., and Posner, E., The effect of the use of calcined alumina in china biscuit placing on the health of the workman. Br. J. Ind. Med., 14, 229, 1957.
7. Posner, E., and Kennedy, M.C.S., A further survey of china clay biscuit placers in Stoke on Trent. Br. J. Ind. Med., 24, 133, 1967.
8. Sutherland, C.L., Meiklejohn, A., and Price, F.N.R., An inquiry into the health hazard of a group of workers exposed to alumina dust. J. Ind. Hyg. Toxicol., 19, 312, 1937.
9. Meiklejohn, A., and Jones, W.W., The effect of the use of calcined alumina in china biscuit placing on health of workmen. A field study in a group of pottery workers in North Staffordshire. J. Ind. Hyg. Toxicol., 30, 160, 1948.
10. Gardner, L.U., Dworski, M., and Delahant, A.B., Aluminum therapy in silicosis: an experimental study. J. Ind. Hyg. Toxicol., 26, 211, 1944.
11. King, E.J., Harrison, C.V., Mohanty, G.P., et al., The effect of various forms of alumina on the lungs of rats. J. Pathol. Bact., 69, 81, 1955.
12. Klosterkotter, W., Effects of ultramicroscopic gamma-aluminum oxide on rats and mice. AMA Arch. Ind. Health, 21, 458, 1960.
13. Stacy, B.D., King, E.J., Harrison, C., et al., Tissue changes in rats' lungs caused by hydroxides, oxides, and phosphates of aluminum and iron. J. Pathol. Bacteriol., 77, 417, 1959.
14. Townsend, M.C., Enterline, P.E., Sussman, N.B., et al., Pulmonary function in relation to total dust exposure at a bauxite refinery and alumina-based chemical products plant. Am. Rev. Respir. Dis., 132, 1174, 1985.
15. Townsend, M.C., Sussman, N.B., Enterline, P.E., et al., Radiographic abnormalities in relation to total dust exposure at a bauxite refinery and alumina-based chemical products plant. Am. Rev. Respir. Dis., 138, 90, 1988.
16. Dick, J.A., Morgan, W.K.C., Muir, D.F.C., et al., The significance of irregular opacities on the chest roentgenogram. Chest, 102, 251, 1992.
17. Morgan, W.K.C., Industrial bronchitis. Br. J. Ind. Med., 35, 285, 1978.
18. Jederlinic, P.J., Abraham, J.L., Churg, A., et al., Pulmonary fibrosis in aluminum oxide workers. Am. Rev. Respir. Dis., 142, 1179, 1990.
19. Abramson, M.J., Wlodarczyk, J.H., Saunders, N.A., et al., Does aluminum smelting cause lung disease? State of the Art. Am. Rev. Respir. Dis., 139, 1042, 1989.
20. Goralewski, G., Zur Symptomatologie der Aluminum-Staublunge. Arch. Gewerbepathol. Gerewbehyg., 10, 384, 1940.
21. Goralewski, G., Die Aluminiumlunge: Eine Klinische Studie Leipzig, Arbeitsmedizin., Suppl. 26, 1950.
22. McLaughlin, A.I.G., Kazantis, G., King, E., et al., Pulmonary fibrosis and encephalopathy associated with the inhalation of aluminium dust. Br. J. Ind. Med., 19, 253, 1962.
23. Koelsch, F., Lederer, E., and Kaestele, L., Die Metallfarbenherstellung und ihre gesundheitliche beurteilung—mit besonderer. Berucksichtigung der Staubgefardung. Arch. Gewerbepathol. Gewerbehyg., 5, 108, 1933.
24. Doese, M., Gewerbemedizinische Studien zur Frage der Gesundheitsschadgungen durch Aluminium, insbesondere der Aluminiumstaublunge. Arch. Gewerbepathol. Gewerbehyg., 8, 501, 1938.
25. Barth, G., Frick, W., and Scheidemandel, H., Die Aluminiumlunge. Deutsch Med. Woehenschr., 81, 1115, 1956.

26. Hunter, D., Milton, R., Perry, M.A., et al., Effects of aluminium and alumina on the lung in grinders of duralumin aeroplane propellers. Br. J. Ind. Med., 1, 159, 1944.
27. Mitchell, J., Pulmonary fibrosis in an aluminium worker. Br. J. Ind. Med., 16, 123, 1959.
28. Mitchell, J., Manning, G.B., and Molyneux, M., Pulmonary fibrosis in workers exposed to fine powdered aluminium. Br. J. Ind. Med., 18, 10, 1961.
29. Jordan, J.W., Pulmonary fibrosis in a worker using an aluminium powder. Br. J. Ind. Med., 18, 21, 1961.
30. Crombie, D.W., Blaisdell, J.L., and MacPherson, G., The treatment of silicosis by aluminum powder. Can. Med. Assoc. J., 50, 318, 1944.
31. Kennedy, M.C.S., Aluminium powder inhalation in the treatment of silicosis of pottery workers and pneumoconiosis of coal miners. Br. J. Ind. Med., 13, 85, 1956.
32. Swensson, A., Nordenfelt, O., Forssman, S., et al., Aluminium dust pneumoconiosis: a clinical study. Arch. Gewerbepathol. Gewerbehyg., 19, 131, 1962.
33. Corrin, B., Aluminium pneumoconiosis. I. In vitro comparison of stamped aluminium powders containing different lubricating agents and granular aluminium powder. Br. J. Ind. Med., 20, 264, 1963.
34. Corrin, B., Aluminium pneumoconiosis. II. Effect on the rat lung of intratracheal injections of stamped aluminium powders containing different lubricating agents and of a granular aluminium powder. Br. J. Ind. Med., 20, 268, 1963.
35. Ueda, M., Mizoi, Y., Maki, Z., et al., A case of aluminium dust lung: a necropsy report. J. Kobe. Med. Sci., 4, 91, 1958.
36. Dinman, B.D., The respiratory condition of potroom workers: Australian experience. In Hughes, J.P., ed., Health Protection in Primary Aluminium Production. London, New Zealand House, 1977, pp. 95–100.
37. Discher, D.P., and Breitenstein, B.D., Prevalence of chronic pulmonary disease in aluminium potroom workers. J. Occup. Med., 18, 379, 1976.
38. Field, G.B., and Smith, M.M., Pulmonary function in aluminium smelters. III. Report of a survey conducted at ALCOA of Australia. International Primary Aluminium Institute. London, New Zealand House, 1977, pp. 76–80.
39. Chan-Yeung, M., Wong, R., MacLean, L., et al., Epidemiologic health study of workers in an aluminium smelter in British Columbia. Am. Rev. Respir. Dis., 127, 465, 1983.
40. Field, G.B., and Owen, P., Airway function in potroom workers. In Hughes, J.P., ed., Health Protection in Primary Aluminium Production, Vol. 2. London, New Zealand House, 1982, pp. 77–84.
41. Morgan, W.K.C., Discussion of respiratory studies in Australia. In Hughes, J.P., ed., Health Protection in Primary Aluminium Production, Vol. 2. London, New Zealand House, 1982, pp. 94–98.
42. Smith, M.M., Asthma in potroom workers. In Hughes, J.P., ed., Health Protection in Primary Aluminium Production, Vol. 2. London, New Zealand House, 1982, pp. 87–89.
43. Kongerud, J., and Samuelsen, S.O., A longitudinal study of respiratory symptoms in aluminium potroom workers. Am. Rev. Respir. Dis., 144, 10, 1991.
44. Gibbs, G.W., Mortality of aluminium reduction plant workers, 1950 through 1977. J. Occup. Med., 27, 761, 1985.
45. Gross, P.R., Harley, A., and De Treville, R.T.P., Pulmonary reactions to metallic aluminium powders. Arch. Environ. Health, 26, 227, 1973.
46. Miller, R.R., Churg, A.M., Hutcheon, M., et al., Pulmonary alveolar proteinosis and aluminium dust exposure. Am. Rev. Respir. Dis., 130, 312, 1984.
47. Herbert, A., Sterling, G., Abraham, J., et al., Desquamative interstitial pneumonia in an aluminium welder. Hum. Pathol., 13, 694, 1982.
48. Chen, W.R., Monnat, J., Chen, M., et al., Aluminium induced pulmonary granulomatosis. Hum. Pathol., 9, 705, 1978.
49. De Vuyst, P., Dumortier, P., Schandene, L., et al., Sarcoidlike lung granulomatosis induced by aluminium dusts. Am. Rev. Respir. Dis., 135, 493, 1987.
50. Shaver, C.G., Pulmonary changes encountered in employees engaged in the manufacture of alumina abrasives: clinical and roentgenologic aspects. Occup. Med., 5, 718, 1948.
51. Shaver, C.G., Further observations of lung changes associated with the manufacturing of alumina abrasives. Radiology, 50, 760, 1948.
52. Jephcott, C.M., Fume exposure in the manufacture of aluminum abrasives. Occup. Med., 5, 701, 1948.
53. Gartner, H., Etiology of corundum smelter's lung. Arch. Ind. Hyg. Occup. Med., 6, 339, 1952.
54. Wyatt, J.P., and Riddell, A.C.R., The morphology of bauxite fume pneumoconiosis. Am. J. Pathol., 25, 447, 1949.
55. Smith, A.R., and Perina, A.E., Pneumoconiosis from synthetic abrasive materials. Occup. Med., 5, 396, 1948.
56. Funahashi, A., Schlueter, D.P., Pintar, K., et al., Pneumoconiosis in workers exposed to silicon carbide. Am. Rev. Respir. Dis., 129, 635, 1984.
57. Bech, A.O., Kipling, M.D., and Zundel, W.E., Emery pneumoconiosis. Trans. Assoc. Ind. Med. Off., 15, 110, 1965.
58. Cooper, D.A., Pendergrass, E.P., Vorwald, A.K., et al., Pneumoconiosis in workers in an antimony industry. Am. J. Roentgen., 103, 495, 1968.

59. McCallum, R.I., Work on an occupational service in environmental control. Ann. Occup. Hyg., 6, 60, 1963.
60. Klucik, I., Juck, A., and Gruberova, J., Respiratory and pulmonary lesions caused by antimony trioxide dust. Pracov. Lek., 14, 363, 1962.
61. McLaughlin, A.I.G., Iron and other radio-opaque dust. *In* King, E.J., and Fletcher, C.M., eds., Industrial Pulmonary Diseases. Boston, Little, Brown & Company, 1960, pp. 146–167.
62. Arrigoni, A., La pneumoconiosis da bario. Clin. Med. Ital., 64, 299, 1933.
63. Arrigoni, A., La pneumoconiosis da bario. Med. Lav., 24, 461, 1933.
64. Pendergrass, E., and Greening, R., Baritosis, report of a case. A.M.A. Arch. Ind. Hyd., 7, 44, 1953.
65. Doig, A.T., Baritosis. *In* XV International Congress on Occupational Health. Vienna, Wiener Medizenische Akademie, Verlag, 1966.
66. Seaton, A., Ruckley, V.A., Addison, J., and Rhind Brown, W., Silicosis in barium miners. Thorax, 41, 591, 1986.
67. Reeves, A.L., and Vorwald, A.J., Beryllium carcinogenesis. II. Pulmonary deposition and clearance of inhaled beryllium sulfate in the rat. Cancer Res., 27, 446, 1967.
68. Hardy, H.L., and Stoeckle, J.D., Beryllium disease. J. Chronic Dis., 9, 152, 1959.
69. Kriebel, D., Sprince, N.L., Eisen, E.A., et al., Beryllium exposure and pulmonary function: a cross sectional study of beryllium workers. Br. J. Ind. Med., 45, 167, 1988.
70. Van Ordstrand, H.S., Hughes, R., De Nardi, J.M., and Carmody, M.G., Beryllium poisoning. J.A.M.A., 129, 1084, 1945.
71. Van Ordstrand, H.S., Acute beryllium poisoning. *In* Vorwald, A.J., ed., Sixth Saranac Symposium (1947). Pneumoconiosis: Beryllium, Bauxite Fumes, Compensation. New York, P.B. Hoeber, 1950, p. 65.
72. De Nardi, J.M., Van Ordstrand, H.S., and Carmody, M.G., Acute dermatitis and pneumonitis in beryllium workers: review of 406 cases in 8-year period with follow-up on recoveries. Ohio State Med. J., 45, 467, 1949.
73. Eisenbud, M., Burghout, C.F., and Steadman, L.T., Environmental studies in plants and laboratories using beryllium: the acute disease. J. Ind. Hyg., 30, 281, 1968.
74. Sprince, N.L., Kanarek, D.J., Weber, A.L., et al., Reversible respiratory disease in beryllium workers. Am. Rev. Respir. Dis., 117, 1011, 1978.
75. Hardy, H.L., and Tabershaw, I.R., Delayed chemical pneumonitis occurring in workers exposed to beryllium compounds. J. Ind. Hyg. Toxicol., 28, 197, 1946.
76. Chesner, C., Chronic pulmonary granulomatosis in residents of a community near a beryllium plant: three autopsied cases. Ann. Int. Med., 32, 1028, 1950.
77. Eisenbud, M., Wanta, R.C., Dunstan, C., et al., Non-occupational berylliosis. J. Ind. Hyg. Toxicol., 31, 282, 1949.
78. Hardy, H.L., Beryllium disease: a continuing diagnostic problem. Am. J. Med. Sci., 142, 150, 1961.
79. Kriebel, D., Brain, J.D., Sprince, N.L., et al., The pulmonary toxicity of beryllium. Am. Rev. Respir. Dis., 137, 464, 1988.
80. Van Ordstrand, H.S., Diagnosis of beryllium disease. A.M.A. Arch. Ind. Health, 19, 157, 1959.
81. Resnick, H., Roche, M., and Morgan, W.K.C., Immunoglobulin concentrations in berylliosis. Am. Rev. Respir. Dis., 101, 504, 1970.
82. Weber, A.L., Stoeckle, J.D., and Hardy, H.L., Roentgenologic patterns in longstanding beryllium disease: report of 8 cases. Am. J. Roentgen., 93, 879, 1965.
83. Wright, G.W., Chronic pulmonary granulomatosis of beryllium workers. Trans. Am. Clin. Climatol. Assoc., 61, 161, 1949.
84. Gaensler, E.A., Verstraeten, J.M., Weil, W.B., et al., Respiratory pathophysiology in chronic beryllium disease. A.M.A. Arch. Ind. Health, 19, 132, 1959.
85. Ferris, B.G., Atfield, J.E., Kriete, H.A., and Whittenberger, J.L., Pulmonary function in patients with pulmonary disease treated with ACTH. A.M.A. Arch. Ind. Hyg., 3, 603, 1951.
86. Curtis, G.H., Cutaneous hypersensitivity due to beryllium. A.M.A. Arch. Derm. Syph., 64, 470, 1951.
87. Sneddon, I.B., Berylliosis, a case report. Br. Med. J., 1, 1448, 1955.
88. Waksman, B.H., The diagnosis of beryllium disease with special reference to the patch test. A.M.A. Arch. Ind. Health, 19, 154, 1959.
89. James, D.G., Dermatological aspects of sarcoidosis. Quart. J. Med., 28, 109, 1959.
90. Dutram, F.R., Cholak, J., and Hubbard, D.M., The value of beryllium determination in the diagnosis of berylliosis. Am. J. Clin. Pathol., 19, 229, 1949.
91. Jones-Williams, W., and Kelland, D., New aid for diagnosing chronic beryllium disease (CBD): laser ion mass analysis. J. Clin. Pathol., 39, 900, 1986.
92. Williams, W.J., A histological study of the lungs in 52 cases of chronic beryllium disease. Br. J. Ind. Med., 15, 84, 1958.
93. Shapley, D., Occupational lung cancer. Government challenged in beryllium proceedings. Science, 198, 898, 1977.
94. The beryllium dispute [Round the World column]. Lancet, 1, 202, 1978.
95. Marx, J.J., Jr., and Burrell, R., Delayed hypersensitivity to beryllium compounds. J. Immunol., 111, 590, 1973.

96. Deodhar, S.D., Barna, B., and Van Ordstrand, H.S., A study of the immunologic aspects of chronic berylliosis. Chest, 63, 309, 1973.
97. Krivanek, N., and Reeves, A.L., The effect of chemical forms of beryllium on the production of the immunologic response. Am. Ind. Hyg. J., 33, 45, 1972.
98. Williams, W.R., and Williams, W.J., Development of beryllium lymphocyte transformation tests in chronic beryllium disease. Int. Arch. Allergy Appl. Immunol., 67, 175, 1982.
99. Kreiss, K., Newman, L.S., Mroz, M.M., et al., Screening blood test identifies subclinical beryllium disease. J. Occup. Med., 31, 603, 1989.
100. Epstein, P.E., Dauber, J.H., Rossman, M.D., and Daniele, R.P., Bronchoalveolar lavage in a patient with chronic berylliosis: evidence for hypersensitivity pneumonitis. Ann. Intern. Med., 97, 213, 1982.
101. Jones, W.W., and Williams, W.R., Value of beryllium lymphocyte transformation tests in chronic beryllium disease and in potentially exposed workers. Thorax, 38, 41, 1983.
102. Chiappino, G., Cirla, A., and Vigliani, E.C., Delayed type hypersensitivity reactions to beryllium compounds. Arch. Pathol., 87, 131, 1969.
103. Stiefel, T., Schulze, K., Zorn, H., and Tolg, G., Toxicokinetic and toxicodynamic studies of beryllium. Arch. Toxicol., 45, 81, 1980.
104. Reeves, A.L., Berylliosis as an autoimmune disorder. Ann. Clin. Lab. Sci., 6, 256, 1976.
105. Schute, H.F., Beryllium, the criteria document. J. Occup. Med., 15, 663, 1973.
106. Harding, H.E., and Oliver, G.B., Changes in the lungs induced by natural graphite. Br. J. Ind. Med., 6, 91, 1949.
107. Gaensler, E.A., Cadigan, J.B., Sasahara, A.A., et al., Graphite pneumoconiosis of electrotypers. Am. J. Med., 41, 864, 1966.
108. Lochtkemper, I., and Teleky, L., Studien uber Staublunge; die in einzelnen besonderen Betrieben und bei besonderen Arbeiten. Arch. Gewerbepath., 3, 600, 1932.
109. Gartner, K., and Brauss, F.W., Russ pneumoconiosis. Med. Welt., 20, 252, 1951.
110. Gloyne, S.R., Marshall, G., and Hoyle, C., Pneumoconiosis due to graphite dust. Thorax, 4, 31, 1949.
111. Meiklejohn, A., In Reports of the 12th International Congress on Occupational Health. Vol. 3. Helsinki, Helsingfors Publications, 1957, p. 335.
112. Koelsch, F., Zum problem der Graphitpneumoconioses. Zentralbl. Arbeitsmed., 8, 1, 1958.
113. Watson, A.K., Black, J., Doig, A.T., and Nagelschmidt, G., Pneumoconiosis in carbon electrode markers. Br. J. Ind. Med., 16, 274, 1959.
114. Miller, A.A., and Ramsden, F., Carbon pneumoconiosis. Br. J. Ind. Med., 18, 103, 1961.
115. Lister, W.B., Carbon pneumoconiosis in a synthetic graphite worker. Br. J. Ind. Med., 18, 114, 1961.
116. Parmeggiani, L., Graphite pneumoconiosis. Br. J. Ind. Med., 7, 42, 1950.
116a. Gardiner, K., Trethowan, N.W., Harrington, J.M., et al., Respiratory effects of carbon black: a survey of European carbon black workers. Br. J. Ind. Med., 50, 1082, 1993.
117. Stewart, M.J., and Faulds, J.S., The pulmonary fibrosis haematite miners. J. Pathol. Bacteriol., 39, 223, 1934.
118. Heath, D., Mool, W., and South, P., The pulmonary vasculature in haematite lung. Br. J. Dis. Chest, 72, 88, 1978.
119. Boyd, J.T., Doll, R., Faulds, J.S., and Leiper, J., Cancer of the lung in iron-ore (haematite) miners. Br. J. Ind. Med., 27, 97, 1970.
120. Roche, A.D., Picard, D., and Vernhes, A., Silicosis of ocher workers (a clinical and anatomo-pathologic study). Am. Rev. Tuberc., 77, 839, 1958.
121. McLaughlin, A.I.G., and Harding, H.E., Pneumoconiosis and other causes of death in iron and steel foundry workers. Arch. Ind. Health, 14, 350, 1956.
122. McLaughlin, A.I.G., Pneumoconiosis in foundry workers. Br. J. Tuberc., 51, 297, 1957.
123. Cordes, L.G., Brink, E.W., Checko, P.J., et al., A cluster of Acinetobacter pneumonia in foundry workers. Ann. Intern. Med., 95, 688, 1981.
124. Harding, H.E., and Massie, A.P., Pneumoconiosis in boiler scalers. Br. J. Ind. Med., 8, 256, 1951.
125. Jones, J.G., and Warner, C.G., Chronic exposure to iron oxide, chromium oxide, and nickel oxide fumes of metal dressers in a steelworks. Br. J. Ind. Med., 129, 169, 1972.
126. Edstrom, H.W., and Rice, D.M.D., "Labrador Lung": an unusual mixed dust pneumoconiosis. Can. Med. Assoc. J., 126, 27, 1982.
127. Agarwal, D.K., Kow, J.L., Srivastava, S.P., and Setth, P.K., Some biochemical and histopathological changes induced by polyvinyl chloride dust in rat lung. Environ. Res., 16, 333, 1978.
128. Richards, R.J., Desai, R., Hext, P.M., and Rose, F.A., Biological reactivity of PVC dust. Nature, 256, 664, 1975.
129. Miller, A., Tiersten, A.S., Chuang, M., et al., Changes in pulmonary function in workers exposed to vinyl chloride and polyvinyl chloride. Ann. N.Y. Acad. Sci., 246, 42, 1975.
130. Lilis, R., Anderson, H., Miller, A., and Selikoff, I.J., Pulmonary changes among vinyl chloride polymerization workers. Chest, 69, 299, 1976.
131. Szende, B., Lapis, K., Nemes, A., and Pinter, A., Pneumoconiosis caused by the inhalation of polyvinylchloride dust. Med. Lav., 61, 433, 1970.
132. Arnaud, A., Pommier De Santi, P., Garbe, L., et al., Polyvinyl chloride pneumoconiosis. Thorax, 33, 19, 1978.

133. Soutar, C.A., Copland, L.H., Thornley, P.E., et al., Epidemiological study of respiratory disease in workers exposed to polyvinyl chloride dust. Thorax, 35, 644, 1980.
134. Zenker, F.A., Ueber Staublinhalationskrankheiten der Lung. Deutch. Arch. Klin. Med., 2, 116, 1866.
135. Doig, A.T., and McLaughlin, A.G., X-ray appearances of the lungs of arc-welders. Lancet, 1, 771, 1936.
136. Harding, H.E., McLaughlin, A.I.G., and Doig, A.T., Clinical, radiographic, and pathological studies of the lungs of electric arc and oxyacetylene welders. Lancet, 2, 394, 1958.
137. Barrie, H.F., and Harding, H.E., Argyro-siderosis of the lungs in silver finishers. Br. J. Ind. Med., 4, 225, 1947.
138. Colleen, M.F.A., A study of pneumonia in shipyard workers with special reference to welders. J. Ind. Hyg., 29, 113, 1947.
139. Doig, A.T., and Duguid, L.N., The health of welders. Ministry of Labour and National Service, London, H.M. Stationery Office, 1951, p. 68.
140. Morgan, W.K.C., and Kerr, H.D., Pathologic and physiologic studies of welder's siderosis. Ann. Intern. Med., 58, 293, 1963.
141. Stern, R.M., Piggott, G.H., and Abraham, J.L., Fibrogenic potential of welding fumes. J. Appl. Toxicol., 3, 18, 1983.
142. Guiodotti, T.L., The higher oxides of nitrogen: inhalation toxicology. Environ. Res., 15, 443, 1978.
143. Challen, P.J.R., Some news on welding and welders. J. Soc. Occup. Med., 24, 38, 1974.
144. Morgan, W.K.C., On welding, wheezing, and whimsy. Am. Ind. Hyg. Assoc. J., 50(2), 59, 1989.
145. McMillan, G.H.G., The health of welders in naval dockyards. Final summary report. J. R. Nav. Med. Serv., 69, 125, 1983.
146. American Welding Society. Fumes and gases in the welding environment. Miami, FL., American Welding Society, 1979.
147. Kalliomaki, P.K., Kalliomaki, K., Korhonen, H., et al., Respiratory studies of stainless steel and mild steel welders. Scand. J. Work Environ. Health, 8(suppl), 1, 117, 1972.
148. Morgan, W.K.C., Industrial bronchitis. Br. J. Ind. Med., 35, 285, 1978.
149. Harries, P.G., Experience with asbestos disease and its control in Great Britain's naval dockyards. Environ. Res., 11, 261, 1976.
150. Hunnicutt, T.N., Cracovaner, D.J., and Myles, J.T., Spirometric measurements in welders. Arch. Environ. Health, 8, 66, 1964.
151. Peters, J.M., Murphy, R.L.H., and Ferris, B.G., Jr., Pulmonary function in shipyard welders. Arch. Environ. Health, 26, 28, 1973.
152. McMillan, G.H.G., Studies of the health of welders in naval dockyards. Ann. Occup. Hyg., 21, 377, 1979.
153. McMillan, G.H.G., and Pethybridge, R.J., A clinical, radiological and pulmonary function case-control study of 135 dockyard welders aged 45 yeras and over. J. Soc. Occup. Med., 34, 3, 1984.
154. McMillan, G.H.G., The health of welders in naval dockyards: welding, tobacco smoking and absence attributed to respiratory disease. J. Soc. Occup. Med., 31, 112, 1981.
155. Meyer, E.C., Kratzinger, S.F., and Miller, W.H., Pulmonary fibrosis in an arc welder. Arch. Environ. Health, 15, 463, 1967.
156. Charr, R., Respiratory diseases among welders. J.A.M.A., 152, 1520, 1953.
157. Charr, R., Respiratory diseases among welders. Am. Rev. Tuberc., 71, 877, 1955.
158. Charr, R., Pulmonary changes in welders. Ann. Intern. Med., 44, 806, 1956.
159. Friede, E., and Rachow, D.O., Symptomatic pulmonary disease in welders. Ann. Intern. Med., 54, 121, 1961.
160. Mann, B.T., and Lecutier, E.R., Arc welder's lung. Br. Med. J., 2, 921, 1957.
161. Morley, R., and Silk, S.J., The industrial hazard from nitrous fumes. Ann. Occup. Hyg., 13, 101, 1970.
162. Harding, H.E., Grout, J.L.A., and Lloyd Davies, T.H., The experimental production of x-ray shadows in the lungs by inhalation of industrial dusts. 1. Iron oxide. Br. J. Ind. Med., 4, 223, 1947.
163. Morgan, W.K.C., Arc welders' lung complicated by conglomeration. Am. Rev. Respir. Dis., 85, 570, 1962.
164. Brun, J., Cassan, G., Kofman, J., and Gilly, J., La sidero-sclerose des soudeurs a l'arc a forme de fibrose interstitielle diffuse et a forme conglomerative pseudo-tumorale. Poumonet Coeur, 28, 3, 1972.
165. Kalliomaki, P.K., Sutinen, S., Kelha, V., et al., Amount and distribution of fume contaminants in the lungs of an arc-welder at post mortem. Br. J. Ind. Med., 36, 224, 1979.
166. Stanescu, D.C., Pilat, L., Gavrilescu, N., et al., Aspects of pulmonary mechanics in welder's siderosis. Br. J. Ind. Med., 24, 143, 1967.
167. Teculescu, D., and Albu, A., Pulmonary function in workers inhaling iron oxide dust. Int. Arch. Arbeitmed., 31, 163, 1973.
168. Morgan, W.K.C., Magnetite pneumoconiosis. J. Occup. Med., 20, 762, 1978.
169. Kleinfeld, M., Messite, J., and Shapiro, J., A clinical, roentgenological and physiological study of magnetite workers. Arch. Environ. Health, 16, 392, 1968.
170. Hoover, H.C., and Hoover, H.L., Footnotes. In Agricola, G., De re Metallica, 1556. In The Mining Magazine, London, 1912, pp. 283–354.

171. Robertson, A.J., The romance of tin. Lancet, 1, 1229, 1289, 1964.
172. Robertson, A.J., Rivers, D., Nagelschmidt, G., and Duncumb, P., Stannosis. Lancet, 1, 1089, 1961.
173. Pendergrass, E.P., and Pryde, A.W., Benign pneumoconiosis due to tin oxide: a case report with experimental investigation of the radiographic density of the tin oxide dust. J. Ind. Hyg., 30, 119, 1948.
174. Bergmann, M., Flance, I.J., and Blumenthal, H.T., Thesaurosis following inhalation of hair spray: a clinical and experimental study. N. Engl. J. Med., 258, 471, 1958.
175. Bergmann, M., Flance, I.J., Cruz., P.T., et al., Thesaurosis due to inhalation of hair spray: a report of 12 new cases, including three autopsies. N. Engl. J. Med., 266, 750, 1962.
176. Edelson, B.G., Thesaurosis following inhalation of hair spray. Lancet, 2, 112, 1959.
177. Nevins, M.A., Stechel, G.H., Fishman, S.I., et al., Pulmonary granulomatoses: two cases associated with inhalation of cosmetic aerosols. J.A.M.A., 193, 266, 1965.
178. Gowdy, J.M., and Wagstaff, M.J., Pulmonary infiltration due to aerosol thesaurosis. Arch. Environ. Health, 25, 101, 1972.
179. Draize, H.J., Nelson, A.A.., Newburger, S.H., et al., Inhalation toxicity studies of six types of aerosol hair sprays. Proc. Sci. Sec. Toilet Goods Assoc., 31, 28, 1959.
180. Calandra, J., and Kay, J.A., The effects of aerosol hair sprays on experimental animals. Proc. Sci. Sec. Toilet Goods Assoc., 30, 41, 1958.
181. Giovacchini, R.P., Becker, G.H., Brunner, M.J., and Dunlap, F.E., Pulmonary disease and hair spray polymers. J.A.M.A., 193, 298, 1965.
182. McLaughlin, A.I.G., and Bidstrup, P.L., The effects of hair lacquer sprays on the lungs. Fed. Cosmet. Toxicol., 1, 171, 1963.
183. Sharma, O.P., and Williams, M.H., Thesaurosis. Arch. Environ. Health, 13, 616, 1966.
184. Larson, R.K., A study of midexpiratory flow rate in users of hair spray. Am. Rev. Respir. Dis., 90, 786, 1964.
185. Palmer, A.A., A morbidity survey of respiratory symptoms and functions among Utah beauticians. Ph.D. dissertation, University of Utah, 1974.
186. Zuskin, E., and Bouhuys, A., Acute airway responses to hair spray preparations. N. Engl. J. Med., 290, 660, 1974.
187. Frank, R., Are aerosol sprays hazardous? Am. Rev. Respir. Dis., 112, 485, 1975.
188. Sjogren, I., Hillerdal, G., Andersson, A., and Zetterstrom, O., Hard metal lung disease: importance of cobalt in coolants. Thorax, 35, 653, 1980.
189. Bech, A.O., Kipling, M.D., and Heather, J.C., Hard metal disease. Br. J. Ind. Med., 19, 239, 1962.
190. Payne, L.R., Hazards of cobalt. J. Soc. Occup. Med., 27, 20, 1977.
191. Cugell, D.W., Morgan, W.K.C., Perkins, D.G., et al., The respiratory effects of cobalt. Arch. Intern. Med., 150, 177, 1990.
192. Davison, A.G., Haslam, P.L., Corrin, B., et al., Interstitial lung disease and asthma in hard metal workers: bronchoalveolar lavage, ultrastructural, and analytical findings and results of bronchial provocation tests. Thorax, 38, 119, 1983.
193. Demedts, M., Gheysens, B., Nagels, J., et al., Cobalt lung in diamond polishers. Am. Rev. Respir. Dis., 130, 130, 1984.
194. Nemery, B., Casier, P., Roosels, D., et al., Survey of cobalt exposure and respiratory health in diamond polishers. Am. Rev. Respir. Dis., 145, 610, 1992.
195. Jobs, H., and Ballhausen, C., Powder metallurgy as a source of dust from the medical and technical standpoint. Vertrauensartz u. Krankenkasse, 8, 142, 1940.
196. Moschinski, G., Jurisch, A., and Reinl, W., Die Lungenveranderungen bei Sinterhartmetallarbeitern. Arch. Gewerbepath., 16, 697, 1959.
197. Fairhall, L.T., Castberg, H.T., Carrosso, N.J., and Brinton, H.P., Industrial hygiene aspects of the cemented tungsten carbide industry. Occup. Med., 4, 371, 1947.
198. Harding, H.E., Notes on the toxicology of cobalt metal. Br. J. Ind. Med., 7, 76, 1950.
199. Delahant, A.B., An experimental study of the effects of rare metals on animal lungs. A.M.A. Arch. Ind. Health, 12, 116, 1955.
200. Kerfoot, E.J., Fredrick, W.G., and Domeier, E., Cobalt metal inhalation studies on miniature swine. Am. Ind. Hyg. Assoc. J., 36, 17, 1975.
201. Griffith, W.H., Paviek, P.L., and Mulford, P.J., The relation of the sulfur amino-acids to the toxicity of cobalt and nickel in the rat. J. Nutr., 23, 603, 1942.
202. Coates, E.O., Jr., and Watson, J.H.L., Diffuse interstitial lung disease in tungsten carbide workers. Ann. Intern. Med., 75, 709, 1971.
203. Coates, E.O., Jr., and Watson, J.H.L., Pathology of the lung in tungsten carbide workers using light and electron microscopy. J. Occup. Med., 15, 280, 1973.
204. Sprince, N.L., Oliver, L.C., Eisen, E.A., et al., Cobalt exposure and lung disease in tungsten carbide production. A cross sectional study of current workers. Am. Rev. Respir. Dis., 138, 1220, 1988.
205. Coates, E.O., Jr., Sawyer, H.J., Rebuck, J.W., et al., Hypersensitivity bronchitis in tungsten carbide workers. Chest, 64, 390, 1973.
206. Kusaka, Y., Yokoyama, K., Sera, Y., et al., Respiratory diseases in hard metal workers: an occupational hygiene study in a factory. Br. J. Ind. Med., 43, 474, 1986.
207. Pimentel, J.C., A granulomatous lung disease produced by bakelite: a clinico-pathologic and experimental study. Am. Rev. Respir. Dis., 108, 1303, 1973.
208. Haley, T.J., Pharmacology and toxicology of rare earth elements. J. Pharm. Sci., 54, 663, 1965.

209. Nappee, J., Bobrie, J., and Lambard, D., Pneumoconioses au cerium. Arch. Med. Profess. Med. Travail Sec. Soc., 33, 13, 1972.
210. Evans, D.J., and Posner, E., Pneumoconiosis in laundry workers. Environ. Res., 4, 121, 1971.
211. Schmitz-Moorman, P., Horlein, H., and Hanefield, F., Lungenveranderungen bei Titandioxyd staub Exposition. Beitr. Silikose Forschung, 80, 1, 1964.
212. Daum, S., Anderson, H.A., Lilis, R., et al., Pulmonary changes among titanium workers [Abstract]. Proc. Roy. Soc. Med., 70, 31, 1977.
213. Chen, J.L., and Fayerweather, W.E., Epidemiologic study of workers exposed to titanium dioxide. J. Occup. Med., 30, 937, 1988.
214. Harding, H.E., and Lloyd Davies, T.H., The experimental production of industrial dust. Part II. Zirconium. Br. J. Ind. Med., 9, 70, 1952.
215. Reed, C.E., A study of the effects on the lungs of industrial exposure to zirconium dusts. A.M.A. Arch. Ind. Health, 13, 578, 1956.
216. McCallum, R.I., The work of an environmental health service in environmental control. Ann. Occup. Hyg., 6, 55, 1953.
217. Sherson, D., Maltblaek, N., and Olsen, O., Small opacities among dental laboratory technicians in Copenhagen. Br. J. Ind. Med., 45, 320, 1988.
218. Rom, W.N., Lockey, J.E., Lee, J.S., et al., Pneumoconiosis and exposures of dental laboratory technicians. Am. J. Public Health, 74, 1252, 1981.
219. Barrett, T.E., Pietra, G.G., Mayock, R.L., et al., Acrylic resin pneumoconiosis: report of a case in a dental student. Am. Rev. Respir. Dis., 139, 841, 1989.
220. Osbern, L.N., and Crapo, R.N., Dung lung: a report of toxic exposure to liquid manure. Ann. Intern. Med., 95, 312, 1981.
221. Golden, E.B., Warnock, M.L., Hulett Jr., L.D., and Churg, A., Fly ash lung: a new pneumoconiosis? Am. Rev. Respir. Dis., 125, 108, 1982.
222. Buchanan, D.R., Lamb, D., and Seaton, A., Punk rocker's lung: pulmonary fibrosis in a drug snorting fire-eater. Br. Med. J., 283, 1661, 1981.

17

Occupational Asthma

Anthony Seaton

Sporadic reports of occupational asthma occur in the early literature; the best known is Ramazzini's description of the breathlessness (and urticarial reactions) that he recognized among grain workers in the 18th century.[1] There is some evidence that allergic diseases, particularly rhinitis, became more common in the Industrial Revolution.[2] In the 19th century, the clinical picture of allergy became a familiar one with the recognition that exposure to many substances, such as animals, hay and grains, pollens, and certain dusts, could provoke attacks of rhinitis and wheeze in a proportion of the population, although the term itself was only coined by van Pirquet in 1906.[3] In the 1920s, Coca and Cooke[4, 5] pointed to the genetic basis of allergy and defined the clinical syndrome of atopy, manifesting itself as asthma and rhinitis and subject to hereditary influence. They demonstrated that first-degree relatives of patients with multiple immediate skin reactions frequently had asthma or hay fever themselves. More recently, molecular genetic studies have shown atopy to be transmitted in some families by a gene situated on chromosome 11q.[6, 7] Such subjects, who may number up to 25% of the population, have been shown to be particularly liable to hypersensitivity to inhaled antigens, particularly those of animal and vegetable origin, in the course of occupational exposure.[8–10] Nevertheless, many people in whom occupational asthma develops are nonatopic; such subjects usually acquire asthma rather later than do atopic patients.

Over the last two decades, occupational asthma has attracted considerable attention. In the 1970s and 1980s, a series of studies of specific causes of occupational asthma in England built on the earlier work of Gandevia in Australia in developing simple, practicable methods of investigation.[11–15] Further studies, notably by Chan-Yeung in Canada,[16–18] drew attention to the widespread nature of the problem in different industries. Work in Finland in the 1970s and 1980s had estimated an annual incidence of occupational asthma of around 70 per 1 million population,[19, 20] and more recent studies in Britain have recorded around 22 per 1 million in that country.[21]

WHAT IS OCCUPATIONAL ASTHMA?

This question is not so straightforward as it might seem. Indeed, it is far from clear what asthma is; most workers who have studied the problem have relied on operational definitions suited to the purpose of their study. The classic presentation of asthma, with intermittent episodes of wheeze, cough, and breathlessness, is easy to recognize, and most definitions emphasize these characteristics. Difficulties arise, however, when the presentation is insidious and less episodic, when cough is the primary symptom, and when the subject has another condition which presents similar features, most notably smoking-induced airway disease. Epidemiologic studies of populations regularly reveal a proportion, round about 5%, who have had asthma diagnosed clinically, a further 15% or so who admit to episodes of intermittent wheeze, and a majority who deny any such symptoms. Specific questions that ask about wheeze after colds or exercise can identify a further proportion with symptoms. This gives rise to the concept of a population not divided into asthmatic and nonasthmatic people but rather distributed on a spectrum of bronchial reactivity. Thus, everyone has the potential to have asthmatic symptoms, but this potential is much greater in some than in others. The potential may be modulated by genetic or environmental factors, and in many cases, both play a role. Of the genetic factors, atopy is the only one that has been clearly recognized. However, since familial asthma may occur in the absence of atopy, others may remain to be discovered. For example, it is not inconceivable that genetic modulation of the lungs' antioxidant defense mechanisms may occur, e.g., there is a genetic basis for regulation of levels of glucose-6-phosphate dehydrogenase, which, in turn, controls the production of reduced glutathione, a major antioxidant.

Much work remains to be done, using modern molecular techniques, on the genetics of atopic and nonatopic asthma. Equally exciting to the researcher, however, is the influence of environmental factors.[22, 23] This is particularly so since there is increasing evidence that asthma is becoming more common within Western society and that it also becomes more prevalent in peoples who migrate to such a society from more primitive ones.[24, 25] Such evidence points to the importance of environmental factors related to industrialization, e.g., tobacco smoke, air pollution, increased exposure to allergens, and alterations in diet as the most obvious contenders. Whatever their relative importance, and the author favors the last of these as being the most plausible,[25a] something in the environment over the last 20 to 30 years seems to have caused a shift in the population's liability to wheeze and have clinical asthma.

Occupational asthma may be defined clinically as wheezy breathlessness occurring after exposure to a sensitizer at work. It should be recognized, however, that this definition is exclusive since it rules out wheezy breathlessness that might follow exposure to toxic gases or fumes or exposure to pharmacological bronchoconstrictors. It also excludes exercise-induced asthma but not subjects with prior asthmatic symptoms whose symptoms subsequently worsen as a consequence of sensitization in the workplace. A broader definition might reasonably include pharmacological asthma and wheezy symptoms after exposure to irritants. These syndromes are also discussed in this chapter.

MECHANISMS

The classic concept is of airway inflammation and smooth muscle constriction occurring as a consequence of an antigen-antibody reaction. The antibody is usually a specific immunoglobulin E (IgE).[26] Little of this is found in the blood of normal subjects, but larger amounts are present in atopic individuals. It is a glycoprotein with a molecular weight of 190,000, and it has a remarkable affinity for mast cells and basophils. Up to 40,000 molecules can bind onto one such cell. A pair of such molecules, bridged by one of antigen, attach to the surface of bronchial mast cells. This alters the membrane properties, allows the intake of calcium into the cell through channels under the control of cyclic adenosine monophosphate, and leads to immediate release of histamine and the synthesis of slower acting mediators of inflammation. This concept is, however, only a partial explanation of a complex series of events which also involves (at least) lymphocytes and eosinophils. A more complete, but still undoubtedly oversimplified, account of the mechanisms has antigen reacting not only with the mast cell but also with submucosal TH_2 lymphocytes.[27] These cells produce interleukins, which attract and prime mast cells, B lymphocytes, and eosinophils. The B lymphocytes produce IgE, and the eosinophils produce a large number of preformed proteins, including major basic protein, and other substances, such as prostaglandins and platelet-activating factor, which act as mediators of airway inflammation.[28] The mast cell produces a range of mediators, including histamine and an eosinophil chemotactic factor. All these events contribute to the pathologic features of asthma, i.e., airway mucosal edema and inflammation characterized by eosinophils and lymphocytes, smooth muscle constriction and hypertrophy, and exudation of protein-rich fluid into the airway's lumen. Two other features should be mentioned: the separation of strips of mucosa from the basement membrane and characteristic thickening of that membrane. This suggests that the action of a protease causes the separation, the thickening being due to secretion of further basement membrane material by regenerating mucosal cells.

These still partly hypothetical concepts allow the establishment of a vicious circle, with airway inflammation causing increased mucosal permeability and, therefore, more ready access of antigen to mediator cells. It is also possible to conceive how airway inflammation *per se,* caused by irritant chemicals, could cause the clinical features of asthma by a local effect on the mucosa and smooth muscle.

Many of the well-known causes of occupational asthma can elicit an IgE-mediated response.[29] Into this category fall the classic animal and plant antigens, such as proteins from domestic pets, laboratory animals, and horses and from grains. In addition, IgE-mediated reactions have been implicated in a number of examples of asthma resulting from low molecular weight chemicals, such as those caused by the acid anhydrides used in epoxy resin systems and by some reactive dyes.[30, 31] In these circumstances, it is likely that the chemical reacts with body proteins to form a hapten, which then acts as the sensitizing agent. In contrast, in a number of cases, no specific IgE has been demonstrated to chemicals that are undoubted sensitizers. These include two of the most common causes of occupational asthma: isocyanates and colophony. Although it is possible that such chemicals act in a different, possibly pharmacological, way, it is more likely that the investigations so far have not produced the relevant antigen, perhaps because the protein combines not with the original compound but with one of its reaction products. At least with respect to colophony, its ability to combine with protein to form a hapten has been shown in mice and guinea pigs.[32]

Two other mechanisms should be discussed, direct pharmacological effects on the airways and acute irritation leading to airway hyperirritability, the so-called reactive airways dysfunction syndrome (RADS).[33] When direct pharmacological effects may be relevant, we might expect a relatively brief bronchoconstrictive episode, mimicking the immediate reaction in a challenge test. Such episodes appear to be rare in practice, although these were the characteristics of the attacks suffered by patients in the population epidemics in Barcelona,[34] which were related to the unloading of soybeans in the docks. It has been suggested that they may have been due to lipoxygenase enzymes, in which soybean is rich, causing release of eicosenoids and thus stimulation of eosinophils to release the bronchoconstrictor lipoxin A_4.[35] If this is the case, it suggests a novel mechanism for some plant-induced asthmas. A less subtle pharmacological cause of asthma may be the inhalation at work of anticholinesterase insecticides, which can have a direct bronchoconstrictive effect.[36]

RADS occurs as a consequence of mucosal damage or inflammation after acute exposure to a toxic chemical.[33] Sensitization is not involved, but the patient is left with airway hyper-reactivity, which is characterized clinically by recurrent wheeze and cough precipitated by nonspecific stimuli, such as tobacco smoke, cold air, strong smells, and taking deep breaths. This is discussed further in the section on clinical features.

Bronchial hyper-responsiveness is present in most subjects with occupational asthma, whatever the cause.[37] Nevertheless, it should be realized that about one third of people with asthma resulting from isocyanates and colophony show no evidence of excessive reactivity of the airways.[38]

EPIDEMIOLOGY

The prevalence or incidence of occupational asthma is not known in most countries, including the United States. One survey of disability by the Social Security Administration in 1978 showed a self-reported diagnosis of asthma in 7.7% of respondents, 15.4% of these attributing their illness to their working conditions.[39] Some attempts have been made to obtain better information, however, in some other countries. Surveys in Finland have shown an annual incidence rate of 71 per 1 million working population.[20] In Britain, since 1989, there has been a voluntary scheme for reporting occupational respiratory diseases in which a high proportion of chest physicians and occupational physicians participate (the so-called SWORD project for surveillance of work-related and occupational respiratory disorders).[21] The definition of an occupational respiratory disease is simple; it is regarded as one by the reporting physician. The reports are therefore based on a clinical diagnosis which does not necessarily require special tests. Over the first 3 years of the project, 1513 cases of occupational asthma were reported (26% of the total of occupational respiratory diseases). There are reasons to believe that this probably underestimates the true total by a factor of three. The annual incidence, calculated from the 1513 cases in a working population of about 26.5 million, is about 23 per 1 million per year in men and 13 per 1 million per year in women. These rates are of course largely influenced by most workers not being exposed to sensitizers at work, and they become more meaningful when individual occupations are examined. Assuming similar working techniques, such figures may give a rough idea of likely incidence in the United States. Some figures from the SWORD project are given in Table 17–1.

The high incidence of occupational asthma in painters and plastics and chemical workers probably reflects the importance of isocyanates and epoxy resins; laboratory animals, grain, and wood dusts are responsible for many of the other high rates. In some industries in which specific studies of incidence have been made, still higher rates have been described, and it should be recalled that these SWORD figures may only represent one third of the true incidence. A recent survey of a random sample of adults in 60,000 households in Great Britain has asked for self-reporting of work-related disease.[40] From the responses, it has been possible to estimate that, in the year of the study, approximately 30,000 people had asthma which they believed was due to their work. This figure represents 1.2 per 1000 of the current British work force and is likely to represent an upper limit of current prevalence.

Over the first 3 years of the SWORD project, many different causes of occupational asthma have been reported. The most common of these are given in

Table 17–1
■
Occupational Asthma in United Kingdom 1989–91: Incidence Rates

Selected Occupational Group	Cases	Rate per Million per Year
Spray painters	108	729
Plastics workers	71	339
Chemical processors	75	337
Bakers	64	285
Laboratory workers	88	220
Metal treatment workers	51	211
Welders/electronics	106	158
Food processors	59	121
Hairdressers	24	81
Other painters	34	53
Farm workers	43	34

Table 17–2
■
Occupational Asthma in United Kingdom 1989–91: Main Causes

Cause	Number	Percentage
Isocyanates	326	22
Flour, grain, hay	108	7
Laboratory animals	87	6
Solder/colophony	85	6
Glues, resins	80	5
Wood	63	4
Other animals	61	4
Metals	58	4
Welding fume	35	2
Glutaraldehyde	30	2
Paints	29	2
Cutting oils	22	1
Inks and dyes	21	1

Table 17–2. The highest proportion of cases, 35%, was attributed to chemicals, followed by 25% attributed to organic substances.

CLINICAL FEATURES

Whereas occupational asthma may occur only after several years of exposure to the relevant sensitizer, it most typically starts within a few weeks or months of first exposure, although only after a symptom-free period. This distinguishes it from RADS, which usually occurs immediately after exposure to high levels of an irritant chemical. The initial symptom is often a tickly dry cough, although in many cases, especially where protein antigens are concerned, rhinitis and itchy conjunctivitis are also common. When taking a history from the patient suspected of having occupational asthma, it is essential to obtain a detailed account of the start of the illness. Typically, in these early stages, the attacks are mild with cough and wheeze occurring toward the end of the working day and remitting at weekends. There may be a history of handling or being exposed to fumes or dust from a known sensitizer, and it is always necessary to ask the patient if there has been exposure to any chemicals, dusts, fumes, or animal or vegetable matter. If there has, the patient may be aware of a relationship in time between the exposure and attacks. This is especially the case if exposure has been intermittent. The patient often notices this relationship, and such information, although it may sometimes be misleading, should never be disregarded by the doctor. Sometimes, with intermittent exposure, the attack may last for several days, and a pattern of recurring attacks over days or even weeks after a single exposure has been described.[41] There may also be a history of others in the workplace being affected, and this information is often extremely useful. In most circumstances, for example, with work forces exposed to isocyanates and laboratory animals, asthma develops in fewer than 10% of those exposed. If a very high proportion of workers have symptoms, the exposure is more likely to be to an irritant, although it should be remembered that several chemicals may be irritant to many but sensitizers to a few, e.g., glutaraldehyde and formaldehyde.

As the condition progresses, usually over a period of several months, the symptoms tend to become more severe, to start earlier and last longer, to wake the patient during sleep, and to impinge on the weekend. If the condition is not recognized and the cause eliminated, continued exposure will often lead to persistent severe asthma indistinguishable from that occurring in a nonoccupational setting. Remissions initially occur on holidays, but even this feature may disappear after sufficiently prolonged exposure.

The patient may have an exquisite sensitivity to the causative sensitizer, especially if this is a reactive chemical, so that exposure to extremely low concentrations may result in an attack. This may be responsible for continued symptoms in some cases in which a worker has been redeployed to another part of the same workplace; walking past a door or meeting colleagues wearing their working clothes in the canteen may be sufficient to provoke an attack. Furthermore, sensitivity persists for a prolonged period, and re-exposure after an interval may provoke severe attacks. Deaths have occurred in these circumstances in relation to exposure to isocyanates and powdered organic dyes.[42, 43]

If the worker is able to avoid further exposure, the natural history of occupational asthma is a gradual improvement in the symptoms. The clinical experience of the author suggests very strongly that the rate of improvement depends on the length of continued exposure after the symptoms first occurred. In those cases, for example, shellfish workers, in whom obvious symptoms of rhinitis and wheeze force the worker to leave work soon after the condition starts, recovery is usually complete and rapid. In others, in whom the onset has been insidious and there has been delay in making the diagnosis, it is usual for symptoms to persist for several years, although there is normally a steady amelioration. This relationship between the length of exposure after symptoms developed and persistence of symptoms has been demonstrated in workers exposed to western red cedar and isocyanates.[44, 45] In some relatively mild cases, it is possible for the employee to stay at work if appropriate precautions are taken and prophylactic drugs are given. Most commonly, however, redeployment to a different process and building is necessary (see Management).

Risk Factors

The major risk factor for occupational asthma is, of course, the extent of exposure to the sensitizer, and workplaces that allow high and frequent exposure of workers to airborne sensitizers may expect a high rate of respiratory problems. Two individual factors have also been shown to be of some importance. With respect to protein antigens, atopy, as defined by positive skin prick tests to common antigens, increases the risk of an individual becoming sensitized and contributes to earlier sensitization.[46, 47] However, since atopic people are generally in the minority and since nonatopic workers are also at some, although lower, risk, it is generally believed that exclusion of atopic workers from a work force makes an insubstantial contribution to solving the problem while unnecessarily penalizing a number of potentially useful workers.[48] (This is discussed under Management.) In contrast, someone who already has clinical manifestations of asthma or allergic rhinitis is probably at sufficient risk of having worsening symptoms to be excluded from work with known sensitizers.

There is now good evidence, at least with respect to platinum refinery and snow crab workers and people exposed to several other sensitizers (including acid anhydrides and ispaghula), that smoking increases the risk of sensitization and the development of IgE antibodies.[49–52] Interestingly, smoking is also reported to have been a factor in the development of attacks of asthma in the soybean epidemics in Barcelona.[35] There is experimental support for the concept that local airway inflammation associated with inhalation of irritants, such as tobacco smoke, ozone, and sulfur dioxide, may increase susceptibility to inhaled antigen.[53, 54]

Reactive Airways Dysfunction Syndrome

Most people exposed transiently to high concentrations of irritant fumes experience a few days of irritant cough and, sometimes, wheeze.[33, 55] A small proportion, however, have more persistent cough and attacks of wheezy breathlessness. These occur typically at night; on exposure to cold air; during exercising or otherwise taking deep breaths; or on exposure to smoke, fumes, or strong smells.

The natural history of the condition is one of gradual improvement, although this may sometimes take years. Occasionally, persistent asthma results.

In RADS, the initial exposure is usually a dramatic episode, and others close by are often affected. In extreme cases, it merges with bronchiolitis obliterans (see Chapter 20). The patient demonstrates bronchial hyperreactivity on testing with histamine or metacholine, but no specific bronchial sensitization is present.

INVESTIGATION OF OCCUPATIONAL ASTHMA

The Patient

The diagnosis of occupational asthma requires several steps. First, does the patient have asthma? Second, is the asthma work related? Third, is the work-related asthma caused by sensitization or some other mechanism? The main problems lie in differentiating work-related asthma from other forms of asthma occurring coincidentally, but RADS and exacerbations of smoking-induced air-flow obstruction may also cause difficulties.

The essential step in the diagnosis is to take a careful history of the onset and early stages of the condition and of any substances that may cause sensitization to which the patient may have been exposed. In many (but not all) cases, the patient has a shrewd idea as to what brings on the symptoms, and the presence of this can be confirmed by an approach to the workplace if necessary (see next section). If the patient does not know but the history suggests work-related disease, questions should be asked about work with animals, vegetable products, dusts, or fumes from chemicals (including pharmaceuticals and food additives) and the use of paints and adhesives.

Physical examination of the patient is unhelpful, except in the negative sense of excluding other disease, and the same applies to chest radiography. However, if the diagnosis is suspected, the implications for the patient in terms of future health and earning capability are so great that further investigation is always necessary. Two such investigations are practicable: documentation of work-related impairment of air flow and demonstration of specific sensitization to the offending antigen.

The first investigative step should normally be to provide the patient with a lightweight portable peak flow meter and a diary card (Fig. 17–1). The patient should be instructed in the use of the meter and asked to record peak flow, as the best of three good blows, at least four times daily. Some authorities suggest that

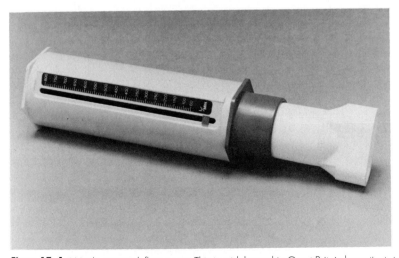

Figure 17–1. Wright minipeak flow meter. This is widely used in Great Britain by patients to monitor the status of their asthma, and is ideal for studies of occupational asthma.

recording every 2 hours is desirable, although in the author's view, this is rarely necessary or achievable in clinical practice. The results should be written down by the patient on the diary card and any symptoms and use of medication recorded. Exposure to any factors suspected of causing asthma should also be noted, and care should be taken to record days on and off work.

The author's preferred method is to ask the patient to make recordings over 1 to 2 weeks while still at work and then to continue over a period off work. The length of this period will depend on the symptoms. In some cases, when the symptoms are of short duration, improvement occurs quickly after leaving work, and 1 week is sufficient (Fig. 17–2). In others, with more long-standing disease, the condition remits only slowly, and several weeks are necessary to show the change (Fig. 17–3). In most circumstances, the patient should then return to work and continue recording, although care should be exercised if the patient is likely to be very sensitive or exposed to high levels of the antigen. In most cases, this simple technique is adequate to demonstrate whether or not work-related asthma is occurring. If clear falls in peak flow occur during the working week, with improvements on days off, it is highly likely that occupational asthma is present, even if the cause is not obvious (Fig. 17–4). If the record shows reasonably normal flow rates and little change, it is equally likely that the patient does not have occupational asthma. Difficulties arise only when there is a very variable and low flow rate without obvious change on days off because this pattern may occur in long-standing severe occupational asthma. Observation over a prolonged period off work may help to resolve this problem, as may tests for specific sensitization.

The tests of specific sensitization consist of skin prick tests, radioallergosorbent (RAST) tests, and bronchial challenge. The first two are only available when specific antigen and IgE antibodies have been identified. It should be noted that they indicate sensitization rather than disease and are therefore only indirect evidence of causation. Nevertheless, positive skin test and/or RAST results to an antigen to which the patient with work-related wheeze is known to be exposed are strong evidence that that substance is to blame. In general, after exposure has ceased skin test and RAST findings may be expected to remain positive for up to 6

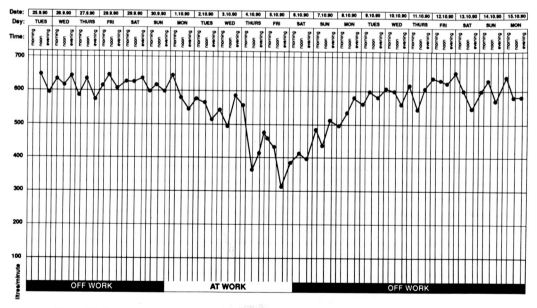

Figure 17–2. Peak flow recordings during a patient sensitized to grain dust. The fall occurred during working in the loading bay of a manufacturer of animal food and remitted when the patient was off work.

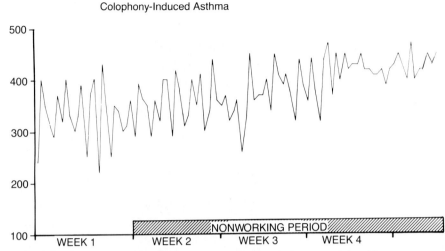

Colophony-Induced Asthma

Figure 17–3. Peak flow recordings by a patient sensitized to colophony. Variability of flow rate was reduced and absolute level rose only slowly after ceasing exposure to soldering fumes.

to 12 months.[56] Bronchial challenge, in contrast, is the only wholly specific diagnostic test. The technique favored by most physicians is that popularized by Pepys and his colleagues at the Brompton Hospital in London, England.[57] In this, patients are exposed to the suspected sensitizer in a way in which they might be exposed at work, although in a setting where symptoms can be controlled and lung function measured (Fig. 17–5). If possible, the concentration of sensitizer in the air the patient breathes should be monitored, and exposure should be controlled by limiting duration. Low exposures should be given initially. Controls should be used, and lung function (plethysmography has no substantial advantages over spirometry) should be measured before the test and every few minutes after for several hours. If no reaction occurs, the test should be repeated on another day, with a higher exposure.

The most usual response to a challenge test is an immediate fall in flow rates, lasting up to about 1 hour. This, in itself, is not diagnostic of sensitization, unless it occurs after a low concentration, since it can result from inhalation of irritants in people with hyper-reactive airways. A later, secondary, fall in flow rates, starting

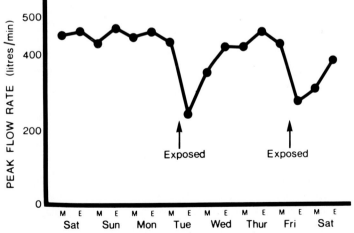

Figure 17–4. Record of peak flow rate kept by patient during a working week. Subsequent investigation revealed the use of isocyanates in the factory on Tuesday and Friday.

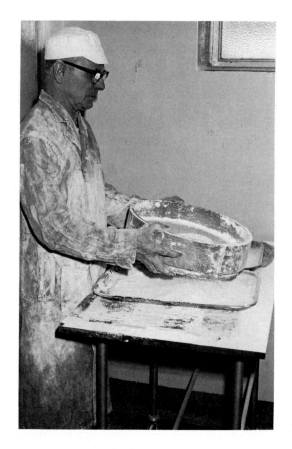

Figure 17–5
Investigation of suspected occupational asthma. The patient, a fitter in a bakery, was suspected of being allergic to flour. Wheezing and a fall in peak flow rates developed after he had spent 15 minutes sieving flour. Similar changes were not recorded after he had sieved sugar.

after about 3 hours and often lasting 12 to 24 hours, is however diagnostic of sensitization. Such a biphasic response to challenge testing (Fig. 17–6) usually follows a rather large exposure, but it should be anticipated in all such tests. The test should therefore be carried out only in a hospital enivronment, and the patient should be kept in for at least 8 hours after the challenge. If a late reaction has not started by then, it is unlikely to occur. However, challenge testing (like occupational exposure) may provoke recurrent subsequent attacks of asthma over several days. The patient should be warned of this possibility and advised what to do and what treatment to take if it does occur.

Inhalation challenge testing is only necessary in a small minority of patients with suspected occupational asthma since the investigations described previously almost always lead to a sufficiently sure diagnosis for action to be taken. In the author's experience, challenge tests have proved useful in the following:

1. When occupational asthma is suspected, but the agent to which the worker is exposed has not previously been recognized as a cause.
2. When the patient is exposed to more than one potential cause.
3. When the diagnosis is in doubt, to confirm that it is safe for the patient to continue working with the suspected agent.
4. In cases in which there appears to be a mixed reaction, with features of both asthma and alveolitis.

Of course, challenge testing has an important part to play (when fully informed consent has been obtained) in research into the mechanisms of occupational asthma. As a test with potentially harmful consequences, however, it does not play a role in coming to a decision purely for medicolegal purposes. It should always be remembered that, first, the medicolegal test of causality, i.e., the balance of probabilities, is considerably less stringent than a test of clinical certainty, and second,

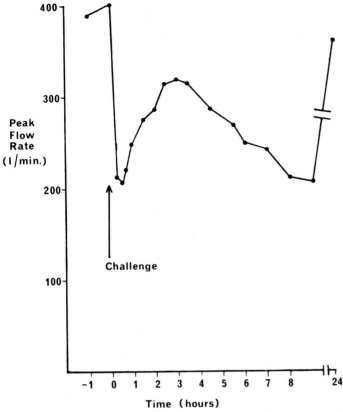

Figure 17–6. Record of peak flow rate of patient before and after a 5-minute challenge with toluene diisocyanate, by using marine varnish. The immediate fall was followed by a later and more prolonged fall.

that potentially harmful investigations should only be carried out if the results hold hope of benefit to the patient's health.

Tests of bronchial hyper-reactivity are of some clinical value in following the course of occupational asthma after exposure has ceased and in the investigation of suspected RADS. Their main role, however, consists in shedding light on the mechanisms of occupational asthma in research studies. Relatively simple tests, using doubling doses of histamine or metacholine until a 20% fall in forced expiratory volume in 1 second has occurred, have proved practicable and reproducible.[58]

The Workplace

The clinician, out of concern for the welfare of the patient, should not forget that occupational disease indicates a problem in a workplace and, therefore, that other workers may also be affected. This puts a rather wider responsibility on the doctor than may be the case with nonoccupational disease. Moreover, occupational asthma always carries the serious implication that, unless something is done about the workplace, the patient may have to give up the job. Doctors sometimes advise this rather lightly; those who do should consider how they would react if someone gave them the same advice!

It follows that, whenever occupational asthma is diagnosed, a workplace visit is desirable. This matter has been discussed in Chapter 2, to which the reader is referred. The visit should be made by someone with appropriate expertise in occupational medicine, who is in a position to give helpful advice to the employer on preventive measures and on legal obligations. Even if, as is often the case, the doctor who is looking after the patient is not in a position to visit the workplace, it is usually necessary to obtain further information about it, especially with respect to possible sensitizers and the way they are handled. The patient may be able to give this and obtain appropriate chemical data sheets, codes of practice, and so on. Alternatively, an approach to the factory medical adviser, personnel manager, or a trade union representative may be helpful. In many countries, a statutory body, including expert doctors, is available to help in these matters (see Chapter 2).

MANAGEMENT

Once occupational asthma has been diagnosed, as a general rule, further exposure of the individual to the causative sensitizer should be prevented. In most cases, the ideal solution is for the patient to be redeployed by the employer to different work in a place where further contact with the sensitizer is not possible. In view of the increasing likelihood of litigation, employers would now be well advised to do all in their power to achieve this desirable end. If this is not possible, in many cases, the patient will need to seek work elsewhere, although this often entails financial hardship and is a stimulus to litigation.

In some cases, the patient is able to continue at work. Physicians should only advise this if the symptoms are relatively mild and reasonably well controlled by appropriate management and if the employer is prepared to take active steps to minimize future exposure.[58a] The principles of this have been discussed in Chapter 2. In brief, consideration should be given (in order of efficiency) to substitution of a less allergenic substance, enclosure of processes, provision of adequate exhaust ventilation, and provision of appropriate respiratory protection. In the case of exposure to organic substances, such as animal antigen and grain or wood dusts, it may be possible to combine good local exhaust ventilation, partial enclosure of processes, and respirator use to reduce exposure sufficiently for the person to continue at work using only inhaled medication. In such circumstances, patients should continue under medical supervision, preferably monitoring their own peak flow on a regular basis. In the case of sensitization to low molecular weight chemicals, such as isocyanates, acid anhydrides, and colophony, such an outcome is less often achievable, and redeployment or change of job is the more usual outcome.

The management should be discussed frankly with the patient, who should be made aware of the need to balance future employment prospects against future risks; ultimately, the patient has to make the decision. This should not be taken, however, without discussion with the employer of preventive measures, including a discussion of risks to other workers. Furthermore, a decision can usually be deferred until after a trial of return to work, taking the measures outlined earlier, including monitoring of peak flow, has taken place. The medical management does not differ from that normally used for asthma, except that, if the asthma is sufficiently severe to require oral steroids, it is most unwise to allow further exposure to occur.

PREVENTION

Prevention of occupational asthma is a problem for governments, employers, and employees.[59] In many countries, including the United States, the condition is not well appreciated by most doctors or employers, and in many cases, the patient simply recognizes that work is causing breathing problems and finds another job. Clearly, governments have a responsibility to inform employers and employees of the risks from exposure to certain substances. Although this can be done by labeling, data sheets, and so on, the real need is for educational publications and probably specific legislation. In Great Britain, under the Control of Substances Hazardous to Health Regulations (see Chapter 2), a Code of Practice on Respiratory Sensitizers has recently been introduced.[60] This gives guidance to employers on the steps to take to prevent sensitization when such substances need to be used in the workplace.

The individual employer should be aware of any substances in the workplace that may be sensitizers and should apply the principles of occupational hygiene (see Chapter 2) to reduce the risks of exposure. Consideration should be given to the surveillance of exposed workers, especially in the first 2 years of work, preferably by a simple questionnaire of nasal and respiratory symptoms. Anyone suspected of early symptoms of occupational asthma should be removed immediately from exposure and investigated by serial peak flow recording.

There has been much debate about the selection of workers. The medical consensus now is that people who already have asthma or allergic rhinitis are better not employed in jobs in which there is a risk of sensitization. However, pre-employment skin testing for atopy and exclusion of workers with positive results is looked on with disfavor. This is because a high proportion (depending on definition) of the normal healthy population is atopic, yet many in whom asthma actually develops are not atopic. Thus, exclusion of atopic workers may unnecessarily remove a large number who would never have asthma without making a substantial impact on the problem.[48] Moreover, such a method of attempting to prevent disease by only employing disease-resistant people detracts attention from the important and effective method of prevention, i.e., control of workplace exposure.

SPECIFIC TYPES OF OCCUPATIONAL ASTHMA

Animal-Derived Antigens

Table 17–3 shows the more important animal causes of asthma. Allergy to household pets and horses has long been recognized in the general population and in others, such as veterinarians and stable hands, who come into contact with animals through their work. However, interest in animal allergy increased considerably with the recognition of the size of the problem in laboratory and food processing workers. Hypersensitivity to small laboratory mammals, especially rats and mice, was recognized as a problem in the early 1970s, and it was subsequently demonstrated that protein in the urine of the animals, rather than dander, was the main cause of sensitization.[61] The syndrome usually presents initially with itchy eyes and rhinitis and progresses to attacks of wheeze and typical asthma.[62] In cross-

Table 17–3
■
Animal Causes of Occupational Asthma

Animal	Occupation
Rats, mice, guinea pigs Rabbits	Laboratory workers, veterinarians
Horses	Veterinarians, stable hands
Prawns, crabs, sea squirt	Shell fish processors
Salmon, trout	Fish processing
Silkworm	Silk culture
Maggots	Fishermen
Storage mites	Farm, grain workers
Screw worm	Biological control work
River fly	Power station workers
Locusts	Laboratory workers
Chicken	Poultry workers
Pigeons, parakeets	Breeders

sectional surveys in typical animal houses, the prevalence has been found to vary between about 3% and 40% of exposed workers.[63, 64] The disease most commonly starts within 1 year of first exposure and progresses in severity; those with manifestations of atopy usually present earlier than those without.[65] The incidence of the disease, which may be as high as 37% of newly exposed workers, can be reduced considerably if appropriate control measures are introduced into animal housing practice. Such measures include careful instruction of the workers in animal handling, appropriate exhaust ventilation, use of nondusty litter, and personal protection by respirators. Skin tests and IgE antibodies to the offending antigen are usually found in affected workers, and IgE titers may be used to monitor exposure of individuals once sensitization has occurred and protective measures are in place.[51]

The shellfish industry has also been responsible for much occupational asthma. Surveys have shown prevalences of between 15% and 40% of workers in crab, prawn, and oyster processing.[50, 66, 67] Again, these patients typically present with eye and nasal symptoms and progress to asthma. The antigen is usually carried in aerosol form from water sprays used in the process of extraction of the meat. Asthma is, in contrast, much less common in fish processing but has recently been recognized to be occurring frequently in the processing of farmed salmon and trout (Douglas, J. M., personal communication 1993). Silk worms and fishermen's maggots, grain and bean weevils, cockroaches, moths, locusts, and various flies have all been recognized as causes of asthma, in some cases very potent.[68–74] A midge in the Sudan, sterile screw flies used for biologic control, and river flies along the Mississippi have caused serious community and occupational outbreaks of asthma.[75–77] The most important animal cause of all, however, the house dust mite, has relatives that are common causes of occupational asthma, the grain mite species *Glycyphagus, Tyrophagus, Acarus,* and *Lepidoglyphus,* which afflict farmers handling stored grain.[78, 79] Many farmers recognize these symptoms and control them by avoiding exposure and, when necessary, wearing respirators. These mites are also responsible for much of the asthma reported in bakers. Finally, birds, although more often thought to cause allergic alveolitis, may occasionally provoke asthma, e.g., pigeons, parakeets, and chickens.[80, 81]

Vegetable-Derived Antigens

The most important antigens derived from plants are given in Table 17–4. Of these, the most frequent causes of asthma are flour and grains and hardwood dusts.

Flour and Grains

Respiratory disease and rhinitis attributable to grains was described by Ramazzini, and its allergic basis was demonstrated by Duke in 1935, when he described

Table 17–4
■
Vegetable Causes of Occupational Asthma

Vegetable	Occupation
Flour	Bakers, millers
Grains	Farmers, distribution workers
Wood dusts	Joiners, sawyers, carpenters
Coffee bean	Processing and distribution workers
Castor bean	Processing and distribution workers
Soybean	Processing and distribution workers
Tea leaves	Processing and distribution workers
Tragacanth	Confectionery, pharmaceuticals
Gum acacia	Confectionery, pharmaceuticals
Latex	Production and use
Fungal spores and antigen	Farmers, biotechnology
Bacterial enzymes	Food technology, washing powder manufacture

four mill workers with asthma caused by an allergen derived from wheat.[82] Workers exposed to grains in harvesting, storage, and transportation and to flour in bakeries are all at risk of sensitization.[83–85] Early studies of bakers showed that approximately 10% of apprentices showed positive skin tests to flour within 1 month of starting work, rising to 20% by the end of 3 years.[8] Later studies have found a prevalence of asthma of up to 30% of bakers, although the condition is often relatively mild and allows the sufferer to continue at work.[86, 87] Spontaneous desensitization has been suggested as an explanation of loss of symptoms with time,[87a] and skin test positivity may also disappear with continued exposure.[8] Although flour allergy is commonly found, so too is allergy to storage mites, and the two often occur together. It has been shown, however, that this is a nonspecific response rather than one specific to work in bakeries.[88] Skin test and IgE results are positive, atopic individuals are at greatest risk, and the development of symptoms correlates with the extent of exposure to flour.

It should be noted that people who handle grains and flour may be exposed to many different antigens, apart from those mentioned. Harvesting is associated with exposure to a wide range of fungal spores, to any of which the worker may become sensitized. Stored grain may contain many insects and particles derived from the small mammals that feed on it. Flour in bakeries may have other allergenic substances, such as enzymes, added to it.[88a]

It is important to recognize the relative mildness of asthma resulting from flour and grains in many cases, such that the sufferer is able to continue at work with some measure of personal protection and medical treatment. This contrasts with the situation among patients with chemical sensitization, and medical advice may be tempered accordingly.

Wood Dusts

The other relatively large group of workers at risk of vegetable asthma are those who work with wood, especially hardwoods.[11, 89–92] The substance studied in greatest detail, first described as a cause of rhinitis and asthma in Japan, is western red cedar, *Thuja plicata*.[93, 94] Workers in sawmills have been shown to have a risk of disease related to the extent of their exposure to dust, and up to 40% may have IgE antibodies to a water-soluble substance found in the wood, plicatic acid (Fig. 17–7), which is combined as a hapten with serum albumin.[95, 96] Symptomatic individuals respond to challenge testing with plicatic acid. Interestingly, atopic subjects are not more susceptible than nonatopic workers, and there is some evidence that smokers are less susceptible than nonsmokers, the reverse of the situation in some other forms of occupational asthma.

The same symptoms may occur in carpenters and joiners, and many other hardwoods have similar effects; among those implicated are redwood, cedar, iroko, oak, walnut, and zebrawood. The symptoms associated with wood dust exposure

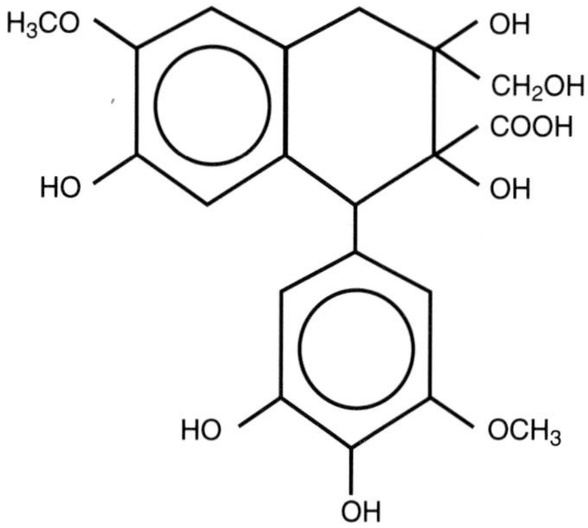

Figure 17–7
Chemical formula of plicatic acid.

are often rather gradual in onset and compatible with continuing exposure for prolonged periods. This is probably why, in many cases, the asthma may continue as an intractable process after exposure has finally ceased. Full recovery is only to be expected if the condition is detected early and further exposure is prevented, regrettably, an outcome that is often difficult to achieve among skilled tradespeople.

Beans

Many other plant-derived antigens have been described as causes of asthma and rhinitis. Dusts from beans in the production of coffee, castor oil, and soy flour seem to be important sensitizers.[97–99] Castor bean dust seems particularly potent; it sensitized workers who handled coffee beans in sacks that previously contained castor beans and also workers who made felt from old sacks that had been used similarly.[100, 101] Soybean dust has been responsible for environmental epidemics of asthma when it has been dispersed over cities from loading points in dockyards, the best known of these being the episodes in Barcelona referred to earlier.[34, 35] Over several years in that city, days occurred on which much increased numbers of patients were seen in emergency rooms with acute and often very severe attacks of asthma. Subsequent epidemiologic investigations showed adult men to be the most affected and children to be spared and the cause to be the dispersal of dust from soybean silos at the docks across the city. Similar epidemics of environmental asthma have been described in other cities, e.g., New Orleans; Birmingham, England; and Brisbane, although the causes have not been identified.[102–104]

Plant Products

Plant-derived substances, such as the gums, tragacanth, and gum acacia (which are used in confectionery, pharmaceuticals, and at one time, printing), and latex (which is used in rubber manufacture) may cause asthma.[105–108] The latex in surgical gloves has been well known to cause dermatitis in surgeons and nurses, but a number of recent reports indicate that proteins in the latex that represent the rubber elongation factor of the original rubber tree may become airborne, perhaps adsorbed onto powder, and cause rhinitis and asthma.[108–111] In one patient seen by the author, asthma was provoked by wearing rubber gloves from a particular batch and not by others; in this case, the offending gloves gave off a vapor containing D-carene which was thought to be the sensitizer.[112] Dust from tea leaves and garlic has also been described as causing asthma.[113]

Microbiological Agents and Enzymes

Allergy to fungal spores is recognized in a nonoccupational setting but may also be a cause of asthma in farmers who are exposed to very high concentrations during mechanized harvesting.[83] The higher actinomycetes and fungal spores associated with moldy hay may also cause asthma and allergic alveolitis. *Aspergillus niger* used in biotechnology is a relatively weak sensitizer,[114, 115] and many other fungal spores have occasionally been described as causing asthma in the working environment.

Aside from sensitization to microbes, asthma has frequently been described in relation to exposure to enzymes derived from biological sources. In the 1960s, an outbreak of asthma was described in workers who handled alcalase, a proteolytic enzyme manufactured by fermentation of *Bacillus subtilis,* that was used as a component of washing powders.[116–118] As in other outbreaks of occupational asthma, sensitization tended to occur relatively early after exposure started, and IgE antibodies have been demonstrated to the enzyme. Some cases of asthma were also suspected in people using the washing powders.[119] The discovery of the cause acted as a stimulus to this major industry to take preventive measures, with careful control of potential exposure of workers and changes in formulation to prevent inhalation of enzyme by users,[120] and the condition is now rarely detected in industrywide health surveillance.

Other enzymes are used in the washing powder industry, food technology, tanning, pharmaceuticals, and laboratories. The author has seen asthma in technicians who prepared microbiological media for bacterial culture, which was probably caused by the enzyme content. Papain (used in many of the aforementioned applications), trypsin, pancreatic extract, and amylase have also been reported to cause asthma.[121–126] It is reasonable to suppose that any enzyme used in the workplace in a form that may be inhalable has this potential.

Chemical Causes

Early reports of asthma resulting from chemicals and pharmaceuticals have included a description of ipecacuanha-induced asthma in pharmacy workers as long ago as 1848,[127] a report of anaphylaxis caused by platinum salts in 1929,[128] and the original report of isocyanate-induced asthma in 1951.[129] These latter compounds have now become the most frequently reported causes of occupational asthma, and they were responsible for a considerable growth in interest in the subject by the medical profession. Other particularly important chemical causes of asthma include the acid anhydrides (used as part of epoxy resin systems), colophony or rosin in multicore solder flux, a large number of pharmaceuticals, various substances used in disinfectants, and several other metals. A list of the main chemicals is given in Table 17–5.

Isocyanates

Isocyanates are widely used in industry in the production of polyurethane, which has applications in the manufacture of plastics, foams, surface coatings (including paints and varnishes), adhesives, synthetic rubber, and fibers.[130] They are therefore found in many industries, sometimes quite unexpectedly. In the British SWORD project, mentioned earlier, the highest rates of occupational asthma reported have been in spray painters and chemical process workers exposed to isocyanates, and these chemicals constitute the single most frequent cause of occupational asthma, i.e., 22% of reported cases.

The reactive diisocyanates (Fig. 17–8) are the substances to blame, particularly

Table 17–5
■
Chemical Causes of Asthma

Chemical	Occupation
Diisocyanates	Plastics, paints, adhesives
Acid anhydrides	Use of epoxy resins
Colophony	Soldering, electronics, metal machining
Amino ethyl ethanolamine	Aluminum jointing
Fluoride	Aluminum refining
Platinum salts	Refining, plating, jewelry
Cobalt and nickel	Hard metal manufacture and use, welding, plating
Chromium	Tanning
Vanadium	Oil-fired boiler cleaning
Antibiotics Laxatives and other drugs }	Manufacture
Powdered organic dyes	Textile dyeing
Paraphenylene diamine	Fur dyeing
Persulfate, henna	Hairdressing
Formaldehyde and glutaraldehyde	Nursing, laboratory work
Azodicarbonamide	Foam manufacture
Cyanoacrylate esters	Adhesive use
Cutting oils	Metal machining

Toluene diisocyanate (TDI)

Diphenyl methane diisocyanate (MDI)

Hexamethylene diisocyanate (HDI)

$$OCN - C - C - C - C - C - C - NCO$$

Naphthylene diisocyanate (NDI)

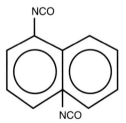

Figure 17–8
Chemical formulae of diisocyanates.

the volatile toluene diisocyanate. Hexamethylene diisocyanate, diphenylmethane diisocyanate, and 1,5 naphthylamine diisocyanate, although less volatile, may also cause asthma if heated or involved in exothermic reactions.[131–133] The vapor of these chemicals is irritant, and some workers may suffer nonallergic symptoms. Up to 10% become sensitized and may become extremely sensitive. Indeed, deaths have been recorded in workers who continued to be exposed after disease developed.[42] In general, people sensitized to isocyanates seem to continue with asthma after exposure has ceased, although usually the disease becomes slowly less troublesome as the years pass.[45] If exposure continues, even in an occasional manner, the patient's condition is likely to deteriorate.

The mechanisms of isocyanate-induced asthma are not clear. IgE antibodies to hapten have not been convincingly demonstrated, but IgG antibodies have been and may play a pathogenic role.[134]

The frequency of isocyanate-caused asthma and the ubiquity of these chemicals put a heavy responsibility on employers to protect workers and on suppliers to provide adequate warnings on their products. Users of two-part paints and varnishes have become sensitized in domestic and do-it-yourself applications.[135] In industry, tight occupational control is required.

Epoxy Resin Systems

Epoxy resins are also widely used in industry and the home in plastics, adhesives, and surface coatings. The resins themselves are long-chain polymers that are converted into hard solids by the addition of reactive chemicals, known as curing agents or hardeners. These are acid anhydrides, including maleic; ethylene diamine; triethylene; tetramine and aminoethyl ethanolamine anhydrides; and phthalic, tetrachlorophthalic, and trimellitic anhydrides (Fig. 17–9). The four most widely used are phthalic, trimellitic, tetrachlorophthalic, and maleic, all of which have caused occupational asthma.[51, 136–139] They act as haptens, and IgE antibodies have been detected. The evidence suggests that smokers and atopic people are at increased risk of sensitization,[51] but according to SWORD statistics, this form of asthma is uncommon, at least in Great Britain. Trimellitic anhydride has also been shown to cause a spectrum of other clinical effects in isolated cases, including pulmonary infiltration, influenza-like symptoms, and hemolytic anaemia, occurring in people exposed to fumes rather than dust.[140, 141] Although the flu-like symptoms may be mild, at least one of the more severe reactions has been fatal.

Soldering

Colophony or rosin fume is probably the second most frequent chemical cause of asthma. It is the solid substance remaining after turpentine has been distilled from pine resin and is used as the major constituent of many solder fluxes and in adhesives, varnishes, and sizes for paper manufacture. It is the component of adhesive skin plasters that commonly causes dermatitis. Colophony is of different chemical composition from different species of pine, but essentially, it is a mixture of abietic resin acids (Fig. 17–10). It is likely that these chemicals (and perhaps their pyrolytic products) are the cause of respiratory sensitization. However, antibodies to colophony have not been demonstrated in humans, although it has been possible to show antibodies to a colophony hapten in mice.[32]

The use of colophony in soldering, particularly in the electronic industry in the production of circuit boards, has caused a great deal of occupational asthma; one early study found about 25% of workers affected.[142–144] Although sensitization often occurs within 2 years of first exposure, in some workers, it may be delayed many years. Atopic individuals and smokers are at greater risk, and the condition may become intractable if not detected early. Since the problem came to light, many electronic employers have taken steps to reduce the exposure of solderers to colophony fumes, but this form of sensitization is still responsible for about 6% of all cases of occupational asthma in Great Britain. Colophony has also been described as a cause of asthma when inhaled in unheated form, either as a dust or in an aerosol of cutting oils.[145, 146] It is also the substance responsible for cutaneous allergic reactions to sticking plaster because it is a component of the adhesive.

Other forms of soldering may cause asthma by exposure to different chemicals. Occasional cases have been described in people who joint aluminum cables using a flux containing amino ethyl ethanolamine, and one case has occurred from inhalation of isocyanates liberated from the polyurethane coating of the wires being soldered.[147–149]

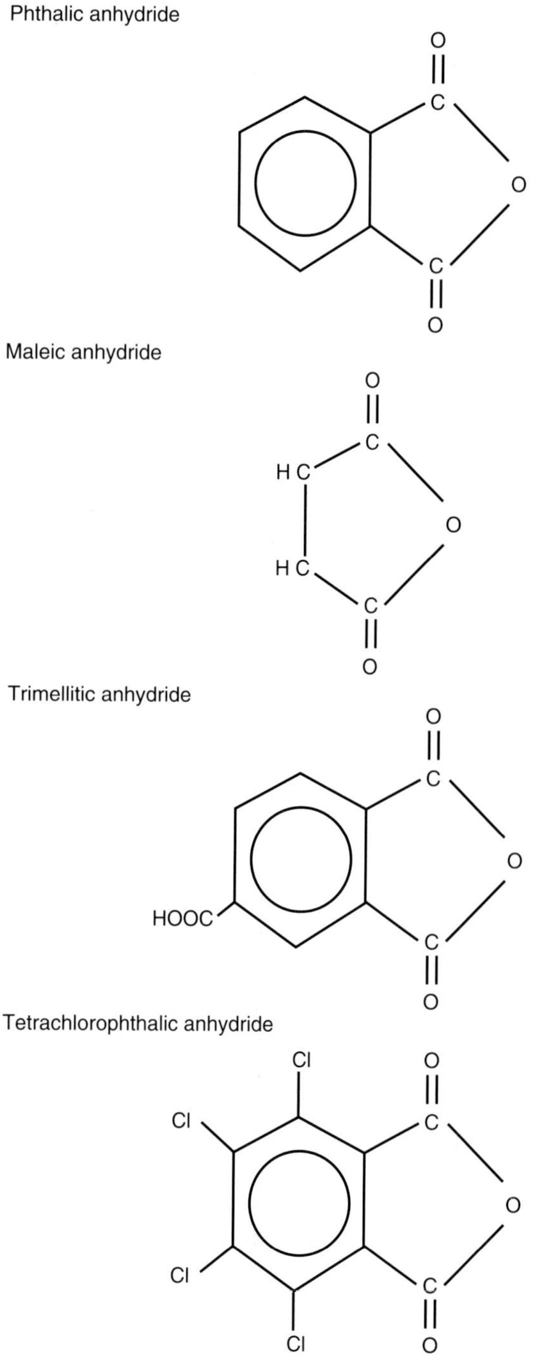

Phthalic anhydride

Maleic anhydride

Trimellitic anhydride

Tetrachlorophthalic anhydride

Figure 17–9
Chemical formulae of acid anhydrides.

Metals and Their Salts

Exposure to metals or their salts is responsible for about 4% of reported cases of occupational asthma in Great Britain. The most frequent reports come from aluminum refineries, so-called pot room asthma.[150, 151] These people suffer headaches, eye irritation, cough, and wheeze, and the symptoms may have an irritant rather than an allergic cause; the fluoride released in the electrolytic process may be responsible.[152] Antibodies have not been found in workers. Aluminum refinery workers may also be at risk of pulmonary fibrosis (see Chapter 16).

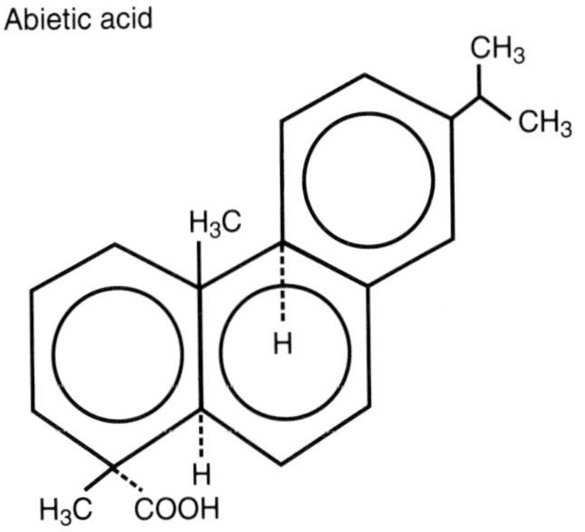

Abietic acid

Figure 17–10
Abietic acid, a major component of colophony.

Platinum and its salts, encountered in refining, jewelry, electroplating, photography, and the production of fluorescent screens and catalytic convertors for automobiles, have been recognized as potent sensitizers, affecting up to 25% of the work force exposed.[49, 128, 153–155] Again, sensitization (characterized by the development of positive skin test findings and IgE antibodies to platinum salts, rhinitis, and asthma) usually occurs within the first year of exposure and is more common in smokers. Although the condition may remit after exposure ceases, long-term asthma may result, and early removal from exposure is desirable.

Hard metal is used for the cutting edges of tools and drill bits. It is made from powdered tungsten carbide, cobalt, and nickel, which are pressed, heated, and shot blasted, prior to brazing and grinding to produce the final product.[156, 157] Dust containing both cobalt and nickel is generated in several parts of this process, and sensitivity to both metals has been described.[158, 159] Cobalt is also present in the coolant used in these processes, and this may also be responsible for sensitization in some cases.[160] Sensitized workers have asthma, but also giant cell interstitial pneumonitis has been well described.[161–163] One case of giant cell lung cancer has also been recorded in a worker.[164] Asthma has also been described in workers exposed to nickel in plating and welding, to chromium in tanning, and to vanadium in hard metal work and in cleaning oil-fired boilers where the residue contains the metal.[165–169]

Other Chemicals and Pharmaceuticals

An ever-increasing number of chemicals have been shown to provoke asthma in occasional cases, and many new causes will be demonstrated in the future. Some of these episodes affect many workers, are recognized, and are controlled by appropriate hygiene measures. The pharmaceutical industry has provided many examples, including various penicillins and cephalosporins, piperazine, psyllium, methyldopa, tetracyclines, spiramycin, and hydralazine,[12, 170–176] but few new cases are currently being reported in Great Britain. Reactive organic dyes (used especially in textiles) may, in the powdered form, cause severe asthma, and a death has occurred as a result of this.[31, 43] Other dyes, persulfates and henna, may be responsible for asthma in hairdressers.[177] Formaldehyde and glutaraldehyde, widely used in laboratories and hospitals, have caused asthmatic symptoms, usually on an irritant basis but, occasionally, probably by sensitization.[178] Paraphenylene diamine in fur dyers, azodicarbonamide (used as a blowing agent in the manufacture of plastic foams), and cyanoacrylate esters in glues have also been incriminated as causes of asthma.[179–181] Finally, asthma after exposure to oils used in machinery and cutting metal and to welding fumes is reported fairly frequently in Great Britain.[147, 182] In the former case, it seems likely that true asthmatic reactions may occur, whereas in the latter, it is more probable that the reactions are usually of an irritant nature.

REFERENCES

1. Ramazzini, B., De morbis artificum diatriba. Written in 1713. Cave, W., translator. Chicago, Wright, 1940.
2. Finn, R., John Bostock, hay fever and the mechanism of allergy. Lancet, 340, 1453, 1992.
3. van Pirquet, C., Allergie. Munch. Med. Wochenschr., 30, 1457, 1906.
4. Coca, A.F., Studies in specific hypersensitiveness: preparation of fluid extracts with solutions for use in diagnosis and treatment of allergies, with notes on collection of pollens. J. Immunol., 7, 163, 1922.
5. Coca, A.F., and Cooke, R.A., Classification of phenomena of hypersensitiveness. J. Immunol., 8, 163, 1923.
6. Cookson, W.O.C.M., Young, R.P., Sandford, A.J., et al., Maternal inheritance of atopic IgE responsiveness on chromosome 11q. Lancet, 340, 381, 1992.
7. Sandford, A.J., Shirakawa, T., Moffatt, M.F., et al., Localisation of atopy and β subunit of high-affinity IgE receptor on chromosome 11q. Lancet, 341, 332, 1993.
8. Herxheimer, H., The skin sensitivity to flour of bakers' apprentices. Acta Allerg., 28, 42, 1973.
9. Venables, K.M., Tet, R.D., Hawkins, E.R., et al., Laboratory animal allergy in a pharmaceutical company. Br. J. Ind. Med., 45, 60, 1988.
10. Topping, M.D., Scarisbrick, D.A., Luczynska, C.M., et al., Clinical and immunological reactions to *Aspergillus niger* among workers at a biotechnology plant. Br. J. Ind. Med., 42, 312, 1985.
11. Gandevia, B.A., and Milne, J., Occupational asthma and rhinitis due to western red cedar. Br. J. Ind. Med., 27, 235, 1970.
12. Pepys, J., Pickering, C.A.C., and Loudon, H.W.G., Asthma due to inhaled chemical agents—piperazine dihydrochloride. Clin. Allergy, 2, 189, 1972.
13. Pickering, C.A.C., Batten, J.C., and Pepys, J., Asthma due to inhaled wood dusts—western red cedar and iroko. Clin. Allergy, 2, 213, 1972.
14. Carroll, K.B., Pepys, J., Longbottom, J.L., et al., Extrinsic allergic alveolitis due to rat serum proteins. Clin. Allergy, 5, 443, 1975.
15. Burge, P.S., O'Brien, I.M., and Harries, M.G., Peak flow records in the diagnosis of occupational asthma due to colophony. Thorax, 34, 308, 1979.
16. Chan-Yeung, M., Barton, G., MacLean, L., and Grzybowski, S., Occupational asthma and rhinitis due to western red cedar (*Thuja plicata*). Am. Rev. Respir. Dis., 108, 1094, 1973.
17. Chan-Yeung, M., Fate of occupational asthma. A follow-up study of patients with occupational asthma due to western red cedar (*Thuja plicata*). Am. Rev. Respir. Dis., 116, 1023, 1977.
18. Chan-Yeung, M., and Lam, S., Occupational asthma. Am. Rev. Respir. Dis., 133, 686, 1986.
19. Keskinen, H., Alanko, K.A., and Saarinen, L. Occupational asthma in Finland. Clin. Allergy, 8, 569, 1978.
20. Keskinen, H., Epidemiology of occupational lung diseases: asthma and allergic alveolitis. *In* Kerr, J.W., and Ganderton, M.A., eds., Proceedings of Invited Symposia, XI International Congress of Allergy and Clinical Immunology. London, Macmillan, 1983, p. 403.
21. Meredith, S.K., Taylor, V.M., and McDonald, J.C., Occupational respiratory disease in the United Kingdom, 1989. Br. J. Ind. Med., 48, 292, 1991.
22. Burney, P., Why study the epidemiology of asthma? Thorax, 43, 425, 1988.
23. Burr, M.L., Epidemiology of asthma. *In* Burr, M.L., ed., Epidemiology of Clinical Allergy. Basel, Karger, 1993, 80.
24. Woolcock, A.J., Dowse, G., Temple, K., et al., Prevalence of asthma in the South Fore people of Papua New Guinea. Eur. J. Respir. Dis., 64, 571, 1983.
25. Van Niekerk, C.H., Weinberg, E.G., Shore, S.C., et al., Prevalence of asthma: a comparative study of urban and rural Xhosa children. Clin. Allergy, 9, 319, 1979.
25a. Seaton, A., Godden, D. J., and Brown, K., The increase in asthma: A more toxic environment or a more susceptible population? Thorax, 49, 171, 1994.
26. Ishizaka, M., Function of IgE antibody and regulation of IgE antibody response. *In* Stein, M., ed., New Directions in Asthma. Park Ridge, IL, American College of Chest Physicians, 1975.
27. Kay, A.B., Lymphocytes in asthma. Respir. Med., 85, 87, 1991.
28. Kroegel, C., Virchow, J.C., Kortsik, C., and Matthys, H., Cytokines, platelet activating factor and eosinophils in asthma. Respir. Med., 86, 375, 1992.
29. Chan-Yeung, M., Occupational asthma. Chest, 98(suppl), 1485, 1990.
30. Newman-Taylor, A.J., Venables, K.M., Ducham, S.R., et al., Acid anhydrides and asthma. Int. Arch. Allergy Appl. Immunol., 82, 435, 1987.
31. Topping, M.D., Foster, H., Ide, C., and Kennedy, F., Respiratory allergy and specific IgE and IgG antibodies to reactive dyes used in the wool industry. J. Occup. Med., 31, 557, 1989.
32. Cullen, R.T., Cherrie, B., Soutar, C.A., Immune responses to colophony, an agent causing occupational asthma. Thorax, 47, 1050, 1992.
33. Brooks, S.M., Weiss, M.A., and Bernstein, I.L., Reactive airways dysfunction syndrome: persistent asthma syndrome after high level irritant exposure. Chest, 88, 376, 1985.
34. Picado, C., Barcelona's asthma epidemics: clinical aspects and intriguing findings. Thorax, 47, 197, 1992.
35. Judd, A., and Docherty, J., Barcelona's asthma epidemics. Thorax, 47, 1086, 1992.
36. Weiner, A., Bronchial asthma due to the organic phosphate insecticides. Ann. Allergy, 19, 397, 1961.

37. Lam, S., Wong, R., and Chang-Yeung, M., Non-specific bronchial reactivity in occupational asthma. J. Allergy Clin. Immunol., 63, 28, 1979.

38. Burge, P.S., Non-specific bronchial hyper-reactivity in workers exposed to toluene di-isocyanate, diphenyl methane di-isocyanate and colophony. Eur. J. Respir. Dis., 63(suppl 123), 91, 1982.

39. Blanc, P., Occupational asthma in a national disability survey. Chest, 92, 613, 1987.

40. Health and Safety Commission, Annual Report 1991/92. London, Her Majesty's Stationery Office, 1992, p. 96.

41. Gandevia, B., and Milne, J., Occupational asthma and rhinitis with western red cedar (*Thuja plicata*) with special reference to bronchial reactivity. Br. J. Ind. Med., 27, 253, 1970.

42. Fabbri, L.M., Danieli, D., Crescioli, S., et al., Fatal asthma in a subject sensitized to toluene diisocyanate. Am. Rev. Respir. Dis., 137, 1494, 1988.

43. Docker, A., Wattie, J.M., Topping, M.D., et al., Clinical and immunological investigations of workers using reactive dyes. Br. J. Ind. Med., 44, 534, 1987.

44. Chan-Yeung, M., Lam, S., and Koerner, S., Clinical features and natural history of occupational asthma due to western red cedar (*Thuja plicata*). Am. Rev. Respir. Dis., 72, 411, 1982.

45. Pisati, G., Baruffini, A., and Zedda, S., Toluene diisocyanate induced asthma: outcome according to persistence or cessation of exposure. Br. J. Ind. Med., 50, 60, 1993.

46. Newhouse, M.L., Tagg, B., Pocock, S.J., and McEwan, A.C., An epidemiological study of workers producing enzyme washing powder. Lancet, 1, 689, 1970.

47. Slovak, A.J.M., and Hill, R., Laboratory animal allergy: a clinical survey of an exposed population. Br. J. Ind. Med., 38, 38, 1981.

48. Slovak, A.J.M., and Hill, R.N., Does atopy have any predictive value for laboratory animal allergy? A comparison of different concepts of atopy. Br. J. Ind. Med., 44, 129, 1987.

49. Venables, K.M., Dally, M.B., Nunn, A.J., et al., Smoking and occupational allergy in workers in a platinum refinery. B.M.J., 299, 939, 1989.

50. Cartier, M., Malo, J.-L., Forest, F., et al., Occupational asthma in snow crab processing workers. J. Allergy Clin. Immunol., 74, 261, 1984.

51. Venables, K.M., Topping, M.D., Howe, W., et al., Interaction of smoking and atopy in producing specific IgE antibody against a hapten protein conjugate. B.M.J., 290, 201, 1985.

52. Zetterstrom, A., Osterman, K., Machado, L., and Johansson, S.G.O., Another smoking hazard: raised serum IgE concentrations and increased risk of occupational allergy. B.M.J., 283, 1215, 1981.

53. Zetterstrom, E., Nordvall, S.L., Bjorksten, B., et al., Increased IgE antibody responses in rats exposed to tobacco smoke. J. Allergy Clin. Immunol., 75, 594, 1985.

54. Biagini, R.E., Moorman, W.J., Lewis, T.R., and Bernstein, I.L., Ozone enhancement of platinum asthma in a primate model. Am. Rev. Respir. Dis., 134, 719, 1986.

55. Brooks, S.M., Occupational asthma. *In* Weiss, E.B., Segal, M.S., Stein, M., eds., Bronchial Asthma. Mechanisms and Therapeutics, 2nd ed. Boston, Little Brown, 1985, p. 477.

56. Venables, K.M., Topping, M.D., Nunn, A.J., et al., Immunologic and functional consequences of chemical (tetrachlorophthalic anhydride)-induced asthma after four years of avoidance of exposure. J. Allergy Clin. Immunol., 80, 212, 1987.

57. Pepys, J., and Hutchcroft, B.J., Bronchial provocation tests in etiologic diagnosis and analysis of asthma. Am. Rev. Respir. Dis., 112, 829, 1975.

58. Lam, S., Wong, R., and Chan-Yeung, M., Non-specific bronchial reactivity in occupational asthma. J. Allergy Clin. Immunol., 63, 28, 1979.

58a. Seaton, A., Management of the patient with occupational lung disease. Thorax, 49, 627, 1994.

59. Venables, K.M., Preventing occupational asthma. Br. J. Ind. Med., 49, 817, 1992.

60. Health and Safety Executive, Advisory Code of Practice. Respiratory Sensitizers. London, Her Majesty's Stationery Office, 1993.

61. Newman-Taylor, A., Longbottom, J.L., and Pepys, J., Respiratory allergy to urine proteins of rats and mice. Lancet, 2, 847, 1977.

62. Cockcroft, A., Edwards, J., McCarthy, P., and Anderson, N., Allergy in laboratory animal workers. Lancet, 1, 827, 1981.

63. Aoyama, K., Ueda, A., Manda, F., et al., Allergy to laboratory animals: an epidemiological study. Br. J. Ind. Med., 49, 41, 1992.

64. Agrup, G., Belin, L., Sjostedt, L., and Skerfving, S., Allergy to laboratory animals in laboratory workers and animal keepers. Br. J. Ind. Med., 43, 192, 1986.

65. Botham, P.A., Davies, G.E., and Teasdale, E.L., Allergy to laboratory animals: a prospective study of its incidence and of the influence of atopy on its development. Br. J. Ind. Med., 44, 627, 1987.

66. Gaddie, J., Legge, J.S., Friend, J.A.S., and Reid, T.M., Pulmonary hypersensitivity in prawn workers. Lancet, 2, 1350, 1980.

67. Jyo, T., Kohmoto, K., Katsutani, T., et al., Hoya (seasquirt) asthma. *In* Frazier, C.A., ed., Occupational Asthma. New York, Van Norstrand Reinhold, 1980, p. 209.

68. Kobayashi, S., Different aspects of occupational asthma in Japan. *In* Frazier, C.A., ed., Occupational Asthma. New York, Van Norstrand Reinhold, 1980, p. 229.

69. Buisseret, P., Seasonal asthma in an angler. Lancet, 1, 668, 1978.

70. Burge, P.S., Edge, G., O'Brien, I.M., et al., Occupational asthma in a research establishment breeding locusts. Clin. Allergy, 10, 355, 1980.

71. Frankland, A.W., and Lunn, J.A., Asthma caused by the grain weevil. Br. J. Ind. Med., 22, 157, 1965.

72. Kino, T., and Oshima, S., Allergy to insects in Japan. 1. The reaginic sensitivity to moth and butterfly in patients with bronchial asthma. J. Allergy Clin. Immunol., 61, 10, 1978.
73. Wittich, F.W., Allergic rhinitis and asthma due to sensitization to the Mexican bean weevil (*Zabrotes subfasciatus Boh*). J. Allergy, 12, 42, 1940.
74. Bernton, H.S., McMahon, T.F., and Brown, H., Cockroach asthma. Br. J. Dis. Chest., 66, 61, 1972.
75. Kay, A.B., McLean, C.M.V., Wilkinson, A.H., et al., The prevalence of asthma and rhinitis in a Sudanese community seasonally exposed to a potent allergen, the green nimitti midge. J. Allergy Clin. Immunol., 71, 345, 1983.
76. Gibbons, H.L., Dille, J.R., and Cowley, R.G., Inhalant allergy to screw worm fly. Arch. Environ. Health, 10, 424, 1965.
77. Figley, K.D., Mayfly (*Ephernerida*) hypersensitivity. J. Allergy, 11, 376, 1940.
78. Cuthbert, O.D., Brostoff, J., Wraith, D.G., and Brighton, W.D., Barn allergy, asthma and rhinitis due to storage mites. Clin. Allergy, 9, 229, 1979.
79. Cuthbert, O.D., Jeffrey, I.G., McNeill, H.B., et al., Barn allergy among Scottish farmers. Clin. Allergy, 14, 197, 1984.
80. Hargreave, F.E., and Pepys, J., Allergic respiratory reactions in bird fanciers, provoked by allergen inhalation provocation tests. J. Allergy Clin. Immunol., 50, 157, 1972.
81. Bar-Sela, S., Teichtal, H., and Lutsky, I., Occupational asthma in poultry workers. J. Allergy Clin. Immunol., 73, 271, 1984.
82. Duke, W.W., Wheat hairs and dust as a common cause of asthma among workers in wheat flour mills. J.A.M.A., 105, 957, 1935.
83. Darke, C.S., Knowleden, J., Lacey, J., and Ward, A.M., Respiratory disease of workers harvesting grain. Thorax, 31, 294, 1976.
84. Chan-Yeung, M., Wong, R., and McLean, L., Respiratory abnormalities among grain elevator workers. Chest, 72, 461, 1979.
85. Hendrick, D.J., Davies, R.J., and Pepys, J., Bakers' asthma. Clin. Allergy, 6, 241, 1976.
86. Thiel, H., and Ulmer, W.T., Bakers' asthma: development and possibility of treatment. Chest, 78(suppl), 400, 1980.
87. Musk, A.W., Venables, K.M., Crook, B., et al., Respiratory symptoms, lung function, and sensitization to flour in a British bakery. Br. J. Ind. Med., 46, 637, 1989.
87a. Gadborg, E., M.D. Thesis, quoted by Bonnevie, P., Occupational Allergy, Leiden, H. E. Stenfert Kroese, 1956, p. 96.
88. Tee, R.D., Gordon, D.J., Gordon, S., et al., Immune response to flour and dust mites in a United Kingdom bakery. Br. J. Ind. Med., 49, 581, 1992.
88a. Cullinan, P., Lowson, D., Nieuwenhuijsen, M. J., et al., Work related symptoms, sensitisation, and estimated exposure in workers not previously exposed to flour. Occ. Environ. Med., 51, 579, 1994.
89. Sossman, A.J., Schlueter, D.P., Fink, J.N., and Barboriak, J.J., Hypersensitivity to wood dust. N. Engl. J. Med., 281, 977, 1969.
90. Greenberg, M., Respiratory symptoms following brief exposure to cedar of Lebanon dust. Clin. Allergy, 2, 219, 1972.
91. Bush, R.K., Junginger, J.W., and Reed, C.E., Asthma due to African zebrawood (*Microberlinia*) dust. Am. Rev. Respir. Dis., 117, 601, 1978.
92. Chan-Yeung, M., and Abboud, R., Occupational asthma due to Californian redwood (*Sequoia sempervirens*) dust. Am. Rev. Respir. Dis., 114, 1027, 1976.
93. Chan-Yeung, M., Lam, S., and Koerner, S., Clinical features and natural history of occupational asthma due to western red cedar (*Thuja plicata*). Am. J. Med., 72, 411, 1982.
94. Milne, J., and Gandevia, B., Occupational asthma and rhinitis due to western red cedar (*Thuja plicata*). Med. J. Aust., 2, 741, 1967.
95. Chan-Yeung, M., Immunologic and nonimmunologic mechanisms in asthma due to western red cedar (*Thuja plicata*). J. Allergy Clin. Immunol., 70, 32, 1982.
96. Chan, H., Tse, H., Oostdam, J., et al., A rabbit model for hypersensitivity to plicatic acid, the agent responsible for red cedar asthma. J. Allergy Clin. Immunol., 79, 762, 1987.
97. Thomas, K.E., Trigg, C.J., Baxter, P.J., et al., Factors relating to the development of respiratory symptoms in coffee process workers. Br. J. Ind. Med., 48, 314, 1991.
98. Kathren, R.L., Price, H., and Rogers, J.C., Air-borne castor-bean pomace allergy. Arch. Ind. Health., 19, 487, 1959.
99. Bush, R.K., and Cohen, M., Immediate and late onset asthma from occupational exposure to soybean dust. Clin. Allergy, 7, 369, 1977.
100. Frigley, K.D., and Rawling, F.F.A., Castor bean: an industrial hazard as a contaminant of green coffee dust and used burlap bags. J. Allergy, 21, 545, 1950.
101. Topping, M.D., Henderson, R.T.S., Luczynska, C.A., and Woodmass, A., Castor bean allergy among workers in the felt industry. Allergy, 37, 603, 1982.
102. Packe, G.E., and Ayres, J.G., Asthma outbreak during a thunderstorm. Lancet, 2, 199, 1982.
103. Morrison, I., It happened one night. Med. J. Aust., 1, 850, 1960.
104. Salvaggio, J., Seabury, J., and Schoenhardt, E.A., New Orleans asthma. V. Relationship between charity hospital asthma admission rates, semiquantitative pollen and fungal spore counts, and total particulate aerometric sampling data. J. Allergy Clin. Immunol., 48, 96, 1971.
105. Fowler, P.B.S., Printers' asthma. Lancet, 2, 755, 1952.

106. Bohner, C.B., and Sheldon, J.M., Sensitivity to gum acacia, with a report of ten cases of asthma in printers. J. Allergy, 12, 290, 1941.

107. Hinaut, G., Blacque-Belair, A., and Buffe, D., L'asthma a la gomme arabique dans un grand atelier de typographia. Fr. Med. Chir. Thorac., 15, 51, 1961.

108. Baur, X., and Jäger, D., Airborne antigens from latex gloves. Lancet, 335, 912, 1990.

109. Sussman, G.L., Tarlo, S., and Dolovich, J., The spectrum of IgE mediated responses to latex. J.A.M.A., 285, 2844, 1991.

110. Marcos, C., Lazaro, M., Fraj, J., et al., Occupational asthma due to latex surgical gloves. Ann. Allergy, 67, 319, 1991.

111. Czuppon, A.B., Chen, Z., and Baur, X., Chemical synthesis of a peptide representing a major latex allergen. Chest, 104, 159s, 1993.

112. Seaton, A., Cherrie, B., and Turnbull, J., Rubber glove asthma. B.M.J., 296, 531, 1988.

113. Uragoda, C.G., Respiratory disease in tea workers in Sri Lanka. Thorax, 35, 114, 1980.

114. Topping, M.D., Scarisbrick, D.A., Luczynska, C.M., et al., Clinical and immunological reactions to *Aspergillus niger* among workers in a biotechnology plant. Br. J. Ind. Med., 42, 312, 1985.

115. Seaton, A., and Wales, D., Clinical reactions to *Aspergillus niger* in a biotechnology plant: an eight year follow up. Occ. Environ. Med., 43, 63, 1994.

116. Flindt, M.L.H., Pulmonary disease due to inhalation of deritatives of *Bacillus subtilis* containing proteolytic enzyme. Lancet, 1, 1177, 1969.

117. Pepys, J., Hargreave, F.E., Longbottom, J.L., and Faux, J., Allergic reactions of the lungs to enzymes of *Bacillus subtilis*. Lancet, 1, 1181, 1969.

118. Newhouse, M.L., Tagg, B., and Pocock, S.J., An epidemiological study of workers producing enzyme washing powders. Lancet, 1, 689, 1970.

119. Falleroni, A.E., and Schwartz, D.P., Immediate hypersensitivity to enzyme detergents. Lancet, 1, 548, 1971.

120. Juniper, C.P., How, M.J., Goodwin, B.F.J., and Kinshott, A.K., *Bacillus subtilis* enzymes: a 7-year clinical, epidemiological and immunological study of an industrial allergen. J. Soc. Occup. Med., 27, 3, 1977.

121. Milne, J., and Brand, S., Occupational asthma after inhalation of dust of the proteolytic enzyme papain. Br. J. Ind. Med., 32, 302, 1975.

122. Tarlo, S.M., Shaikh, W., Bell, B., et al., Papain-induced allergic reactions. Clin. Allergy, 8, 207, 1978.

123. Novey, H., Keenan, W.J., Fairshter, R.D., et al., Pulmonary disease in workers exposed to papain: clinicophysiological and immunological studies. Clin. Allergy, 10, 721, 1980.

124. Dolan, T.F., and Meyers, A., Bronchial asthma and allergic rhinitis associated with inhalation of pancreatic extracts. Am. Rev. Respir. Dis., 110, 812, 1974.

125. Colten, H.R., Polakoff, P.L., Weinstein, S.F., and Strieder, D.J., Immediate hypersensitivity to hog trypsin resulting from industrial exposure. N. Engl. J. Med., 292, 1050, 1975.

126. Flindt, M.L.H., Allergy to alpha-amylase and papain. Lancet, 1, 1407, 1979.

127. Seaton, A., Ipecacuanha asthma: an old lesson. Thorax, 45, 974, 1990.

128. Valléry-Radot, L., and Blamoutier, R., Sensibilisation au chloroplatinité de potassium. Accidents graves de choc survenus à la suite d'une cutiréaction avec le cel. Bull. Mem. Soc. Med. Hop. Paris, 45, 222, 1929.

129. Fuchs, S., and Valade, P., Étude clinique et éxperimentale sur quelques cas d'intoxication par de desmondur T. Arch. Mal. Prof., 12, 191, 1951.

130. Vandenplas, E., Malo, J.-L., Saetta, M., et al., Occupational asthma and extrinsic alveolitis due to isocyanates: current status and perspectives. Br. J. Ind. Med., 50, 213, 1993.

131. O'Brien, I.M., Harries, M.G., Burge, P.S., and Pepys, J., Toluene diisocyanate induced asthma. I. Reactions to TDI, MDI, HDI and histamine. Clin. Allergy, 9, 1, 1979.

132. Tanser, A.R., Bourke, M.P., and Blandford, A.G., Isocyanate asthma. Respiratory symptoms caused by diphenylmethane isocyanate. Thorax, 28, 596, 1973.

133. Harries, M.G., Burge, P.S., Samson, M., et al., Isocyanate asthma: respiratory symptoms due to 1:5 naphthylene diisocyanate. Thorax, 34, 762, 1979.

134. Cartier, A., Grammer, L., Malo, J.-L., et al., Specific serum antibodies against isocyanates: association with occupational asthma. J. Allergy Clin. Immunol., 84, 507, 1989.

135. Peters, J.M., and Murphy, R.L.H., Hazards to health—do-it-yourself polyurethane foam. Am. Rev. Respir. Dis., 184, 432, 1971.

136. Newman Taylor, A.J., Venables, K.M., Durham, S.R., et al., Acid anhydrides and asthma. Int. Arch. Allergy Appl. Immunol., 82, 435, 1987.

137. Maccia, C.A., Bernstein, I.L., Emmett, E.A., and Brooks, S.M., In vitro demonstration of specific IgE in phthalic anhydride sensitivity. Am. Rev. Respir. Dis., 113, 701, 1976.

138. Lee, H.S., Wang, Y.T., Cheong, T.H., et al., Occupational asthma due to maleic anhydride. Br. J. Ind. Med., 48, 283, 1991.

139. Schleuter, D.P., Banaszak, E.F., Fin, J.N., and Barboriak, J., Occupational asthma due to tetra-chlorophthalic anhydride. J. Occup. Med., 20, 183, 1978.

140. Zeiss, C.R., Wolkonsky, P., Chacon, R., et al., Syndromes in workers exposed to trimellitic anhydride: a longitudinal clinical and epidemiologic study. Ann. Intern. Med., 98, 8, 1983.

141. Zeiss, C.R., Patterson, R., Pruzonsky, J.J., et al., Trimellitic anhydride induced airways syndromes: clinical and immunologic studies. J. Allergy Clin. Immunol., 60, 96, 1977.

142. Burge, P.S., Harries, M.G., O'Brien, I.M., and Pepys, J., Respiratory disease in workes exposed to solder flux fumes containing colophony (pine resin). Clin. Allergy, 8, 1, 1978.

143. Burge, P.S., Perks, W.H., O'Brien, I.M., et al., Occupational asthma in an electronics factory. Thorax, 34, 13, 1979.

144. Burge, P.S., Perks, W.H., O'Brien, I.M., et al., Occupational asthma in an electronics factory: a case control study to evaluate aetiological factors. Thorax, 34, 300, 1979.

145. Burge, P.S., Wieland, A., Robertson, A.S., and Weir, D., Occupational asthma due to heated colophony. Br. J. Ind. Med., 43, 559, 1986.

146. Hendy, M.S., Beattie, B.E., and Burge, P.S., Occupational asthma due to an emulsified oil mist. Br. J. Ind. Med., 42, 51, 1985.

147. Pepys, J., Pickering, C.A.C., and Hughes, E.G., Asthma due to inhaled chemical fumes—amino-ethyl ethanolamine in aluminium soldering flux. Clin. Allergy, 2, 197, 1972.

148. Sterling, G.M., Asthma due to aluminium soldering flux. Thorax, 22, 533, 1967.

149. Pepys, J., Pickering, C.A.C., Breslin, A.B.X., and Terry, D.J., Asthma due to inhaled chemical agents—toluene diisocyanate. Clin. Allergy, 2, 225, 1972.

150. Saric, M., and Marelja, J., Bronchial hypersensitivity in potroom workers and prognosis after stopping exposure. Br. J. Ind. Med., 48, 653, 1991.

151. Kongerud, J., and Samuelsen, S.O., A longitudinal study of respiratory symptoms in aluminium potroom workers. Am. Rev. Respir. Dis., 144, 10, 1991.

152. Soyseth, V., and Kongerud, J., Prevalence of respiratory disorders among aluminium potroom workers in relation to exposure to fluoride. Br. J. Ind. Med., 49, 125, 1992.

153. Roberts, A.E., Platinosis. A five-year study of soluble platinum salts on employees in a platinum laboratory and refinery. Arch. Ind. Hyg., 4, 549, 1951.

154. Pepys, J., Pickering, C.A.C., and Hughes, E.G., Asthma due to inhaled chemical agents—complex salts of platinum. Clin. Allergy, 2, 391, 1972.

155. Cleare, M.J., Hughes, E.G., Jacoby, B., and Pepys, J., Immediate (type 1) allergic responses to platinum compounds. Clin. Allergy, 9, 99, 1979.

156. Kusaka, Y., Yokoyama, K., Sera, Y., et al., Respiratory diseases in hard metal workers: an occupational hygiene study in a factory. Br. J. Ind. Med., 43, 474, 1976.

157. Kusaka, Y., Kumagai, S., Kyono, H., et al., Determination of exposure to cobalt and nickel in the atmosphere in the hard metal industry. Ann. Occup. Hyg., 36, 497, 1992.

158. Shirakawa, T., Kusaka, Y., Fujimura, N., et al., Hard metal asthma: cross immunological and respiratory activity between cobalt and nickel? Thorax, 45, 267, 1990.

159. Shirakawa, T., Kusaka, Y., and Morimoto, K., Specific IgE antibodies to nickel in workers with known reactivity to cobalt. Clin. Exp. Allergy, 22, 213, 1992.

160. Sjörgen, I., Hillerdal, G., Anderson, A., and Zetterström, O., Hard metal lung disease: importance of cobalt in coolants. Thorax, 35, 653, 1980.

161. Miller, C.W., Davis, M.W., Goldman, A., and Wyatt, J.P., Pneumoconiosis in the tungsten carbide tool industry. Arch. Ind. Hyg., 8, 453, 1953.

162. Sprince, N.L., Chamberlin, R.I., Hales, C.H., et al., Respiratory disease in tungsten carbide production workers. Chest, 86, 549, 1984.

163. Davison, A.G., Haslam, P.L., Corrin, B., et al., Interstitial lung disease and asthma in hard metal workers: bronchoalveolar lavage, ultrastructural and analytical findings and results of bronchial provocation tests. Thorax, 38, 119, 1983.

164. Kusaka, Y., Kuwabara, O., and Kitamura, H., A case of diffuse lung disease associated with lung cancer in a hard metal worker. Jpn. J. Thorac. Dis., 22, 804, 1984.

165. McConnell, L.H., Fink, J.N., Schleuter, D.P., and Schmidt, M.G., Asthma caused by nickel sensitivity. Arch. Intern. Med., 78, 888, 1973.

166. Sunderman, F.W., and Sunderman, F.W., Jr., Loffler's syndrome associated with nickel sensitivity. Arch. Intern. Med., 107, 405, 1961.

167. Smith, A.R., Chrome poisoning with manifestations of sensitization: report of a case. J.A.M.A., 97, 95, 1931.

168. Joules, H., Asthma from sensitisation to chromium. Lancet, 2, 182, 1932.

169. Williams, N., Vanadium poisoning from cleaning oil-fired boilers. Br. J. Ind. Med., 9, 50, 1952.

170. Davies, R.J., Hendrick, D.J., and Pepys, J., Asthma due to inhaled chemical agents: ampicillin, benzyl penicillin, 6 amino penicillanic acid and related substances. Clin. Allergy, 4, 227, 1974.

171. Coutts, I.I., Dally, M.B., Newman Taylor, A.J., et al., Asthma in workers manufacturing cephalo-sporins. B.M.J., 283, 950, 1981.

172. Malo, J.-L., Cartier, A., L'Archeveque, J., et al., Prevalence of occupational asthma and immuno-logic sensitization to psyllium among health personnel in chronic care hospitals. Am. Rev. Respir. Dis., 142, 1359, 1990.

173. Harries, M.G., Newman Taylor, A.J., Wooden, J., and MacAuslan, A., Bronchial asthma due to alpha methyl dopa. B.M.J., 1, 1461, 1979.

174. Menon, M.P.S., and Das, A.K., Tetracycline asthma. Clin. Allergy., 7, 285, 1977.

175. Davies, R.J., and Pepys, J., Asthma due to inhaled chemical agents—the macrolide antibiotic spiramycin. Clin. Allergy, 5, 99, 1975.

176. Perrin, B., Malo, J.-L., Cartier, A., et al., Occupational asthma in a worker exposed to hydralazine. Thorax, 45, 980, 1990.

177. Pepys, J., Hutchcroft, B.J., and Breslin, A.B.X., Asthma due to inhaled chemical agents: persul-phate salts and henna in hairdressers. Clin. Allergy, 6, 399, 1976.

178. Hendrick, D.J., and Lane, D., Formalin asthma in hospital staff. B.M.J., 1, 607, 1975.
179. Silberman, D.E., and Sorrell, A.H., Allergy in fur workers with special reference to paraphenyl diamine. J. Allergy, 30, 11, 1959.
180. Slovak, A.J.M., Occupational asthma caused by plastics blowing agent, azodicarbonamide. Thorax, 36, 906, 1981.
181. Lozewicz, S., Davison, A., Hopkirk, A., and Burge, P.S., Occupational asthma due to methyl methacrylate and cyanoacrylates. Thorax, 40, 836, 1985.
182. Gannon, P.F.G., and Burge, S., A preliminary report of a surveillance scheme of occupational asthma in the West Midlands. Br. J. Ind. Med., 48, 579, 1991.

18

Byssinosis and Related Conditions

W. Keith C. Morgan

■

Relatively early in the 19th century Kay described a respiratory disease that affected cotton workers.[1] He correctly attributed the symptoms to excessive cotton dust exposure. Because of the onset of chest tightness and fever on Monday morning, it became known as Monday morning fever. The condition has been described in cotton, flax, and hemp workers and is known as byssinosis, a term derived from the Greek βυσσοζ, meaning linen or fine flax.

Ramazzini in his treatise *De Morbis Artificum Diatriba* mentioned the chronic cough of combers of flax and hemp. Greenhow described chronic bronchial irritation in a group of about 100 English flax workers.[2] The 19th century cotton famine in England resulted in a great increase in the size and prosperity of the Irish linen industry. Flax spinning, formerly carried out in the crofter homes, was now carried out mainly in Belfast flax mills. Shortly afterward, reports of chronic cough and shortness of breath in mill operatives began to make their appearance. The problems of the early Irish flax operatives have been well described by Schilling.[3] Similar problems were later described in hemp workers.[4]

Byssinosis has been described in all countries of the world where cotton, flax, and hemp are spun and processed. Much of the early clinical investigation was carried out in Great Britain, and for many years, byssinosis was assumed to be peculiar to Lancashire and Ulster. Over the past four decades, a significant prevalence has been reported from Spain, Egypt, the Netherlands, India, Sweden, and the United States,[5–9] but no matter where the disease is described, the symptoms are the same. Somewhat similar chest symptoms have been reported in jute, wool, and sisal workers, but doubt exists as to whether these textiles cause byssinosis.

THE MANUFACTURE OF COTTON

A series of processes are involved in the manufacture of cotton yarn. First, the cotton lint has to be separated from the seed. Until Eli Whitney invented the cotton gin, this had to be done by hand, and the ginners came into intimate contact with the dust. Since Whitney's time, further strides toward mechanization of cotton ginning have taken place, although even now there is evidence that byssinosis may still be occurring in cotton ginners. Seed cotton is first cleaned before being passed to the gin stand, where the lint is separated from the seed. The latter is then transported to the oil mill for separation into linters, oils, and meats. When the lint has been separated by pneumatic suction, it is carried pneumatically into a chamber. There it is compressed into bales, which are then transported to cotton mills.

At the mill, the cotton bale is first divided up and the cotton cleaned. This is effected by running the cotton through the cotton chamber, blowing room, and carding room. The cotton is first broken out of the bales and fed by hand into a

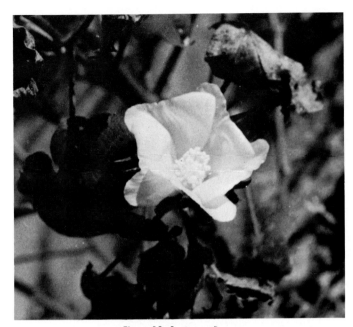

Figure 18–1. Cotton flower.

machine known as the hopper bale opener. It then passes into the blowing room, where it undergoes a series of processes the purpose of which is to open out and separate the compressed cotton fibers. Treatment of the cotton in the blowing room is designed to ensure that the impurities are removed and that the different qualities of fiber are completely mixed. In general, the machines used in the blowing room are protected so that they do not generate much dust. They have to be cleaned, however, and this is a dusty job and should not be done unless those involved are suitably clad and wearing respirators. Byssinosis is as common in the blowing room as it is in the carding room, although fewer workers are at risk.[10]

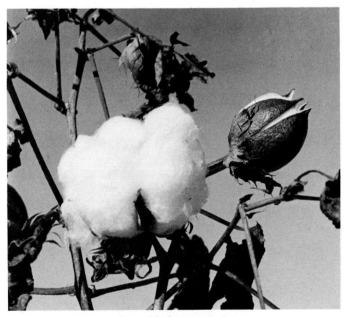

Figure 18–2. Cotton boll.

From the blowing room, the cotton is taken to the carding room. Carding involves the final removal of impurities and the aligning of the fibers. The term carding is derived from the Latin *cardus,* meaning thistle. At one time, the dried prickly cotton bracts were used for carding, but today, the process is done by a carding machine (Fig. 18–3). This consists of a metal cylinder on which are set numerous steel-wire teeth. The cylinder rotates against a separate series of teeth set in the opposite direction. As a result, the cotton is combed into line, and the short lengths are removed. Each carding engine has to be cleaned by vacuum several times a day and then later "brush stripped." After prolonged use, the carding cylinder's teeth become dull and deformed and must be reshaped and sharpened. The men who carry out these tasks are known as strippers and grinders, and it is they, rather than the other employees of the carding room, who are most affected. Although carding room processes and the machines used tend to differ according to the country in which the cotton is being processed, carding itself is universal. The respiratory symptoms that occur in carding-room workers have long been known as "stripper's asthma."

From the carding room, the cotton is twisted into threads before being made into the fabric. The final stages, i.e., spinning, weaving, and finishing, are relatively free from dust, although byssinosis has been reported in spinners.

THE MANUFACTURE OF FLAX

Certain of the processes involved in the manufacture of yarn from flax differ from those used in the cotton industry. The fibers of the flax plant are 3 to 3.5 cm long and occur in their natural state as compound fibers that have to be separated from the woody part of the stem by a process known as scutching. This involves beating bundles of the plant after they have been softened by allowing bacteria to act on them while they are immersed in water, a process known as retting. Instead of bacteria, molds and fungi can be used to ret the fibers, in which circumstances the fibers are exposed above ground in a dry state. This is known as dew retting. A third process is also sometimes used in which the fibers are retted in a tank to which chemicals have been added; this is known as tank retting. After the fibers have been retted, they can be separated from the stem by beating. The various

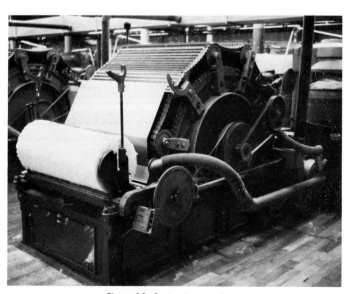

Figure 18–3. Carding machine.

procedures and jobs involved in the preparation of flax have been well described by Elwood et al.[11]

Flax fibers are first combed to separate them and to rid them of dirt and other impurities. The separated tow is carded to form a sliver. The slivers are repeatedly drawn through rows of "gills," in contrast to the cotton fiber, which is drawn through parallel pressure rollers. Spinning of the coarse flax yarn is similar to that of cotton fibers, but when fine linen yarn is needed, the flax slivers have to be softened in hot water, a process known as wet spinning. Byssinosis may be found in all stages of the manufacture of flax, although it is rare in wet spinners. It is most prevalent in flax preparers, namely, those involved in the mixing and carding of the tow.

MORTALITY AND MORBIDITY DATA

Despite the fact that byssinosis has been recognized for many years and is known to occur on every continent, adequate mortality and morbidity data are scarce. Although mortality statistics in textile workers have been available in Britain for some time, many of the data have been contradictory, and to date, no one has demonstrated that byssinosis is associated with an increased standardized mortality ratio (SMR) or that cotton textile workers have an increased death rate from occupationally acquired respiratory disease. The Registrar General of Great Britain's report of 1897 showed that cotton, linen, and flax workers had excessive death rates.[12] In 1923, 1927, and 1938, the Registrar General published specific data on the death rates for strippers, grinders, spinners, and weavers for three triennia (1910–1912, 1921–1923, and 1930–1932).[13–15] In each 3-year period, strippers and grinders had an excess mortality from respiratory disease, although the mortality declined appreciably between the 1921–1923 and the 1930–1932 triennia. In the late 1940s, it was suggested that cotton workers suffered an excess of cardiovascular disease; however, this claim was largely spurious because cor pulmonale secondary to airways obstruction was being certified as a primary circulatory disease.[16] In addition, it is now apparent that the excess mortality rate in textile workers in the three triennia arose from a variety of different causes, including tuberculosis, pneumonia, and other nonbyssinotic causes of airways obstruction. The Registrar General's Decennial Supplement for 1951 showed an excess mortality rate for bronchitis and myocardial degeneration in cotton spinners; however, the mortality rate for rheumatic disease was also increased in cotton weavers,[17] an unexpected anomalous finding. In the latest Decennial Supplement (1970–1972), which was published in 1978, no excess death rates from respiratory disease were noted in fiber preparers.[18] Twenty deaths were expected from bronchitis, asthma, and emphysema, whereas 24 occurred, a negligible and statistically insignificant difference. Unfortunately, the Decennial Supplement is no longer published, and many useful mortality data relating to occupation are no longer available.

In the United States, Henderson and Enterline used cotton workers as controls for asbestos workers in a mortality study, and in doing so, they showed that the cotton workers had no excess deaths from respiratory disease.[19] A later study of mortality rates of textile workers in two North Carolina cotton mills likewise showed no surfeit of respiratory deaths, and indeed for the most part, cotton workers had a normal life expectancy.[20]

Berry and Molyneux also described the findings of a mortality study in 16 Lancashire textile mills.[21] They found that, in many instances, the death rates were lower than expected, and this was equally true for strippers and grinders. They did, however, stress that the number of deaths was relatively few, that the results described were preliminary, and that before definitive conclusions could be drawn further follow-up was necessary. A comprehensive follow-up study of 2528 flax workers has also been published. Both male and female deaths were fewer than expected, and the most dust-exposed workers had no increased death rate. These data make it clear that any effect on occupational mortality associated with byssinosis is, at the worst, extremely small.[22] Suffice it to say, at the present time, there is no evidence to indicate that cotton or flax workers have an increased death rate from respiratory disease.

CLINICAL FEATURES

Byssinosis was originally recognized by a set of characteristic symptoms that occur in cotton workers, namely, chest tightness and shortness of breath that develop on returning to work each Monday. Lee thinks that the term tightness does not do justice or fully describe the symptoms experienced by subjects who have byssinosis.[23] He quotes Kay's description of the chest disease that affects cotton spinners: "[The affected worker] experiences a diffuse and obscure sensation of uneasiness beneath the sternum. On sudden exertion a pectoral oppression occurs as if it were from an inability to dilate the chest fully in ordinary inspiration." Kay's somewhat rococo description is not quite the mode of expression used by patients who have byssinosis and who seem almost invariably to complain of chest tightness. Epidemiological studies in cotton, flax, and hemp workers have made it apparent that those exposed to these textiles in addition may develop a variety of respiratory symptoms that differ from the typical symptoms of chest tightness and shortness of breath. It is now evident that exposure to cotton, hemp, and flax dust may be associated with four responses:

1. The development of chest tightness and shortness of breath on first returning to work.
2. A decline in ventilatory capacity over the first work shift of the week.
3. An increased prevalence of bronchitis, as manifested by persistent cough and sputum.
4. A clinical syndrome known as mill fever that usually occurs when a worker first starts working or on returning from a prolonged absence. Mill fever is characterized by the onset of fever and aches and pains, symptoms closely resembling those induced by a gram-negative endotoxin.

With the exception of mill fever, all of these conditions are often loosely referred to as byssinosis. There are, nonetheless, compelling arguments to limit the term byssinosis to the acute response, i.e., the chest tightness that develops on first returning to work, and possibly the decrement in ventilatory capacity. Although there is some concordance between the symptoms of chest tightness and the acute shift decrement, this relationship is often far from exact. In the case of the more chronic syndrome of bronchitis, this is apparently unrelated to the acute symptoms. Moreover, the previously widely held belief that the acute response, when it occurs over a prolonged period, slowly evolves into chronic irreversible airways obstruction and emphysema is suspect and probably incorrect.[24]

Acute Effects

Although some subjects may experience chest tightness on the first occasion they are exposed to cotton dust, more commonly, the employee has been working for several years before symptoms develop.[3, 25] Those persons who react on the first day of exposure are likely to leave the job and seek employment elsewhere within 1 to 2 months of starting work. To begin with, symptoms usually occur only on the first shift after a subject returns to work, and because this is usually a Monday, the normal history is one of Monday morning chest tightness. Should the subject work over the weekend and have days off in the middle of the week, then the symptoms will develop the day work is resumed. Initially, the chest tightness and wheeze last for a few hours and then disappear, but with increasing exposure, some subjects notice that the symptoms either recur or persist on Tuesdays and occasionally for the rest of the working week.[3-10]

Epidemiological surveys to detect the prevalence of byssinosis in working populations have, to a large extent, relied on the Medical Research Council of Great Britain (MRC) questionnaire on respiratory symptoms.[26] The usefulness of this questionnaire has been greatly enhanced by the addition of some supplementary questions on chest tightness. By means of the responses to the questionnaire, a useful grading system for byssinosis has evolved: grade ½, occasional tightness on Mondays or the day on which work is resumed; grade 1, chest tightness and/or difficulty in breathing on Monday or the day on which work is resumed; and grade 2, chest tightness and difficulty breathing not only on Mondays but on other days of the week. Although the questionnaire is a useful approach to quantifying the prevalence of byssinosis, it has to be administered in an objective fashion. Unless the interviewer is careful, bias may result from framing the questions in a tendentious fashion.

The acute symptoms of chest tightness can be duplicated by inhalational challenges with both cotton dust and aqueous extract of cotton bract.[9] Not all workers react, however. Those at risk can be divided into reactors and nonreactors, with the former in the majority and usually constituting up to 65% to 75% of the total. The prevalence of symptoms of byssinosis also appears to be influenced by smoking habits. In many surveys, smokers have been shown to have a greater prevalence of byssinosis.[27, 28]

Although it has been suggested that allergic diathesis or atopy play a role in the development of byssinosis,[29] convincing evidence is not yet available to support this contention. In some relatively recent studies, it has been claimed that most byssinotic subjects have bronchial reactivity, even though atopy was no more prevalent in byssinotic patients than in those cotton operators who did not have byssinosis.[29, 30] It was suggested, moreover, that bronchial hyperreactivity may be an index of susceptibility to inhaled cotton dust and that it predisposes to the development of byssinosis. This observation does not necessarily follow. Bronchial hyperreactivity may be acquired with the passage of time from exposure to cotton dust or other irritants.

The role of atopy and skin reactivity to cotton antigens is uncertain, and more work needs to be done in this field. Jones et al. studied 255 workers in a cotton seed crushing mill.[31] Atopy was determined by prick tests using common inhalant allergens. Atopic workers were subsequently shown to have greater falls in the forced expiratory volume in 1 second (FEV_1) than nonatopic workers. The investigators believed that certain types of cotton dust led to a more positive response in atopic subjects. Thus, it was shown that atopic workers showed a greater fall in FEV_1 over a work shift. The authors concluded that atopy may well interact with the effects of exposure to a particular type of cotton dust to accentuate the acute bronchoconstrictor response. The possibility exists, however, that the fall in FEV_1 may be nonspecific and is not necessarily related to cotton fibers but that is a manifestation of bronchial hyperreactivity that is gradually acquired in subjects who have been repeatedly exposed to nonspecific irritants. Earlier studies have shown that nonasthmatic responders to cotton bract (byssinotics) do not react to histamine in the same overly sensitive fashion as do asthmatics.[32]

In subjects challenged with cotton extract, the acute response may take several hours to develop. In this way, it differs from typical immunoglobulin E (IgE)-mediated asthma and the characteristic rapid onset of the response seen in asthmatic patients who are challenged with either methacholine or histamine.[32-34] Challenge experiments have been carried out for periods up to 4 hours, a finding which suggests that factors other than smooth muscle contraction may play a role in the development of the acute byssinotic response. The acute response can be attenuated or averted by prior administration of atropine, cromolyn sodium, and chlorpheniramine, but it is enhanced by propranolol.[35-37] The prevalence of byssinosis also varies from mill to mill, and such differences cannot be explained by a single variable, such as dust exposure.[38]

Changes in Ventilatory Capacity

Acute

A degree of biological variability is inherent in all tests, and this is particularly true of tests of ventilatory capacity. Part of the variability is related to the diurnal variation in ventilatory capacity that occurs in both normal persons and those with respiratory disease. It therefore becomes difficult to establish definite criteria for what constitutes an acute response. For want of something better, it is suggested that any shift decrement in the FEV_1 of between 5% and 10% should be regarded as strongly suggestive of byssinosis; any change of greater than 10% should be regarded as diagnostic. Alternatively, should there be a fall in the FEV_1 of greater than 200 ml, the shift decrement should be regarded as strongly suggestive of the presence of byssinosis. The highest of three acceptable FEV_1s, all of which should be within 5% of each other, should be accepted as the subject's value. Although other tests of ventilatory capacity, e.g., maximal flows, FEF_{25-75}, and closing volume, have been suggested as being more sensitive in the detection of byssinosis, these tests are less reproducible and are affected by changes in lung volume. For this reason, the FEV_1 is preferred.[39] The forced vital capacity (FVC) also often shows a change over a shift, but as a test, it is less sensitive than the FEV_1 in the diagnosis of byssinosis (Fig. 18–4). In testing subjects, it is important to remember that the pre- and postventilatory studies should always be done on the first morning the subject returns to work, whether that be a Monday or any other day, since the back-to-work decrement is usually appreciably larger on that day than on subsequent days of the week.

The National Institute of Occupational Safety and Health (NIOSH)-recommended standard for cotton dust contains an appendix that describes the requirements and criteria that should be, and now have to be, met when carrying out serial pulmonary function tests in textile workers.[40] In general, the regulations seem appropriate, with the exception that they permit a 10% difference between the two larger FEV_1s and FVCs. Such a large difference is too lax and can only lead to dubious results, which will detract from the medical surveillance program.

A number of other indices of lung function have been used to study the acute effects of cotton dust exposure. These include the measurement of lung volumes, diffusing capacity, and arterial blood gases.[41, 42] Small increases in residual volume may occur following acute exposure, but the total lung capacity, for the most part, is unaffected. The diffusing capacity remains unchanged over a work shift. Significant falls in partial arterial oxygen pressure (Pa_{O_2}) and oxygen saturation have also been reported in active and retired hemp workers following challenges with hemp fibers.[41] The decrement in the Pa_{O_2} is the consequence of worsening of ventilation/perfusion mismatching. Guyatt and coworkers have also made a study of lung

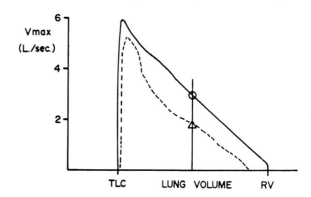

Figure 18–4. Flow volume loops before and after exposure to cotton dust. Vertical lines with circle and triangle represent flow at 50% of vital capacity, assuming that total lung capacity (TLC) is not significantly changed. The FEV_1 fell 14%. RV increased 12.5%.

mechanics in subjects with byssinosis.[43] They concluded that there was a loss of elastic recoil in affected subjects, and in part, this contributed to the decreased flows observed in cotton workers with chronic airways obstruction. Unfortunately, the subject selection in the study was less than optimal, and there may have been appreciable bias. Moreover, the results for smokers and nonsmokers were considered together, thereby, to a large extent, making it difficult to separate the effects of dust exposure from those of smoking. Furthermore, only six of the 23 subjects included in the study were nonsmokers. Bouhuys and Van de Woestijne carried out detailed studies of lung mechanics in hemp workers and suggested that two responses to the offending agent are seen.[44] They termed the first a flow rate response and suggested that this is seen in subjects with typical byssinotic symptoms, i.e., chest tightness. In these subjects, there is a decrement in the FEV_1 and flow rates. Although the FVC may also decrease to a limited extent, the subject's airways conductance remains unchanged. These authors attributed the decline in the flow rates to a pharmacologically induced bronchoconstriction taking place in the small airways. The second type of response was seen in those subjects who, after the challenge, had no symptoms. These subjects showed no decrement in the FEV_1, vital capacity, or maximal flows but did show a decrease in their airways conductance. The latter response was attributed to a reflex or a mechanical effect on the large airways. It was noted that both types of response could be abolished by the prior administration of bronchodilators.

In the study of 645 cotton operators alluded to earlier, 85 subjects complained of respiratory symptoms that could possibly be related to occupation.[29] The investigators found that only 23 of the 85 subjects could be definitely categorized as having byssinosis; the other 62 subjects had symptoms of a nonspecific nature that could be caused by other exposures, including smoking. These two groups were matched with 84 asymptomatic operatives. All three groups had a reduced FEV_1, but the byssinotic subjects had the lowest mean FEV_1 value. Only the byssinotic patients, however, had a reduced FVC. The three groups were by no means well matched, at least for height, weight, and smoking habits, and unfortunately, no data were given in regard to these confounding factors. The significance of the reduced FVC remains dubious and is probably due to encroachment of the residual volume (RV) on the FVC in those subjects who had the most obstruction. Without better matching, few inferences can be drawn in regard to the effects of byssinosis and atopy on this group of cotton operators.

Long-Term Effects

For many years, it was presumed that the acute response to cotton dust portended the development of irreversible airways obstruction. It was assumed that the acute response gradually became less evident and slowly evolved into a more chronic condition that was characterized by continuous shortness of breath, cough, and sputum. It was further assumed that chronic exposure eventually led to emphysema and irreversible obstruction, but a number of recent studies have shown that there is either a poor or, more commonly, no relationship between the acute response and the development of the chronic syndrome. Although certain studies have demonstrated an unusually high decrement in the ventilatory capacity of textile workers, such findings have been inconsistent and are not wholly convincing for a variety of reasons.[28, 45] Moreover, studies of the pathological findings of the condition have shown that, although bronchitis and bronchiolitis occur more commonly in the lungs of textile workers, whether smokers or not, emphysema was observed only in the lungs of smokers.[46] Morphological evidence of bronchitis and bronchiolitis was to be found in the lungs of nonsmoking textile workers. Even in textile workers with dust-associated bronchitis, the relationship between cumulative dust exposure or the duration of dust exposure and the presence of bronchitis is sadly deficient. Much the same situation exists for the annual change in FEV_1. Some studies have suggested that the annual rate of decline of the FEV_1 is greater in cotton mill workers than in workers in mills that process synthetic fibers, but the rate of decline was unrelated to symptoms of byssinosis, to past or current dust levels, or to the postshift decline in the FEV_1.[27, 28, 47] One such study reported a FEV_1 decrement of "54 ml/yr (expected 25 ml/year)" in a group of Lancashire mill workers.[47] Those processing synthetic fibers had a decrement of 32 ml/year. However, only two synthetic mills were included in the study, one of which seemed to be mainly responsible for the overall relatively normal rate of decline observed in the noncotton textile workers. Whether these two mills represent the general population of noncotton-exposed textile workers is doubtful. Furthermore, dust sampling was carried out only at the time of the survey and not over a longer period. Similar studies in retired mill workers in South Carolina have shown an increased annual decrement in the FEV_1, but it has been impossible to exclude geographical and other selection biases.[48] In this study, a survivor population of active and retired cotton workers was shown to have a lower mean FEV_1 and FVC than did the reference population who came from Connecticut.[48] Whether the latter group can be regarded as comparable to the study group is a moot point because of the geographical difference. Another study showed that the FEV_1 of nonbyssinotic cotton workers was below the predicted value for all durations of employment beyond 2 years.[49] Incongruously, however, the nonsmoking byssinotic workers with the longest employment had the best ventilatory capacity, making it difficult to reconcile dust exposure with any chronic decline in lung function. This study probably had a greater than normal percentage of black subjects included in it, and no obvious effort was made to correct for the smaller lung volumes of the black subjects. In another widely quoted study, the purpose of which was to detect the effect of steam treating cotton, the study population was deliberately chosen so as to include a high proportion of byssinotic subjects with heavy exposure to low-grade cotton.[50] The decline in the FEV_1 over an observation period of 10 months was 192 ml, but the observation period in this study was too short. Were this the usual rate of decline in the FEV_1, it would be difficult to explain why such a rapid deterioration in lung function would not be reflected in increased mortality figures.

A more recent study of 66 cotton textile workers who were followed from 1970 to 1985 claimed to have demonstrated an increasing prevalence of respiratory symptoms and impairment of lung function over the period of observation.[51] The group consisted of 35 nonsmoking female and 31 smoking male workers. The average annual decline in the FVC for the male workers was less in those who had symptoms of byssinosis than in those who did not (0.043 L *versus* 0.068 L). The annual decline in the FEV_1 for those with and without byssinotic symptoms was the same. In the women with byssinosis, there was a minimally greater annual decline in both the FVC and FEV_1 (0.07 L and 0.01 L); however, the figures did not differ significantly from those in subjects without byssinosis. Although the annual decline in the FEV_1 as a whole, irrespective of symptoms, was slightly greater than expected in the general population, the study population was drawn mainly from rural Serbia, and no epidemiological reference data were available from this region. As far as this study is concerned, the increased rate of decline in lung function in men may be entirely a consequence of smoking, but whether the same can be said of the women is debatable.

It is reasonably clear that, although byssinosis, whether acute or chronic, may be associated with some impairment of ventilatory capacity, the overall decrement in lung function is small. Thus, Elwood et al. found a 2% to 8% reduction in ventilatory capacity in ex-cotton workers compared with that in controls.[52] A small effect on the FEV_1 with increasing dust exposure was noticed. This small reduction in ventilatory capacity, however, would not be expected to affect the SMR for respiratory disease in cotton workers.

Although the ventilatory capacity of flax, hemp, and cotton workers has repeatedly been demonstrated to be lower than that of comparable controls, it is often difficult to separate the effects of the acute response from the more chronic effects. The decreased ventilatory capacity that characterizes the acute response is seen, for the most part, in carders, pickers, and those involved in early processing of cotton. It has also been observed that workers with symptoms of byssinosis—in this instance, chest tightness and wheeze—have significantly lower spirometric values than do asymptomatic workers,[28, 45] but again, it is not known whether the lower FEV_1 is permanent and irreversible or simply a delayed manifestation of acute exposure that is likely to resolve completely when exposure ceases. Other studies have shown that cough and sputum are more common in textile workers than in nonexposed workers, but the exact implications of these symptoms are not clear. The clinical significance of the increased prevalence of cough and sputum is debatable, but there is excellent evidence to indicate that these symptoms do not necessarily portend the onset of irreversible obstruction.[53] Indeed, such symptoms are present in numerous dust-exposed populations, and most evidence points to the fact that the symptoms are of little moment. When it comes to comparing ventilatory capacity in exposed and nonexposed populations, there have been problems in the selection of the control or reference population. Differing smoking habits; differing types of fibers, whether coarse or fine; and the different ethnic origins of the workers surveyed all may play a role in introducing bias. Moreover, the results of many of these studies have been conflicting. There is ample morphological and epidemiological evidence to indicate that bronchitis and bronchiolitis occur more frequently in those exposed to cotton dust, but the same cannot be said for emphysema, which appears to be limited to textile workers who smoke.[24, 46]

Whether byssinosis predisposes to the development of progressive chronic airflow limitation has not been fully settled, but it is clear that, if there are any effects, they are minor. At this juncture, it seems that there is a slight increase in the rate of decline of the FEV_1 in cotton mill workers as a whole, but this is not necessarily related to byssinosis and may well be attributable to industrial bronchitis, which may be induced by a variety of nonspecific dusts.[53, 54] Moreover, it needs to be borne in mind that similar effects have been noted in woolen mills.[55]

A 5-year longitudinal study of 611 workers at six cotton mills claimed to have shown a significant association between the acute and chronic effects of exposure to cotton dust.[55a] Both dust exposure and across-shift change were said to be predictors of excess annual declines in the FEV_1. Such effects were present even when cotton dust exposure was less than 200 g/m³, i.e., below the TLV. While this was true for the entire group of cotton workers, the decline in the FEV_1 varied according to the shift worked (shift 1, 7 AM to 3 PM; shift 2, 3 PM to 11 PM; and shift 3, 11 PM to 7 AM). In some instances the annual across-shift changes were greatest in those who were exposed to the least dust, and both the annual decline and shift change were significantly influenced by smoking. Moreover, there were three times as many workers with bronchitis in shift 1 as there were in shift 3. Thus, the greater annual decline and across-shift change in the workers in shift 1 may be related to the fact that they were heavier smokers and could also have increased bronchial hyperreactivity as a result of their smoking habits.

The specificity of cotton dust as the agent responsible for so-called chronic byssinosis must remain *sub judice*. There is a need for longer prospective studies that investigate the decline in ventilatory capacity to cotton dust levels and other variables, including smoking and the cotton fiber type. It must be borne in mind, however, that the cotton industry has significantly contracted in Europe and North America over the past 15 years.

BYSSINOSIS IN HEMP AND FLAX WORKERS

Exposure to hemp dust is associated with the same effects as is exposure to cotton dust. It occurs usually in soft hemp spinners. Carey et al. found that Ulster flax workers who complained of byssinotic symptoms had a lower average FEV_1 than did nonbyssinotic workers.[56] The highest prevalence of symptoms occurred in those exposed to retted flax.[57] The decrease in ventilatory capacity occurs most commonly in preparers; spinners and polishers are much less likely to be affected. Bronchitis is a common finding in flax mill operatives.

Byssinosis is also found in cottonseed mills in which the raw cottonseed is separated into short cotton fibers or linters, hulls, and meats; the latter is the source of cottonseed oil.[58] The process of separation is often dusty, and there is some evidence that byssinosis occurs in around 2% to 3% of the workers.

PATHOLOGICAL FINDINGS

Until recently, there have been few descriptions of the morphological changes found in the lungs of textile workers, and the few observations that have been made have generally been nonspecific or suggested the presence of emphysema. Moreover, little attempt was made to relate postmortem findings to premortem dust exposure, smoking habits, and pulmonary function tests.

It has been suggested that chronic byssinosis is associated with a loss of elastic recoil, presumably caused by emphysema,[43] and that the latter may account for the airways obstruction noted in cotton workers. This seems unlikely in that Edwards and coworkers examined the heart and lungs of 43 subjects who, in life, had been diagnosed as having byssinosis and, subsequently, were awarded compensation.[54] Although some emphysema was found at the postmortem examination, there appeared to be no relationship between the presence of this condition and prior cotton dust exposure. In contrast, bronchitis and bronchiolitis were found more frequently in the textile workers than in the general population. Neither right ventricular hypertrophy nor pulmonary vascular abnormalities were noted. In addition, a study found that emphysema is not associated with exposure to cotton dust *per se,* and when observed in a cotton worker postmortem, it is almost certainly a consequence of the individual's smoking habits.[24] Further careful studies carried out by Rooke demonstrated similar findings.[46] He was unable to show any evidence of fibrosis or emphysema in the lungs of textile workers and likewise could not demonstrate emphysema unless the subjects were cigarette smokers. These findings are supported by an extensive and well-controlled investigation in which the diffusing capacity of 153 English female textile workers was measured. A reduction of the diffusing capacity was present only in those subjects who were or had been smokers.[59] Rooke also made the observation that so-called byssinotic bodies were uncommon in the lungs of textile workers.[46] Byssinotic bodies are rounded aggregates of debris with a central black core that is surrounded by yellowish material and are composed for the most part of degenerated alveolar macrophages.

ETIOLOGICAL FACTORS

Before the late 1940s, little attention had been given to the investigation of the etiology of byssinosis; however, the situation has changed radically. Many hypotheses have been put forward to explain the airway changes seen in byssinosis, but none is entirely satisfactory. There is little doubt that the agent or agents responsible for the bronchoconstriction are located in the cotton bract; however, their identity remains unknown.

Early observers noted the similarity between the symptoms of byssinosis and those of asthma, and for years, byssinosis was believed to be a form of asthma. Nevertheless, there are features of byssinosis that are completely different from those of asthma. Extrinsic asthma is associated with an immediate response that develops in 10 to 30 minutes. Such a reaction is brought on by exposure to antigenic proteins. In contrast, the symptoms of byssinosis develop slowly over several hours and improve as the week goes by, despite continued exposure. Subjects with byssinotic symptoms do not demonstrate the acute response to histamine or methacholine challenge. Furthermore, some subjects with byssinosis have undergone repeated challenges with antigen for periods up to 4 hours, a procedure that would be quite intolerable in asthmatic patients. Another difference is that, in contrast to asthma, byssinosis affects a large proportion of those exposed to the offending agent, usually well over 50%. Likewise, asthmatic attacks occur unpredictably and may remit in an equally unpredictable fashion. The absence of both a family history and the allergic diathesis in byssinosis serves to distinguish the two conditions. Such differences seem a most telling argument against considering byssinosis to be a form of asthma.

A variety of pathophysiological mechanisms have been put forward to explain the symptoms and decrement in ventilatory capacity that are seen in byssinotic patients. At least three of these can be dismissed fairly summarily. At one time, the symptoms and ventilatory decrement were thought to be a consequence of an inert dust reaction; however, cotton dust produces a response at much lower concentrations (roughly one thirtieth to one fiftieth) of coal and other inert dusts. Moreover, washed cotton dust and other fibers, such as polyesters, do not have the same effect on the FEV_1. Other persons have suggested that cotton dust contains agents that act directly on the airways and induce bronchoconstriction. Included in this category are histamine and serotonin, which are present, albeit in minute quantities insufficient to induce bronchoconstriction. The third hypothesis is that byssinosis is an immediate asthmatic reaction to an allergen. Reasons have already been stated for rejecting this theory.

Several other more likely theories of the pathogenesis of byssinosis exist, including the following hypotheses.[60]

1. **Pharmacological release of histamine or other mediators.** There is no doubt that cotton dust can cause liberation of histamine.[61] Similar observations have been made with cotton extracts. Inhalation experiments with cotton dust and aqueous extracts of cotton bract have been shown to induce a fall in the FEV_1, which can be prevented by the prior administration of antihistamines.[34, 62] Extracts of cotton dust will liberate histamine from platelets.[63] An increase of histamine metabolites has been shown to occur in the urine of subjects exposed to cotton dust, but the site of histamine release has not been established.[33] Although the histamine hypothesis has a certain meretricious appeal, there are certain weaknesses to it. First, the time course of the reaction with reference to the changes in ventilatory capacity is inappropriate and cannot be explained by histamine alone. Second, the evidence from the use of histamine antagonists is nonspecific and questionable.

   The possibility that mediators other than histamine are important in the pathogenesis of byssinosis needs further study. It is known that slow-reacting substance of anaphylaxis (SRS-A) not only induces bronchoconstriction but is also an eosinophil chemotaxin. SRS-A is released from several cells that are commonly found in the lung, including polymorphonuclear leukocytes. In addition, it has been shown that aqueous extract of cotton dust will mobilize polymorphonuclear leukocytes in lung tissue. Leukotrienes C and E are derivatives of arachidonic acid and are released by the cell surfaces of polymorphonuclear leukocytes, mononuclear phagocytes, and basophils, and as such are 200 to 2000 times more powerful than histamine in inducing smooth muscle contraction.[64] Other potential mediators include platelet-activating factors, which also may be released in the lung under certain circumstances and can induce bronchoconstriction.[65, 66]

2. **Chemotactic mechanisms.** It has been suggested that the induction of chemotaxis by cotton dust may play a role in the pathogenesis of byssinosis. Certain polyphenolic extracts of cotton trash and quercetin have been shown to recruit polymorphonuclear leukocytes into hamsters' airways, Lancinilene C and lancinilene E-7 methyl ether have been isolated from water extracts of the cotton bract and have been demonstrated to be chemotactic.[67] Even so, the mechanism whereby chemotaxis might induce acute bronchoconstriction is unclear, and the exact role of chemotaxis, if any, in the induction of the acute byssinotic reaction

is not known. Rohrbach et al. observed that the inhalation of cotton mill dust or condensed tannin, which is a prime component of cotton mill dust, will induce an acute inflammatory lung response associated with the ingress of neutrophils into the airways.[68] These investigators claimed that the effect of tannin on alveolar macrophages leads to the secretion of neutrophil chemotactic factor, and they suggest this may be responsible for the development of the acute neutrophil alveolitis found after the inhalation of cotton dust.

3. **Endotoxin activity.** A group of Italian workers showed that the inhalation of purified *Escherichia coli* endotoxin will induce a fall in the ventilatory capacity and that an associated febrile response was frequently absent.[69, 70] The levels of endotoxin were roughly equal to those that are found in exposed cotton mill workers. Rylander and Lundholm have extended these observations and showed that symptoms of byssinosis correlate better with endotoxin levels that occur in cotton dust than they do with measurements of respirable dust.[71] It is also abundantly clear that cotton plants are invariably contaminated with gram-negative organisms, and the same can be said for the air of most cotton mills. Gram-negative bacilli contain a particularly toxic substance that is known as lipopolysaccharide (LPS). This consists of hydrophilic and lipid-rich fractions. The hydrophilic fraction consists of a polysaccharide chain with repeating units, constituting the somatic O antigens and a core polysaccharide. The lipid-rich fraction consists of phosphate groups, diglucosamine, and fatty acids and is probably the active fraction.[71–72] It seems that the lower the LPS content of cotton dust, the less likely are exposed subjects to react.[73] While the role of endotoxin as a cause of byssinosis is by no means certain, further investigations, including human challenges with LPS, would seem desirable in investigating the role of endotoxin in the etiology of byssinosis. It has been shown in animal experiments that it is possible to induce parenchymal lesions in the lungs of hamsters by the intratracheal instillation of cotton dust, cellulose, and endotoxin. The lesions have a composite feature of emphysema and fibrosis, but their relevance to human byssinosis is tenuous.[74] Other investigators have suggested that cotton dust may impair surfactant activity.[75]

4. **Antigen-antibody reaction.** Various workers have put forward the hypothesis that byssinosis is a type III hypersensitivity reaction, but there is little scientific evidence in support of this notion. Massoud and Taylor reported that cotton bract extracts produce lines of precipitation in sera from byssinotic patients, but the presence of antibody was subsequently shown to be nonspecific precipitation of IgG.[76] In later work, Taylor et al. isolated a polyphenyl, 5,7,3,4,tetrahydroxy-flavan 3,4 diol (THF) that they suggested was the agent responsible.[77] In a double-blind trial, although challenges with THF induced symptoms of byssinosis, it did not induce a drop in the FEV_1.[77] Firm evidence that THF has a role in the cause of byssinosis is lacking, and the type III hypothesis has been examined in more detail by Kutz et al. and found unconvincing.[78] They are of the opinion that true precipitating antibodies do not exist.

It is thus apparent that there is a great divergence of opinion as to the causative agent of byssinosis.[79] Various groups of workers with a vested interest in a particular agent have become unduly preoccupied with that agent to the extent that they tend to dismiss other hypotheses too summarily. At the present time, it seems probable that several agents may play a role or that there may be a multicomponent cause, with various agents enhancing the effects of one another. Most evidence suggests that cotton dust contains an agent or agents that will induce both chest tightness and an associated decrement in ventilatory capacity. Such a response appears to involve the liberation of mediators that will contract bronchial smooth muscle. For reasons previously stated, this seems unlikely to be related to any specific immunological reaction. Such a nonspecific response might originate, first, as a result of an inhaled component of cotton dust activating complement components that have been synthesized by activated macrophages with the formation of

C3a and C5a anaphylatoxins, or second, as a result of two or more constituents of the inhaled dust-activating lymphocytes, macrophages, mast cells, or basophils in a polyclonal and nonimmune fashion. The second hypothesis appears to be more likely.

Host Factors

A variety of host factors have been suggested as possibly predisposing to the development of byssinosis. These include atopy, aspirin sensitivity, and airways hyperreactivity. Most such suggestions do not bear close examination. Histocompatibility antigen (HLA) frequency has been investigated in flax workers with byssinosis, with the finding that HLA-B27 predisposes to the development of byssinosis, but this observation has little importance, since byssinosis occurs so frequently with other HLA types.[80]

PREVENTION

Dust Measurement

A number of different instruments have been used in the measurement of cotton dust[40] (see also Chapter 9). These include the cascade impactor, the high-volume total dust sampler, the vertical elutriator, and the horizontal elutriator. The vertical elutriator excludes all particles with an aerodynamic diameter greater than 14.5 microns; the horizontal elutriator of Roach segregates particles into coarse, medium, and fine. In the United States, the recommended instrument is the vertical elutriator, and the dust concentration is expressed as milligrams per cubic meter (mg/m^3).

Cotton Dust Standard

The current United States Cotton Dust Standard, which took effect in 1984, is 0.2 mg/m^3.[81] The standard was introduced gradually, with a progressive decline in the allowable concentration. The 0.2-mg/m^3 limit applies only to the picking, carding, and spinning areas, whereas in the slashing and weaving stages, the allowable concentration is 0.750 mg/m^3. The standard does not apply to cotton ginners.

Several problems exist with the recommended standard other than those relating to its financial impact on industry. The standard is based largely on the results of one or two United States cross-sectional studies,[82] the conclusions of which have repeatedly been questioned. Nowhere is it apparent which of the features of byssinosis the standard has been designed to control, the impression being that the standard will be equally effective in controlling both the acute and chronic effects of cotton dust.

Other recommendations included in the United States Cotton Dust Standard are as follows:

1. A preplacement examination to include a history, FVC, and FEV_1. The history is to include a respiratory questionnaire and is based on Schilling's modification of the British MRC questionnaire.[26]
2. Each newly employed cotton mill worker will have a repeat FVC and FEV_1 within 6 months of starting employment.
3. Periodic testing of ventilatory capacity will take place on the first day after return to work and shall be performed both before and following an exposure for at least 6 hours. These tests will be repeated at varying intervals, and specific criteria are laid down for those persons who showed a ventilatory decrement. The Occupational Safety and Health Administration standard also suggests that the FEV_1 variation should not exceed 10%; however, this would seem to be

unduly generous since a 5% to 10% drop in FEV$_1$ strongly suggests the presence of byssinosis.

Treatment of Cotton to Remove Bronchoconstrictor Agents

A variety of approaches have been used in the attempt to reduce the prevalence of byssinosis[50, 83] including cotton steaming to reduce the biological effects of cotton dust. Another approach relies on washing the cotton prior to carding and processing. An ingenious process was recently devised in which a small quantity of cotton was harvested before the opening of the boll. This was compared with standard cotton collected when the boll had already opened.[84] Cotton dust from the closed boll had a lesser effect on ventilatory capacity than the dust derived from the open boll.

These modifications have resulted in a lesser decrement in expiratory flow per milligram of cotton dust exposure. The effects on the FEV$_1$, for the most part, occurred in those subjects working in areas where dust levels were highest.

ACUTE NONBYSSINOTIC RESPIRATORY ILLNESS IN COTTON AND OTHER TEXTILE WORKERS

There have been frequent reports of outbreaks of acute respiratory illness among cotton workers. The symptoms and signs of these illnesses suggest that they are distinct from those of byssinosis; however, the clear-cut distinction that was formerly made between byssinosis and mill fever may not be as justifiable, as was believed in the recent past. No single factor appears to be concerned in their pathogeneses, and a variety of agents have been implicated. Molds and vegetable allergens are among those incriminated, and in particular, the dust of the tamarind seed (*Tamarindus indica*) has been thought to be responsible for some outbreaks. In 1913, an outbreak of cough and respiratory illness among Lancashire weavers was described by Collis.[85] The condition was characterized by bronchoconstriction, cough, purulent sputum, and shortness of breath. The material woven was cotton that had been sized with a mixture of flour, tallow, and china clay. At the time of the outbreak, the warp threads were observed to be mildewed, and furthermore, the outbreak disappeared when dry threads were substituted. The recurrence of mildew in the threads led to a further outbreak of the illness. The air over the looms was found to contain many mycelia and conidia. *Penicillium, Aspergillus,* and *Mucor* were identified in the loom dust.

In 1954, Vigliani and associates reported an epidemic of bronchoconstriction among cotton weavers.[86] The cotton yarn had been sized with locust bean gum and potato starch. About half the weavers were affected by wheezing, breathlessness, and a dry irritative cough. The symptoms were worse on Mondays, and the illness lasted between 2 and 6 months. Skin tests with molds of *Aerobacter aerogenes* produced positive results in many of the affected subjects, but the organism was never definitely implicated.

An outbreak of similar respiratory symptoms was reported in a group of Indian workers involved in the sizing of jute and cotton.[87] The weavers had started using tamarind seed a short time previously. No effect occurred with the first exposure, but with repeated exposure, sensitization seemed to take place. In some of the affected workers, but not in controls, inhalational challenges using tamarind powder produced acute symptoms of the syndrome.

A few cotton and hemp workers suffer from chills, fever, nausea, and vomiting when they first return to work after a prolonged absence. This complaint is known as mill fever or hemp fever and usually disappears in a few days. Although the term mill fever is often used as if it were a distinct entity and separate from byssinosis, some doubt remains as to whether this distinction is justifiable. In practice, although mill fever is uncommon in cotton workers, this is less true in mattress workers. Most subjects with byssinosis have characteristic symptoms, in particular, chest tightness. This is much less marked in subjects who complain of mill fever. There is evidence to indicate that *Aerobacter cloacae* is one of the responsible agents. This bacterium is found as a normal soil inhabitant and as a contaminant of cotton in cold and wet seasons. The studies of Rylander and Lundholm have shown that cotton products are contaminated by many gram-negative bacteria, particularly *Enterobacter, Pseudomonas,* and *Agrobacterium* species.[71] These bacteria are also present in the cotton plant itself. Exposure to inhaled endotoxins may lead to the development of fever, chills, and malaise and also to a decrement in the FEV_1. Gram-negative bacteria are frequently found in the air of cotton mills, and the concentration of endotoxin dust from cotton mills has been shown to range from 0.2 to 1.6 mg/g of dust—with the higher level being greatly in excess of that at which symptoms will develop in exposed workers.[88] Endotoxins can also activate complement and liberate anaphylatoxins and chemotaxins. Tolerance to endotoxin follows prolonged exposure.[89] Thus, the possibility still exists that mill fever and byssinosis are just variants of the same condition, with both being due to endotoxins.

RESPIRATORY DISEASE IN SISAL AND JUTE WORKERS

Sisal is a hard fiber produced from the leaves of *Agave sisalana,* a species of amaryllis. First found in Yucatan, Mexico, it is now grown in the United States, Europe, and Africa. It is used in the manufacture of ropes, coarse textiles, carpets, and twine. The leaves are first removed from the sisal plant. After the fibers have been extracted, they are combed and carded in a fashion similar to cotton fibers.

A byssinosis-like condition has been described in sisal workers,[90] reportedly affecting the combers more often than the drawers and spinners. Significant mean reductions in ventilatory capacity over a work shift have been recorded. This has been attributed to sisal dust causing histamine release, with its associated broncho-constriction.[91] More recently, lung function was measured in 66 workers in a sisal rope-making factory and in a matched control population.[92] A major contaminant found in the air was a lubricant used to soften the fiber. At the start of the work shift, comparison of lung function in the control and exposed groups showed no significant difference between them. However, those exposed to sisal did not change their lung function over the shift, although the control group showed the usual and expected increase in FEV_1. Baker and colleagues suggested that perhaps the lubricant and softeners used were responsible for the effect on ventilatory capacity.[92] A further study involved 77 sisal spinners and 83 sisal brushers working in six Tanzanian sisal factories.[93] Symptoms of byssinosis were low in the spinners but relatively high in those workers employed in the brushing departments. As has been observed with other textile workers, sisal workers who smoked were more prone to have symptoms of byssinosis.[27, 28] Acute changes in the FVC and FEV_1 occurred over the work shift, but in some instances acute falls in the FEV_1 were not accompanied by symptoms. Unfortunately, no dust measurements were available at the time of the survey, although prior measurements showed that brushers were exposed to higher levels than spinners.

The prevalence of symptoms of byssinosis in two groups who were exposed simultaneously to jute or hemp has been compared. Classical symptoms of byssinosis did not occur in those exposed to jute.[94] Although most studies have shown no effect from jute processing,[95, 96] Popa and coworkers suggested that byssinosis could result from exposure to jute.[97] A study of the ventilatory capacity of 46 workers exposed to jute dust likewise showed a significant decrease in the FEV_1 on the first day of work.[98] A subsequent study carried out by Valic and Zuskin compared the effects of cotton and jute dust on respiratory symptoms and respiratory function in 60 cotton and 91 jute nonsmoking female workers of similar age and similar length of dust exposure.[99] They showed that cotton workers had a significantly higher prevalence of byssinosis and of dyspnea than did jute workers. None of the jute workers had the characteristic symptoms of byssinosis. Both cotton and jute caused a significant reduction in ventilatory capacity on the first working shift in the week; however, cotton dust had a significantly greater effect. Thus, it would seem that jute probably induces a shift decrement in the FEV_1, but its effect is much less than that of cotton and flax and may be nonspecific.

REFERENCES

1. Kay, J.P., Trades producing phthisis. N. Engl. J. Med., 1, 357, 1831.
2. Greenhow, E.H., Report of the Medical Officer of the Privy Council, 1860. Appendix VI. London, H.M. Stationery Office, 1861.
3. Schilling, R.S.F., Byssinosis in cotton and other textile workers, Lancet, II, 319, 1956.
4. Jimenez Diaz, C., and Lahoz, C., La cannobosis (enfermedad de los trabajadores del canamo). Rev. Clin. Esp., 14, 366, 1944.
5. Bouhuys, A., Barbero, A., Lindell, S.-E., et al., Byssinosis in hemp workers. Arch. Environ. Health, 14, 533, 1967.
6. El Batawi, M.A., Byssinosis in cotton industry in Egypt. Br. J. Ind. Med., 19, 126, 1962.
7. Lammers, B., Schilling, R.S.F., and Walford, J., A study of byssinosis, chronic respiratory symptoms and ventilatory capacity in English and Dutch cotton workers, with special reference to atmospheric pollution. Br. J. Ind. Med., 21, 124, 1964.
8. Belin, L., Bouhuys, A., Hoekstra, W., et al., Byssinosis in cardroom workers in Swedish cotton mills. Br. J. Ind. Med., 22, 101, 1965.
9. Bouhuys, A., Heaphy, L.J., Jr., Schilling, R.S.F., and Welborn, J.W., Byssinosis in the United States. N. Engl. J. Med., 277, 170, 1967.
10. Schilling, R.S.F., Hughes, J.P.W., Dingwall-Fordyce, I., et al., Epidemiological study of byssinosis among Lancashire cotton workers. Br. J. Ind. Med., 12, 217, 1955.
11. Elwood, P.C., Pemberton, J., Merrett, J.D., et al., Byssinosis and other respiratory symptoms in flax workers in Northern Ireland. Br. J. Ind. Med., 22, 27, 1965.
12. Registrar General, Supplement to 55th Annual Report for England and Wales 1891. London, H.M. Stationery Office, 1897.
13. Registrar General, Supplement to 75th Annual Report for England and Wales 1910–12. London, H.M. Stationery Office, 1923.
14. Registrar General, Decennial Supplement, England and Wales for 1921. London, H.M. Stationery Office, 1927.
15. Registrar General, Decennial Supplement, England and Wales for 1931. London, H.M. Stationery Office, 1938.
16. Schilling, R.S.F., and Goodman, N., Cardiovascular disease in cotton workers: part 1. Br. J. Ind. Med., 8, 77, 1951.
17. Registrar General, Decennial Supplement, England and Wales 1951. Occupational Mortality, Part II, Vol. 1. London, H.M. Stationery Office, 1958.
18. Registrar General, Decennial Supplement (1970–1972). Occupational Mortality. London, H.M. Stationery Office, 1978, pp. 87–88.
19. Henderson, V.L., and Enterline, P.E., An unusual mortality experience in cotton textile workers. J. Occup. Med., 15, 717, 1973.
20. Merchant, J.A., and Ortmeyer, C.E., Mortality of employees of two cotton mills in North Carolina. Chest, 79(suppl.), 6, 1981.
21. Berry, G., and Molyneux, M.K.B., A mortality study of workers in Lancashire cotton mills. Chest, 79(suppl.), 11, 1981.
22. Elwood, P.C., Thomas, H.F., Sweetman, P.M., and Elwood, J.H., Mortality of flax workers. Br. J. Ind. Med., 39, 18, 1982.
23. Lee, W.R., Clinical diagnosis of byssinosis. Thorax, 34, 287, 1979.
24. Pratt, P.C., Vollmer, R.T., and Miller, J.A., Epidemiology of pulmonary lesions in non textile and cotton workers. Arch. Environ. Health, 35, 133, 1980.
25. Schilling, R.S.F., Byssinosis in the British cotton textile industry. Br. Med. Bull., 7, 52, 1950.
26. Roach, S.A., and Schilling, R.S.F., A clinical and environmental study of byssinosis in the Lancashire cotton industry. Br. J. Ind. Med., 17, 1, 1960.
27. Fox, A.J., Tombleson, J.B.L., Watt, A., and Wilkie, A.G., A survey of respiratory disease in cotton operatives. Part II. Symptoms, dust estimations and the effect of smoking habit. Br. J. Ind. Med., 30, 48, 1973.
28. Berry, G., Molyneux, M.K.B., and Tombleson, J.B.L., Relationship between dust level and byssinosis and bronchitis in Lancashire cotton mills. Br. J. Ind. Med., 31, 18, 1974.
29. Fishwick, D., and Pickering, C.A.C., Byssinosis—a form of occupational asthma. Thorax, 47, 401, 1992.
30. Fishwick, D., Fletcher, A.M., Pickering, C.A.C., et al., Lung function, bronchial reactivity, atopic status and dust exposure in Lancashire cotton mill operatives. Am. Rev. Respir. Dis., 145, 1103, 1992.

31. Jones, R.N., Butcher, B.T., Hammad, Y.Y., et al., Interaction of atopy and exposure to cotton dust in the bronchoconstrictor response. Br. J. Ind. Med., 37, 141, 1980.

32. Massoud, A.A.E., Altounyan, R.C., Howell, J.B.L., and Lane, R.E., Effect of histamine aerosol in byssinotic subjects. Br. J. Ind. Med., 24, 38, 1967.

33. Edwards, J., McCarthy, P., McDermott, M., et al., The acute physiological pharmacological effects of inhaled cotton dust in normal subjects. J. Physiol. (Lond.), 298, 63, 1970.

34. Bouhuys, A., Lindell, S.E., and Lundin, G., Experimental studies on byssinosis. B.M.J., 1, 32, 1960.

35. Valic, F., and Zuskin, E., Pharmacological prevention of acute ventilatory capacity reduction in flax dust exposure. Br. J. Ind. Med., 30, 381, 1973.

36. Schachter, E.N., Brown, S., Zuskin, E., et al., The effect of mediator modifying drugs in cotton bract induced bronchospasm. Chest, 79 (suppl.), 73, 1981.

37. Zuskin, E., and Bouhuys, A., Protective effect of disodium cromoglycate against airway constriction induced by hemp dust extract. J. Allergy Clin. Immunol., 57, 473, 1976.

38. Jones, R.N., Diem, J.E., Glindmeyer, H., et al., Mill effect and dose-response relationships in byssinosis. Br. J. Ind. Med., 36, 305, 1979.

39. Fairman, P., Hankinson, J.L., Lapp, N.L., and Morgan, W.K.C., A pilot study of closing volume in byssinosis. Br. J. Ind. Med., 32, 235, 1974.

40. National Institute of Occupational Safety and Health, Occupational Exposure to Cotton Dust. Publication no. (NIOSH) 75–118. Washington, D.C., U.S. Government Printing Office, 1974.

41. Merino, V.L., Lombart, R.L., Marco, R.F., et al., Arterial blood gas tension and lung function during acute responses to hemp dust. Am. Rev. Respir. Dis., 107, 809, 1973.

42. Zuskin, E., Valic, F., Butkovic, D., and Bouhuys, A., Lung function in textile workers. Br. J. Ind. Med., 32, 283, 1975.

43. Guyatt, A.R., Douglas, J.S., Zuskin, E., and Bouhuys, A., Lung static recoil and airway obstruction in hemp workers with byssinosis. Am. Rev. Respir. Dis., 108, 1111, 1973.

44. Bouhuys, A., and Van de Woestijne, K.P., Respiratory mechanics in dust exposure in byssinosis. J. Clin. Invest., 49, 106, 1970.

45. Bouhuys, A., Schoenberg, J.B., Beck, G.J., and Schilling, R.S.F., Epidemiology of chronic lung disease in cotton mill community. Lung, 154, 167, 1977.

46. Rooke, G.B., The pathology of byssinosis. Chest, 79(suppl.), 67, 1981.

47. Berry, G., McKerrow, C.W., Molyneux, M.K.B., et al., A study of the acute and chronic changes in ventilatory capacity in Lancashire cotton mills. Br. J. Ind. Med., 30, 25, 1973.

48. Beck, G.J., Schachter, E.N., Maunder, L.R., and Bouhuys, A., The relation of lung function to subsequent employment status and mortality in cotton textile workers. Chest, 79(suppl.), 26, 1981.

49. Imbus, H.R., and Suh, M.W., Byssinosis: a study of 10,133 textile workers. Arch. Environ. Health, 26, 183, 1973.

50. Merchant, J.A., Lumsden, J.C., Kilburn, K.H., et al., Intervention studies of cotton steaming to reduce biological effects of cotton dust. Br. J. Ind. Med., 31, 261, 1974.

51. Zuskin, E., Ivankovic, E., Schachter, E.N., et al., A ten year follow up study of cotton textile workers. Am. Rev. Respir. Dis., 143, 301, 1991.

52. Elwood, P.C., Sweetman, P.M., Bevan, C., et al., Respiratory disability in ex-cotton workers. Br. J. Ind. Med., 43, 580, 1986.

53. Morgan, W.K.C., Industrial bronchitis. Br. J. Ind. Med., 35, 285, 1978.

54. Edwards, C., Macartney, J., Rooke, G., and Ward, F., The pathology of the lung in byssinosis. Thorax, 30, 612, 1975.

55. Zuskin, E., Valic, F., and Bouhuys, A., Effect of wool dust on respiratory function. Am. Rev. Respir. Dis., 114, 705, 1976.

55a. Glindmeyer, H.W., Lefante, J.J., Jones, R.N., et al., Cotton dust and across shift change in FEV₁ as predictors of annual change in FEV₁. Am. J. Respir. Crit. Care Med., 149, 584, 1994.

56. Carey, G.G.R., and Merrett. J.C., Changes in ventilatory capacity in a group of flax workers in Northern Ireland. Br. J. Ind. Med., 22, 121, 1965.

57. Zuskin, E., and Valic, F., Respiratory changes in two groups of flax workers with different exposure patterns. Thorax, 28, 579, 1973.

58. Jones, R.N., Carr, J., Glindmeyer, H., et al., Respiratory health and dust levels in cotton seed mills. Thorax, 32, 281, 1977.

59. Honeybourne, D., and Pickering, C.A.C., Physiological evidence that emphysema is not a feature of byssinosis. Thorax, 41, 6, 1986.

60. Edwards, J., Mechanisms of disease induction. Chest, 79(4)(Supplement), 38, 1981.

61. Antweiler, H., Histamine liberation by cotton dust extract. Br. J. Ind. Med., 18, 130, 1961.

62. Davenport, A., and Paton, W.D.M., The pharmacological activity of extracts of cotton dust. Br. J. Ind. Med., 19, 19, 1962.

63. Hitchcock, M., In vitro histamine release from human lungs as a model for the acute response to cotton dust. Ann. N.Y. Acad. Sci., 221, 124, 1974.

64. Murphy, R.C., Hammarstrom, S., and Samuelsson, B., Leukotriene C.: A slow reacting substance from murine mastocytoma cells. Proc. Nat. Acad. Sci. U.S.A., 76, 4275, 1979.

65. Ainsworth, S.K., Neuman, R.E., and Harley, R.A., Histamine release from platelets for assay of byssinogenic substances in cotton mill dust and related materials. Br. J. Ind. Med., 36, 35, 1979.

66. Knauer, K.A., Lichtenstein, L.M., Adkinson, N.F., and Fish, J.E., Platelet activation during antigen induced airways reactions in asthmatic subjects. N. Engl. J. Med., 304, 1404, 1981.

67. Lynn, W.C., Munoz, S., Campbell, J.A., and Jeffs, P.M., Chemotaxis and cotton extracts. Ann. N. Y. Acad. Sci., 221, 163, 1974.

68. Rohrbach, M.S., Kreofsky, T., Rolstad, R.A., and Russell, J.A., Tannin mediated secretion of a neutrophil chemotactic factor from alveolar macrophages. Am. Rev. Respir. Dis., 139, 39, 1989.

69. Pernis, B., Vigliani, E.C., Cavagna, C., and Finulli, M., The role of bacterial endotoxins in occupational disease caused by inhaling vegetable dust. Br. J. Ind. Med., 18, 120, 1967.

70. Cavagna, C., Foa, V., and Vigliani, E.C., Effects in men and rabbits of inhalation of cotton dust or extracts and purified endotoxins. Br. J. Ind. Med., 26, 314, 1969.

71. Rylander, R., and Lundholm, M., Bacterial contamination of cotton and cotton dust and effects on the lung. Br. J. Ind. Med., 35, 204, 1978.

72. Burrell, R., and Rylander, R., Further studies of inhaled endotoxin containing bacteria. Environ. Res., 27, 325, 1982.

73. Castellan, R.M., Olenchock, S.A., Kinsley, K.B., and Hankinson, J., Inhaled endotoxin and decreased spirometric values: an exposure response relationship for cotton dust. N. Engl. J. Med., 317, 605, 1987.

74. Milton, D.K., Godleski, J.J., Feldman, H.A., et al., Toxicity of intratracheally instilled cotton dust, cellulose and endotoxin. Am. Rev. Respir. Dis., 142, 184, 1990.

75. Delucca, A.J. II, Brogden, K.A., Catalano, E.A., and Morris, N.M., Biophysical alteration of lung surfactant by extracts of cotton dust. Br. J. Ind. Med., 48, 41, 1991.

76. Massoud, A.A.E., and Taylor, G., Byssinosis: antibodies to cotton antigens in normal subjects and in cotton cardroom workers. Lancet, 2, 607, 1966.

77. Taylor, G., Massoud, A.A.E., and Lucas, F., Studies in aetiology of byssinosis. Br. J. Ind. Med., 28, 143, 1971.

78. Kutz, S.A., Mentnech, S., Olenchock, S., and Major, P.C., Immune mechanisms of byssinosis. Chest, 79(suppl.), 53, 1981.

79. Morgan, W.K.C., Vesterlund, J., Burrell, R., et al., Pulmonary perspective: Byssinosis: some unanswered questions. Am. Rev. Respir. Dis., 126, 354, 1982.

80. Middleton, D., Logan, J.S., Magennis, B.P., and Nelson, S.D., HLA antigen frequencies in flax byssinosis patients. Br. J. Ind. Med., 36, 123, 1979.

81. Occupational Safety and Health Administration (OSHA), Cotton Dust Standard. Federal Register, 43, 27394, June 23rd, 1978.

82. Merchant, J.A., Lumsden, J.C., Kilburn, K.H., et al., I. An industrial study of the biological effects of cotton dust and cigarette smoke exposure. II. Dose response studies in cotton textile workers. J. Occup. Med., 15, 212 and 222, 1973.

83. Imbus, H.R., and Suh, M.W., Steaming of cotton to prevent byssinosis. Br. J. Ind. Med., 31, 209, 1974.

84. Boehlecke, B., Cocke, J., Bragge, K., et al., Pulmonary function response to dust from standard and closed boll harvested cotton. Chest, 79(suppl.), 77, 1981.

85. Collis, E.L., Annual report of chief inspector of factories, 1953. Public Health, 28, 252, 1915.

86. Vigliani, E.C., Parmeggiani, L., and Sassi, C., Studio di un'epidemìa tessitura di cotone. Med Lav., 45, 349, 1954.

87. Murray, R., Dingwall-Fordyce, I., and Lane, R.E., An outbreak of weaver's cough associated with tamarind seed powder. Br. J. Ind. Med., 14, 105, 1957.

88. Rylander, R., Bacterial toxins and the etiology of byssinosis. Chest, 79(suppl.), 34, 1981.

89. Wolff, S.M., Biological effects of bacterial endotoxins in man. In Kass, E.H., and Wolff, S.M., eds., Bacterial Lipopolysaccharides. Chicago, Chicago University Press, 1973, p. 251.

90. Munt, D.F., Gauvain, S., Walford, J., et al., Study of respiratory symptoms and ventilatory capacities among rope workers. Br. J. Ind. Med., 22, 196, 1965.

91. Nicholls, P.J., Evans, E., Valic, F., et al., Histamine-releasing activity and bronchoconstricting effects of sisal. Br. J. Ind. Med., 30, 142, 1973.

92. Baker, M.D., Irwig, L.M., Johnston, J.R., et al., Lung function in sisal ropemakers. Br. J. Ind. Med., 36, 216, 1979.

93. Mustafa, K.Y., Lakha, A.S., Milla, M.H., et al., Byssinosis, respiratory symptoms and spirometric lung function tests in Tanzanian sisal workers. Br. J. Ind. Med., 35, 123, 1978.

94. El Ghawabi, S.H., Respiratory function and symptoms in workers exposed simultaneously to jute and hemp. Br. J. Ind. Med., 35, 16, 1978.

95. Mair, A., Smith, D.H., Wilson, W.A., et al., Dust diseases in Dundee textile workers. Br. J. Ind. Med., 17, 272, 1960.

96. Siddhu, C.M.S., Nath, J., and Mehotra, R.K., Byssinosis amongst cotton and jute workers in Kanpur. Indian J. Med. Res., 54, 980, 1966.

97. Popa, V., Gavrilescu, N., Preda, N., et al., An investigation of allergy in byssinosis: sensitization to cotton, hemp, flax and jute antigens. Br. J. Ind. Med., 26, 101, 1968.

98. Gandevia, B., and Milne, J., Ventilatory capacity on exposure to jute dust and the relevance of productive cough and smoking to the response. Br. J. Ind. Med., 22, 187, 1965.

99. Valic, F., and Zuskin, E., A comparative study of respiratory function in female nonsmoking cotton and jute workers. Br. J. Ind. Med., 28, 364, 1971.

Industrial Bronchitis and Other Nonspecific Conditions Affecting the Airways

19

W. Keith C. Morgan

Although the harmful effects of dust on the lungs have been known since the 15th century and even before, it was the observations of Ramazzini in the late 17th and early 18th centuries and of Thackrah and Greenhow in Victorian times in Great Britain that called attention to the magnitude of the problem.[1, 2] The increased frequency of lung disease in grinders, textile workers, weavers, tailors, and potters was noted by Thackrah. In a series of monographs and pamphlets, he effectively called the attention of Parliament to the sorry state of health that existed in workers at the time of the Industrial Revolution. Unfortunately, Thackrah died at the age of 38, and it was left to Greenhow and others to carry on his mission.

The recognition of dust as a hazard in the mid-19th century led to the introduction in Great Britain and Europe of attempts to control its effects through the application of industrial hygiene measures. In the United States, a comparable program did not come into existence until the pioneering efforts of Alice Hamilton in the first two decades of this century. In her autobiography, *Exploring the Dangerous Trades,* she describes the Fourth International Congress on Occupational Accidents and Diseases that took place in Brussels in 1910.[3] Her chagrin and disappointment at the absence of a program in the United States for the control of occupational disease, especially when compared with the various European nations, did something to bring the deficiencies to the attention of legislators and the public and, to some extent, helped eliminate the complacency of industry in the United States. To use her phrase, "It (the Congress) was not an occasion for national pride." In 1914, as a result of her proselytizing, the United States Public Health Service set up the Office of Industrial Hygiene and Sanitation. The efforts of this office were the stimulus to the development of a program for the prevention of occupationally related diseases in the United States.

It is now clear that the so-called dust-induced diseases, that variously were referred to as grinders' rot, miners' phthisis, bronchitis, and other names, included a number of distinct diseases that it is now possible to diagnose with certainty. Not all were a consequence of the inhalation of dust. Included among them were tuberculosis, emphysema, bronchitis, silicosis, coal workers' pneumoconiosis (CWP) and other pneumoconioses, and lung cancer. It was not until the turn of this century that the discovery of x-rays and their application to the diagnosis of disease, along with advances in bacteriólogy, pathology, and epidemiology, made it possible to separate with any precision the various diseases and conditions mentioned previously. Much of what is now known about the relationship of airways obstruction to occupation has come about through detailed studies of specific diseases that affect certain workers, i.e., CWP, silicosis, asbestosis, and byssinosis.

Early in this century, Haldane made the observation that coal miners had fewer bronchitic symptoms and a lower mortality rate than did metal miners.[4] At that time, cigarette smoking played a small role in the induction of bronchitis and respiratory impairment. Between 1925 and 1940, British coal mines became mechanized, and the dust levels to which coal miners were exposed rose significantly. Concomitant with the rise in the dust levels was an increase in the incidence and prevalence of respiratory disease. Much of the increased frequency of respiratory disease was subsequently found to be a consequence of CWP. This prompted the government of the day to establish the Pneumoconiosis Research Unit (PRU) of the Medical Research Council (MRC).

In 1961, a 5% sample of the entire population of Great Britain was surveyed by the Ministry of Pensions and National Insurance. The results of this survey indicated that bronchitis was an important cause of absenteeism in the working classes and that miners and quarrymen were particularly affected. Subsequently, the Ministry of Pensions asked the MRC of Great Britain to set up a committee to study the cause of bronchitis, with particular emphasis on the role played by occupation.

In 1966, the MRC committee published a report that examined the role of bronchitis as a cause of respiratory disability.[5] The committee noted that chronic bronchitis had a multifactorial cause and that cigarette smoking, air pollution, social class, and dust exposure all apparently played a role. The committee noted that, since the symptoms of bronchitis were the same whatever the cause, it was not possible to apportion the contribution of a particular exposure or factor or to know whether any impairment that might be present was a consequence of occupational or other factors. The committee concluded that, although the dusty occupations had a greater incidence and prevalence of bronchitis (and, in this regard, it was apparent that coal miners and foundry workers had greater morbidity and mortality rates from bronchitis), it was difficult to show a direct cause-and-effect relationship between dust exposure and either morbidity or death. Thus, the wives of coal miners and foundry workers were also noted to have more cough and sputum and, on occasion, a lower ventilatory capacity than did the wives of nonminers. This suggested that factors other than occupation were important contributory factors to the bronchitis of miners and foundry men. The committee suggested that dust played only a limited role in the induction of bronchitis and respiratory disability; however, they recommended that the situation be kept under review. The MRC committee's report occasioned several critical responses, but the arguments used to rebut the committee's conclusions seemed based on clinical impression and political ideology rather than objective evidence.[6-8]

RESPIRATORY SYMPTOMS, VENTILATORY IMPAIRMENT, AND EXPOSURE TO DUST

Compared with a comparable reference population, workers in the dusty trades have an increased prevalence of bronchitis, as manifested by the presence of cough and sputum.[9, 10] Although many of the initial observations in this regard were made in coal miners,[9-11] over the years, similar findings have been noted in steel workers,[12, 13] foundry men,[14] textile workers,[15] gold miners,[16] cement workers,[17, 18] and in those who work with bauxite.[19] The increased prevalence of cough and sputum, in many instances, has been accompanied by a slight reduction in ventilatory capacity. This is reflected as a lower forced expiratory volume in 1 second (FEV_1) in the presence of a relatively normal or only slightly reduced forced vital capacity (FVC). Such a reduction in the ventilatory capacity may be seen in coal miners and those exposed to silica in the absence of conglomerate silicosis or progressive massive fibrosis (PMF).[16, 20]

A number of studies have been carried out in coal miners which make it clear that the ventilatory defect does not appear to be related to the presence or severity of simple CWP (Fig. 19–1).[21, 22] Similar studies have shown a like situation in silica-exposed populations, i.e., a reduced ventilatory capacity may be seen in both

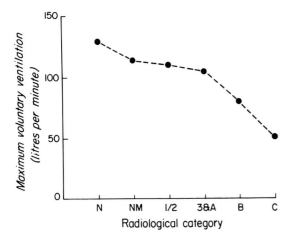

Figure 19-1
The relationship of ventilatory capacity to radiographic category in a group of coal miners and of a comparable reference population. N, nonminers; NM, miners with category 0; 1/2, miners with category 1 and 2; 3 and A, miners with category 3 and complicated A; B and C, miners with complicated B and C pneumoconiosis. (Data from Gilson, J.C., and Higgins, I.T.T., Industrial Pulmonary Diseases. Boston, Little, Brown, 1960.)

those with and without simple silicosis.[16] The reduction in ventilatory capacity that occurs in such subjects can be explained in two ways.

1. There exists a condition that is associated with airflow obstruction which is peculiar to the dusty trades and which affects miners with and without simple pneumoconiosis. This condition could be either emphysema or bronchitis or both.
2. Differential migration is responsible. When new workers are recruited to the industry, if the fitter and younger men subsequently leave the industry within months or a few years of starting work, those who remain in the mines would be likely to have a lower ventilatory capacity and would not be representative of the total population who started work.

It was noted sometime back that, during hard times and when unemployment was high in the coal industry, those who left the industry and sought employment elsewhere tended to be both fitter and younger.[21] Over the last 20 to 30 years, however, this has not been the case, and indeed a study by McClintock of new entrants into coal mining in Great Britain showed that it was the more muscular and probably fitter recruits who stayed in the industry.[23] This perhaps might also explain why coal miners with categories 2 and 3 simple pneumoconiosis often have a higher ventilatory capacity than those with category 1 and those with normal chest x-ray findings. Thus, the increased prevalence of cough and sputum and of increased airways obstruction cannot be explained by selective migration and would seem to be related to the development of either emphysema or chronic bronchitis, or both.

DEFINITION AND PATHOLOGICAL FINDINGS OF BRONCHITIS

Until recently, a diagnosis of bronchitis implied a condition characterized by cough and sputum and usually associated with a reduction in ventilatory capacity or likely to lead to one.[24] The typical bronchitic subject was a cigarette smoker who presented with breathlessness plus cough and sputum and a chest radiograph showing an absence of parenchymal opacification and nodulation. In such a subject, a diagnosis of chronic bronchitis and emphysema was made, a practice that implied that these two conditions were invariably associated and were part and parcel of the same process. At the time the MRC published its statement on occupation and bronchitis, it was evident that not all subjects with cough and sputum necessarily had a decrement in their FEV_1, but the committee did not at that time define bronchitis.[5] Prior to that, however, the Ciba Foundation had defined chronic bronchitis as a condition of chronic or recurrent excess of mucus secretion in the bronchial tree.[25] Subsequently, the MRC classified bronchitis into (1) chronic simple bronchitis, i.e., a chronic or recurrent increase in the volume of mucoid secretions sufficient to be associated with cough; (2) chronic mucopurulent bronchitis, i.e., chronic bronchitis in which the sputum is persistent or intermittently mucopurulent and which is not related to localized destructive pulmonary disease; and (3) chronic obstructive bronchitis, i.e., persistent widespread narrowing of the intrapulmonary airways on expiration which caused airways obstruction.[26] This statement and the work of Fletcher et al.[27] provided the stimulus for a definition of bronchitis that depended solely on the basis of cough and sputum without reference to lung function. The present generally accepted definition of chronic bronchitis is cough and sputum for 3 months of the year for 2 consecutive years.[26–28]

The seminal studies of Lynne Reid at the Brompton Hospital characterized the pathological features of bronchitis.[29] She showed that there was an increase in the depth and number of mucus-secreting glands in the airways. In humans, the mucus glands of the large airways are mostly responsible for mucus secretion. The goblet cells which are present in the smaller airways also tend to increase in number, but the changes in them are less evident. The ratio of the depth of the mucous glands (gland thickness) to the bronchial wall thickness, measured from the surface of the respiratory epithelium to the cartilage, is known as the Reid index and provides a most useful way of quantifying the degree and severity of bronchitis (Fig. 19–2).

Bronchitis and mucous gland hypertrophy may occur as a result of long continued exposure to any number of chronic irritants. These include cigarette smoke, dust, and air pollutants, be they particulates or gaseous.[30] Continued exposure to sulfur dioxide, ozone, or ammonia may produce chronic bronchitis. When attempting to study the prevalence of bronchitis in a working population and trying to determine the cause of the bronchitis, there are two important confounding factors, namely, cigarette smoking and age. In cigarette smokers, the effects of cigarette smoking overwhelm the effects of air pollution, dust, and other factors. In women, the prevalence of bronchitis frequently does not show the same clear-cut relationship to smoking and often appears to be related to social class.[31] This is a consequence of the fact that women in the professional classes tend to be reluctant to admit that they cough up sputum.

BRONCHITIS, EMPHYSEMA, AND CIGARETTE SMOKING

It is now apparent that cigarette smoking may lead to both bronchitis and emphysema and that the two are distinct and unrelated responses with vastly different effects.[27, 32] Chronic bronchitis, as described by Reid, mainly involves the glands of the larger airways, although the goblet cells of the smaller airways are to some extent affected.[29] It tends to be reversible, and after a subject has stopped smoking for 6 to 9 months, the cough and sputum usually clear up. Fletcher et al., as a result of their long-term studies in a cigarette-smoking population, clearly indicated that bronchitis is distinct from emphysema and, moreover, is associated

Figure 19–2

Diagrammatic representation of the Reid index. A represents the depth of the glands, and B is the distance from the mucosal surface to the bronchial cartilage. The index is A/B.

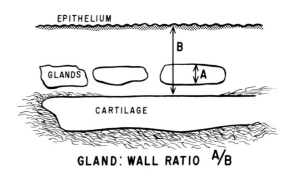

with little in the way of ventilatory impairment.[27] They term the presence of cough and sputum in the absence of localized parenchymal destruction as bronchial hypersecretion. Some degree of bronchial hypersecretion is found in virtually every smoker of more than 10 cigarettes a day who has been smoking for more than 5 years. In contrast, emphysema has been defined as an anatomical alteration of the lungs characterized by an abnormal enlargement of the air spaces distal to the terminal bronchiole and associated with destruction of the alveolar walls.[28] The initial lesion in centrilobular (centriacinar) emphysema is located in the smaller airways and, to be more precise, the second division of the respiratory bronchioles. In some instances, the disease extends to the more distal parts of the acinus and involves the alveoli. It is associated with irreversible obstruction and clearly cannot be expected to improve when the subject stops smoking. More importantly, as is evident from the studies of Fletcher et al.,[27] Peto et al.,[32] Bates,[33] Thurlbeck et al.,[34] and Jamal et al.,[35] chronic bronchitis neither causes significant airways obstruction nor portends the development of chronic irreversible airways obstruction. The latter develops in only 12% to 15% of those who are cigarette smokers. Although the presence or absence of airways obstruction is not an all-or-none attribute and it is clear that a spectrum of susceptibility exists, nevertheless, there seem to be two contrasting groups, namely, the susceptible subjects, who in their normal life span may become disabled by obstruction if they happen to be smokers, and the nonsusceptible, who will not have obstruction irrespective of smoking habit.[32]

If we compare the mean FEV_1 of smokers and nonsmokers, in most instances, a sizable disparity is not evident. This results from the fact that the real effect of smoking on the FEV_1 occurs only in the susceptible minority and is more or less obscured by the virtually normal FEV_1 of the majority. Nevertheless, among the susceptible minority, some are severely affected and suffer premature disability and death. It is also abundantly evident that those who are cigarette smokers and who happen to have airways obstruction tend to underestimate their cigarette consumption or have reduced their cigarette consumption because of their symptoms and relay their reduced consumption as if it were their lifetime average cigarette consumption.[32]

EMPHYSEMA, AIRWAYS OBSTRUCTION, AND DUST EXPOSURE

First, it is necessary to point out that, in the aging population, emphysema is found frequently at the postmortem examination without any obvious cause and such subjects may show no impairment of ventilatory capacity.[36] It is also abundantly clear from the work of Ryder and others that at least 15% of the lungs needs to be involved before the subject is likely to complain of shortness of breath or have a reduced ventilatory capacity.[37] Minor degrees of emphysema therefore do not lead to symptoms or breathlessness.

A series of articles from South Wales put forward the proposition that coal miners have a higher prevalence of emphysema than do nonminers.[38-41] The authors of these reports attempted to relate emphysema demonstrated at postmortem examination to antemortem measurements of lung function and radiographic category. The subjects included in these studies had been referred to a pneumoconiosis medical panel. All were claiming or had been awarded compensation, and most had undergone serial pulmonary function tests performed as a result of their claim for compensation. Emphysema was quantified by point counting. The investigators claimed to have demonstrated a relationship between the presence of simple and complicated CWP and antemortem pulmonary impairment, as diagnosed by a reduction in the ventilatory capacity, as measured by the FEV_1.[38, 39] They suggested that the p type of opacity is associated with emphysema more frequently than the larger q and r types. The statement that ''there is no reason why these deaths should not provide a true sample of experience of men with this disease,'' i.e., CWP, appeared in their article.[38] This would imply that the sample of subjects was representative of coal miners not only in Wales but throughout Great Britain and, indeed, the rest of the world. The notion that disability claimants can be regarded as a random and unbiased sample was disputed by Gilson and Oldham.[42] By the same token, Ryder et al. attempted to relate the presence of emphysema and airways obstruction to the radiographic category of pneumoconiosis and in doing so made no distinction between those subjects who had simple and complicated disease.[38] Since categories B and C complicated CWP are known to lead to airways obstruction and emphysema in the absence of smoking, such an assumption introduced significant bias. In their second article, these authors still chose not to separate their subjects with simple CWP from those with PMF, and again they were criticized by Oldham and Berry.[43] Moreover, when an attempt was made to relate the size of the decrements in FEV_1 to the radiographic category, it was evident that those with category 2 and 3 simple CWP had a lesser decrement (0.8 L below the predicted value) than did those who had a clear chest x-ray finding (1.25 L below the predicted value).

Although there is no doubt that, during life and also at postmortem examination, coal miners with CWP can be shown to have an increased prevalence of emphysema,[44–48] it is also apparent that the emphysema that occurs in nonsmoking pneumoconiotic miners is seldom, if ever, associated with significant or disabling airways obstruction.[46, 47] Similarly, it is well accepted that the higher categories of simple pneumoconiosis are associated with increased dust deposition in the lung.[44–47, 49–51] It has likewise been shown that the severity of the category of simple pneumoconiosis increases concomitantly with the extent of focal emphysema.[44–46] Thus, if emphysema were the cause of the airways obstruction in coal miners, an increasing category of simple CWP would be associated with a decrement in ventilatory capacity. This is not the case.

Further studies have related the presence of right ventricular hypertrophy in coal miners to the presence of simple and complicated CWP and to the miners' smoking habits during life.[52] Right ventricular hypertrophy and cor pulmonale did not occur in coal miners unless they had been cigarette smokers or had PMF. This has been previously demonstrated elsewhere.[53–55] By the same token, if emphysema were the cause of the airways obstruction, then in simple CWP there should be a reduction of the alveolocapillary surface. This would be associated with a concomitant and significant reduction in the diffusing capacity. This is not the case.[56]

Early studies of simple CWP suggested that the type of emphysema that occurred in this condition was different from that seen in smokers. Gough[51] and Heppleston[57] both referred to the condition as focal dust emphysema or focal emphysema. In 1968, Gough wrote that "in a young coal miner with a short exposure to dust dying of an accident, there is an accumulation of coal dust specifically related to the terminal and respiratory bronchioles. The lungs can evidently withstand this deposition without harm for some years. Emphysema then develops and in miners who have been exposed for 20 years or more, some degree of dilatation of the proximal order of respiratory bronchioles is usual and may be marked. After 40 years of dust exposure, the majority of miners will show focal dust emphysema, although there is a surprising range in the quantity of dust deposited and the degree of emphysema noted in miners working under similar conditions."[51] Heppleston[57] and Gough[51] went on to suggest that cigarette smoke–induced centrilobular emphysema, although occurring in a similar site to focal emphysema, tended to extend to the alveoli more often and, in addition, was associated with bronchiolitis. Some pathologists, however, now dispute that any distinction can be made between the centrilobular emphysema seen in cigarette smokers and focal dust emphysema. In the cigarette-smoking miner, both are obviously likely to coexist. Ruckley et al. demonstrated a relationship between emphysema and exposure to respirable coal dust, but this is evident only in the lungs of those miners with parenchymal fibrosis.[45] It is clear, however, that focal emphysema and overdistention may be present in the absence of impairment of ventilatory capacity.[22, 47, 58] This is not true of the subject who has extensive small airways disease and centrilobular emphysema caused by cigarette smoking. More-over, many other relatively inert dusts may lead to the presence of focal emphy-sema, including hematite, stannic oxide, and the common air pollutants.[30, 59] A cogent argument against the likelihood of emphysema being responsible for the airways obstruction that occurs specifically in coal miners is the fact that similar decrements in lung function have been observed in those exposed to silica[16] and asbestos.[60] Such obstruction is independent of radiographic change. In simple sili-cosis, there is no excess emphysema, except in smokers.[61, 61a] In asbestosis, the characteristic lesions are of interstitial fibrosis in which the lungs become stiffer than normal, i.e., the antithesis of emphysema in which the lungs are exceptionally compliant.

It has also been shown that the ventilatory capacity, lung volumes, and diffus-ing capacity of coal miners with the various types of small, rounded opacity differ little, except insofar as those miners with simple CWP and the p type of opacity tend to have a slightly reduced diffusing capacity.[62] If significant emphysema leading to obstruction were present in miners with the p type of opacity, the residual volume (RV) and total lung capacity (TLC) might be expected to be significantly increased compared with those in miners with the q and r types of opacities, but such changes have not been consistently demonstrated. Moreover, a large epidemi-ological study in a group of working coal miners has shown that miners with and without simple CWP have a slight increase in TLC and RV and that an increasing category of simple CWP was associated with a concomitant increase in RV.[22] These findings suggest either that there is a slight loss of elastic recoil in miners with simple CWP or that coal miners often have obstruction of the small airways produced by a dust-induced bronchiolitis. Moreover, Waters et al. showed that the p type of opacity is not associated with decreased longevity.[63] If disabling emphy-sema were present and associated with a lower ventilatory capacity, it could reason-ably be expected that miners with the p type of opacity would show a decreased life expectancy. Hankinson and colleagues measured air space size and, in miners with CWP, showed there is a dilatation of either or both the alveoli and the respiratory bronchioles which was greater in those with p-type opacities.[64] They were, however, unable to detect any differences in ventilatory function between those miners with the p, q, and r types of opacities.

In conclusion, although coal miners with simple CWP undoubtedly have an increased prevalence of focal emphysema, unless the miner happens to be a smoker, this is not associated with significant airways obstruction nor a significant loss of the diffusing capacity. Focal emphysema is associated with a somewhat abnormal distribution of inspired gas, a slight loss of elastic recoil in the lungs, an increased RV, and minor ventilation perfusion inequalities,[47] but none of these explains the slight loss of ventilatory capacity that is found in a proportion of coal miners.[30, 47] A most compelling argument against emphysema being the cause of the reduced ventilatory capacity in coal miners is the poor relationship between the FEV_1 and the extent of emphysema, as is clear from Figure 19–3, which is reproduced from the Ruckley et al. monograph.[46] Thus, only 40 of 257 of their subjects had a FEV_1 below 1.2 L but no significant emphysema, while only 18 subjects with a FEV_1 of below 1.2 L had more than 20% of the lung involved.

THE EFFECTS OF DUST-INDUCED BRONCHITIS

Most studies that have related the prevalence of bronchitis to dust exposure have been carried out in coal miners. As a population, coal miners offer many advantages in that they are usually a well-defined and relatively homogeneous group who, throughout most of their life, tend to work in the same occupation. Although many of the observations and inferences that follow have been derived from studies of coal miners, there is no reason to believe that the dust-induced bronchitis of coal miners differs in any way from the bronchitis that is seen in

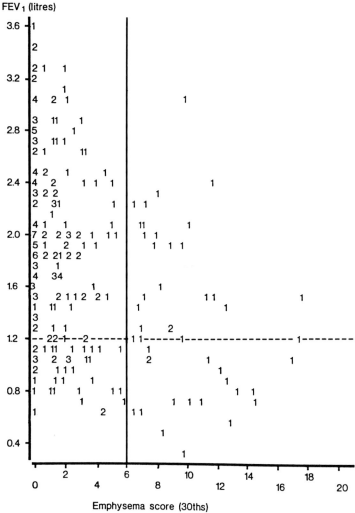

Figure 19–3. Shows the association in 257 coal workers between the FEV₁ measured during life and the postmortem emphysema score in thirtieths of the lungs. The numbers greater than 1 indicate coincident points for more than one subject. Those with less than 20% involvement, i.e., six-thirtieths, would not be expected to have any symptoms. (Courtesy of Dr. V. Ruckley and the Institute of Occupational Medicine, Edinburgh.)

workers exposed to silica, bauxite, or any other mineral or gaseous occupational pollutants.

A number of studies have shown that the prevalence of bronchitis increases with cumulative dust exposure.[65–67] In Great Britain, it has been possible to relate cumulative coal mine dust exposure to the prevalence of bronchitis,[66] but long-term dust measurements have been lacking in the United States until recently. In an early study in the United States, Kibelstis et al. related cough and sputum to surrogate measures of dust exposure and also to cigarette smoking.[67] They were able to show that nonsmoking coal miners who worked at the face had a greater prevalence of bronchitis than did those in the less dusty jobs. This effect was evident in virtually all age groups. In smoking miners, however, the effects of cigarette smoke overwhelmed those of dust. Similar observations have been reported in Belgian coal miners.[68]

Rogan et al. demonstrated in British coal miners that ventilatory capacity was inversely related to lifetime cumulative exposure to coal dust.[69] The presence of pneumoconiosis did not lead to an additional decrement of ventilatory capacity above and beyond those decrements caused by cumulative dust exposure, smoking habits, and stature. Although smokers showed a more rapid decline in the FEV_1 than did nonsmokers, an effect of dust exposure was apparent in both smoking and nonsmoking miners. Among nonsmokers, the FEV_1 was generally lower in the most exposed subjects compared with the less dust–exposed miners; however, the rate of decline of the FEV_1 remained the same in nonsmoking miners from age 30 to 60 whether they were exposed to high or low dust levels. At the same time, Kibelstis et al. were similarly able to show a dust-induced effect on the ventilatory capacity of nonsmoking miners.[67] As mentioned earlier, the investigators subdivided their cohort according to their job, i.e., face workers, those employed on transportation, those in miscellaneous other jobs, and finally, those working on the surface. The years worked in each particular job were also known. They were also able to show that the FEV_1 of the nonsmoking surface workers, when expressed as a percentage of the predicted value, was statistically significantly greater than that of the nonsmoking face workers. The difference, however, was relatively small (4.3%). When expressed as a percentage of the predicted, a significant difference existed between the FEV_1 values of the smoking and the nonsmoking face workers (6%) and also between those of the smoking surface workers and the nonsmoking surface workers (10.6%). Cigarette consumption, as we might expect, was appreciably higher in the surface workers than it was in the face workers since the latter were not permitted to smoke while underground. Similarly, airways obstruction was found to be three times more common in smokers than in nonsmokers.

A West German study of some 7000 workers from a variety of dusty trades related respiratory symptoms and lung function to dust exposure, smoking habits, and other factors.[70] Age and smoking habits were the most important factors related to the prevalence of bronchitis and airways obstruction. There was an additive effect of smoking, age, and dust in the younger workers, the combined decrement of all three variables equaled the sum of their separate effects.

Hankinson et al.[48, 71] compared the type of respiratory impairment associated with dust-induced bronchitis with the type of impairment induced by cigarette smoking. They used the same cohort of more than 9000 working coal miners that had been studied by Kibelstis.[56] In this study, the ventilatory capacity had been assessed with flow volume curves, and in addition, dynamic lung volumes had been measured. The TLC was calculated using a radiological method.[72] The RV was calculated by subtracting the FVC from the TLC. Thus, it was possible to express flow rates as a percentage of vital capacity, of total lung capacity, and also at absolute lung volumes. Hankinson et al. selected four age- and height-matched groups, according to whether or not they had bronchitis and whether or not they were cigarette smokers.[48] In each group, 428 subjects were included. The mean flow volume curves are shown in Figures 19–3 to 19–5. It is evident from the figures that cigarette smoking led to a reduction of flows at all lung volumes. In the subjects who were nonsmokers and had bronchitis, flows were reduced mainly at high lung volumes, although there was some effect at low lung volumes, suggesting that the small airways had not entirely been spared. Flows at absolute lung volumes revealed similar findings, but more importantly, it was noted that smokers, as a whole, had an increased RV and TLC. The increase in TLC that occurred in smokers was statistically highly significant and indicated that there was a loss of elastic recoil in the lungs, presumably caused by the presence of subclinical emphysema. The TLC of subjects with dust-induced bronchitis, on the other hand, was within the normal range. Thus, it would seem that there is little doubt that dust may induce bronchitis and that this is associated with a small reduction in the ventilatory capacity, in particular, in the FEV_1 and in flows at high lung volumes.[48, 71]

Although these data, in the main, have been derived from coal miners, it is noteworthy that, between 1958 and 1972, Brinkman et al. carried out a well-planned series of epidemiological investigations in an industrial population who were exposed to various dusts, some of which were inert, but some of which

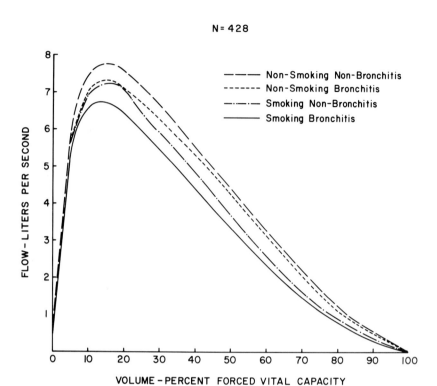

Figure 19–4. Maximal expiratory flows of the four groups of coal miners expressed as a percentage of vital capacity. (From Hankinson, J.L., Reger, R.B., and Morgan, W.K.C., Maximal expiratory flows in coal miners. Am. Rev. Respir. Dis., 116, 175, 1977.)

contained a reasonably high percentage of free silica, although few, if any, had silicosis.[73–75] As in other studies, they came to the conclusion that the main factors affecting the rate of decline of ventilatory capacity were age and cigarette smoking and that any contribution from dust was relatively small.

A recent study by Kreiss et al. showed that hard rock mining exposures affected smokers and nonsmokers differently.[76] In smokers, flow rates were decreased at all lung volumes, and the TLC and RV were increased. In nonsmokers, dust exposure was associated with decreased lung volumes and increased flow rates. The authors further stated that their results differed from those of Hankinson et al. who had expressed the opinion that "industrial bronchitis is limited to the large airways."[48] In practice, Hankinson and colleagues showed that, although flows in the large airways were predominantly affected, there was also a reduction in flows in the small airways. The apparent disparities in the findings of the two groups of investigators can be easily reconciled. Kreiss et al. studied hard rock miners exposed to silica.[76] Exposure to the latter leads to nodular fibrosis and increased stiffness of the lungs, with decreased lung volumes. The opposite situation prevails in coal miners. The focal dust emphysema that affects them, especially those with CWP, leads to an increased TLC and an increased RV.[72, 77] It is well recognized that maximal expiratory flow rates depend on (1) the elastic recoil of the lungs, (2) the frictional resistance of the small airways, and (3) the cross-sectional area of the large airways. Thus, in a dust-exposed population, flow rates are influenced by the effects of both parenchymal and tracheobronchial dust deposition. Moreover, the lung parenchyma may become either more or less compliant with dust exposure (CWP *versus* asbestosis or silicosis). The effects of industrial bronchitis on expiratory flow rates at various lung volumes are, therefore, influenced significantly by the elastic properties of the lung parenchyma, and these differ significantly in CWP and silicosis. Nevertheless, the predominant effect of

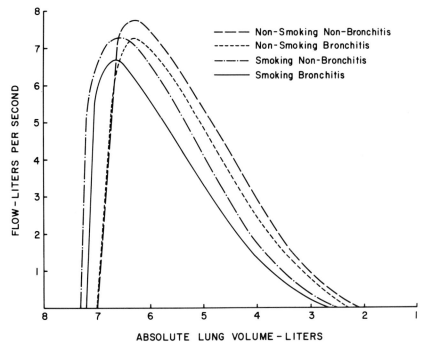

Figure 19–5. Maximum flows of the four groups of miners expressed as absolute lung volumes. (From Hankinson, J.L., Reger, R.B., and Morgan, W.K.C., Maximal expiratory flows in coal miners. Am. Rev. Respir. Dis., 116, 175, 1977.)

industrial bronchitis is on the large airways, just as it is in cigarette smoke–induced bronchitis.[32] Cotes et al.[78] claimed that they have been unable to duplicate the findings of Hankinson and colleagues[48, 71] and argued that the effects of industrial bronchitis are not predominantly located in the large airways. However, they expressed their flows as a percentage of vital capacity in the absence of any knowledge of TLC or RV. As indicated earlier, this may be misleading and introduces error.

In those exposed to mineral dusts, ventilatory impairment occurs as frequently in those with radiographic evidence of CWP or silicosis as it does in those who have a clear chest x-ray film. Since the radiologic category of both silicosis and CWP is related to the weight of dust retained in the lung parenchyma,[29, 79] it is reasonable to infer that the reduction in the FEV_1 that is seen in dust-exposed workers, and which is independent of the radiographic category, originates from dust deposition in the dead space, i.e., bronchitis. The apparent lack of association between bronchitis and the presence of silicosis or CWP suggests that the particles responsible for the two conditions probably differ in size with those responsible for bronchitis being somewhat larger than those responsible for pneumoconiosis.[30] The particles responsible for bronchitis are mainly deposited as a result of inertial impaction and are removed by the mucociliary escalator; those responsible for pneumoconiosis are more likely to be deposited by sedimentation. There is, moreover, no indication that industrial bronchitis predisposes in any way to the development of the type of small airways disease and bronchiolitis that leads to emphysema. Whether the cessation of exposure leads to an improvement in the symptoms of industrial or occupationally induced bronchitis is unknown; however, it is likely that this is the case.

DUST VERSUS CIGARETTE SMOKE: RELATIVE CONTRIBUTIONS TO VENTILATORY IMPAIRMENT

A few longitudinal studies of decrements in lung function with cumulative dust exposure have been carried out in coal miners[80, 81] and in those exposed to silica.[82] Most such studies have shown that the mean effects of dust are about equal to one third to one fifth of those of cigarette smoke.

Some 1677 miners from five British collieries were studied over a period of 11 years by Love and Miller.[80] The FEV_1 loss was related to cumulative dust exposure after correction for age, smoking, and colliery effect. The cohort was divided according to whether they were nonsmokers, ex-smokers, or current smokers, and some adjustments were made for the duration and intensity of smoking. The authors showed that cigarette smoking had roughly three times the effect of dust; however, there were a number of problems with the study, including the fact that smoking was treated as a static unchanging variable such as height. Obviously, this is not the case, and the effects of cigarette smoking increase with the number of pack-years and age. Attfield described his findings subsequently in a 9-year follow-up of coal miners in the United States.[81] Here again, only about one quarter of the population were available to be included in the final analysis. It was noted that those who left coal mining tended to be older, showed more evidence of bronchitis and ill health, and were more likely to be smokers. Because much of the difference between those who remained at work and those who left could be accounted for by age, he decided to include only those miners between 29 and 49 years of age. Unfortunately, the older age groups would consist of those subjects who were most likely to show the greatest effects of cigarette smoking. He likewise found that cigarette smoking had three to four times the effects of coal dust exposure. It is interesting to note, however, that the dust exposures in coal miners in the United States were significantly less than they were during the comparable period in Great Britain, despite relatively similar effects on ventilatory capacity. However, the dust data collected during a significant time over the period of observation were inaccurate.[83, 84]

An additional study of the previously described cohort of British miners puts forward the proposition that chronic bronchitis is associated with a loss of lung function that may be severe.[85] The authors noted ''that men with bronchitic symptoms have evidence of airways obstruction more often than do men without symptoms,'' an observation that has been made repeatedly and was to be expected since cigarette smoking is known to be the most common cause, not only of bronchitis, but also of irreversible airways obstruction. Later, they maintain that the ''dust related increase in symptom prevalence may be regarded as indicators to dust induced impairment of respiratory function,'' but then, they subsequently add that ''they do not claim that chronic bronchitis leads to significant disabling obstruction.'' If bronchitis does not lead to the obstruction, the only other possibility would seem to be emphysema. The arguments against this thesis have already been rejected for a variety of reasons. Similarly, it is also stated that their interpretation of the results is supported by the demonstration of an increase in mortality rate in coal miners in the absence of PMF who have had relatively high dust exposures, an observation that several other studies using data that were collected prospectively have not confirmed.[86–88]

A series of reports from France claimed that occupational exposure leads to a bronchitis which is associated with a significant reduction in the ventilatory capacity sufficient to cause disabling impairment.[89] However, the cohort studied by these investigators consisted of multiple occupations with varied exposures and included metallurgists, chemists, printers, and flour millers. Some of those employed in the flour mill would be expected to develop asthma rather than irreversible obstruction; those in the sector described as ''chemistry'' would be exposed to paints, varnishes, and plastics. Here again, occupational asthma may have been a problem. More importantly, of the original population of 1002 men, only 780 were examined 11 years later. Of this group, only 556 had satisfactory spirometric tracings, i.e., 29% of those retested had unsatisfactory tracings, an inordinately high failure rate. A further article on miners in the United States purported to show that cigarette smoking and dust exposure had roughly the same effect on ventilatory capacity.[90] Unfortunately, the dust measurements used in this study,[90a] as in their previous study, were invalid, and furthermore, there was only a small residue of the original cohort available for study.

Oxman et al. reviewed all of the studies that had been carried out of the various forms of pneumoconiosis in which an attempt had been made to relate dust exposure and impairment of ventilatory capacity.[91] They decided to include only longitudinal studies in which both measurements and ventilatory capacity had been measured. They also decided that certain criteria must be fulfilled. Thus, it was required that dust exposure must have been measured quantitatively, and a quantitative relationship between dust exposure and one of the outcomes was calculated while controlling at least for smoking and age. They were able to find three cohorts of coal miners who, in their judgment, fulfiled these criteria and, in addition, one cohort of gold miners who were exposed mainly to silica. In general, although the highest coal dust exposures had the greatest effect on ventilatory capacity, it was evident that only in those with lifetime exposures of 350 gh/m^3 did a significant likelihood of disabling impairment appear. However, there were a number of anomalies. The effect of dust in gold miners was three times as large as it was in coal miners. Moreover, the dust measurements made in the solitary study in the United States were invalid. When mild respiratory impairment attributable to dust was analyzed, it was apparent that there were more nonsmokers with a dust-induced decrement, i.e., a FEV_1 below 80%, than there were smokers with an equivalent reduction. Such an observation makes one question the validity of the data included in the analysis.

A number of problems exist in regard to comparisons made between the mean decrement in FEV_1 induced by cigarette smoking and that induced by dust.[92] While only 12% to 13% of cigarette smokers have airways obstruction, around 40% to 50% of nonsmoking miners who have worked for 20 or more years underground complain of cough and sputum and are likely to show a minor decrement in FEV_1. Thus, to compare the mean decrement in FEV_1 in cigarette smokers with the equivalent in nonsmokers is misleading in that, of the smokers in whom airways obstruction develops, a significant proportion will have a disabling decrement in ventilatory capacity. In contrast, a far greater percentage of nonsmoking coal miners will have bronchitis and a concomitant but much smaller dust-induced decrement in FEV_1. The 11-ml decrement noted by Love and Miller occurs solely in the 12% to 13% of cigarette-smoking coal miners who are susceptible and who develop airways obstruction.[80] If the whole population smoked 20 cigarettes a day, the resultant mean reduction in the FEV_1 would be minor, because the effects are skewed, with 87% to 88% of subjects showing a normal age-related decline in FEV_1. Thus, the decrement induced by cigarette smoking will lead to severe impairment in a minority, while the decrement that occurs in a greater percentage of the nonsmoking miners who have dust-induced bronchitis is slight and nondisabling. Ryder et al. graphically illustrate this point in Figure 6 of their article on the prevalence of emphysema found at postmortem examination with regard to age and cigarette smoking.[37] The fact that only 19 of the 106 smokers' lungs that were examined by Ryder and his colleagues showed more than 20% involvement makes it evident that most smokers do not develop emphysema.

Other problems also exist with longitudinal studies, including the healthy worker effect. It is frequently assumed that workers leave their occupation prematurely because of exposure to dust or other occupationally related hazards. In reality, the percentage of nonsmokers, ex-smokers, and smokers in the various age groups changes gradually over the working lifetime.[92] Thus, in the older workers, there is a greater percentage of nonsmokers and ex-smokers compared with that in younger employees. This is especially true of coal miners.[67] Moreover, Attfield showed that it was the smokers who tended to drop out prematurely rather than the nonsmokers.[81] Thus, it would be reasonable to infer that the smokers who leave the work force do so because of premature disability, and those who continue working are likely to be relatively resistant to the effects of cigarette smoking.

Numerous studies have shown that bronchitis is associated with an increased mortality rate from malignant and nonmalignant respiratory disease.[93] When an attempt, however, is made to control for the effect of the reduced ventilatory capacity in subjects who have bronchitis, then it becomes evident that cough and sputum alone do not lead to decreased longevity from respiratory disease other than that caused by lung cancer.[32, 88] Thus, the increased death rate associated with bronchitis is a reflection of cigarette smoking and not an effect of bronchitis.

Most mortality studies in working coal miners have shown a normal life expectancy.[94, 95] Miller and Jacobsen have shown that British coal miners, as a whole, have a 13% lower general mortality rate than do men from the same region.[96] By selecting specific subgroups and by relying on the interpretation of the initial radiograph when many miners continued to work for another 20 or so years (by which time their subsequent radiographs had shown progression, in some instances to PMF), these authors concluded that miners with chronic bronchitis and certain categories of CWP had an increased mortality rate. In practice, the latest radiograph should have been chosen. Moreover, cigarette smoking is the most common cause of chronic bronchitis, and since cigarette smoking leads to numerous life-threatening diseases, it is not surprising that those with cough and sputum show an increased standardized mortality ratio (SMR). Since bronchitis has been shown by Fletcher et al.[27] and by Foxman et al.[88] to have little or no effect on lung function, it is difficult to see why bronchitic subjects should die prematurely, at least of airways obstruction. Moreover, Ortmeyer and coworkers,[87] in a prospective study carried out on a randomly selected population of coal miners and ex-miners in the United States, were unable to show any effect of dust exposure in the absence of PMF on life expectancy. In contrast, the effects of cigarette smoking stood out like a sore thumb. Elmes comprehensively reviewed the relative effects of cigarette smoking and dust in the induction of irreversible airways obstruction and concluded that cigarette smoking is a far more serious hazard.[97]

It has been claimed that a miner's risk of having the lung involved by emphysema is related to cumulative exposure to dust and to a reduction of FEV_1. This relationship was said to be present in both smokers and nonsmokers.[98] The proponents of this argument also maintain that, as in cigarette smokers, there is a susceptible minority who are extremely sensitive to dust.[90, 99] The argument against this is the almost complete absence of significant ventilatory impairment in disability claimants who are nonsmokers and who do not suffer from PMF.[100, 101] Thus, Lapp et al. found only one of 611 subjects who claimed disability had a significant reduction in the FEV_1, i.e., below 60% of the predicted figure. The decrement in this subject was not disabling in the true sense of the word and did not meet the United States Department of Labor's criteria for total disability.[101]

The incrimination of bronchitis as the cause of the decreased ventilatory capacity observed in coal miners in the absence of PMF and smoking, and in other dust-exposed workers, partly depends on the exclusion of emphysema as the responsible agent. The most compelling reason for the indictment of bronchitis is the fact that, during the first few years of employment, there is a rapid decline in the FEV_1 but this is followed by no additional loss of function for the next 10 to 15 years. This observation was made by Cochrane et al.[21] and has recently been rediscovered.[102] It is clear that emphysema could not appear so rapidly and that the rapid induction of bronchitis provides a more plausible explanation for the early decrease in ventilatory capacity.

RESPIRATORY EFFECTS OF GRAIN DUST

Ramazzini in 1700 described ''diseases of sifters and measurers of grain.''[103] He recognized that exposure to grain dust had both acute and chronic effects. Over the past several years, there has been a spate of investigations designed to look into the hazards of those exposed to grain dust. Most of these have taken place in Canada and the United States, and it is becoming increasingly evident that the effects of grain dust inhalation are far more complex than was originally thought.

Grain dust contains not only the plant matter of the various grains (which range from wheat and rye to rapeseed and sunflower seeds) but numerous other contaminants. The latter include fungal spores, such as *Cladosporium* and *Aspergillus,* animal matter (including weevils, bird and rodent droppings, and mites); fertilizers, and pesticides, not to mention various soils and dust, some of which contain free silica.

Work Force

Those exposed to grain dust include (1) farmers; (2) workers in grain elevators, which include country, terminal, and transfer elevators; (3) dock workers; and (4) feed, flour, and seed mill workers. In the United States, it is estimated that there are about 500,000 grain workers; the comparable Canadian figure is around 30,000.[104] In addition, there are around 1.5 to 2 million farmers and farm workers who are exposed to grain at work. Farmers and dock workers for the most part are exposed intermittently.

Grain processing takes place in three different elevators: country, terminal, and transfer. The country elevator is the site where the grain is graded, cleaned, and stored before being shipped to local mills or terminal elevators. Ventilation is often poor at local elevators. The terminal elevator is where the grain is unloaded from railroad cars and trucks prior to processing and storing in concrete silos. From the terminal elevator, the grain is loaded onto grain ships. Transfer elevators store grain prior to shipment to local mills, breweries, and abroad.

Acute Effects

The acute effects of exposure to grain dust include conjunctivitis and rhinitis.[105] In addition, in some subjects, grain asthma develops.[106, 107] This latter condition has been described elsewhere in Chapter 17. The onset of grain asthma may be immediate or delayed for several hours.[107, 108] It is associated with the rapid development of bronchial hyperreactivity.[109] Recurrent nocturnal asthma has likewise been described, and there is a suggestion that the grain mite, *Glycyphagus destructor,* might be an important allergen, although skin and precipitin test results are usually negative.[110, 111] The Canadian storage mite, *Lepidoglypus destructor,* has also been implicated as a cause of grain asthma.[111] Surveys of workers in grain elevators show a lower than normal prevalence of asthma, presumably because, in the most susceptible subjects, asthma develops shortly after first exposure and they cannot continue working in the elevators. A syndrome akin to asthma also occurs in a proportion of grain workers. In this case, there is an acute decrease in the FEV_1 over a work shift.[104] As such, the fall in the FEV_1 may or may not be associated with symptoms. Falls between 100 and 290 ml in the FEV_1 have been reported over a work shift,[112] but smaller decrements are much more common.[113] Diurnal variation in peak respiratory flows have been demonstrated in grain workers and generally occur among those who smoke and in those who have pulmonary symptoms.[114] The duration of occupation had no independent effect on the diurnal variation of the peak flow, whereas cold and exposure to grain dust did.[114]

Aside from asthma, in certain workers, an acute febrile response develops, with rigors, chills, and sundry aches and pains.[105-107] This is known as grain fever and is associated with a fall in dynamic lung volumes but not in the diffusing capacity.[115] Alveolitis does not occur, and there is an absence of precipitin antibodies in the serum.[104] Although the cause of grain fever is unknown, gram-negative endotoxins must be considered to be a likely etiological factor. Extrinsic allergic alveolitis also occasionally occurs in those exposed to grain, usually farmers, and is probably due to a number of fungi, including aspergilli. It is not, as was formerly believed, caused by *Sitophilus granarius.*

Chronic Effects

The chronic effects of grain dust are less well understood. There seems little doubt that prolonged high exposure can induce both cough and sputum. This may be regarded as a form of industrial bronchitis, since it seems to be a nonspecific response to dust.[116, 117] Studies of pulmonary function in grain workers have yielded conflicting results but, for the most part, seem to suggest that smoking exaggerates the effects of exposure to grain dust. Generally, nonsmokers appear to have normal or near-normal pulmonary function.[105, 116–118]

Many of the studies of lung function have relied on so-called sensitive tests of ventilatory capacity, such as the FEF_{25-75}, closing volume, and forced expiratory flow (FEF) at low lung volumes.[118] The significance of these tests in regard to the prediction of permanent disability is either dubious or nonexistent. Broder et al. showed that absence from work because of temporary layoffs is associated with a decrease in the symptoms of cough and sputum.[119] Continued exposure, however, usually led to a gradual increase in the prevalence and severity of these symptoms. Those who continued to work also tended to have lower maximal expiratory flow rates. Rehiring of those who were initially laid off was associated with a marked increase in the symptoms and a corresponding fall in the ventilatory capacity. Further studies by the same group suggested that acute exposure may lead to minor restrictive impairment. The changes induced by exposure are small but affect both the TLC and the FVC.[120] The concomitant reduction in the FVC that is seen may be a consequence of the RV encroaching on the FVC in the absence of an increase in TLC.

There is nevertheless some evidence that continued exposure to grain dust causes an increased prevalence of cough, phlegm, wheeze, and shortness of breath, along with a greater than average decrement in ventilatory capacity.[104, 109] It is more difficult to show a consistent effect from high concentrations of grain dust on the prevalence of symptoms, especially in nonsmokers. In cross-sectional studies, it has been suggested that grain dust leads to a greater decrement in the FVC than in the FEV_1 and does so by damaging the lung parenchyma.[120] The FEV_1 is also affected, but the FEF_{25-75} is not. This hypothesis, however, should be treated with some skepticism, especially in view of the difficulties in obtaining complete FVC maneuvers in different populations and in longitudinal studies. The prevalence of wheeze appears not to be related to the level of dust.

Perhaps of more interest is the fact that, in grain workers, the rate of decline in lung function is most rapid in the first 6 years and then decreases with the passage of time, so that by 12 years, the rate of decline in the civic workers and the grain workers was the same.[104] This would go along with the findings of studies of industrial bronchitis occurring in coal miners since, during the first 3 years, there is a fairly steep decline in the FEV_1 but the annual decrement gradually tails off. Within a few years, the decline is small or negligible.[21, 102] Given the similarity of the initial response in miners and the fact that coal is not asthmogenic, it seems reasonable to attribute the initial rapid decline in ventilatory capacity that occurs in grain workers to industrial bronchitis rather than to asthma or some other specific effect that damages the lung parenchyma.

It has become increasingly clear that both farmers and those who are exposed to grain may have a number of diverse respiratory conditions. Since the etiology of some of these conditions remains unknown, prevention is often difficult or impractical at the present time, and the effects of a reduced exposure to grain dust have had little effect. Indeed, in many instances, the annual decline in the ventilatory capacity in grain workers has been no different or sometimes less than that in the control or reference populations.[104, 120]

RESPIRATORY HAZARDS OF FIREFIGHTING

During the course of their work, firefighters are exposed to a multiplicity of potentially toxic fumes, gases, and particulates. While firemen are dealing with minor fires, occasionally explosions or conflagrations take place. If those exposed are not wearing masks or self-contained breathing units, severe flash burns of the upper and, sometimes, of the lower respiratory tract may occur. Nevertheless, it must be borne in mind that life-threatening respiratory injuries can occur in the absence of thermal burns.[121, 122] It is useful to divide the respiratory problems encountered as a result of firefighting into those that are acute and those that are chronic.

Acute Effects

Aside from smoke, which for the most part consists of carbon and other particles, a wide variety of other agents may be incinerated during a fire.[123, 124] These include textiles, such as cotton and wool; various plastics and similar substances, including polymers, polyurethane,[125] polyvinyl chloride (PVC); sundry chemicals, including methyl isocyanate, as in Bhopal;[126] lumber; hay; and straw. The acute response largely depends on the agent that is undergoing combustion.

The breakdown products of most fires depend on whether the agents at the site of the fire are undergoing combustion (a process in which organic materials undergo thermal decomposition in an atmosphere containing sufficient oxygen to permit combustion) or, alternatively, pyrolysis (in which thermal decomposition takes place either when oxygen is absent or severely depleted). Incomplete combustion liberates excessive quantities of carbon monoxide and frequently occurs when fires break out in buildings without adequate ventilation or when the building's ventilation system ceases to function during a fire. Aside from carbon monoxide, other gases may be encountered in the building and include the oxides of nitrogen; hydrochloric acid vapor and hydrogen chloride from the incineration of PVC; and vaporized isocyanates and their breakdown products, which include hydrogen cyanide, aldehydes, and sundry amines.

Respiratory burns may occur after the inhalation of extremely hot smoke and fumes in the absence of overt burns on the face and lips and lead to severe injury of the respiratory tract.[121, 127] Shortly after the inhalation of extremely hot fumes and particulates, and regardless of whether respiratory burns are present, cough, soreness of the throat, and a retrosternal burning sensation develop. In less severe exposures, these symptoms may be relatively transient and disappear after a few hours only to return in 24 to 36 hours. By the time they return, cough has become distressing and is frequently productive of thick and often blood-stained tenacious mucus. In the most severely exposed subjects, breathlessness develops rapidly along with crackles and wheezes. Pulmonary edema is a frequent complication. Radiographic abnormalities also occur commonly. These include edema and patchy atelectasis. Severe infection often supervenes within 42 to 72 hours. Life-threatening airways obstruction requiring intubation is fairly frequent.[127] In those subjects with burns, severe hypoxemia and markedly elevated carboxyhemoglobin levels are common unless the subject has been wearing a protective breathing apparatus.

Bronchoscopically, the airways are hyperemic and edematous. They often show mucosal sloughing and a purulent exudate. Many of these effects are not due to direct thermal burns but are indirect effects of inhaling the fumes produced, often at sufficiently high temperatures to burn or cause necrosis of the respiratory mucosa.

Acute exposures often lead to small but usually reversible changes in ventilatory capacity.[122, 124] Some investigators have claimed to show that more persistent defects may arise after exposure.[128–130] Airways responsiveness has been shown to be increased after smoke exposure; however, this is to be expected.[131] An excellent study of lung function in subjects with thermal injury and smoke inhalation is to be found in an article by Whitener et al.[132]

Chronic Effects

Several cross-sectional studies have demonstrated an association between fire-fighting, lung disease, and decrements in lung function.[129, 133–135] In one study of a cohort of Boston firemen who were followed for 1 year, an increased rate of decline for the FVC and FEV_1 was demonstrated.[131] Repeat studies 3 years later showed no such decline.[136] A longitudinal study of 168 firefighters and 1476 controls was carried out by Sparrow et al.[137] The authors found that the firefighters had a greater annual loss of pulmonary function than did the reference group, and the occupational effects could not be explained by smoking habits, age, height, or other factors. Firemen also tended to have more symptoms than did the reference group. Unfortunately, this study relied on current smoking habits rather than pack-years, and as mentioned previously, although bronchitis correlates well with this index of smoking, ventilatory capacity is far better related to lifelong cigarette consumption, as measured by pack-years. A follow-up study of a group of 30 firemen over a period of 15 months showed some suggestion that the FVC and FEV_1 of those exposed were declining at a more rapid rate than that in the matched controls.[129] In contrast, a well-controlled longitudinal study of London firemen showed that, for the most part, the rate of decline of ventilatory capacity was normal, except in cigarette smokers.[138] In this regard, it must be borne in mind that the prevalence of smoking used to be extremely high in firefighters, although it appears that it is now decreasing.

In reviewing the published evidence, it would seem that firemen tend to have more chronic respiratory symptoms than do nonexposed reference groups. Acute and usually transient decrements in ventilatory capacity are common after the inhalation of smoke and dense fumes, but whether there is an increased annual decrement in ventilatory capacity is unsettled. Although some studies have produced limited circumstantial evidence in favor of this belief, at least in selected groups of firemen, the effect on ventilatory capacity is likely to be small since it is not reflected in the SMR of firemen, at least for respiratory disease.[139, 140] More recent studies of mortality data in firemen have suggested that the increased risk may have been missed in previous studies because of the limitations of using a general reference population without a comparable cohort.[141] Even with the use of a comparable cohort, the increase in the SMR is relatively small and could easily be explained by different smoking habits and other factors.[141, 142]

REFERENCES

1. Thackrah, C.T., The Effects of Arts, Trades and Professions and of Civic States and Habits of Living on Health and Longevity, 2nd ed. London, Longman, 1932.
2. Greenhow, E.H., Report of the Medical Officer of the Privy Council. Appendix VI. London, H.M. Stationery Office, 1861.
3. Hamilton, A., Exploring the Dangerous Trades. Boston, Little Brown & Co., 1943.
4. Haldane, J.S., Historical Review of Coal Mining. London, Fleetway Press, 1925, p. 266.
5. Medical Research Council, Chronic bronchitis and occupation. B.M.J., 1, 101, 1966.
6. Gough, J., Chronic bronchitis and occupation. B.M.J., 1, 480, 1966.
7. McLaughlin, A.I.G., Chronic bronchitis and occupation. B.M.J., 1, 354, 1966.
8. Pemberton, J., Occupational lung disease. B.M.J., 1, 609, 1966.
9. Higgins, I.T.T., and Cochrane, A.L., Population studies of miners, foundry workers and others in Staveley, Derbyshire. Br. J. Ind. Med., 16, 255, 1958.
10. Higgins, I.T.T., An approach to the problem of bronchitis in industry: studies in agricultural, mining, and farming communities. In King, E.J., and Fletcher, C.M., eds., Industrial Pulmonary Disease. London, J & A Churchill Limited, 1960, pp. 195–207.
11. Gilson, J.C., Occupational bronchitis. Proc. R. Soc. Med., 63, 857, 1970.
12. Lowe, C.R., Chronic bronchitis and occupation. Proc. R. Soc. Med., 61, 98, 1968.
13. Lowe, C.R., Campbell, H., and Khosla, T., Bronchitis in two integrated steel works II. Respiratory symptoms and ventilatory capacity related to atmosphere pollution. Br. J. Ind. Med., 27, 121, 1970.

14. Lloyd Davies, T.A., Respiratory disease in foundrymen. Report of a survey. Department of Employment. London, H.M. Stationery Office, 1971.
15. Pratt, P.C., Vollmer, R.T., and Miller, J.A., Epidemiology of pulmonary lesions in non-textile and cotton textile workers. A retrospective autopsy analysis. Arch. Environ. Health, 35, 133, 1980.
16. Irwig, L., and Rocks, P., Lung function and respiratory symptoms in silicotic and nonsilicotic gold miners. Am. Rev. Respir. Dis., 117, 429, 1978.
17. Kalacic, I., Chronic nonspecific lung disease in cement workers. Arch. Environ. Health, 26, 78, 1973.
18. Kalacic, I., Ventilatory lung function in cement workers. Arch. Environ. Health, 26, 84, 1973.
19. Townsend, M., Enterline, P.E., Sussman, N.B., et al., Pulmonary function in relation to total dust exposure at a bauxite refinery and alumina-based chemical products plant. Am. Rev. Respir. Dis., 132, 1174, 1985.
20. Higgins, I.T.T., Chronic respiratory disease in mining communities. Ann. N. Y. Acad. Sci., 200, 197, 1972.
21. Cochrane, A.L., Higgins, I.T.T., and Thomas, J., Pulmonary ventilatory function of coal miners in various areas in relation to x-ray category of pneumoconiosis. Br. J. Prev. Soc. Med., 15, 1, 1961.
22. Morgan, W.K.C., Handelsman, L., Kibelstis, J., et al. Ventilatory capacity and lung volumes of U.S. coal miners. Arch. Environ. Health, 28, 182, 1974.
23. McClintock, J.S., The selection of juvenile entrants to mining. Br. J. Ind. Med., 28, 45, 1971.
24. Fletcher, C.M., Elmes, P.C., Fairbairn, A.S., and Wood, C.M., The significance of respiratory symptoms and the diagnosis of chronic bronchitis in the working population. B.M.J., 2, 257, 1969.
25. Ciba Foundation Guest Symposium, Terminology, definition, and classification of chronic pulmonary emphysema and related conditions. Thorax, 16, 286, 1959.
26. Medical Research Council Committee on the Aetiology of Chronic Bronchitis, Definition and classification of chronic bronchitis for clinical and epidemiological purposes. Lancet, 1, 775, 1965.
27. Fletcher, C.M., Peto, R., Tinker, C., and Speizer, F.C., The Natural History of Chronic Bronchitis and Emphysema. Oxford, Oxford University Press, 1976.
28. American Thoracic Society, Statement on definitions and classifications of chronic bronchitis, asthma, and pulmonary emphysema. Am. Rev. Respir. Dis., 85, 762, 1962.
29. Reid, L., Measurement of bronchial mucous gland layer: a diagnostic yardstick in chronic bronchitis. Thorax, 15, 132, 1960.
30. Morgan, W.K.C., Industrial bronchitis. Br. J. Ind. Med., 35, 285, 1978.
31. Enterline, P.E., and Lainhart, W.S., The relationship between coal mining and chronic nonspecific respiratory disease. Am. J. Public Health, 57, 484, 1967.
32. Peto, R., Speizer, F.E., Cochrane, A.L., et al., The relevance in adults of airflow obstruction, but not of mucus hypersecretion, to mortality from chronic lung disease. Am. Rev. Respir. Dis., 128, 491, 1983.
33. Bates, D.V., The fate of the chronic bronchitic: report of the ten year followup in the Canadian Department of Veterans Affairs coordinated study of chronic bronchitis. Am. Rev. Respir. Dis., 108, 1043, 1973.
34. Thurlbeck, V.M., Henderson, J.A.M., Fraser, R.G., and Bates, D.V., Chronic obstructive lung disease. A comparison between the clinical, roentgenologic, functional and morphological criteria in chronic bronchitis, asthma, and bronchiectasis. Medicine, 49, 81, 1970.
35. Jamal, K., Cooney, T.P., Fleetham, J.A., and Thurlbeck, W.M., Chronic bronchitis: correlation of morphologic findings to sputum production and flow rates. Am. Rev. Respir. Dis., 129, 719, 1984.
36. Heard, B.E., and Izukawa, T., Pulmonary emphysema in 50 consecutive male necropsies in London. J. Pathol. Bacteriol., 88, 423, 1964.
37. Ryder, R.C., Dunnill, M.S., and Anderson, J.S., A quantitative study of bronchial mucus gland volume, emphysema, and smoking in a necropsy study. J. Pathol. Bacteriol., 106, 59, 1971.
38. Ryder, R.C., Lyons, J.P., Campbell, H., and Gough, J., Emphysema in coal workers' pneumoconiosis. B.M.J., 3, 481, 1970.
39. Lyons, J.P., Ryder, R., Campbell, H., and Gough, J., Pulmonary disability in coal workers' pneumoconiosis. B.M.J., 1, 713, 1972.
40. Lyons, J.P., and Campbell, H., Evolution of disability in coal workers' pneumoconiosis. Thorax, 31, 527, 1976.
41. Cockcroft, A.E., Wagner, J.C., Seal, R.M.E., and Campbell, M.J., Irregular opacities in coal workers' pneumoconiosis: correlation with pulmonary function and pathology. Ann. Occup. Hyg., 26, 767, 1982.
42. Gilson, J.C., and Oldham, P.D., Coal workers' pneumoconiosis. B.M.J., 4, 305, 1970.
43. Oldham, P.D., and Berry, G., Coal miner's pneumoconiosis. B.M.J., 2, 292, 1970.
44. Heppleston, A.G., The pathogenesis of simple pneumoconiosis in coal workers. J. Pathol. Bacteriol., 67, 51, 1954.
45. Ruckley, V.A., Gauld, S.J., Chapman, J.S., et al., Emphysema and dust exposure in a group of coal workers. Am. Rev. Respir. Dis., 129, 528, 1984.
46. Ruckley, V.A., Fernie, J.M., Campbell, S.J., et al., Causes of disability in coal miners: a clinicopathological study of emphysema, airways obstruction and massive fibrosis. Report no. TM 89/05. Edinburgh. Institute of Occupational Medicine, May 1989.
47. Morgan, W.K.C., and Lapp, N.L., Respiratory disease in coal miners: State of the art. Am. Rev. Respir. Dis., 113, 531, 1976.

48. Hankinson, J.L., Reger, R.B., and Morgan, W.K.C., Maximal expiratory flows in coal miners. Am. Rev. Respir. Dis., 116, 175, 1977.
49. Caswell, C., Bergman, I., and Rossiter, C.E., The relation of radiological appearance in simple pneumoconiosis of coal workers to the content and composition of the lung. *In* Walton, W.H., ed., Inhaled Particles II., Vol. 2. London, Unwin Brothers, 1970, p. 713.
50. Rossiter, C.E., Evidence of a dose-response relation in pneumoconiosis. Trans. Soc. Occup. Med., 22, 83, 1972.
51. Gough, J., The pathogenesis of emphysema. *In* Liebow, A., and Smith, D.R., eds., The Lung. Baltimore, Williams and Wilkins, 1968, p. 109.
52. Fernie, J.M., Douglas, A.N., Lamb, D., and Ruckley, V.A., Right ventricular hypertrophy in a group of coal workers. Thorax, 38, 436, 1983.
53. Wells, A.L., Pulmonary vascular changes in coal workers' pneumoconiosis. J. Pathol., 68, 573, 1954.
54. Thomas, A.J., Right ventricular hypertrophy in the pneumoconiosis of coal miners. Br. Heart. J., 13, 1, 1951.
55. James, W.R.L., and Thomas, A.J., Cardiac hypertrophy in coalworkers' pneumoconiosis. Br. J. Ind. Med., 13, 24, 1956.
56. Kibelstis, J.A., Diffusing capacity in bituminous coal miners. Chest, 63, 501, 1973.
57. Heppleston, A.G., The pathological recognition and pathogenesis of emphysema and fibrocystic disease of the lung with special reference to coal workers. Ann. N. Y. Acad. Sci., 200, 347, 1972.
58. Morgan, W.K.C., Burgess, D.B., Lapp, N.L., et al., Hyperinflation of the lungs in coal miners. Thorax, 26, 585, 1971.
59. Morgan, W.K.C., and Reger, R.B., Chronic airflow limitation and occupation. *In* Cherniack, N. ed., Chronic Obstructive Pulmonary Disease. Philadelphia, W.B. Saunders Co., 1991.
60. McDonald, J.C., Becklake, M.R., Fournier-Massey, G., and Rossiter, C.E., Respiratory symptoms in chrysotile asbestos mine and mill workers in Quebec. Arch. Environ. Health, 24, 358, 1972.
61. Kinsella, M., Muller, N., Vedal, S., et al., Emphysema in silicosis: a comparison of smokers with nonsmokers using pulmonary function testing and computed tomography. Am. Rev. Respir. Dis., 141, 1497, 1990.
61a. Hnizdo, E., Sluis-Cremer, G.K., Baskind, E., et al., Emphysema and airway obstruction in nonsmoking South African gold miners with long exposure to silica dust. Occup. Environ. Med., 51, 557, 1994.
62. Seaton, A., Lapp, N.L., and Morgan, W.K.C., Relationship of pulmonary impairment in simple coal workers' pneumoconiosis to type of radiographic opacity. Br. J. Ind. Med., 29, 50, 1972.
63. Waters, W.E., Cochrane, A.L., and Moore, F., Mortality in punctiform type of coal workers' pneumoconiosis. Br. J. Ind. Med., 31, 196, 1974.
64. Hankinson, J.L., Palmes, E.D., and Lapp, N.L., Pulmonary air space size in coal miners. Am. Rev. Respir. Dis., 119, 391, 1979.
65. Ashford, J.R., Morgan, D.C., Rae, S., and Sowden, R.R., Respiratory symptoms in British coal miners. Am. Rev. Respir. Dis., 102, 370, 1970.
66. Rae, S., Walker, D.D., and Attfield, N.D., Chronic bronchitis in dust exposure in British coal miners. *In* Walton, W.H., ed., Inhaled Particles II. Old Woking, Surrey, UK, Unwin, 1971, p. 883.
67. Kibelstis, J.A., Morgan, E.J., Reger, R.B., et al., Prevalence of bronchitis and airway obstruction in American bituminous coal miners. Am. Rev. Respir. Dis., 108, 886, 1973.
68. Vuylsteek, K., and Depoorter, A.M., Smoking, occupational dust exposure and chronic nonspecific lung disease. Broncho-Pneumologie, 28, 31, 1978.
69. Rogan, J.M., Attfield, M.D., Jacobsen, M., et al., Role of dust in the working environment in development of chronic bronchitis in British coal miners. Br. J. Ind. Med., 123, 372, 1973.
70. Deutsche Forschungsgemeinschaft, Research Report on Chronic Bronchitis and Occupational Dust Exposure. Boppard, Germany, Harold Boldt Verlag KG, 1978.
71. Hankinson, J.L., Reger, R.B., Fairman, R.P., et al., Factors influencing expiratory flow rates in coal miners. *In* Walton, W.H., ed., Inhaled Particles IV. Oxford, Pergamon Press, 1977, p. 737.
72. Morgan, W.K.C., Burgess, D.B., Lapp, N.L., et al., Hyperinflation of the lungs in coal miners. Thorax, 26, 585, 1971.
73. Brinkman, G.L., and Coates, E.O., The prevalence of chronic bronchitis in an industrial population. Am. Rev. Respir. Dis., 86, 47, 1962.
74. Brinkman, G.L., and Block, D.L., The prognosis in chronic bronchitis. JAMA, 197, 71, 1966.
75. Brinkman, G.L., Block, D.L., and Cress, C., The effects of bronchitis on occupational pulmonary ventilation over an 11-year period. J. Occup. Med., 14, 615, 1962.
76. Kreiss, K., Greenburg, L.M., Kogut, S.J.H., et al., Hard-rock mining exposures affect smokers and nonsmokers differently. Results of a community prevalence study. Am. Rev. Respir. Dis., 139, 1487, 1989.
77. Nemery, B., Veriter, C., and Brasseur, L., Impairment of ventilatory function and pulmonary gas exchange in nonsmoking miners. Lancet, 2, 1427, 1987.
78. Cotes, J.D., Feinmann, E.L., Male, V.G., et al., Respiratory symptoms and impairment in shipyard welders and caulker/burners. Br. J. Ind. Med., 46, 292, 1989.
79. Nagelschmidt, G., The study of lung dust in pneumoconiosis. Am. Ind. Hyg. Assoc. J., 26, 1, 1965.
80. Love, R.G., and Miller, B.G., Longitudinal study of lung function in coal miners. Thorax, 37, 193, 1982.

81. Attfield, M.D., Longitudinal decline in FEV_1 in United States coal miners. Thorax, 40, 132, 1985.
82. Glover, J.R., Bevan, C., Cotes, J.E., et al., Effects of exposure to slate dust in North Wales. Br. J. Ind. Med., 37, 152, 1980.
83. National Bureau of Standards; An Evaluation of the Accuracy of the Coal Mine Dust Sampling Program Administered by the Department of the Interior. A Final Report to the Senate Committee on Labour and Public Welfare. Washington, D.C., Department of Commerce, 1975.
84. Comptroller General of the United States, Report to Congress. Improvements Still Needed in Coal Mine Dust Sampling Program and Penalty Assessment and Collections. Red-76-75. Washington, D.C., Department of Health, Education and Welfare, December 31, 1975.
85. Marine, W.M., Gurr, D., and Jacobsen, M., Clinically important respiratory effects of dust exposure and smoking in British coal miners. Am. Rev. Respir. Dis., 137, 106, 1988.
86. Cochrane, A.L., Haley, T.J.L., Moore, F., et al., The mortality of men in the Rhondda Fach, 1950–1970. Br. J. Ind. Med., 36, 15, 1979.
87. Ortmeyer, C.E., Costello, J., Morgan, W.K.C., et al., The mortality of Appalachian coal miners, 1963–1971. Arch. Environ. Health, 29, 67, 1974.
88. Foxman, B., Higgins, I.T.T., and Oh, M.S., The effects of occupation and smoking on respiratory disease mortality. Am. Rev. Respir. Dis., 134, 649, 1986.
89. Kauffman, K., Drouet, D., Lellouch, J., et al., Occupational exposure and 12 year spirometric changes among Paris area workers. Br. J. Ind. Med., 39, 221, 1982.
90. Attfield, M.D., and Hodous, T.K., Pulmonary function of U.S. coal miners related to dust exposure estimates. Am. Rev. Respir. Dis., 145, 605, 1992.
90a. Lapp, N.L., and Morgan, W.K.C., Pulmonary function of U.S. coal miners related to dust exposure. Am. Rev. Respir. Dis., 147, 237, 1993.
91. Oxman, A.D., Muir, D.C.F., Shannon, H.S., et al., Occupational dust exposure and chronic obstructive pulmonary disease. A systematic overview of the evidence. Am. Rev. Respir. Dis., 148, 38, 1993.
92. Morgan, W.K.C., On dust, disability, and death. Am. Rev. Respir. Dis., 134, 639, 1986.
93. Public Health Service, Office of the Assistant Secretary for Health, Office on Smoking and Health, A Report of the Surgeon General. DHEW publication no. (PHS) 79–50066. Washington, D.C., Department of Health, Education, and Welfare, 1979.
94. Morgan, W.K.C., Coal workers' pneumoconiosis. *In* Morgan, W.K.C., and Seaton, A., eds., Occupational Lung Diseases. Philadelphia, W.B. Saunders Co., 1984.
95. Surgeon General, The Health Consequences of Smoking. Cancer and Chronic Obstructive Lung Disease in the Workplace. A Report of the Surgeon General. Rockville, MD, Office on Smoking and Health, 1985, pp. 300–304.
96. Miller, B.G., and Jacobsen, M., Dust exposure, pneumoconiosis and mortality of coal miners. Br. J. Ind. Med., 42, 723, 1985.
97. Elmes, P.C., Relative importance of cigarette smoking in occupational lung disease. Br. J. Ind. Med., 38, 1, 1981.
98. Seaton, A., Coal mining, emphysema, and compensation. Br. J. Ind. Med., 47, 433, 1990.
99. Hurley, J.F., and Soutar, C.A., Can exposure to coal mine dust cause a severe impairment of lung function? Br. J. Ind. Med., 43, 150, 1986.
100. Morgan, W.K.C., Coal mining, emphysema and compensation revisited. Br. J. Ind. Med., 50, 1051, 1993.
101. Lapp, N.L., Morgan, W.K.C., and Zaldivar, G., Airways obstruction, coal mining and disability. Occup. Environ. Med., 51, 234, 1994.
102. Seixas, N.S., Robins, T.G., Attfield, M.D., et al., Longitudinal and cross sectional analyses of exposure to coal mine dust and pulmonary function in new miners. Br. J. Ind. Med., 50, 929, 1993.
103. Ramazzini, B., De Morbes Artificum Diatriba 1713. Translated by W.C. Wright. Chicago, University of Chicago Press, 1940.
104. Chan-Yeung, M., Enarson, D.A., and Kennedy, S.M., The impact of grain dust on respiratory health. State of the art. Am. Rev. Respir. Dis., 145, 476, 1992.
105. Becklake, M., Grain dust and health. State of the art. *In* Dosman, J.A., and Cotton, L., eds., Occupational Lung Diseases. New York, Academic Press, 1980, pp. 180–201.
106. Williams, N., Skoulas, A., and Merrimen, J., Exposure to grain dust. I. A survey of health effects. J. Occup. Med., 6, 319, 1964.
107. do Pico, G., Reddan, W., Flaherty, D., et al., Respiratory abnormalities among grain handlers. A clinical, physiologic and immunologic study. Am. Rev. Respir. Dis., 115, 915, 1977.
108. Davies, R.J., Green, M., and Schofield, N.M., Recurrent nocturnal asthma after exposure to grain dust. Am. Rev. Respir. Dis., 114, 1011, 1976.
109. James, A.L., Zimmerman, M.J., Ee, H., et al., Exposure to grain dust and changes in lung function. Br. J. Ind. Med., 47, 466, 1990.
110. Chan-Yeung, M., Wong, R., and MacLean, L., Respiratory abnormalities among grain elevator workers. Chest, 75, 461, 1979.
111. Warren, C.P.W., Holford-Strevens, V., and Singha, R.N., Sensitization in a grain handler to the storage mite *Lepidoglypus destructor* (shrank). Ann. Allergy, 50, 30, 1983.
112. Gandevia, B., and Ritchie, B., Relevance of respiratory symptoms and signs to ventilatory capacity. Changes after exposure to grain dust and phosphate rock dust. Br. J. Ind. Med., 23, 181, 1966.

113. Chan-Yeung, M., Schulzer, M., MacLean, L., et al., Epidemiological health survey of grain elevator workers in British Columbia. Am. Rev. Respir. Dis., 121, 329, 1980.

114. Revsbech, P., and Andersen, G., Diurnal variation in peak flow rate among grain elevator workers. Br. J. Ind. Med., 46, 566, 1989.

115. do Pico, G.A., Flaherty, D., Bhansali, P., et al., Grain fever syndrome induced by inhalation of airborne grain dust. J. Allergy Clin. Immunol., 69, 435, 1982.

116. Chan-Yeung, M., Wong, R., and MacLean, L., Respiratory abnormalities among grain elevator workers. Chest, 75, 461, 1979.

117. Dosman, J., Chronic obstructive pulmonary disease and smoking in grain workers. Ann. Intern. Med., 87, 784, 1977.

118. Broder, I., Mintz, S., Hutcheon, M., et al., Comparison of respiratory variables in grain elevator workers and civic outside workers of Thunder Bay, Canada. Am. Rev. Respir. Dis., 119, 193, 1979.

119. Broder, I., Mintz, S., Hutcheon, M., et al., Effect of lay-off and rehire on respiratory variables of grain elevator workers. Am. Rev. Respir. Dis., 122, 601, 1980.

120. Chan-Yeung, M., Dimichi-Ward, H., Enarson, D., et al., Five cross-sectional studies of grain elevator workers. Am. J. Epidemiol., 136, 1269, 1992.

121. Hampton, T.R.W., Acute inhalation injury. J. R. Nav. Med. Serv., 57, 4, 1971.

122. Landa, J., Avery, W., and Sackner, M.A., Some physiologic observations in smoke inhalation. Chest, 61, 62, 1972.

123. Musk, A.W., Smith, T.J., and McLaughlin, E., Pulmonary function and fire fighters: acute changes in ventilatory capacity and their correlates. Br. J. Ind. Med., 36, 29, 1972.

124. Brandt-Rauf, P.W., Cosman, B., Fallon, L.F., Jr., et al., Health hazards of firefighters: acute pulmonary effects after toxic exposures. Br. J. Ind. Med., 46, 209, 1989.

125. Le Quesne, P.M., Axford, A.T., McKerrow, C.B., et al., Neurological complications after a single severe exposure to toluene di-isocyanate. Br. J. Ind. Med., 33, 72, 1976.

126. Anderson, N., Kerr-Muir, M., Mehra, V., et al., Exposure and response to methyl isocyanate: results of a community based survey in Bhopal. Br. J. Ind. Med., 45, 1469, 1988.

127. Wanner, A., and Cutchavaree, A., Early recognition of upper airways obstruction following smoke inhalation. Am. Rev. Respir. Dis., 108, 1421, 1973.

128. Tashkin, D.P., Genovesi, M.G., Chopra, S., et al., Respiratory status of Los Angeles firemen, one month follow-up after inhalation of dense smoke. Chest, 71, 445, 1977.

129. Unger, K.M., Snow, R.M., Mestas, J.M., et al., Smoke inhalation in firemen. Thorax, 35, 838, 1980.

130. Horsfield, K., Cooper, F.M., and Buckman, M.P., Respiratory symptoms in firemen. Br. J. Ind. Med., 45, 251, 1988.

131. Chia, K.S., Jeyaratnam, J., Chan, T.B., et al., Airways responsiveness in firefighters after smoke exposure. Br. J. Ind. Med., 47, 524, 1990.

132. Whitener, D.R., Whitener, L.M., Robertson, K.J., et al., Pulmonary function measurements in patients with thermal injury and smoke inhalation. Am. Rev. Respir. Dis., 122, 731, 1980.

133. Peters, J.M., Theriault, B.P., Fine, L.J., et al., Chronic effect of fire-fighting on pulmonary function. N. Engl. J. Med., 291, 1320, 1974.

134. Sidor, R., and Peters, J.M., Prevalence rates of nonspecific respiratory disease in fire-fighters. Am. Rev. Respir. Dis., 109, 1421, 1974.

135. Sidor, R., and Peters, J.M., Fire-fighting and pulmonary function. Am. Rev. Respir. Dis., 109, 249, 1974.

136. Musk, A.W., Peters, J.M., and Wegman, D.H., Lung function in fire-fighters: a three year follow-up of active subjects. Am. J. Public Health, 67, 626, 1976.

137. Sparrow, D., Bosse, R., Rosner, B., et al., The effect of occupational exposure on pulmonary function. A longitudinal evaluation of firefighters and non-firefighters. Am. Rev. Respir. Dis., 125, 319, 1982.

138. Douglas, D.B., Douglas, R.B., Oakes, D., et al., Pulmonary function of London firemen. Br. J. Ind. Med., 42, 55, 1985.

139. Mastromatteo, E., Mortality in city firemen II. A study of mortality in firemen of a city health department. Arch. Ind. Health, 20, 227, 1959.

140. Musk, A.W., Monson, R.R., Peters, J.M., et al., Mortality among Boston fire-fighters. Br. J. Ind. Med., 35, 104, 1978.

141. Rosenstock, L., Demers, P., Heyer, N.J., et al., Respiratory mortality among firefighters. Br. J. Ind. Med., 47, 462, 1990.

142. Hansen, E.S., A cohort study on the mortality of firefighters. Br. J. Ind. Med., 47, 805, 1990.

20

Hypersensitivity Pneumonitis

David M.F. Murphy

W. Keith C. Morgan

Anthony Seaton

The inhalation of organic particles or gases may lead to a number of different pulmonary responses. The best understood of these is asthma, characterized by increased resistance to flow in the airways and usually mediated by reaginic antibody (see Chapter 17). Less common is a reaction involving the lung acinus, including the bronchioles, and known as allergic alveolitis or allergic bronchiolo-alveolitis.[1] There is still considerable debate about the immunological mechanisms involved in this disease, and indeed, the different clinical patterns seen in various manifestations of allergic alveolitis suggest that several mechanisms may be involved. In addition to these diseases, there are also several even less well-understood conditions in which the lung may be involved as part of a response to an organized antigen. Humidifier fever, sewage worker's disease, and grain fever are examples. Finally, an occasional patient may present with a dual reaction at both the bronchial and acinar level. This may occur with exposure to gases or fumes, such as isocyanates and cobalt, and to particulate organic matter. In view of the variety of pulmonary responses to inhaled organic material and the uncertainties surrounding their pathogenesis, this chapter has been given the rather general heading of hypersensitivity pneumonitis so as to include other less well-defined syndromes.

ALLERGIC ALVEOLITIS

Epidemiology

Although many different causes of allergic alveolitis have been identified (Table 20–1), epidemiological studies describing the prevalence of these conditions are relatively few in number. This may reflect difficulties in establishing generally accepted diagnostic criteria,[2] although Terho proposed criteria which are more clinically useful.[3]

Precipitins which were once regarded as the *sine qua non* of the disease are now more useful in establishing evidence of exposure to specific antigens.[4] Where symptom-based criteria have been used to detect the prevalence of farmer's lung, the rates reported range from 1.3% in Italy[5] to 8.6% in Ayrshire, Scotland.[6] Rates from East Lothian, Scotland (2.3%) are similar to those in the west of Ireland (2.6%).[7] In Wisconsin, a rate of 3.9% has been recorded.[8] Building-associated alveolitis involves isolated outbreaks with rates varying from 10% to 50%,[9, 10] whereas in the sugar cane (bagasse) industry, rates as high as 49% have been recorded from some parts of the world.[11] In the United States, improvements in industrial practice have resulted in virtual disappearance of bagassosis.[12]

When asymptomatic farmers have been studied, the prevalence of positive

Table 20–1

■

Recognized Types of Allergic Alveolitis

	Condition	Antigen
Fungal causes	Farmer's lung	Thermophilic actinomycetes
	Air conditioner lung	″ ″
	Bagassosis	″ ″
	Mushroom worker's lung	″ ″
	Malt worker's lung	*A. clavatus*
	Cheese washer's lung	*P. casei*
	Maple bark stripper's disease	*C. corticale*
	Sequoiosis	*A. pullulans*
	Woodworker's disease	*C. corticale*
	Suberosis	*P. frequentans*
	Paprika splitter's lung	*Mucor*
	Dry rot lung	*M. lacrymans*
	"Dog house disease"	*A. versicolor*
	Lycoperdonosis	*Lycoperdon*
Animal causes	Bird breeder's lung	Avian protein, bloom
	Rat handler's lung	Rat protein
	Wheat weevil disease	Wheat weevil
	Furrier's lung	Animal fur
	Pituitary snuff taker's lung	Ox and pork protein
Chemical causes	Isocyanate lung	TDI, MDI, HDI
	Pauli's reagent lung	Pauli's reagent
	Vineyard sprayer's lung	Bordeaux mixture
	Hard metal disease	Cobalt
	Cromolyn sodium lung	Cromolyn sodium
Bacterial causes	Washing powder lung	*B. subtilis* enzymes
	B. subtilis alveolitis	*B. subtilis*
	B. cereus alveolitis	*B. cereus*
Uncertain	Sauna lung	Lake water (?)
	New Guinea lung	Hut thatch (?)
	Ramin lung	Ramin wood (?)
	Insecticide lung	Pyrethrum (?)

precipitin reactions against thermophilic *Actinomyces* ranges from 8% in Quebec[13] to 22% in Finland.[14] In asymptomatic employees of buildings in which allergic alveolitis has been identified, studies have revealed a prevalence of 12%.[10]

Clinical Features

The factors that determine the manner of clinical presentation are little understood. There is little to support a dose-response relationship, although theoretically, a variety of factors, including the concentration of organic antigen, duration of exposure, frequency of exposure, particle size, antigen solubility, respiratory protection, and differences in work practice, should all influence the type of presentation and the possible outcome.[15]

The classical acute episode of allergic alveolitis starts with fever, muscular aches, and general malaise some 4 to 8 hours after exposure to the antigen. Occasionally, this is preceded or accompanied by wheeze or tightness in the chest and a dry cough. Shortness of breath is a feature of more severe attacks and may occasionally be dramatic and disabling or even fatal. The symptoms typically reach a peak at about 8 to 12 hours after exposure and then improve over another 12 to 24 hours in the absence of further exposure. The physical signs during such an attack are fever, tachycardia, and tachypnea. The last sign may be detected only in mild cases if the patient is exercised. Auscultation of the lungs invariably reveals repetitive mid- and end-inspiratory crackles. Wheeze may uncommonly be heard also and should not exclude the diagnosis. In general, the symptoms might be described as nonwheezy dyspnea. Acute attacks are sometimes associated with leukocytosis and a relative lymphopenia in the peripheral blood.

Such an acute attack usually resolves rapidly, but occasionally, it may persist much longer and require the patient's admission to the hospital (Fig. 20–1). These episodes may cause diagnostic difficulties if the physician does not ask about the patient's job and recent activities. The most frequent condition with which it may be confused is a mycoplasmal or another atypical pneumonia. This confusion may be confounded by the anamnestic rise in viral antibody titers that may occur in

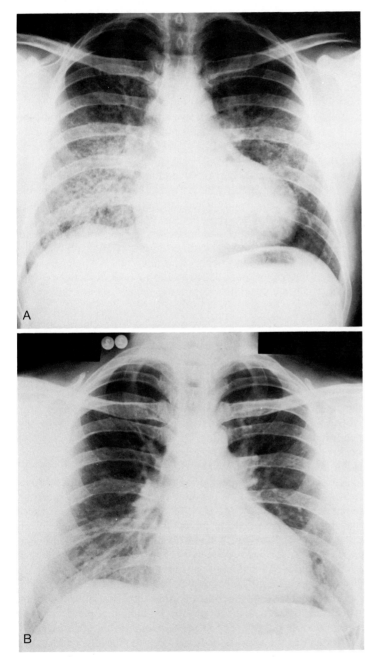

Figure 20–1. *A,* Radiograph of patient with his first attack of acute farmer's lung, showing diffuse ground-glass opacification. *B,* Same patient 5 weeks later. Slow resolution has taken place, but some residual shadowing remains.

acute allergic alveolitis.[16] Even more confusing is the finding of spurious false-positive precipitins to farmer's lung antigen in mycoplasmal pneumonia.[17] In such difficult cases, the diagnosis initially depends on a careful history of the patient's exposure.

A third way in which allergic alveolitis may manifest itself is as a recurrent, subacute illness. In this case, patients complain of general malaise, cough, wheeze or shortness of breath, laryngitis, and other symptoms, none of which is specific or dramatic. He or she may have consulted their physicians repeatedly for what both the patient and doctor believe to be upper respiratory tract infections, and in some instances, there may even have been thoughts of involving a psychiatrist. Such patients usually respond promptly to removal of the antigen. This type of presentation is found most frequently among people exposed to relatively low doses of an antigen on a regular basis, such as keepers of parakeets or pigeons.

It should be pointed out that, although age may modify the body's immune response to antigen, allergic alveolitis may occur at any age. Children who help their parents on farms and with racing pigeons are at risk, and it is important that pediatricians be aware of this, since permanent lung damage may occur. Besides age, another factor that may modify the response to inhaled antigen is cigarette smoking, and there is now good evidence that smokers are less susceptible to allergic alveolitis than are nonsmokers.[18, 19] This should not, of course, be used as an argument in favor of smoking!

It is likely that any acute attack of allergic alveolitis causes some scarring of the acinar structures. However, the patients who are most likely to have irreversible pulmonary fibrosis are those with the recurrent subacute attacks. Such patients may have clinical evidence of pulmonary fibrosis, with retraction of the upper lobes and widespread crackles. Finger clubbing is unusual but occurs. A proportion of patients with chronic allergic alveolitis have airways obstruction that is clinically indistinguishable from emphysema.[20] Any nonsmoker who presents with emphysema should be carefully questioned about possible exposure to organic antigens. In a few patients with chronic allergic alveolitis, respiratory failure and cor pulmonale may ultimately develop.

Radiographic Features

The radiographic appearance of allergic alveolitis is variable.[20] In the acute episode, there may be a dramatic bilateral acinar filling process indistinguishable from pulmonary edema (Fig. 20–2) or a diffuse miliary mottling (Fig. 20–3). There is often an irregular linear component to the shadowing in the lower zones (Fig. 20–4), and Kerley B lines may be seen. The shadowing is usually diffuse and shows no preference for any regions of the lung.

In the subacute type of allergic alveolitis, radiographic changes may be minimal or absent, even in the presence of profuse inspiratory crackles on auscultation (Fig. 20–5). As the disease becomes chronic, the irregular linear and cystic shadows associated with fibrosis occur, usually in the upper zones. The upper zones contract with upward retraction of the pulmonary arteries (Fig. 20–6). The final appearances may be indistinguishable from those seen in tuberculosis, sarcoidosis, ankylosing spondylitis, or histiocytosis X, all of which figure in the differential diagnosis of upper zone fibrosis.

When high-resolution computed tomography (CT) has been used to study patients with extrinsic allergic alveolitis, no single pathognomic feature identifying the condition has been recognized.[21] However, in most subjects with a subacute presentation, diffuse parenchymal opacification with or without a poorly defined alveolar component is found. In this phase of the disease, routine chest radiography usually shows the lower half of the lungs to be more affected, but CT demonstrates a uniform increase in density of the lung parenchyma with no sparing of the extended lung bases and no differential involvement between the central and peripheral parts of the lung. A nodular or reticular pattern also may be seen, with or

Text continued on page 533

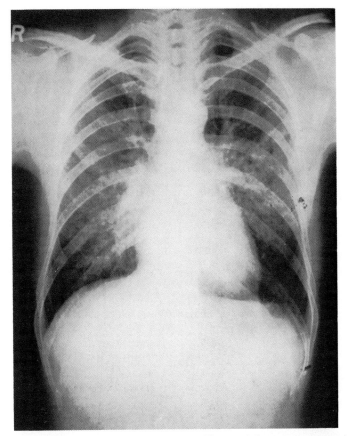

Figure 20–2. Farmer's lung. Acute episode of fever and dyspnea occurring 4 hours after the patient had forked moldy hay for feeding cattle. Radiograph shows a fine nodular infiltrate, confluent toward the hila and sparing of the periphery. Patient recovered rapidly with steroid treatment. (Courtesy of Dr. J. Meek.)

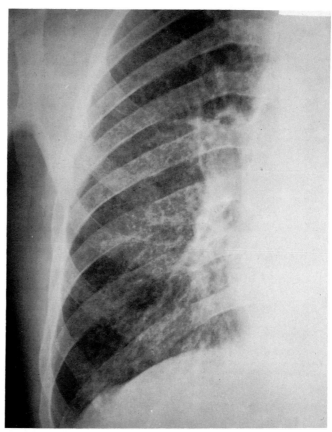

Figure 20–3. Acute farmer's lung. Macroradiograph of lower right lung to show the typical pattern of fine miliary mottling. (Courtesy of Dr. J. Meek.)

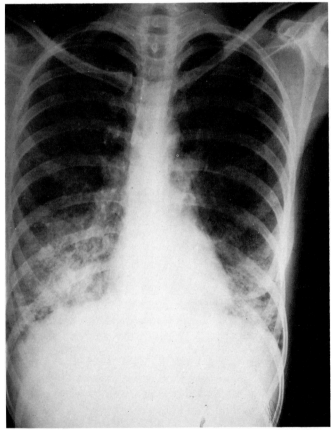

Figure 20–4. Acute farmer's lung in farmer's wife after feeding cattle with hay. Radiograph shows a pattern of miliary mottling with a linear component at the bases. (Courtesy of Dr. J. Meek.)

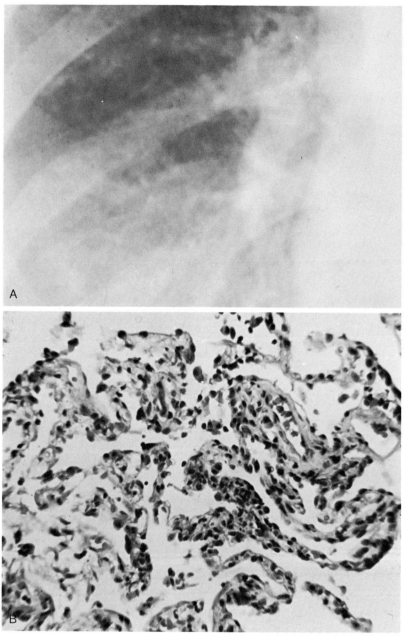

Figure 20–5. *A,* Right mid zone of radiograph of shopkeeper exposed to parakeets, showing possible diffuse nodularity. *B,* Needle lung biopsy specimen from same patient, showing nonspecific alveolitis.

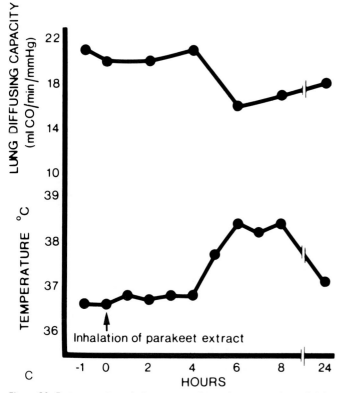

Figure 20–5 *Continued C,* Challenge test with parakeet serum showed delayed rise in temperature and fall in diffusing capacity, diagnostic of allergic alveolitis.

without diffuse air space consolidation in the middle and lower lung zones in about 50% of patients.[21]

Pulmonary Function

During the acute attack, the subject's lung volumes and, in particular, the vital capacity are reduced. Although there are regional changes in the distribution of ventilation and perfusion, airways resistance remains normal. The diffusing capacity (transfer factor) is reduced, and the lungs have a reduced compliance.[20, 22] Blood gas analysis at this stage shows arterial oxygen desaturation, which may be profound. The arterial carbon dioxide tension is usually slightly reduced because of alveolar hyperventilation, although renal compensation for this respiratory alkalosis tends to keep the pH normal (Table 20–2). In the acute attack, exercise testing is usually impracticable, but when it becomes possible, it usually causes a further fall in arterial oxygen tension. Neither does the diffusing capacity rise as expected on exercise at this stage. The administration of 100% oxygen produces complete saturation, and the arterial oxygen tension rises to a level sufficient to indicate that the basic defect responsible for desaturation is an inequality in ventilation/perfusion ratios. Concomitant with the hyperventilation and desaturation is an increase in the ratio of physiological dead space to tidal volume. Some studies have suggested that the reduction in diffusing capacity is related to a fall in the membrane component rather than the pulmonary capillary blood volume.[20, 22] Pulmonary artery pressure and vascular resistance may, however, be slightly elevated in the acute stages, an increase possibly related to the fall in arterial oxygen tension.

In the typical acute attack, these abnormalities resolve over a few days. Prolonged attacks may, however, be associated with severe reductions of lung

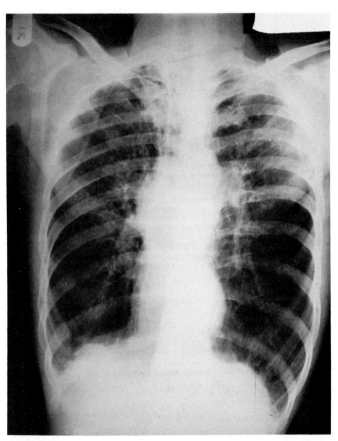

Figure 20–6. Chronic farmer's lung. This farmer was exposed over many years to moldy hay dust and had several previous episodes of shivering and dyspnea after exposure. Now he is persistently short of breath on moderate exertion with lung function tests showing a mixed pattern of restriction and obstruction. Radiograph shows linear shadows extending into contracted upper lobes and compensatory emphysematous changes in lower zones. (Courtesy of Dr. J. Meek.)

Table 20–2

■

Pulmonary Function Changes in a Subject with Acute Farmer's Lung

	Predicted	Observed	3 Weeks Later	6 Months Later
Lung Volumes				
VC (L)	5.10	3.80	4.20	5.30
RV (L)	1.50	1.90	1.80	1.80
TLC (L)	6.60	5.70	6.00	7.10
Mechanics				
FEV$_1$ (L)	4.08	3.04	3.21	4.20
MVV (L/m)	145	95	107	144
Static compliance				
(L/cm H$_2$O)	0.20	0.045	0.10	0.21
Gas diffusion				
Carbon monoxide diffusing capacity (steady state)				
(ml/min/ mm Hg)	37.00	18.00	22.00	34.00
Arterial Po$_2$ (mm Hg)	95.00	52.00	75.00	92.00
Arterial Pco$_2$ (mm Hg)	38.0–42.0	34.00	38.00	39.00
pH	7.38–7.42	7.44	7.40	7.40

VC, vital capacity; RV, residual volume; TLC, total lung capacity; FEV$_1$, forced expiratory volume in 1 second; MVV, maximum voluntary ventilation; Po$_2$, partial oxygen pressure; Pco$_2$, partial carbon dioxide pressure.

volumes and of the diffusing capacity which last for several weeks. In some patients, these abnormalities may persist indefinitely as chronic disease. In the subacute cases, diffusing capacity and lung compliance changes may be the only abnormalities found. It should also be remembered that up to one third of chronic cases show an obstructive pattern, sometimes with raised residual volume and a low diffusing capacity mimicking emphysema.[20]

Pathological Findings

The pathological findings in extensive allergic alveolitis depend on the stage of the disease. The appearance of the acute condition is strikingly different from that of the chronic fibrotic end stages of the condition. In the acute stage, the macroscopic appearance is of a reddish gray consolidated lung, whereas in the chronic fibrotic stage, the lung is firm and rubbery in texture.

Often the most characteristic feature of the pathological results of allergic alveolitis is its centrilobular distribution (Fig. 20–7). There is frequently an inflammatory reaction in the bronchiolar wall, and this may be intense. Occasionally, the alveolar wall is also involved (Fig. 20–8). Another conspicuous feature of the pathological findings of the acute disease is the presence of numerous noncaseating sarcoid-like granulomata, usually associated with giant cells and, again, located predominantly in the center of the acinus. The giant cells may be of both Langhans and foreign body types (see Fig. 20–7). The alveolar walls are typically thickened by edema and infiltration with monocytes, predominantly lymphocytes, plasma cells, and histiocytes.[23, 24] Alveolar macrophages may be profuse and, especially in bird breeder's lung, have a foamy appearance. In very acute severe cases, alveolar edema may be present with macrophage aggregations within alveoli.[25] Bronchiolitis obliterans occurs in 50% of subjects.[23, 26] When a lung biopsy is performed a month or more after an acute attack, the granulomas have usually resolved, unlike sarcoidosis, in which they typically become hyalinized.

While some alveolar wall fibrin may be seen in the acute phase (Fig. 20–9), collagenous fibrosis is an important feature in chronic disease.[23] Macroscopically, irregular fibrosis and honeycombing are present, predominantly in the upper zones

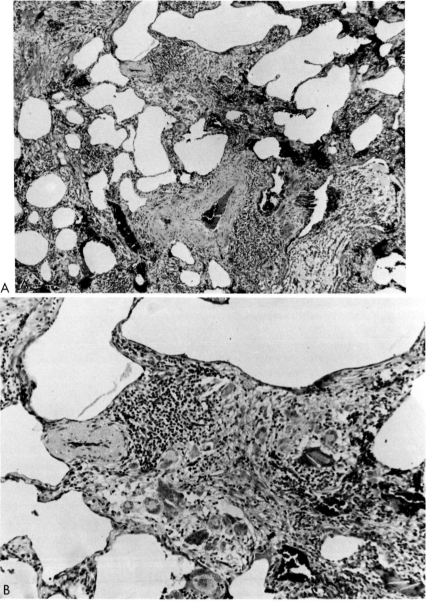

Figure 20–7. *A*, Low-power photomicrograph of lung biopsy in acute farmer's lung, showing extensive inflammatory changes in centrilobular areas, bronchiolitis (bottom right), and thickening of related pulmonary arteries. There is an interstitial mononuclear inflammatory infiltrate (alveolitis), and a perivascular giant cell granuloma is present (top center). The disease in this patient progressed to chronic fibrosis in spite of treatment with steroids. *B*, Higher-power photomicrograph of the perivascular granuloma in *A*, showing epithelioid cells, giant cells of both Langhans and foreign body type (with inclusions in the latter), and focal collections of lymphocytes.

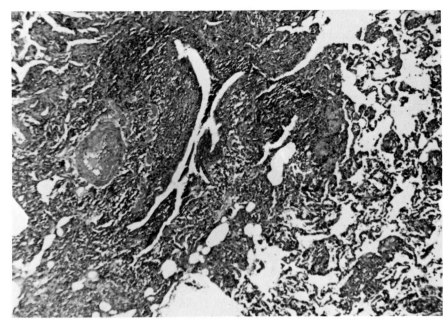

Figure 20–8. Low-power photomicrograph of biopsy specimen from patient with acute farmer's lung, showing proliferative bronchiolar changes, ballooning of arteriolar endothelial cells, and mononuclear infiltration maximal in the center of the lobule; the peripheral alveolar septa are less involved.

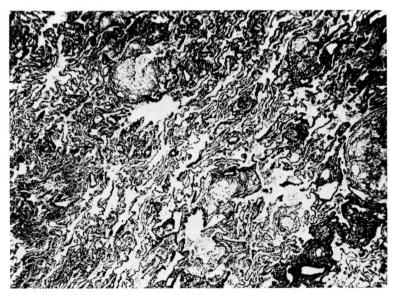

Figure 20–9. Low-power photomicrograph (reticulin stain) showing generalized increase in reticulin and three epithelioid tubercles. This biopsy was taken from a 20-year-old farmer after his second attack of farmer's lung. He has made a complete recovery and has normal lung function tests 20 years later.

(Figs. 20–10 and 20–11). Microscopically, focal fibrosis is found around bronchioles and the small bronchi (Fig. 20–12). Alveolar septa are thickened with collagen, and in the vicinity of bronchioles, the alveolar architecture may be totally destroyed. Pulmonary hypertensive changes may be seen in the vessels, and in such cases, right ventricular hypertrophy will be evident. Occasionally, chronic cases may be seen in which emphysema is the main pathological finding but in which microscopy reveals this to be associated with a fine interstitial fibrosis (Fig. 20–13). It is probable that such changes, as well as those of extensive peribronchiolar fibrosis, are responsible for the airways obstruction found in a proportion of patients with chronic allergic alveolitis.

Pathogenesis

The pathogenesis of allergic alveolitis begins with the inhalation of particulate organic matter sufficiently small in aerodynamic diameter to reach the lung acinus. In many instances, this means the inhalation of fungal spores. These particles are present in the normal atmosphere throughout the year,[27] often in large numbers, and may sometimes provoke asthma in atopic subjects. However, the much larger numbers of particles associated with profuse growth on dead organic matter stored at an appropriate temperature and suitable humidity are necessary in most cases for sensitization of the allergic alveolitis type to occur.[28] Other organic particles that may be sufficiently small to cause acinar disease may be derived from feathers and animal dander and animal excreta. In a few instances, a similar reaction has also been recorded after inhalation of organic vapor or even inorganic fumes, presumably as a result of hapten formation within the lung.

Pepys et al. were the first to propose that serum precipitins played a role in the pathogenesis of allergic alveolitis.[29] They reported on bronchial inhalational challenge tests which showed a delayed response coming on 4 to 8 hours after exposure with timing similar to the Arthus reaction. There is now little evidence that precipitins are responsible for the pathogenesis of extrinsic allergic alveolitis.[4] Notwithstanding, these antibodies are usually detected in the presence of acute disease and may persist for up to 3 years after antigen exposure ceases.[30] Although antibody combined with antigen as immune complexes can induce local granulomata, the usual pathological response is a vasculitis, which is rarely found in allergic alveolitis.[26] However, vasculitic-like lesions have occasionally been reported in the earliest stages of the condition. This may be explained by complement activation, since C5a, a chemotaxin, has been detected in the bronchoalveolar lavage (BAL) fluid obtained in acute stages of the condition,[31, 32] which suggests activation of the alternative pathway of complement, leading to chemotaxis of neutrophils and increased vascular permeability.[33] This is also in keeping with the finding of neutrophils in the BAL fluid of the acute phase of the disease.[34]

In the classification of hypersensitivity responses first proposed by Coombs et al.,[35] a type III hypersensitivity response is one associated with immune complex–mediated injury. The immune complexes consist of antigen, antibody of the immunoglobulin IgG or IgM class that has been generated against the offending antigen, and complement. Release of the chemotactic complement factor C5a attracts polymorphonuclear leukocytes to the area, and liberation of their lysosomal enzymes causes tissue injury. This response is associated with a particular skin test, the Arthus reaction,[36] which comes on 4 to 6 hours after the intradermal injection of antigen and mimics the delay in the onset of symptoms associated with the response. The characteristic histological picture associated with the response is a vasculitis.

Since our understanding of the role of precipitins in the pathogenesis of allergic alveolitis has changed with the recognition that precipitins can be detected against potential disease-inducing antigens in a significant percentage of exposed but asymptomatic subjects, attempts to relate extrinsic allergic alveolitis to the type III response have been questioned.[4] In particular, the usual histological finding of

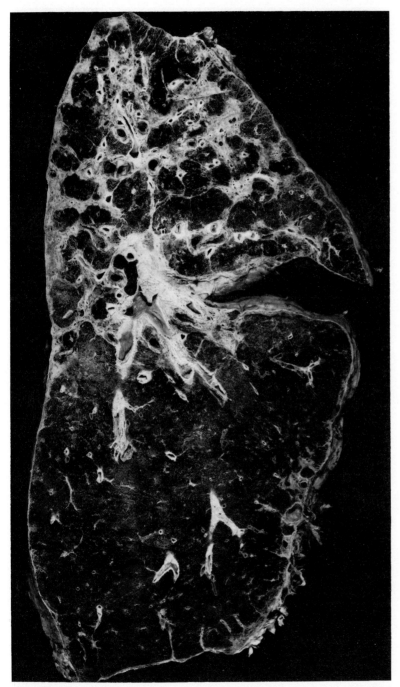

Figure 20–10. Barium sulfate impregnation specimen of left lung of patient who died in the chronic stage of farmer's lung, illustrating the more extensive involvement of the upper lobe with areas of focal fibrosis and interlacing communications. (From Seal, R.M.E., Hapke, E.J., Thomas, G.O., et al., The pathology of the acute and chronic stages of farmer's lung. Thorax, 23, 469, 1968.)

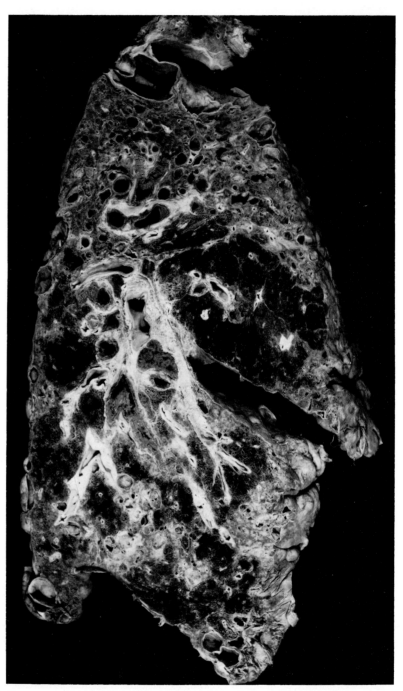

Figure 20–11. Barium sulfate impregnation specimen of left lung of patient who died of chronic farmer's lung, showing generalized disease, accentuation in the upper lobe and extensive honeycomb change. (From Seal, R.M.E., Hapke, E.J., Thomas, G.O., et al., The pathology of the acute and chronic stages of farmer's lung. Thorax, 23, 469, 1968.)

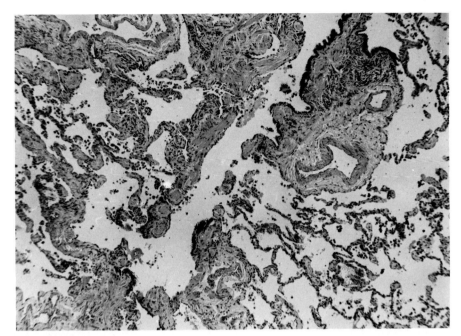

Figure 20–12. Low-power photomicrograph of biopsy from a patient with chronic farmer's lung, showing fibrosis maximal around the respiratory bronchiole but occurring also in peripheral alveolar walls.

loosely formed granulomata in allergic alveolitis is more in keeping with the type IV hypersensitivity response described by Coombs et al.[35] Similarly, when the condition has been reproduced in animal models using appropriate specific antigens, a granulomatous histological response results.[37] Although the delayed onset of symptoms fits a type III response, complement is not consumed,[38] and vasculitis rarely is found.[26] The cellular response is usually an interstitial infiltrate of lymphocytes, plasma cells, and histiocytes, although recent BAL studies have revealed that polymorphonuclear leukocytes are also present in the acute stage.[34] Thus, although there are some features of a type III response in the early acute phase, in the subacute and chronic stages, most features suggest a type IV hypersensitivity response.

Recently, the use of BAL in human subjects has provided information which has advanced our understanding of the pathogenesis of the condition. Whereas BAL findings in normal subjects reveal the majority of cells recovered to be macrophages,[39] studies in asymptomatic subjects exposed to the offending antigen reveal increased numbers of lymphocytes.[40] While activated T lymphocytes are usually absent, increased levels of albumin, fibronectin, and angiotensin-converting enzyme can be detected.[41] These studies indicate that, even in exposed healthy subjects, a subclinical alveolitis may develop.

When subjects in the acute stage of the condition undergo BAL, increased numbers of neutrophils, eosinophils, and mast cells are detected. Complement-derived chemotactic factors are also apparently present.[34] Other studies have shown increased levels of hyaluronic acid and procollagen 3N terminal peptide in the lavaged fluid.[42] Since hyaluronic acid has the ability to trap water, it may contribute to pulmonary function impairment by inducing interstitial edema.

In the earliest stages of the acute phase of the condition, although immune complex formation and complement activation may play a role, the presence of activated T lymphocytes indicates a localized immune process, i.e., a lymphocytic alveolitis with its intensity modulated by the extent of the exposure.[43] Prolonged follow-up studies have revealed increases in both suppressor T lymphocytes and

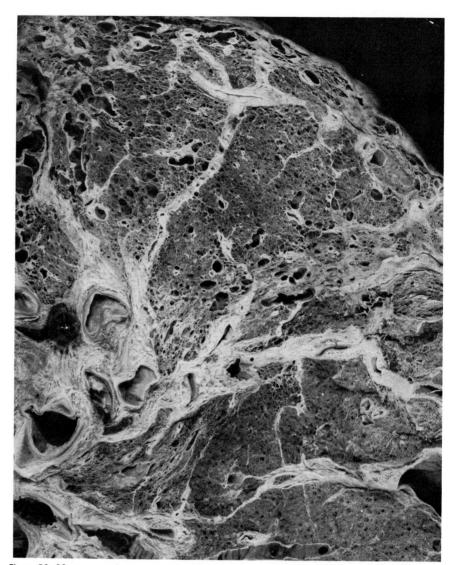

Figure 20–13. Barium sulfate–impregnated lung slice from farmer followed from his second acute attack of farmer's lung 18 years previously. He had minimal radiographic changes but a severely obstructed pattern of lung function and died in respiratory failure. The appearances illustrate fine interstitial fibrosis and dilated air spaces that many might interpret as emphysema. (Courtesy of Dr. R.M.E. Seal.)

natural killer cells.[44] After cessation of exposure to the agent, the helper T-cell population recovers.[40]

To understand the significance of the findings from BAL, it is necessary to appreciate the complex interaction between helper/inducer and suppressor/cytologic lymphocytes and lung macrophages.[39] At present, it is believed that alveolar macrophages originate from circulating monocytes under the influence of vitamin D metabolites and differentiate in the interstitial spaces, later to appear within the alveoli. When activated, macrophages release mediators (cytokines) that affect the function of other cells. These include chemotactic factors, such as leukotriene B_4, fibronectin, and fibroblastic growth which affect fibroblast replication. Interleukin-1 (IL-1) is also liberated and attracts lymphocytes into the area. The macrophage also serves in the role of antigen presenter, since it can display a processed antigen on its surface for attachment to a T-lymphocyte antigen receptor. On activation of the receptor, a variety of mediators (monokines) are released such as migration inhibition factor (MIF), which act on macrophages to hold them on station. In addition, activated lymphocytes can release their own mediators (lymphokines) that affect other lymphocytes. Of particular importance is interleukin-2 (IL-2), which stimulates T cells to replicate and increase in number by enlarging a clone of cells. Natural killer lymphocytes can also be activated, and B lymphocytes can be stimulated to secrete immunoglobulins.

With an understanding of cellular interaction, the results of BAL studies in allergic alveolitis may be interpreted. In the earliest stage of the disease, the chemotactic cytokines released from activated macrophages may lead to an accumulation of inflammatory cells, including neutrophils, eosinophils, and mast cells. In the acute stage, the characteristic lymphocytic alveolitis may be explained by expansion of a clone of T cells along with activation of natural killer lymphocytes under the influence of the IL-2 released from activated helper T lymphocytes. The increase in immunoglobulins that is usually detected may result from stimulation of B lymphocytes. Later in the disease, another cytokine, fibroblastic growth factor, may contribute to the development of interstitial fibrosis.

Clearly, in spite of much research, the pathogenesis of allergic alveolitis is not yet completely understood.[45] It should be remembered that the clinical spectrum of the disease is wide, ranging from the acute, but rarely fatal, attack to the chronic fibrosing type. The histological appearances vary according to the stage of the disease. In clinical practice, atypical cases are seen. It seems likely that a number of different pathogenic mechanisms are at work, and it may be unwise to attempt at this stage to fit all clinical and experimental features into one hypothesis of pathogenesis.

Diagnosis

The diagnosis of allergic alveolitis often presents an interesting challenge to the physician. For example, although the typical acute case of farmer's lung poses no particular problems, many patients present with rather nonspecific symptoms and may easily be thought to have other diseases, such as bronchitis, asthma, idiopathic pulmonary fibrosis, sarcoidosis, drug-induced lung disease, or even a psychogenic illness. As suggested in Chapters 2 and 3, when lung disease is investigated it is useful to start from the premise that the cause comes from the external environment. Beginning with that suspicion, the route to confirmation of the diagnosis of allergic alveolitis is described next.

History

A careful note should be made of the patient's occupation and of any organic or chemical aerosols to which the individual may have been exposed. In acute attacks, a history of what the patient was doing some hours prior to falling ill is essential. The relationship of symptoms to periods at work and while the patient is on vacation is less clear in allergic alveolitis than in occupational asthma and, in subacute and chronic cases, may be frankly misleading. In addition, the patient's recreational pursuits should be investigated, and contact or exposure to birds, damp molds, or air conditioners in the home or place of work should be noted. In puzzling cases, a visit to the patient's home or workplace may be necessary. Any drugs the patient may be taking should be recorded, since drug-induced lung disease is often an important differential diagnosis. Other occupational lung diseases which may cause diagnostic difficulties are silo filler's disease, which may mimic farmer's lung; Legionnaires' disease, which may also be spread by aerosol in the workplace; and occupational asthma of the chronic type. Physical examination and further investigation will usually allow these to be differentiated.

Examination

The only sign on examination of most patients is the presence of bilateral, gravity-dependent, repetitive mid- and end-inspiratory crackles, although tachypnea may be present in acute and subacute forms. The absence of other abnormalities, such as finger clubbing or signs of left ventricular disease, should raise the suspicion of an extrinsic alveolitis, whether caused by an inhaled or ingested antigen. The signs seldom distinguish allergic alveolitis from atypical pneumonia or toxic pneumonitis.

Radiographic Findings

The chest radiograph shows nonspecific features but, combined with clinical examination and other tests, may be of considerable help. For example, an apparently normal radiograph in someone with basal crackles and a low diffusing capacity is more likely to be a sign of allergic alveolitis than anything else. A change in the radiograph after a challenge test is strong evidence of the condition, although challenge testing should be used cautiously, since severe reactions may occur.

Immunological Findings

The most useful diagnostic test is that which detects precipitating antibodies to the suspected antigen in the patient's serum. As noted previously, this may be misleading; precipitins are absent in some patients with the disease and present in some exposed but well individuals. Nevertheless, when present in someone with appropriate clinical findings, this is usually the only test necessary. A simple test by Ouchterlony gel diffusion is sufficient in many cases, but a more sensitive radioimmunoassay based on a modification of the radioallergosorbent test (RAST) is available for quantitation of the antibody. Some authorities find this more valuable as a diagnostic test.[46] It is certainly advisable to use such a test if the simple one shows no precipitin lines in the serum of a patient with a clinical picture consistent with allergic alveolitis.

The demonstration of precipitins to a particular antigen depends on the appropriate selection of relevant antigens. More sophisticated testing using enzyme-linked immunosorbent assays for the detection of antibodies may result in better characterization of the immune response in both serum and BAL fluid.[47]

In some subjects, it will be necessary to make extracts of suspected antigens collected from home or work to carry out testing for an antibody. The same extracts, in suitable concentration, can be used for intradermal skin testing to look for an Arthus reaction (an indurated tender swelling at 4 hours which lasts about 24 hours) and for pulmonary challenge.

Lung Function Testing

In the typical acute case, lung function testing usually confirms the expected reduction in lung volumes, diffusing capacity, and arterial oxygen tension. In obscure cases, its main value lies in demonstrating that restrictive and diffusion abnormalities are present. Although this is of no help *per se* in the differential diagnosis, it is useful in conjunction with other findings, such as basal crackles or dubious radiographic changes, in making a decision on whether further investigation is necessary. Lung function testing, however, has its greatest value in monitoring the progress of the disease and its response to treatment.

Challenge Testing

A challenge test is necessary only when the diagnosis of allergic alveolitis remains in doubt and the clinical and immunological findings are equivocal. Thus, it has proved useful in the investigation of previously undescribed causes of the disease and in confirming the diagnosis in patients with suggestive clinical findings without serum precipitins.

The simplest such test is to expose the patient to the suspected harmful environment for a limited period and observe changes in temperature, white blood cell count, lung volumes, and diffusing capacity. The period of observation may vary from a few minutes to a work shift and should be determined by the patient's history. Alternatively, the patient may be asked to bring the suspected agent to the laboratory so exposure can occur. A third and widely used method for investigating soluble organic antigens is to make an extract of the suspected antigen and to expose the patient to a nebulized extract. Again, the strength of the solution and length of exposure must be estimated from the patient's history. Generally, a relatively light exposure should be used initially with a gradual increase in concentration if no reaction occurs. The characteristic response includes fever; dyspnea; basal crackles; a rise in the exercise minute ventilation and neutrophil count; and a fall in lymphocytes, vital capacity, and the diffusing capacity.

Hendrick et al. investigated these responses to challenge.[48] They found a specificity of 95% and sensitivity of 45% to 85%, for a combination of six responses, namely, an increase of 15% or more in exercise ventilation and a rise in temperature by more than 37.2°C, of neutrophils by 2500/mm³ or more, and of exercise respiratory rate by 25% or more with a fall in lymphocytes of 500/mm³ or more and vital capacity by 15% or more. These authors also pointed out that changes in lung volumes, diffusing capacity, the presence of crackles, and radiographic changes are not sufficiently sensitive to be useful, although it would seem likely that such changes, when provoked, are highly specific. It is probably better, when possible, to carry out challenge tests with a dose that produces minor and less distressing symptoms to avoid a more severe attack that could lead to permanent sequelae.

It needs to be emphasized that a challenge test may provoke a dual obstructive and alveolar response,[49] and the obstructive response may have immediate and delayed components (Fig. 20–14).[50] Such a mixed immunological response necessitates watchfulness to avoid serious alveolar damage.

Lung Biopsy

Lung biopsy is neither necessary nor justifiable in most cases of allergic alveolitis. However, the disease may occasionally be suspected but no allergen identified. In such cases, a biopsy may be necessary to prove the diagnosis or to exclude other possible diseases. Open biopsy produces the best specimens from the pathologist's point of view but is a major procedure for the patient. Transbronchial biopsies often provide pieces too small for a confident diagnosis to be made. Percutaneous drill biopsy may be the best compromise, although the relatively nontraumatic transbronchial procedure is now often tried first. It has the additional marginal advantage that it can be preceded by BAL, a procedure that holds some hope as a means of monitoring the course of the disease. In the authors' view, however, it is really valuable only as a means of understanding the immune and other processes involved and is more a research than a clinical tool.[51] Studies of animal models of allergic alveolitis using BAL have shown increased proportions of T lymphocytes in the fluid.[52, 53]

Treatment

Although death during an acute attack of allergic alveolitis is uncommon, it is by no means unknown.[25] As corticosteroids are known to reverse the effect of the inhaled antigen, their use in all but the mildest attack is justified. During the acute attack, arterial oxygen desaturation should be relieved by the use of oxygen, which may be given by any convenient means sufficient to raise the arterial oxygen

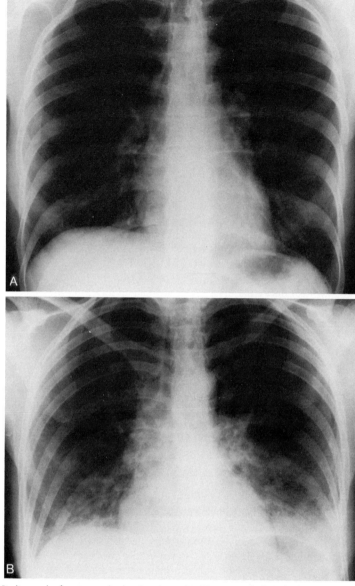

Figure 20-14. *A,* Radiograph of patient with alveolitis due to Pauli's reagent before challenge. *B,* Same patient after challenge test mixing reagents in laboratory.

tension to between 60 and 100 mm Hg. There is no risk of provoking carbon dioxide retention in the acute attack since alveolar hypoventilation is not a feature unless the patient already has chronic airways obstruction. In exceptional cases, if the lungs are very stiff and the patient cannot achieve a sufficient oxygen saturation without excessive respiratory effort, mechanical ventilation may be required. Should this become necessary, nasal endotracheal intubation is preferable to tracheostomy since the disease almost always responds rapidly to treatment with corticosteroids.

In a proportion of acute attacks, the response is delayed even when adequate doses of prednisone (40 mg daily) are given. Occasionally, it may be several weeks before recovery is complete. In such cases, the slow response may cause diagnostic

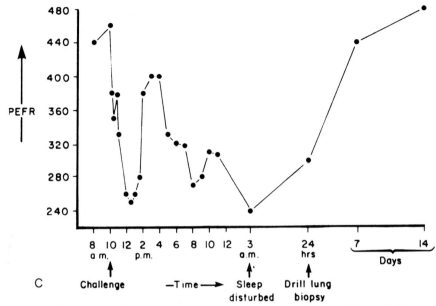

Figure 20–14 *Continued C,* Recording of peak flow rate during challenge test, showing both immediate and delayed obstructive patterns in addition to interstitial disease apparent on radiograph and also seen on biopsy. (From Evans, W.V., and Seaton, A., Hypersensitivity pneumonitis in a technician using Pauli's reagent. Thorax, 34, 767, 1979.)

uncertainty, and this constitutes a situation in which lung biopsy should be considered.

Recent clinical studies both on farmer's lung[54] and avian hypersensitivity pneumonitis[55] have shown that continued exposure to the relevant antigen does not always lead to progression of the disease. This finding confirms the observation that animals that have been sensitized to repeated antigen challenge and have a chronic granulomatous inflammatory response can later become desensitized, with resolution rather than progression of the mononuclear cell infiltrate.[56] Usually, removal from exposure results in improvement of the condition with the disappearance of the acute recurrent symptoms.[9]

The effect of corticosteroids on the progression of allergic alveolitis recently has been shown to be effective only in the early stages of the condition. Follow-up after 5 years showed no statistically significant difference between treated and untreated groups.[57] In practice, a tendency for recurrence was observed in the group treated with corticosteroids. This may be a consequence of the tendency for workers who feel better to return to work, thereby undergoing re-exposure to the offending antigen. Corticosteroids may have some value in preventing fibrosis in one subset of patients who have serum markers that presage progression to irreversible impairment.[58]

The chronic form of the disease responds less well to treatment, especially if the obstructive element predominates. It is essential that the patient be removed from contact with the offending antigen, and it should always be assumed that at least a part of the disease is potentially reversible. If the patient is unable to be removed from possible exposure, respirators are available that will reduce the exposure to a level that is relatively safe.[59, 60] Steroids should be given, and their efficacy should be monitored by serial measurements of vital capacity and diffusing capacity. The collagenous component of chronic allergic alveolitis will not respond to therapy, and once this has become the predominant feature of the disease, only symptomatic therapy is useful. This includes oxygen when necessary, antibiotics for acute infections, and a regimen for cor pulmonale.

Specific Types of Allergic Alveolitis

Any account of the causes of allergic alveolitis must be incomplete, since new ones are constantly being described and no doubt many remain to be discovered. However, the causes may be grouped under general headings on the assumption that other potential antigens in these categories, in due course, will be shown to cause disease. Thus, it is convenient to consider the causes of allergic alveolitis as follows: fungi, animal materials, low molecular weight chemicals, and bacteria. In addition, a number of outbreaks have occurred in which the cause has not been clearly identified (see Table 20–1).

DISEASES OF FUNGAL ORIGIN

Farmer's Lung

The first detailed description of farmer's lung was published in 1932, and the relationship of the condition to the inhalation of hay dust was recognized.[61] The disease was initially thought to be due to fungal infection of the lung. Further and more complete descriptions were given by Fawcett in 1936[62] and Fuller in 1953.[63] A similar condition occurs in cattle and is known as fog fever.

In the early case reports, it was apparent that farmer's lung occurred mostly in wet summers, and in many instances, there was an obvious relationship between exposure to moldy hay and the onset of symptoms. In some outbreaks, barley or oats that had stood in wet weather and been threshed before they were completely dry were implicated. It is now appreciated that if hay is stored in a damp state, i.e., with a moisture content greater than 30%, heat is generated. This encourages the growth of thermophilic microorganisms. Of these, the most important from the point of view of farmer's lung are *Micropolyspora faeni* and *Thermoactinomyces vulgaris*. These organisms produce vast numbers of spores that are liberated into the air when the hay is raked or turned over (Fig. 20–15). The farm worker inhales these spores, and an attack usually develops a few hours later. Attacks are now seen most commonly in winter because baled hay is often stored in barns for winter fodder. During the winter, the bales are broken, and the hay is forked into appropriate portions for the cattle. This is usually done inside the barn, and mild attacks may occur every time the worker handles the hay.

Outbreaks of a disease similar to farmer's lung have also been described in association with exposure to air conditioners, humidifiers, and heating systems contaminated by thermophilic *Actinomyces*.[64–66] This emphasizes the fact that these organisms are widely distributed and may grow and sporulate whenever the temperature and humidity are appropriate. The relationship of this condition to humidifier fever is discussed later in this chapter.

The clinical features of farmer's lung may range from the most acute attack to a slowly progressive pulmonary fibrosis, probably depending on the individual's pattern of exposure and natural susceptibility. Although acute attacks have been recognized most frequently, it is likely that more insidious disease, without all the classical symptoms, develops in a high proportion of exposed subjects.

The immunology of the disease has been studied in great detail. Originally, Williams showed that aerosols of aqueous extracts of moldy hay would produce the clinical picture of farmer's lung.[67] Subsequently, Pepys and Jenkins showed that extracts of *M. faeni* had a similar effect.[68] No such reactions were produced by extracts prepared from *Aspergillus* or *Pencillium* species, nor by *Mucor* or other fungi found in hay and grass dust. Dry hay was likewise inert. The reactions developed several hours after the challenge and were associated with a fall in vital capacity and diffusing capacity and a rise in temperature. Hyperventilation also occurs but in the absence of airways obstruction.

The antigens were extracted in a variety of ways from moldy hay or grain.[69, 70] Barbee et al. showed that they were soluble in trichloroacetic acid.[71] Scratch tests

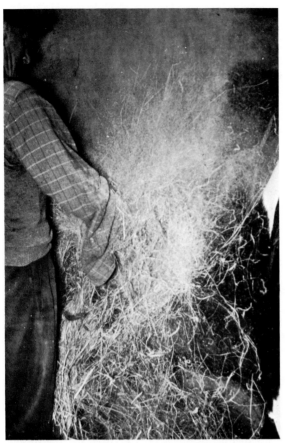

Figure 20-15. Farmer shaking bale of moldy hay. The haze in the upper part of the picture is a cloud of dust containing respirable spores of thermophilic actinomycetes.

with the antigen rarely produced a reaction, but intradermal injections of extracts may produce a typical late type III response.

The first demonstration of precipitating antibodies in the sera of subjects with farmer's lung was made by Pepys and his colleagues in the early 1960s.[70, 72, 73] Simple carbol-saline extracts were prepared and tested against the sera of farmers with and without the clinical condition. These workers employed a double-diffusion technique. They showed first that the titer of antibodies in different sera varied and, second, that not all hay extracts were equally antigenic. A number of other fungal extracts were also shown to produce precipitin lines. Challenge of the subject with these extracts did not produce a clinical response, with the exception of that prepared from *T. vulgaris,* which occasionally produced a reaction similar to that of *M. faeni.*[73]

Studies of the prevalence of farmer's lung are confounded by the difficulty of deciding on diagnostic criteria. The presence of precipitins in the sera of farm workers, a test that does not correlate very well with clinical disease but is at least an indication of exposure, varies greatly. In the United States, the prevalence is highest in Wisconsin and Pennsylvania; in Canada, in Manitoba;[74] and in Great Britain, in Scotland[6] and the southeast. Studies of the prevalence of clinical disease have indicated figures of about 3% to 5% in both the United States and Great Britain.[8] These represent between one half and one sixth of those subjects with positive precipitin tests. There is no evidence that patients are genetically predisposed to the disease,[75] although cigarette smoking clearly may have a protective effect.[19]

The management of farmer's lung often requires the use of steroids for an acute attack. The disease may largely be prevented by care in the making and use of hay, especially in reducing its water content and allowing free ventilation. Subjects who have had an attack should attempt to avoid exposure completely, if necessary by changing jobs, since the risk of further attacks and the production of chronic disease is high.[76] The number of spores inhaled may be reduced by wearing an appropriate respirator.[59] This, together with expert advice on proper hay making (which can be provided by agricultural scientists in many farming communities), is the best and most helpful approach because farmers are rarely in a position to change jobs.

In Great Britain, farmer's lung has been compensatable as an industrial disease since 1964. In many Western countries and in most states in the United States, patients affected by the disease are still not covered by workers' compensation acts, a situation that is very far from satisfactory.

Bagassosis

This condition bears many resemblances to farmer's lung. Bagasse is a fiber, derived from dried sugar cane, that is used in the manufacture of paper, cardboard, and building materials. The disease is a result of exposure to moldy, stored bagasse and is seen in the southern United States, the West Indies, India, Italy, Peru, and even Great Britain.[77] The outbreak that occurred in Great Britain was related to exposure to bales of bagasse that had been imported from Louisiana.[78]

This disease develops in approximately 50% of subjects exposed to moldy bagasse. The available evidence suggests that thermophilic actinomycetes are responsible, and precipitins are frequently present in the subject's serum in the acute stages of the disease. Systemic and pulmonary reactions have been produced by inhalation challenges of moldy bagasse.[79] The response usually appears 3 to 6 hours after the challenge. The same subjects, when challenged with extracts of *M. faeni,* did not respond, and it seems likely that the main antigens are from *T. vulgaris* and *Thermoactinomyces sacchari.*

The clinical, radiologic, and pathological features of bagassosis are essentially the same as those of farmer's lung. Thus, the presenting symptoms are shortness of breath, fever, chest discomfort, anorexia, and sweating. Although complete recovery is the rule, repeated lesser exposures can lead to a chronic form of the disease. The acute stage is characterized by pulmonary function evidence of interstitial lung involvement, while in the chronic form of the disease airways obstruction is also seen.[80] Although cessation of exposure to bagasse results in a remission of symptoms, restrictive lung function lasting up to 10 years after the acute attack has been described.[81]

Mushroom Worker's Lung

This condition, like bagassosis, is a variant of farmer's lung. It was first described by Bringhurst and colleagues.[82]

The common mushroom, *Agaricus hortensis,* is grown on compost whose main constituents are usually straw and horse droppings. The compost is usually allowed to "ferment" in the open for 2 to 3 weeks. It is then exposed to a moist heat of no more than 60°C for several days in special chambers. This process eliminates many of the organisms that interfere with the growth of the mushrooms and also provides an ideal medium for the growth of *M. faeni* and thermophilic actinomycetes. The compost is later dried and seeded with mushroom mycelia. The latter process involves mechanical mixing of the mushroom spawn with the compost. The compost is then spread on trays, which are placed in mushroom houses where the temperature is kept at 15°C and the humidity at 90%. The first crop of mushrooms usually appears in 3 to 4 weeks.

Subjects in whom mushroom worker's lung develops have usually worked in the sheds in which spawning is effected and where the compost and spawn are mechanically mixed. Occasionally, the condition occurs after emptying and cleaning of the mushroom sheds. Precipitins against *M. faeni* and *T. vulgaris* have been reported in the serum of the subjects with this condition.[83]

Malt Worker's Lung

A further cause of allergic alveolitis was described in 1968 by Riddle et al.[84] The subject was a malt worker who had developed a farmer's lung–like respiratory illness. The illness was associated with low-grade fever, dyspnea, and cough. All the symptoms cleared while he was away from work, only to recur when he returned. When seen after the recurrence of symptoms, he was found to have basal crackles and impairment of his diffusing capacity along with a restrictive ventilatory defect. He was treated with steroids, with a good response.

In the malting process, fresh farm barley is first dried in kilns and then stored for 2 months in a silo. It is next rehydrated over 36 hours and is then treated with hypochlorite to rid the barley of fungi. It is then allowed to germinate in a hot and humid atmosphere, where both the heat and humidity are controlled. The malt is turned regularly to release carbon dioxide. It is then dried once again in kilns, and afterward, the rootlets are removed. Lastly, the malt is taken to the distillery.

As his main job, the subject in whom allergic alveolitis developed turned the malt on open floors, thereby producing a spore-laden dusty atmosphere. The patient's sputum grew a mix fungal flora, as did samples of the maltings. However, *Aspergillus clavatus* was grown both from the patient's sputum and from nearly every sample of the maltings. Moreover, this was the only fungus that could be repeatedly isolated from both his sputum and the maltings.

Precipitating and complement-fixing antibodies against *A. clavatus* were demonstrated in the subject's serum. An intradermal injection of an extract of the antigen produced an Arthus-type skin reaction, and an inhalational challenge duplicated the respiratory symptoms of the naturally occurring disease. Subsequent studies showed that approximately 5% of workers in the malting industry had symptoms of the disease, although in most cases it was relatively mild.[85] Modern methods of malting, especially in which a closed drum rather than an open floor process is used, are associated with a much lower incidence of disease.

Cheese Washer's Disease

This condition was described in Switzerland in 1969.[86] In the process of making some cheeses, aging is carried out in damp cellars. A mold forms on the surface of the cheese, and cheese workers are required to wash this off periodically. Some of these subjects developed a disease similar to farmer's lung and were found to have serum precipitins against *Penicillium casei*. Subsequent investigation of the epidemiology of the disease revealed precipitins in 21% of exposed workers and in 55% of those with a history of symptoms. Lung function study results, not usually performed in acute attacks, were mostly normal in this study, suggesting that the disease is usually mild and reversible. It is thought that most cheese producers in the United States avoid the risk of causing this disease by wrapping the cheese in foil during aging.[87]

Maple Bark Stripper's Disease

Maple bark disease was first described by Tower et al. in 1932.[88] The condition affected lumber workers whose job it was to strip the bark from maple logs. Further outbreaks of maple bark stripper's disease have been reported by Emanuel et al.[89, 90] The fungus that is responsible is known as *Cryptostroma corticale* and grows beneath the bark of the tree; it affects both the hard maple and the sycamore.

The processes and operations that are involved in the lumber mill have been thoroughly described by Wenzel and Emanuel.[91] The maple logs are brought into the wood room on a continuous chain and are first cut in half. The logs then are debarked on a series of drums. The drums have a tumbling action and are sprayed with water. After the bark has been removed, the log is carried to a chipper, which cuts it into small chips. The latter are shaken on a screen, and the remnants of the bark are removed. The chips are then taken on a conveyer belt to a silo in which they are stored.

C. corticale produces ovoid spores of 4 to 5 μm in length. They are brownish red in color but, when present in large numbers, appear black. Maple logs that are affected by the fungus show large blackened areas underneath the bark. Removal of the bark during the stripping process liberates the spores into the air, and high spore counts were observed in the wood room, especially in winter, when the doors of the room were kept closed because of the cold.

The clinical features of this condition are very similar to those of farmer's lung. Cough, fever, and shortness of breath are common. Rigors and marked cyanosis with severe arterial oxygen desaturation occur. Subacute forms of the disease are also seen in which the fever is low grade and symptoms of chronic shortness of breath and loss of weight predominate. Eosinophilia is unusual. The radiographic findings vary according to the stage of the disease. The subject with acute disease usually shows an extensive confluent acinus filling process; however, reticulonodulation and stringy infiltrates are seen in the more chronic forms of the disease and during the convalescent stage.

Emanuel et al. carried out lung biopsies in some of their subjects.[90] The appearances resembled those of farmer's lung in that an extensive granulomatous pneumonitis was present with frequent foreign body giant cells. With silver methenamine fungal stains, in a few instances, the spores could be recognized in the lung parenchyma and, indeed, were initially mistaken for *Histoplasma capsulatum*. Cultures of resected lung tissue are often successful, and the organism appears as a white mycelial growth. Despite the presence of the spores in the lung, there is no real evidence that the disease is infectious in origin. Precipitins against extracts of the spores can be demonstrated not only in affected subjects but also in some exposed workers who have no overt disease. Intracutaneous tests with an extract of the antigen cause an immediate wheal that persists for up to 8 hours.

Most subjects with the condition improve rapidly when exposure to the spores ceases. As they become convalescent, their antibody titers decline. Since the complete description of the disease by Emanuel et al.,[90] the lumber mill in which the subjects worked has introduced preventive measures to lessen the spore counts in the sawing area and wood room by continuous spraying of the logs as they are debarked, by isolation of the chipper, and by improved ventilation. Immediately after these measures were introduced, there was a decline in the incidence of this condition.

Sequoiosis

A subject with granulomatous pneumonitis associated with redwood dust inhalation has been described by Cohen et al.[92] The man had worked for 17 years as a sawyer in a redwood lumber mill. The patient was first seen with dyspnea and a chest radiograph showing a ''ground-glass'' pattern. The symptoms and radiographic findings disappeared spontaneously when he was in the hospital. With further exposures to redwood dust, the symptoms returned, dyspnea developed, and crackles were found in his chest. Pulmonary function testing revealed evidence of interstitial disease. Biopsy of the lung showed septal thickening, lymphocytic and plasma cell infiltration, and a granulomatous pneumonitis. He was given steroids, which produced marked improvement.

Skin tests with redwood extracts produced no immediate reaction, although precipitins against redwood sawdust extract were present in the patient's serum. Precipitins were present only rarely in other workers exposed to the redwood dust and not at all in controls. Culture of the sawdust grew several species of fungi, but only *Graphium* and *Aureobasidium pullulans* showed antigens with immunological identity to the redwood antigen. It was therefore concluded that the latter were probably responsible for the condition.

Woodworker's Disease

Hypersensitivity to wood dust has been described on several occasions.[93, 94] A respiratory illness resembling hypersensitivity pneumonitis has been described in two subjects who worked at a paper mill.[95] Although the clinical and occupational history suggested maple bark disease, inhalation challenge tests with extracts of *C. corticale* did not confirm the diagnosis. The first subject presented with recurrent episodes of dyspnea, chills, and fever. Persistent radiographic abnormalities developed, and a lung biopsy was interpreted as showing chronic interstitial pneumonitis and fibrosis. He was subsequently challenged with an extract of *Alternaria,* with the development of all the acute symptoms and signs of extrinsic alveolitis. Steroids had to be given because of the severity of the reaction, but within 24 hours, the patient's signs and symptoms had resolved. The other patient had a similar but shorter history, and he likewise had a positive inhalation test result when challenged with an extract of *Alternaria.* In both of these subjects, a type I reaction with an immediate reduction in ventilatory capacity occurred after the challenge in addition to the type III response. Moreover, the serum of one of the subjects contained rheumatoid factor. Precipitins which reacted against an extract of *Alternaria* were present in the sera of both subjects.

A similar illness, called suberosis, has been described in workers who produce bottle stoppers and disks from cork.[96] Although initially it was thought that this condition, which may have asthmatic features or may be typical of allergic alveolitis, was due to hypersensitivity to cork itself, the evidence now suggests that it results from exposure to moldy cork bark. The mold that is probably responsible is *Penicillium frequentans.*[97] Finally, allergic alveolitis has been described in a woodworker exposed to ramin (*Gonystylus bancanus*) dust. In this case, the wood itself rather than fungi appeared to be responsible for the disease.[98]

Paprika Splitter's Lung

Capsicum annuum longum, red pepper or paprika, has long been cultivated for medical purposes. It is grown mainly in Hungary and Yugoslavia. The fruit of the plant is about 4 to 5 inches long and was usually split open by women workers to remove the "ribs" of the plant. The latter were then thrown away since they contain an excess of capsaicin. Late in the year, paprika fruits are often parasitized by *Mucor* species, and the air of the workroom in which the women worked used to be grossly contaminated with spores. Respiratory complaints were common in the paprika splitters but not in the workers who handled the finished product.[99]

The clinical features of the disease are cough and loss of weight. Fever and "bronchiectasis" may develop. The development of bronchiectasis must be doubted and is probably explained by the fact that bronchography, when performed in subjects with established interstitial fibrosis, often shows shortening and a tuberous appearance in the segmental bronchi.[100] The chest film shows consolidation and stringy infiltrates. Death may occur from right heart failure. It is probable that this disease is an allergic alveolitis, but it is now seldom, if ever, seen. Selective breeding has evolved a plant in which the ribs contain little capsaicin; hence, workers are no longer employed to split the paprika fruit.

Dry Rot Lung

A typical case of allergic alveolitis has been described in a patient exposed to the dry rot fungus *Merulius lacrymans* in a house.[101]

Dog House Disease

The development of acute, very severe interstitial lung disease in a woman who was exposed to moldy straw has been described by Rhudy et al.[102] She was admitted to a hospital *in extremis* with a history of having been well until a few hours before admission. At the time of her admission, she was cyanotic, with gross hypoxia, and was semicomatose. Despite oxygen supplements, she required mechanical ventilation. Her chest radiograph showed a diffuse acinus filling process throughout both lungs. She was treated with oxygen, assisted ventilation, and steroids and, in spite of the development of other complications, made a recovery.

She kept two dogs which slept on straw in her basement. The bale of straw that she had been using for their bedding in the week prior to admission had been damp and moldy. It was her custom to spread fresh straw out every day. Culture of the moldy straw grew a mixed fungal flora, but *M. faeni* and *T. vulgaris* could not be isolated, despite several attempts to do so. Among the several fungi present was *Aspergillus versicolor.* It was later shown that the patient's serum contained precipitins against an extract prepared from this fungus. As the patient improved and became convalescent, her antibody titer fell. Three months after the illness, precipitins were no longer demonstrable. An inhalation challenge was thought inadvisable because of the severity of the patient's illness and because of the difficulty in titrating the dose.

Lycoperdonosis

A respiratory disease caused by the inhalation of large numbers of puffball spores was described by Strand et al. in 1967.[103] *Lycoperdon* is the genus of fungi to which most puffballs belong. They grow in woods and forests on decaying logs and stumps and sometimes in fields. Within the puffball wall, vast numbers of clavate spores are contained. Because of their styptic action, these have been used to stop nosebleeds. With the inhalation of large numbers of spores, nausea, fever, dyspnea, and lung crackles appear, and the chest film shows miliary mottling. No attempt has been made to see whether the serum of such patients contains precipitins.

DISEASES OF ANIMAL ORIGIN

Allergic Alveolitis Caused by Birds

The first reports of allergic alveolitis caused by birds were published in 1960 and recorded the disease in duck pluckers and people exposed to parakeets.[104, 105] Soon afterward, the disease was reported in pigeon breeders[106–109] and, more recently, in people farming chickens[110] and turkeys.[111] Cockateels and other birds may also be responsible. The spectrum of symptoms and signs in these patients is the same as is other types of allergic alveolitis, although with a tendency for fewer of the acute cases to occur. Most cases fall into the category of recurrent, nonacute disease. This is especially true of those who keep parakeets in their home. Children with the disease may present with nonspecific symptoms and failure to thrive. The lung function findings are of a restrictive type with low diffusing capacity,[112, 113] although raised residual volume and obstructive findings may predominate.[49] In acute recurrent cases, lung function may be normal between attacks. Studies of the prevalence of the condition are again confused by the difficulty of defining a case and by unsatisfactory population sampling. However, studies among pigeon fanciers suggest that the prevalence of clinical disease may be between 10% and 20% of those regularly exposed in the lofts.[114]

Affected individuals often have serum precipitins to bird serum, feathers, egg white, and droppings.[115] It is likely that sensitization has occurred to the birds' serum globulin. In pigeons at least, IgA seems to be the predominant antigen, although patients probably become sensitized to one or more of a range of antigens.[116]

The route of sensitization is presumably inhalational, and challenge testing uses bird serum administered by this route. Bird droppings, which contain protein, have been considered a likely source of the aerosol, but they tend to be hygroscopic and do not dry out easily. Exposure to feathers may be a more important source of antigen, and recent work has confirmed that bloom, a waxy material composed of fine 1-μm particles of keratin coated with IgA, is a potential source of antigen.[117] Bloom is produced in large amounts by flying birds, especially pigeons in peak condition, and this may explain why such birds as pigeons and parakeets seem to be more potent sensitizers than chickens and turkeys. Although bird fancier's disease is most commonly seen in those exposed to the droppings of pigeons, parakeets, and parrots, it must be remembered that the disease may result from exposure to more exotic birds. We recently saw a subject who had four to five attacks of the sudden onset of fever, breathlessness, and restrictive impairment accompanied by an acinus filling process in the chest radiograph. On each occasion, when he was admitted to the hospital, his symptoms and signs cleared up. Although an occupational history was taken at the peripheral hospital to which he was admitted, no enquiries were made about his avocation. It subsequently became apparent that he kept 250 Australian finches, which he bred and sold (Fig. 20–16).

The diagnosis of allergic alveolitis in people exposed to birds is made more difficult by the relatively high proportion of subjects who have no precipitins when tested by standard gel diffusion. However, the use of more sensitive tests increases the possibility of diagnosing some cases without the need for challenge testing.[116]

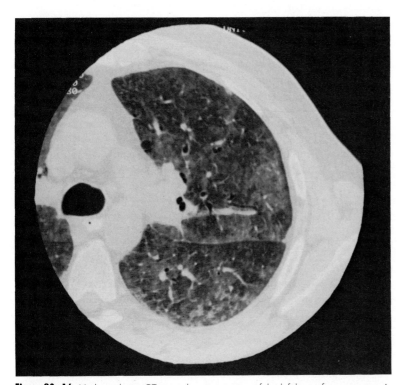

Figure 20–16. High-resolution CT scan showing section of the left lung of a carpenter. As an avocation, he kept and bred 250 Australian finches. He presented with recurrent bouts of fever, shortness of breath, and an acinus filling pattern on the chest radiograph. He was admitted to the hospital on four occasions and treated with antibiotics. On each occasion his symptoms and chest radiograph improved. The scan of the left lung shows a diffuse ground-glass or acinus filling pattern. Pleuroscopic biopsy of the lung showed slightly atypical features of extrinsic allergic alveolitis.

The disease should be managed by the prevention of exposure, generally by avoiding contact with birds. If this is not possible, an efficient respirator should be worn.[60] Cross reactivity between species occurs, and the authors have seen patients who, having got rid of their pigeons, became ill on exposure to friends' or relatives' parakeets. We have also seen a patient who had typical disease, proved by challenge test, simply from exposure to feathers in the cushions of her three-piece furniture suite!

A comment should be made on two possible diagnostic pitfalls with respect to bird breeder's lung. First, false-positive viral complement fixation tests may be found in pigeon fanciers with allergic alveolitis, caused either by a polyclonal stimulation of antibody formation[118] or by a reaction with antigens in the hen's egg on which the virus was grown.[119] Confusion with influenzal or other viral pneumonias may therefore become a real problem. Secondly, patients with celiac disease frequently have precipitins in their blood to avian antigens, probably derived from egg protein in their food.[120] Since celiac disease is occasionally accompanied by a diffuse pulmonary fibrosis unrelated to bird exposure,[121] diagnostic confusion may occur, especially when the patient keeps a parakeet.[122] Such problems may require a challenge test to resolve.[123]

Allergic Alveolitis Caused by Small Mammals

Laboratory rats are well described as a cause of occupational asthma and rhinitis, and there is strong evidence that protein excreted in their urine is an important antigen. One case of typical allergic alveolitis caused by exposure to rats has been described in a research assistant.[124] This patient had typical symptoms and signs, precipitating antibody, and responses to work and laboratory challenges. A similar case has been described following exposure to gerbils.[125]

Wheat Weevil Disease

Asthmatic reactions to the wheat weevil, *Sitophilus granarius,* were first described by Jiminez-Diaz et al. in 1947.[126] Subsequent studies showed that the wheat weevil produced asthma in subjects exposed to it in the laboratory and that the affected subjects had positive skin and inhalation tests. Control subjects did not react when similarly challenged.[127, 128]

In a few of the challenged workers, the immediate response was followed by a delayed reaction several hours later. Associated with the latter was a fall in the gas-diffusing capacity. Precipitins against an extract of the weevil were present in the subjects' sera.

Furrier's Lung

The antigenic properties of animal hairs were recognized in 1928 by Vallery-Radot and Giroud.[129] It has also been claimed that animal hairs can produce interstitial pulmonary disease.[130] Biopsy showed that the process was a granulomatous interstitial pneumonia, although the patient's serum was not examined for precipitating antibodies. This remains a very dubious entity.

Pituitary Snuff Taker's Lung

The development of pulmonary infiltrates as a result of the inhalation of bovine and porcine pituitary snuff was first reported in the British literature.[131] Since that time, there have been further reports from Europe[132] and the United States.[133] Pituitary snuff used to be used in the treatment of diabetes insipidus, and the method of administration avoids the need for repeated injections. The snuff is prepared from finely ground mixtures of dried bovine and porcine posterior pituitary; the particles usually are smaller than 50 μm, with some in the respirable range. Snuff prepared from the pituitary glands of animals has been superseded by synthetic vasopressin. While pituitary snuff taker's lung has not been described except in patients who used pituitary snuff, in theory at least, those who manufactured it were at risk.

In the subjects described by Mahon et al., a generalized reticulonodulation of the lungs developed.[131] Bronchospasm and eosinophilia may also occur. The symptoms, signs, and impairment are not so acute or so severe as those in farmer's lung and resemble bird fancier's lung more closely.

Immunological studies have demonstrated the presence of precipitins in the serum of affected subjects. The precipitins develop not only against porcine and bovine serum proteins but also against the pituitary antigens themselves. The offending antigen in the patient described by Harper et al. was identified as a hormone constituent of the pituitary rather than the specific antigens of the animals from which the snuff was prepared.[133] The serum of this patient also did not react with synthetic lysine 8-vasopressin, probably because the low molecular weight of this substance would make it a hapten and it would not be large enough to form a lattice with a homologous antibody.

DISEASE CAUSED BY LOW MOLECULAR WEIGHT CHEMICALS

Isocyanate Alveolitis

The uses of isocyanates are described in Chapter 17 because these chemicals are potent causes of occupational asthma. Several subjects, however, have been reported to have pulmonary shadowing and a restrictive type of lung function abnormality after exposure. The initial report described four toluene diisocyanate (TDI) workers with radiographic changes.[134] Three of these patients also had asthma. Subsequently, the cases of four patients with restrictive lung function— one of whom had signs of consolidation on chest radiography, biopsy changes of diffuse alveolitis, and an Arthus skin reaction to TDI—were described.[135]

Three of these subjects had been exposed to TDI and one to hexamethylene diisocyanate (HDI). The patients responded to treatment with corticosteroids. Challenge tests with TDI-albumin in sensitized rabbits produced changes of allergic alveolitis, whereas controls challenged with albumin showed no such changes.[135] Since then, there have been reports of three more subjects developing alveolitis after exposure to isocyanates.[136–138] Two were workers exposed to diphenylmethane diisocyanate (MDI) and one was a man exposed to TDI.

Disease Caused by Pauli's Reagent

Pauli's reagent, sodium diazobenzenesulfonate, is widely used in laboratories for identifying arylamines and phenols. A laboratory technician working in a medical school developed symptoms and signs of allergic alveolitis after her work in making and using this reagent in a defective fume cupboard. An occupational-type challenge produced immediate and delayed asthmatic reactions and also signs and biopsy evidence of allergic alveolitis. Skin tests showed evidence of atopy and also an immediate response to Pauli's reagent (see Fig. 20–14).[50]

Vineyard Sprayer's Lung

A granulomatous alveolitis has been described in workers spraying vines with Bordeaux mixture, a 1% to 2% solution of copper sulfate neutralized with lime.[139] The histological changes described seem typical of a hypersensitivity pneumonitis, with lymphocytes, plasma cells, and histiocytic granulomata that tend to fibrose. The lesions contain copper and tend to regress radiologically when exposure ceases. A somewhat atypical feature is the occasional development of massive fibrosis similar to that seen in silicosis. It has been suggested that these patients have an increased risk of lung cancer, although the evidence for this is flimsy because the patients were selected partly on the basis of having lung tumors.[140] The evidence for the existence of this condition is not entirely convincing.

Other Chemical Causes

Many drugs taken orally may cause a hypersensitivity pneumonitis; the best known of these probably are sulfasalazine[141] and nitrofurantoin.[142] A discussion of these is outside the scope of this book, but it is possible that workers who produce these drugs may become sensitized. Drugs taken by inhalation may, like pituitary snuff, cause an alveolitis, and hypersensitivity to cromolyn sodium, which must be exceedingly rare, has been described.[143] Cobalt, used as a coolant in the grinding of tungsten carbide, presumably binds with protein to act as a hapten and has been shown to cause allergic alveolitis (see Chapter 16).[144]

Other Causes of Allergic Alveolitis

There have been occasional reports of allergic alveolitis after exposure to bacteria or the proteolytic enzymes derived from them. Early reports of respiratory disease in detergent workers exposed to *Bacillus subtilis* enzyme stressed the occurrence of asthma and rhinitis but also hinted that an alveolitis might develop.[145, 146] Certainly, precipitins were found in exposed workers, although their significance is dubious. More recently, *B. subtilis* was clearly implicated as the cause of allergic alveolitis in six members of a family who were exposed to dust from decaying wood.[147] *Bacillus cereus* has also been implicated as a cause of allergic alveolitis caused by a humidifier.[148]

In other outbreaks of allergic alveolitis, the precise cause has not been identified. One community outbreak in Finland was spread by tap water in baths and saunas, with the water coming from a local lake.[149] A subject who had worked for 20 years in a coffee-roasting factory was described as having chronic allergic alveolitis, with precipitins to coffee bean dust and compatible biopsy findings. However, long-term follow-up revealed that the patient in fact had pulmonary fibrosis in association with rheumatoid disease.[150] A chronic lung disease in Papuans, termed New Guinea lung, has been ascribed to a hypersensitivity reaction to the thatch roofing of their huts, and precipitins have been found to extracts of the thatch.[151] Prolonged and heavy exposure to the pyrethrins in insecticides has caused allergic alveolitis in one individual.[152]

Finally, many lists include smallpox handler's lung as an allergic alveolitis. Follow-up of the original patients with this, it is to be hoped, now extinct disease suggested that it was a smallpox pneumonia modified by vaccination (see Chapter 23).[153]

SYNDROMES RELATED TO ALLERGIC ALVEOLITIS

Organic Dust Toxic Syndrome

The term *organic dust toxic syndrome* (ODTS) was first used at a workshop on Health Effects of Organic Dusts in the Farm Environment held in Sweden in 1985 to describe a febrile condition distinct from hypersensitivity pneumonitis.[154] This syndrome had been recognized in 1975 by Emanuel et al. who used the term mycotoxicosis to describe the fever and cough which occurred in a group of Wisconsin dairy farmers after exposure to moldy silage.[155] At open lung biopsy, the loosely formed granulomata so characteristic of hypersensitivity pneumonitis were absent, and the histopathological findings identified acute inflammation with the presence of fungal elements. None of the 10 patients had positive precipitin reactions against farmer's lung antigens. In retrospect, this clinical picture was similar to that of a patient described in 1974 as having "seronegative" farmer's lung.[33] This patient was one of three workers who had a febrile illness after heavy exposure to grain dust. Several other reports have mentioned similar febrile seronegative conditions after the uncapping or unloading of silos.[156, 157]

Similar reports from Sweden have observed the condition to occur most commonly in the autumn after the patient worked with hay, straw, woodchips, or grain.[158] The symptoms are very similar to those seen in polymer fume fever or metal fume fever and after exposure to contaminated cotton yarn. These include shivering, myalgias, breathlessness, cough, headache, nausea, and chest tightness. The symptoms usually clear up after a few days, and, unlike extensive allergic alveolitis, ODTS has a benign course without long-term effects.[159]

Mycotoxicosis, as the condition was first called, usually occurs after massive exposure to fungal spores or the offending agent, and unlike farmer's lung, in most of those exposed, the disease develops. Significant restriction may occur along with a reduction in the diffusing capacity, but this is by no means invariable and is not as common as it is in extrinsic allergic alveolitis.[159] Bronchoconstriction may also occur. Leukocytosis up to $20,000/mm^3$ may be found but usually subsides within 24 to 48 hours.[159, 160] When BAL is performed in ODTS, the findings are usually those of an increase in the number of neutrophils with a normal lymphocyte count.[160, 161] The clinical features of farmer's lung and ODTS are similar, and the two conditions are often confused. However, ODTS probably deserves to be regarded as a distinct entity since there are important distinctive features (Table 20–3). It has been suggested that ODTS is a result of activation of the alternative pathway of complement in unsensitized individuals by dust that contains mycotoxins rather than by a direct effect of fungal toxins.[33, 151] May et al. were unable, however, to find measurable mycotoxin in a silo where ODTS occurred.[162] The role of bacterial endotoxins rather than mycotoxins, however, needs to be considered.[163, 164] Experimental inhalation of isolated endotoxin or endotoxin attached to bacteria derived from *Enterobacter* species can induce symptoms of

Table 20–3
■
Acute Inhalation Disease in Agricultural Workers: Causes of and Differential Diagnoses

	Chemical Alveolitis (Silo Filler's Disease)	Extrinsic Allergic Alveolitis	ODTS	Delayed Asthma
Exposure	Oxides of nitrogen	Hay, silage, bedding	Moldy dust, grain, wood chips, etc.	Grain
Dose	Large	Varies	Large or massive	Varies
Onset	Occasionally immediate More often 4 to 6 hours	4 to 8 hours	May be immediate or delayed 1 to 8 hours	4 to 12 hours
Symptoms	Cough, breathlessness	Aches, pains, breathlessness, fever, cough	Flu-like, fever, cough, myalgias	Wheezing, breathlessness
Signs	Crackles	Crackles, wheezes (rare)	May or may not be crackles	Wheezes
Lung function	Restriction (always)	Restriction (nearly always)	Restriction (occasionally)	Obstruction
Histological findings	Edema, alveolitis	Alveolitis, bronchitis, granulomas	Alveolitis in some, no change in others	?
BAL fluid	?	Lymphocytes ↑ CD4/CD8 ↓ Mast cells ↑ Macrophages ↑	Neutrophils ↑, macrophages ↑	Eosinophils ↑

ODTS, occupational dust toxic syndrome; BAL, bronchoalveolar lavage.

airways irritation, chest tightness, headache, arthralgias, and myalgias. The forced expiratory volume in 1 second may fall, and there may be increase in bronchial reactivity and a fall in the diffusing capacity. No specific treatment is known, and spontaneous recovery is the rule.

Humidifier Fever

The inhalation of organic material suspended as an aerosol in fine water droplets has been recognized for many years as an important means of spread of infectious disease and has recently come into prominence again in association with Legionnaires' disease (see Chapter 23). There are many situations within workplaces in which the opportunity exists to inhale aerosols dispersed by humidifying systems or by processes that require the spraying of water. If that water is recycled through a sump, and this is often the case for reasons of economy or convenience, it will inevitably become contaminated by microorganisms unless specific steps are taken to sterilize it.[165] The organisms grow in the sump or in any container in which water is allowed to lie. The precise species and their abundance presumably depend on the basic substance in the water and on the temperature, pH, presence or absence of sunlight, and so on. It is not surprising, therefore, that a number of different syndromes have been described in association with humidifiers and that several different microorganisms have been shown to produce symptoms. The syndromes range from a dramatic and sometimes fatal pneumonia in which *Legionella pneumophilia* is the predominant organism, through typical allergic alveolitis provoked by thermophilic *Actinomyces*[64, 66] to an ill-defined feeling of malaise, fever, cough, and myalgia with a tendency to be worse at the beginning of the working week, a syndrome that has been called humidifier fever.[165]

The first reports of humidifier fever came from Switzerland and Great Britain.[166, 167] Apparently, similar episodes in the United States were subsequently shown to be a form of allergic alveolitis caused by *T. vulgaris, Thermoactinomyces candidus, M. faeni, A. pullulans,* and *Aspergillus fumigatus,* among other theromophilic and mesophilic organisms.[9, 10, 65, 66] The sources of the aerosol included industrial humidifiers and air conditioners, home central heating and humidifiers, and a cool-mist domestic vaporizer.[9, 10, 65, 66] The clinical, radiographic, immunological, and histological features of these diseases were all typical of allergic alveolitis. Curiously, however, when the condition in Great Britain was investigated, a different pattern was observed.[168–171]

Although the symptoms of malaise, myalgia, fever, cough, and chest tightness were similar to those of allergic alveolitis, the occurrence of symptoms early in the week with improvement as the week went on and the absence of radiological abnormalities suggested that this was a different disease. Furthermore, no consistent pattern of sensitization to thermophilic actinomycetes emerged on challenge testing, although precipitins were frequently found in the blood of patients. The workplaces in which outbreaks occurred in Great Britain were a printing works, a rayon factory, and a stationery factory (all of which employed cellulose as a substrate) and a hospital operating room.

Even in this small group of outbreaks, different patterns were described. Challenge testing with the contaminated water sometimes caused fever and a fall in diffusing capacity,[169] but sometimes only systemic symptoms and a slight fall in vital capacity.[172] A possible clue as to etiological factor has come from the demonstration of amebae, *Naegleria gruberi* and *Acanthamoeba,* in the water from all outbreaks and of antibodies to these amebae in the blood of exposed individuals.[173] These organisms live on gram-negative bacteria, and it is possible that inhalation of amebic or bacterial antigen is the cause of the syndrome of humidifier fever. So far, it has not been possible to perform challenge tests with pure amebic extracts, but tests with humidifier water have shown the reaction to be immunological rather than caused by an endotoxin and yet not mediated by complement activation.[174] The last chapter in this interesting story has yet to be written.

In the investigation of outbreaks of febrile illness in the workplace, care should be taken to consider all the possible mechanisms of disease. Moreover, it is reasonable to suppose that other organisms that cause similar syndromes will be identified in the near future. Humidifier fever may be diagnosed from the clinical history, the presence of precipitins to extracts of the water or sludge from sumps or baffle plates, and if necessary, the reproduction of symptoms by challenge testing or by exposure to the suspected water either at work after a break or in the laboratory. As far as is presently known, typical humidifier fever is not progressive and does not cause chronic lung disease. It is preventable by stopping exposure, ideally by changing the system so that water does not recirculate or by injection of steam rather than cold water into humidifiers.[175] These solutions may often be expensive, and investigations of biocidal agents and the use of ultraviolet light are under way. The efficacy of preventive measures may be monitored by testing the water for antigen against the serum of patients known to contain antibody.

Sewer Sludge Fever

A disease similar to humidifier fever has been described in workers in sewage treatment plants.[174, 175] The symptoms of fever, malaise, and myalgia followed by a general feeling of tiredness do not have any special periodicity but follow unusually high exposures to aerosolized sewage sludge or the dust of dried sludge. The sludge contains large numbers of gram-negative bacteria, and it has been suggested that the disease is a response to inhalation of bacterial endotoxin. To date, no long-term or specific pulmonary effects have been described.

Grain Fever

As pointed out in Chapter 19, exposure to grain dust involves inhalation of not only cereal matter but also bacteria, fungi, and antigenic material from mites, weevils, and even small mammals.[126] Asthma is well recognized in such workers, and allergic alveolitis may occur in appropriate circumstances. There is also much discussion as to whether chronic airways obstruction may also be a consequence of prolonged exposure, although to date the epidemiological studies have not successfully separated the effects of dust from those of smoking. In addition to these possible problems, a syndrome of fever, myalgia, and malaise, known as grain fever, has been described in workers after massive exposure, particularly on first working in an elevator or after a period off work.[176, 177]

Whether this syndrome is related to inhaled endotoxin, complement activation, or some other mechanism has not been determined. The effects of exposure to grain have been recently reviewed in detail (see Chapter 19).[178]

Animal Confinement–Related Diseases

Intensive farming has led to the raising of large numbers of animals and birds in confined and limited spaces. The pigsties, barns, and so forth, used for this purpose have controlled humidity, temperature, ventilation, feeding, watering, and waste removal. Large numbers of workers are now employed in the raising of swine, poultry, and beef under such conditions, and a number of respiratory hazards to both the animals and workers have been described.[159]

Hydrogen sulfide, carbon monoxide, methane, ammonia, and formaldehyde are emitted, especially when pig or poultry manure undergo disturbance as they are removed from animal quarters.[159] Ammonia levels tend to be high, both in mammal and avian housing. Endotoxin levels are also elevated, especially in pigsties. Symptoms may develop within a few minutes, or they may develop over several hours, depending on the concentration of the particular hazardous agent.[159]

Rhinitis and tracheitis along with cough are usually the first to appear. Watering of the eyes, chest tightness, wheezing, and breathlessness may also occur.[179]

Asthma may occur but is uncommon. Smokers are more affected than nonsmokers. A small and clinically insignificant fall in the ventilatory capacity may occur. Attempts to relate changes in pulmonary function to the levels of endotoxin, ammonia, and total dust have produced disparate findings.[159, 180, 181]

No risk of irreversible airways obstruction has been demonstrated, but long-term studies are not available to confirm that this type of farm work does not lead to this type of impairment.

REFERENCES

1. Pepys, J., Hypersensitivity diseases of the lungs due to fungi and organic dusts. Monogr. Allergy, 4, 1, 1969.
2. Lopez, M., and Salvaggio, J.E., Epidemiology of hypersensitivity pneumonitis/allergic alveolitis. Monogr. Allergy, 21, 70, 1987.
3. Terho, E.O., Diagnostic criteria for farmer's lung disease. Am. J. Ind. Med., 10, 329, 1986.
4. Burrell, R., and Rylander, R., A critical review of the role of precipitins in hypersensitivity pneumonitis. Eur. J. Respir. Dis., 62, 332, 1981.
5. Mastrangelo, G., Reggio, O., Zambun, P., and Saia, B., Screening delle Bronchopneumonalie in Agriculture: Aspetti Epidemiologici and Ambientati. Presented at Cremona, Italy, January 6, 1981, p. 43.
6. Grant, I.W., Blyth, W., Wardrop, V.E., et al., Prevalence of farmer's lung in Scotland. A pilot survey. Br. Med. J., 1, 530, 1972.
7. Shelley, E., Dean, G., Collins, D., et al., Farmers' lung. A study in North West Ireland. J. Irish Med. Assoc., 72, 261, 1979.
8. Madsen, D., Klock, L.E., Wenzel, F.J., et al., The prevalence of farmer's lung in an agricultural population. Am. Rev. Respir. Dis., 113, 171, 1976.
9. Woodard, E.D., Friedlander, B., Lesher, R.J., et al., Outbreak of hypersensitivity pneumonitis in an industrial setting. JAMA, 259, 1963, 1988.
10. Ganier, M., Lieberman, P., Fink, J., et al., Humidifier lung. An outbreak in office workers. Chest, 77, 183, 1980.
11. Bayonet, N., and Lavergne, R., Respiratory disease of bagasse workers. A clinical analysis of 69 cases. Ind. Med. Surg., 25, 519, 1960.
12. Lehrer, S.B., Turer, E., Weill, H., et al., Elimination of bagassosis in Louisiana paper manufacturing plant workers. Clin. Allergy, 8, 15, 1978.
13. Cormier, Y., Belanger, J., and Durand, P., Factors influencing the development of serum precipitins to farmer's lung antigen in Quebec dairy farmers. Thorax, 40, 138, 1985.
14. Terho, E.O., Husman, K., Vohlonen, I., et al., Serum precipitins against microbes in mouldy hay with respect to age, sex, atopy, and smoking of farmers. Eur. J. Respir. Dis., 152(suppl.), 115, 1987.
15. Rose, C., and King, T., Controversies in hypersensitivity pneumonitis [editorial]. Am. Rev. Respir. Dis., 145, 1, 1992.
16. Boyd, G., Clinical and immunological studies in pulmonary extrinsic allergic alveolitis. Scott. Med. J., 23, 267, 1978.
17. Davies, B.H., Edwards, J.H., and Seaton, A., Cross reacting antibodies to *Micropolyspora faeni* in mycoplasma pneumonia. Clin. Allergy, 5, 217, 1975.
18. Boyd, G., Madkour, M., Middleton, S., et al., Effect of smoking on circulating antibody levels to avian protein in pigeon breeder's disease. Thorax, 32, 651, 1977.
19. Morgan, D.C., Smyth, J.T., Lister, R.W., et al., Chest symptoms in farming communities with special reference to farmer's lung. Br. J. Ind. Med., 32, 228, 1975.
20. Hapke, E.J., Seal, R.M.E., and Thomas, G.O., Farmer's lung. Thorax, 23, 451, 1968.
21. Hansell, D.M., and Moskovic, E., High resolution computed tomography in extrinsic allergic alveolitis. Clin. Radiol., 43, 8, 1991.
22. Rankin, J., Kobayashi, M., Barbee, R.A., and Dickie, H.A., Pulmonary granulomatoses due to inhaled organic antigens. Med. Clin. North Am., 51, 459, 1967.
23. Seal, R.M.E., Hapke, E.J., Thomas, G.O., et al., The pathology of the acute and chronic stages of farmer's lung. Thorax, 23, 469, 1968.
24. Emanuel, D.A., Wenzel, F.J., Bowerman, C.I., and Lawton, B.R., Farmer's lung. Clinical, pathologic, and immunologic study of 24 patients. Am. J. Med., 37, 392, 1964.
25. Barrowcliff, D.F., and Arblaster, P.G., Farmer's lung: a study of an early acute fatal case. Thorax, 23, 490, 1968.
26. Reyes, C.N., Wenzel, F.J., Lawton, B.R., et al., The pulmonary pathology of farmer's lung disease. Chest, 81, 142, 1982.
27. Mullins, J., and Seaton, A., Fungal spores in lung and sputum. Clin. Allergy, 8, 525, 1978.
28. Mullins, J., Harvey, R., and Seaton, A., Sources and incidence of airborne *Aspergillus fumigatus* (*Fres*). Clin. Allergy, 6, 209, 1976.
29. Pepys, J., Riddell, R.W., Citron, K.M., et al., Clinical and immunologic significance of *Aspergillus fumigatus* in the sputum. Am. Rev. Respir. Dis., 80, 167, 1959.

30. Cormier, Y., and Belanger, J., The fluctuant nature of precipitating antibodies in dairy farmers. Thorax, 44, 469, 1989.
31. Kreutzer, D.L., McCormick, J.R., Thrall, R.S., et al., Elevation of serum chemotactic factor inactivator activity during acute inflammatory reactions in patients with hypersensitivity pneumonitis. Am. Rev. Respir. Dis., 125, 612, 1982.
32. Yoshizawa, Y., Nomura, A., Ohdama, S., et al., The significance of complement activation in the pathogenesis of hypersensitivity pneumonitis: sequential changes of complement components and chemotactic activities in bronchoalveolar lavage fluids. Int. Arch. Allergy Appl. Immunol., 87, 417, 1988.
33. Edwards, J.H., Baker, J.T., and Davies, B.H., Precipitin test negative farmer's lung—activation of the alternative pathway of complement by mouldy hay dust. Clin. Allergy, 4, 379, 1974.
34. Haslam, P.L., Dewar, A., Butchers, P., et al., Mast cells, atypical lymphocytes and neutrophils in bronchoalveolar lavage in extrinsic allergic alveolitis: Comparison with other interstitial lung disease. Am. Rev. Respir. Dis., 135, 35, 1987.
35. Coombs, R.P., Gell, P.G., and Laehman, P.J., eds., The Classification of Allergic Reactions Underlying Disease. Clinical Aspects of Immunology. Oxford, Blackwell, 1962, p. 761.
36. Pepys, J., Riddell, R.W., Citron, K.M., et al., Clinical and immunologic significance of *Aspergillus fumigatus* in the sputum. Am. Rev. Respir. Dis., 80, 167, 1959.
37. Salvaggio, J.E., Phanuphak, P., Bice, D., et al., Experimental production of granulomatous pneumonitis. J. Allergy Clin. Immunol., 56, 364, 1975.
38. Salvaggio, J.E., and deShazo, R.D., Pathogenesis of hypersensitivity pneumonitis. Chest, 89, 190S, 1986.
39. Reynolds, H.Y., Hypersensitivity pneumonitis. Correlation of cellular and immunological changes with clinical phases of disease. Lung, 166, 189, 1988.
40. Cormier, Y., Belanger, J., Beaudoin, J., et al., Abnormal bronchoalveolar lavage in asymptomatic dairy farmers—study of lymphocytes. Am. Rev. Respir. Dis., 130, 1046, 1984.
41. Larsson, K., Malmberg, P., Eklund, A., et al., Exposure to microorganisms, airway inflammatory changes and immune reactions in asymptomatic dairy farmers: bronchoalveolar lavage evidence of macrophage activation and permeability changes in the airways. Int. Arch. Allergy Appl. Immunol., 87, 127, 1988.
42. Larsson, K., Eklund, A., Malmberg, P., et al., Hyaluronic acid (hyaluronan) in BAL fluid distinguishes farmers with allergic alveolitis from farmers with asymptomatic alveolitis. Chest, 101, 109, 1992.
43. Cormier, Y., Belanger, J., and Laviolette, M., Prognostic significance of bronchoalveolar lymphocytosis in farmer's lung. Am. Rev. Respir. Dis., 135, 692, 1987.
44. Leatherman, J.W., Michael, A.F., Schwartz, B.A., et al., Lung T cells in hypersensitivity pneumonitis. Ann. Intern. Med., 100, 390, 1984.
45. Roberts, R.C., and Moore, V.L., Immunopathogenesis of hypersensitivity pneumonitis. Am. Rev. Respir. Dis., 116, 1075, 1977.
46. Neilsen, K.H., Parratt, D., Boyd, G., and White, R.G., Use of a radiolabelled antiglobulin for quantitation of antibody to soluble antigens rendered particulate: application to pigeon fancier's lung syndrome. Int. Arch. Allergy Appl. Immunol., 47, 339, 1974.
47. Sandoval, J., Banales, J.L., Cortes, J.J., et al., Detection of antibodies against avian antigens in bronchoalveolar lavage from patients with pigeon fancier's disease: usefulness of enzyme linked immunosorbent assay and enzyme immunotransfer blotting. J. Clin. Lab. Anal., 4, 81, 1990.
48. Hendrick, D.J., Marshall, R., Faux, J.A., et al., Positive "alveolar" responses to antigen inhalation provocation tests: their validity and recognition. Thorax, 35, 415, 1980.
49. Warren, C.P.W., Tse, K.S., and Cherniack, R.M., Mechanical properties of the lung in extrinsic allergic alveolitis. Thorax, 33, 315, 1978.
50. Evans, W.V., and Seaton, A., Hypersensitivity pneumonitis in a technician using Pauli's reagent. Thorax, 34, 767, 1979.
51. Bernardo, J., Hunninghake, G.W., Gadek, J.E., et al., Acute hypersensitivity pneumonitis: serial changes in lung lymphocyte subpopulations after exposure to antigen. Am. Rev. Respir. Dis., 120, 985, 1979.
52. Godard, P., Clot, J., Jonquet, O., et al., Lymphocyte subpopulations in bronchoalveolar lavages of patients with sarcoidosis and hypersensitivity pneumonitis. Chest, 80, 447, 1981.
53. Reynolds, H.Y., Fulmer, J.D., Kazmeirdwski, J.A., et al., Analysis of cellular and protein content of bronchoalveolar lavage fluid from patients with idiopathic pulmonary fibrosis and chronic hypersensitivity pneumonitis. J. Clin. Invest., 59, 165, 1977.
54. Cuthbert, O.D., and Gordon, M.F., Ten year follow-up of farmers with farmer's lung. Br. J. Ind. Med., 40, 173, 1983.
55. Bourke, S.J., Banham, S.W., Carter, R., et al., Longitudinal course of extrinsic allergic alveolitis in pigeon breeders. Thorax, 44, 415, 1989.
56. Richerson, H.B., Richards, D.W., Swanson, P.A., et al., Antigen-specific desensitization in a rabbit model of acute hypersensitivity pneumonitis. J. Allergy Clin. Immunol., 68, 226, 1981.
57. Kokkarinen, J.I., Tukiainen, H.O., and Terho, E.O., Effect of corticosteroid treatment on the recovery of pulmonary function in farmer's lung. Am. Rev. Respir. Dis., 145, 3, 1992.
58. Anttinen, H., Terho, E.O., Myllyla, R., et al., Two serum markers of collagen biosynthesis as possible indicators of irreversible pulmonary impairment in farmer's lung. Am. Rev. Respir. Dis., 133, 88, 1986.

59. Gourley, C.A., and Braidwood, G.D., The use of dust respirators in the prevention of recurrence of farmer's lung. Trans. Soc. Occup. Med., 21, 93, 1971.
60. Hendrick, D.J., Marshall, R., Faux, J.A., et al., Protective value of dust respirators in extrinsic allergic alveolitis: clinical assessment using inhalation provocation tests. Thorax, 36, 917, 1981.
61. Campbell, J.M., Acute symptoms following work with hay. Br. Med. J., 2, 1143, 1932.
62. Fawcett, R., Fungoid conditions of the lung. I and II. Br. J. Radiol., 9, 172, 1936.
63. Fuller, C.J., Farmer's lung—a review of present knowledge. Thorax, 8, 59, 1953.
64. Banaszak, E.J., Thiede, W.H., and Fink, J.N., Hypersensitivity pneumonitis due to contamination of an air conditioner. N. Engl. J. Med., 283, 271, 1970.
65. Fink, J.N., Banaszak, E.J., and Thiede, W.H., Interstitial pneumonitis due to hypersensitivity to an organism contaminating a heating system. Ann. Intern. Med., 74, 80, 1971.
66. Fink, J.N., Banaszak, E.J., Barboriak, J.J., et al., Interstitial lung disease due to contamination of forced air systems. Ann. Intern. Med., 84, 406, 1976.
67. Williams, J.V., Inhalation and skin tests with extracts of hay and fungi in patients with farmer's lung. Thorax, 18, 182, 1963.
68. Pepys, J., and Jenkins, P.A., Precipitin (F.L.H.) test in farmer's lung. Thorax, 20, 21, 1965.
69. LaBerge, D.E., and Stahmann, M.A., Antigens from mouldy hay involved in farmer's lung. Proc. Soc. Exp. Biol. Med., 121, 463, 1966.
70. Pepys, J., Riddell, R.W., Citron, K.M., et al., Precipitins against extracts of hay and fungi in the serum of patients with farmer's lung. Acta Allergy, 16, 76, 1961.
71. Barbee, R.A., Dickie, H.A., and Rankin, J., Pathogenicity of specific glycopeptide antigen in farmer's lung. Proc. Soc. Exp. Biol. Med., 118, 546, 1965.
72. Pepys, J., Riddell, R.W., Citron, K.W., et al., Precipitins against extracts of hay and moulds in the serum of patients with farmer's lung, aspergillosis, asthma, and sarcoidosis. Thorax, 17, 336, 1962.
73. Pepys, J., Jenkins, P.A., Festenstein, G.N., et al., Farmer's lung: thermophilic actinomycetes as a course of "farmer's lung hay" antigens. Lancet, 2, 607, 1963.
74. Wenzel, F.J., Gray, R.L., and Emanuel, D.A., Farmer's lung—its geographic distribution. J. Occup. Med., 12, 493, 1970.
75. Flaherty, D.K., Braun, S.R., Marx, J.J., et al., Serologically detectable HLA-A, B, and C loci antigens in farmer's lung disease. Am. Rev. Respir. Dis., 122, 437, 1980.
76. Braun, S.R., doPico, G.A., Tsiatis, A., et al., Farmer's lung disease: long-term clinical and physiologic outcome. Am. Rev. Respir. Dis., 119, 185, 1979.
77. Buechner, H.A., Prevatt, A.L., Thompson, J., et al., Bagassosis: review with further historical data, studies of pulmonary function, and results of adrenal steroid therapy. Am. J. Med., 25, 234, 1958.
78. Hunter, D., and Perry, K.M.M., Bronchiolitis from industrial handling of bagasse. Br. J. Ind. Med., 3, 64, 1946.
79. Hearn, C.E., and Holford-Strevens, B., Immunological aspects of bagassosis. Br. J. Ind. Med., 25, 283, 1968.
80. Weill, H., Buechner, H.A., Gonzalez, E., et al., Bagassosis: a study of pulmonary function in 20 cases. Ann. Intern. Med., 64, 737, 1966.
81. Miller, G.J., Hearn, C.E., and Edwards, R.H., Pulmonary function at rest and during exercise following bagassosis. Br. J. Ind. Med., 28, 152, 1971.
82. Bringhurst, L.S., Byrne, R.N., and Gershon-Cohen, J., Respiratory disease of mushroom workers. JAMA, 171, 15, 1959.
83. Sakula, A., Mushroom worker's lung. Br. Med. J., 2, 708, 1967.
84. Riddle, H.F.V., Channell, S., Blyth, W., et al., Allergic alveolitis in a malt worker. Thorax, 23, 271, 1968.
85. Grant, I.W.B., Blackadder, E.S., Greenberg, M., et al., Extrinsic allergic alveolitis in Scottish malt workers. Br. Med. J., 1, 490, 1976.
86. DeWeck, A.L., Gutersohn, J., and Bütikofer, E., La maladie des laveurs de fromage:une forme particuliere du syndrome du poumon du fermier. Schweiz Med. Wochenschr., 99, 872, 1969.
87. Schlueter, D.P., Cheesewasher's disease: a new occupational hazard? Ann. Intern. Med., 78, 606, 1973.
88. Tower, J.W., Sweaney, H.C., and Huron, W.H., Severe bronchial asthma apparently due to fungus spores found in maple bark. JAMA, 99, 453, 1932.
89. Emanuel, D.A., Lawton, B.R., and Wenzel, F.J., Maple bark disease. N. Engl. J. Med., 266, 333, 1962.
90. Emanuel, D.A., Wenzel, F.J., and Lawton, B.R., Pneumonitis due to *Cryptostroma corticale* (maple bark disease). N. Engl. J. Med., 274, 1413, 1966.
91. Wenzel, F.J., and Emanuel, D.A., The epidemiology of maple bark disease. Arch. Environ. Health, 14, 385, 1967.
92. Cohen, H.I., Merigan, T.C., Kosek, J.C., et al., Sequoiosis; A granulomatous pneumonitis associated with redwood sawdust inhalation. Am. J. Med., 43, 785, 1967.
93. Michaels, L., Lung changes in woodworkers. Can. Med. Assoc. J., 96, 1150, 1967.
94. Sosman, A.J., Schlueter, D.P., Fink, J.H., et al., Hypersensitivity to wood dust. N. Engl. J. Med., 281, 977, 1969.
95. Schlueter, D.P., Fink, J.N., and Hensley, G.T., Wood-pulp worker's disease. A hypersensitivity pneumonitis caused by Alternaria. Ann. Intern. Med., 77, 907, 1972.
96. Avila, R., and Villar, T.G., Suberosis, respiratory disease in cork workers. Lancet, 1, 620, 1968.

97. Avila, R., and Lacey, J., The role of *Penicillium frequentans* in suberosis (respiratory disease in workers in the cork industry). Clin. Allergy, 4, 109, 1974.
98. Howie, A.D., Boyd, G., and Moran, F., Pulmonary hypersensitivity to ramin (*Gonystylus bancanus*). Thorax, 31, 585, 1976.
99. Hunter, D., The Diseases of Occupations, 4th ed. London, English Universities Press, 1969, p. 1081.
100. Livingston, J.L., Lewis, J.G., Reid, L., et al., Diffuse interstitial pulmonary fibrosis. Q. J. Med., 33, 71, 1964.
101. O'Brien, I.M., Bull, J., Creamer, B., et al., Asthma and extrinsic allergic alveolitis due to *Merulius lacrymans*. Clin. Allergy, 8, 535, 1978.
102. Rhudy, J., Burrell, R.G., and Morgan, W.K.C., Yet another cause of allergic alveolitis. Scand. J. Respir. Dis., 52, 177, 1971.
103. Strand, R.D., Neuhauser, E.B.D., and Sornberger, C.F., Lycoperdonosis. N. Engl. J. Med., 277, 89, 1967.
104. Plessner, M.M., Une maladie de trieurs de plumes: la fievre de canard. Arch. Mal. Prof., 21, 67, 1960.
105. Pearsall, H.R., Morgan, E.G., Tesluk, H., et al., Parakeet dander pneumonitis. Acute psittaco-kerato-pneumoconiosis. Report of a case. Bull. Mason. Clinic, 14, 127, 1960.
106. Barboriak, J.J., Sosman, A.J., and Reed, C.E., Serological studies in pigeon breeder's disease. J. Lab. Clin. Med., 65, 600, 1965.
107. Reed, C.E., Sosman, A., and Barbee, R.A., Pigeon breeder's lung. JAMA, 193, 261, 1965.
108. Villar, T.G., Avila, R., and Araugo, J., O "pulmao dos criadores de pombos." A proposito de un case de un plano. J. Soc. Ciencias Med. Lisboa, 130, 181, 1966.
109. Hargreave, F.E., Pepys, J., Longbottom, J.H., et al., Bird breeder's (fancier's) lung. Lancet, 1, 445, 1966.
110. Warren, C.P.W., and Tse, K.S., Extrinsic allergic alveolitis owing to hypersensitivity to chickens—significance of sputum precipitins. Am. Rev. Respir. Dis., 109, 672, 1974.
111. Boyer, R.S., Klock, L.E., Schmidt, C.D., et al., Hypersensitivity lung disease in the turkey raising industry. Am. Rev. Respir. Dis., 109, 630, 1974.
112. Schlueter, D.P., Fink, J.N., and Sosman, A.J., Pulmonary function in pigeon fancier's disease. A hypersensitivity pneumonitis. Ann. Intern. Med., 70, 457, 1969.
113. Allen, D.H., Williams, G.V., and Woolcock, A.J., Bird breeder's hypersensitivity pneumonitis: progress studies of lung function after cessation of exposure to the provoking antigen. Am. Rev. Respir. Dis., 114, 555, 1976.
114. Christensen, L.T., Schmidt, C.D., and Robbins, L., Pigeon breeder's disease—a prevalence study and review. Clin. Allergy, 5, 417, 1975.
115. Barboriak, J.J., Sosman, A.H., and Reed, C.E., Serological studies in pigeon breeder's disease. J. Lab. Clin. Med., 65, 600, 1965.
116. Boyd, G., McSharry, C.P., Banham, S.W., et al., A current view of pigeon fancier's lung. A model for extrinsic allergic alveolitis. Clin. Allergy, 12(suppl.), 53, 1982.
117. Banham, S.W., McKenzie, H., McSharry, C., et al., Antibody against a pigeon bloom extract: a further antigen in pigeon breeder's lung. Clin. Allergy, 12, 173, 1982.
118. Boyd, G., Dick, H.W., Lorimer, A.R., et al., Bird breeder's lung. Scott. Med. J., 12, 69, 1967.
119. Taylor, A.J., Taylor, P., Bryant, D.H., et al., False positive complement fixation tests with respiratory virus preparations in bird fanciers with allergic alveolitis. Thorax, 32, 563, 1977.
120. Faux, J.A., Hendrick, D.J., and Anand, B.S., Precipitins of different avian serum antigens in bird fancier's lung and coeliac disease. Clin. Allergy, 8, 101, 1978.
121. Hood, J., and Mason, A.M.S., Diffuse pulmonary disease with transfer defect occurring with coeliac disease. Lancet, 1, 445, 1970.
122. Berrill, W.T., Fitzpatrick, P.F., Macleod, W.M., et al., Bird fancier's lung and jejunal villous atrophy. Lancet, 2, 1006, 1975.
123. Hendrick, D.J., Faux, J.A., Anand, B., et al., Is bird fancier's lung associated with coeliac disease? Thorax, 33, 425, 1978.
124. Carroll, K.B., Pepys, J., Longbottom, J.L., et al., Extrinsic allergic alveolitis due to rat serum proteins. Clin. Allergy, 5, 443, 1975.
125. Korenblat, P., Slavin, R., Winzenburger, P., et al., Gerbil keeper's lung—a new form of hypersensitivity pneumonitis. Ann. Allergy, 38, 437, 1977.
126. Jiminez-Diaz, C., Lahoz, C., and Cento, G., The allergens of mill dust. Asthma in millers, farmers, and others. Ann. Allergy, 5, 519, 1947.
127. Frankland, A.W., and Lunn, J.A., Asthma caused by the grain weevil. Br. J. Ind. Med., 22, 157, 1965.
128. Lunn, J.A., and Hughes, D.T.D., Pulmonary hypersensitivity to the grain weevil. Br. J. Ind. Med., 24, 158, 1967.
129. Vallery-Radot, L., and Giroud, P., Sporomycose des pelleteuers de grains. Bull. Mem. Soc. Hop. Paris, 52, 16, 1928.
130. Pimentel, J.C., Furrier's lung. Thorax, 25, 387, 1970.
131. Mahon, W.E., Scott, D.J., Ansell, G., et al., Hypersensitivity to pituitary snuff with miliary shadowing in the lungs. Thorax, 22, 13, 1967.
132. Butikoffer, E., DeWeck, A.L., and Scherrer, M., Pituitary snufftaker's lung. Schweiz. Med. Wochenschr., 100, 97, 1970.

133. Harper, L.O., Burrell, R.G., Lapp, N.L., et al., Allergic alveolitis due to pituitary snuff. Ann. Intern. Med., 73, 581, 1970.

134. Fuchs, S., and Valade, P., Étude clinique et expérimentale sur quelques cas d'intoxication par le desmodur T (diisocyanate de tolulene 1-214 et 1-216). Arch. Mal. Prof., 12, 191, 1951.

135. Charles, J., Bernstein, A., Jones, B., et al., Hypersensitivity pneumonitis after exposure to isocyanates. Thorax, 31, 127, 1976.

136. Fink, J.N., and Schlueter, D.P., Bathtub refinisher's lung: an unusual response to toluene diisocyanate. Am. Rev. Respir. Dis., 118, 955, 1978.

137. Zeiss, C.R., Kanellakes, T.B., Bellone, J.D., et al., Immunoglobulin E-mediated asthma and hypersensitivity pneumonitis with precipitating anti-hapten antibodies due to diphenyl dimethane diisocyanate. J. Allergy Clin. Immunol., 65, 346, 1980.

138. Malo, J.L., and Zeiss, C.R., Occupational hypersensitivity pneumonitis after exposure to diphenylmethane diisocyanate. Am. Rev. Respir. Dis., 125, 113, 1982.

139. Pimentel, J.C., and Marques, F., Vineyard sprayer's lung: a new occupational disease. Thorax, 24, 678, 1969.

140. Villar, T.G., Vineyard sprayer's lung. Clinical aspects. Am. Rev. Respir. Dis., 110, 545, 1974.

141. Thomas, P., Seaton, A., and Edwards, J., Respiratory disease due to sulphasalazine. Clin. Allergy, 4, 41, 1974.

142. Rosenow, E.C., DeRemee, R.A., and Dines, D.E., Chronic nitrofurantoin pulmonary reaction. N. Engl. J. Med., 279, 1258, 1968.

143. Burgher, L.W., Kass, I., and Schenken, J.R., Pulmonary allergic granulomatosis: a possible drug reaction in a patient receiving cromolyn sodium. Chest, 66, 84, 1974.

144. Sjogren, I., Hillerdal, G., Andersson, A., et al., Hard metal lung disease: importance of cobalt in coolants. Thorax, 35, 653, 1980.

145. Newhouse, M.L., Tagg, B., Pocock, S.J., et al., An epidemiological study of workers producing enzyme washing powders. Lancet, 1, 689, 1970.

146. Franz, T., McMurrain, K.D., Brooks, S., et al., Clinical immunologic and physiologic observations in factory workers exposed to B. subtilis enzyme dust. J. Allergy, 47, 170, 1971.

147. Johnson, C.L., Bernstein, I.L., Gallagher, J.S., et al., Familial hypersensitivity pneumonitis induced by Bacillus subtilis. Am. Rev. Respir. Dis., 122, 339, 1980.

148. Kohler, P.F., Gross, G., Salvaggio, J., et al., Humidifier lung: hypersensitivity pneumonitis related to thermotolerant bacterial aerosols. Chest, 69(suppl.), 294, 1976.

149. Muittari, A., Kuusisto, P., Virtanen, P., et al., An epidemic of extrinsic allergic alveolitis caused by tap water. Clin. Allergy, 10, 77, 1980.

150. Van den Bosch, J.M., Van Toorn, D.W., and Wagenaar, S.S., Coffee workers' lung: reconsideration of a case report. Correspondence. Thorax, 38, 720, 1983.

151. Blackburn, C.R., and Green, W., Precipitins against extracts of thatched roofs in the sera of New Guinea natives with chronic lung disease. Lancet, 2, 1396, 1966.

152. Carlson, J.E., and Villaveces, J.W., Hypersensitivity pneumonitis due to pyrethrum. JAMA, 237, 1718, 1977.

153. Ross, P., Seaton, A., Foreman, H.M., et al., Pulmonary calcification following smallpox handler's lung. Thorax, 29, 659, 1974.

154. Rylander, R., Lung diseases caused by organic dusts in the farm environment. Am. J. Ind. Med., 10, 221, 1986.

155. Emanuel, D.A., Wenzel, F.J., and Lawton, B.R., Pulmonary mycotoxicosis. Chest, 67, 293, 1975.

156. May, J.J., Stallones, L., Darrow, D., et al., Organic dust toxicity (pulmonary mycotoxicosis) associated with silo unloading. Thorax, 41, 919, 1986.

157. Pratt, D.S., Stallones, L., Darrow, D., et al., Acute respiratory illness associated with silo unloading. Am. J. Ind. Med., 10, 238, 1986.

158. Rask-Andersen, A., Organic dust toxic syndrome among farmers. Br. J. Ind. Med., 46, 233, 1989.

159. DoPico, G.A., Hazardous exposure and lung disease among farm workers. Clin. Chest Med., 13, 311, 1992.

160. Lecours, R., Laviolette, M., and Cormier, Y., Bronchoalveolar lavage in pulmonary mycotoxicosis (organic dust toxic syndrome). Thorax, 41, 924, 1986.

161. Emanuel, D.A., Marx, J.J., Ault, B., et al., Organic dust toxic syndrome (pulmonary mycotoxicosis). In Dosman, J.A., Cockcroft, D.W., eds., Principles of Health and Safety in Agriculture. Boca Raton, FL, CRC Press, 1989, p. 72.

162. May, J.J., Pratt, D.S., Stallones, L., et al., A study of dust generated during silo opening and its physiologic effect on workers. In Dosman, J.A., and Cockcroft, D.W., eds., Principles of Health and Safety in Agriculture. Boca Raton, FL, CRC Press, 1989, pp. 58–61.

163. DoPico, G.A., Flaherty, D., Bhansali, P., et al., Grain fever syndrome induced by the inhalation of airborne grain dust. J. Allergy Clin. Immunol., 69, 435, 1982.

164. Rylander, R., Bake, B., Fischer, J.J., et al., Pulmonary function and symptoms after inhalation of endotoxin. Am. Rev. Respir. Dis., 140, 981, 1989.

165. MRC Symposium, Humidifier fever. Thorax, 32, 653, 1977.

166. Pestalozzi, C., Febrile Gruppener Krankungen in einer Modellsch reinerei durch inhalation von mit Schimelpilzen Kontaminierten Befeuchteawasser. Schweiz. Med. Wochenschr., 89, 710, 1959.

167. H.M. Chief Inspector of Factories, Annual Report 1969. London, H.M. Stationery Office, 1970, p. 72.

168. Pickering, C.A.C., Moore, W.K.S., Lacey, J., et al., Investigation of a respiratory disease associated with an air-conditioning system. Clin. Allergy, 6, 109, 1976.
169. Friend, J.A.R., Gaddie, J., Palmer, K.N.V., et al., Extrinsic allergic alveolitis and contaminated cooling water in a factory machine. Lancet, 1, 297, 1977.
170. Edwards, J.H., Microbial and immunological investigations and remedial action after an outbreak of humidifier fever. Br. J. Ind. Med., 37, 55, 1980.
171. Cockcroft, A., Edwards, J., Bevan, C., et al., An investigation of operating theatres staff exposed to humidifier fever antigens. Br. J. Ind. Med., 38, 144, 1981.
172. Edwards, J.H., and Cockcroft, A., Inhalation challenge in humidifier fever. Clin. Allergy, 11, 227, 1981.
173. Edwards, J.H., Griffiths, A.J., and Mullins, J., Protozoa as sources of antigen in "humidifier fever." Nature, 264, 438, 1976.
174. Rylander, R., Anderson, K., Belin, L., et al., Sewage worker's syndrome. Lancet, 2, 478, 1976.
175. Mattsby, I., and Rylander, R., Clinical and immunological findings in workers exposed to sewage dust. J. Occup. Med., 20, 690, 1978.
176. Williams, N., Skonlas, A., and Merriman, J.E., Exposure to grain dust. I. A survey of the effects. In Dosman, J.A., and Cotton, D.S., eds., Occupational Pulmonary Disease. Focus on Grain Dust and Health. New York, Academic Press, 1980, p. 367.
177. Tse, K.S., Warren, P., Janusz, M., et al., Respiratory abnormalities in workers exposed to grain dusts. Arch. Environ. Health, 27, 74, 1973.
178. Chan-Yeung, M., Enarson, D.A., and Kennedy, S., The impact of grain dust on respiratory health. Am. Rev. Respir. Dis., 145, 476, 1992.
179. Dosman, J.A., Graham, B.L., and Hall, D., Respiratory symptoms and pulmonary function in farmers. J. Occup. Med., 29, 38, 1987.
180. Donham, K.J., Ravala, D.C., and Merchant, J.A., Acute effects of work environment on pulmonary functions of swine confinement workers. Am. J. Ind. Med., 5, 367, 1984.
181. Zhou, C., Muller, R., and Barber, E., Shift changes in lung function in swine farmers. Am. Rev. Respir. Dis., 143A, 439, 1991.

21

John A. S. Ross

Anthony Seaton

W. Keith C. Morgan

Toxic Gases and Fumes

■

The danger to life of gases and fumes in mining has been appreciated since the earliest times. Pliny the Elder in Book 33 of his *Natural History* wrote: "But for that the vapour and smoke that ariseth from thence, by the means, may stifle and choke them within those narrow pits and mines, they are forced to give over such fire-work and betake themselves often-times to great mattocks and pickaxes." This referred to the practice in gold mining of cracking rocks with fire. Silver miners were also at risk from naturally generated vapors: "And yet there is a damp or vapour breathing out of silver mines, hurtful to all living creatures and to dogs especially." Apart from asphyxiation, it was appreciated that poisoning could occur from absorption of toxic matter from dust and fumes, and Pliny described the use of masks made from bladders for the prevention of mercury poisoning in vermilion workers. Agricola in Book 6 of *De re Metallica* gave details of many poisonous fumes encountered in the mine atmosphere and described apparatus for minimizing the danger by ventilation.

Toxic gases and fumes continue to cause such problems in industry. The United Kingdom Health and Safety Commission reported the recent annual incidence of carbon monoxide poisoning to be 164 with 32 fatalities, and it was stated that this was likely to be a substantial underestimation. The annual incidence of injury due to poisoning and gassings was 729 with 24 fatalities.[1] Further insight into the agents involved in industrial inhalation injury has been given by the SWORD (Surveillance of Work-related and Occupational Respiratory Disorders) study described in Chapter 17. In 1990, 285 inhalation accidents were reported to the study. The most common agents were chlorine (35 cases) and phosphine (33), with perchloroethylene (15), sulfur dioxide (14), zinc compounds (14), nitrogen oxides (13), and trichloroethylene (10) also being important. Other agents reported were triethylamine, hydrogen sulfide, carbon monoxide, and combustion products.

PRINCIPLES OF ACTION

Harmful airborne material may be present as a gas or suspended in a solid or liquid form in air. Within the particular sphere of occupational medicine, it has become accepted usage to call a fine solid particulate, often formed by the vaporization and oxidation of a metal, a *fume* and the gaseous form of a substance which is liquid if enclosed at normal temperature and pressure a *vapor*. Nevertheless, the reader should be aware that these words are used interchangeably in broader, nontechnical texts, and when the physical nature of an inhaled substance is important, it should be described.

The behavior of such matter when inhaled depends on its physical and chemical properties and its velocity in the respiratory tract. Particulate matter falls out of the breathing gas stream when it comes into contact with a lung surface. This is influenced primarily by sedimentation and impaction, both of which are increased by increasing velocity and particle size but are reduced by increased airway diameter. As particles become smaller, brownian diffusion becomes more important and is significant at particle diameters of 1 μm and less. Large particles, of 15 to 20 μm in diameter, tend to be deposited in the nose, smaller ones in the trachea and bronchi, and those between 0.5 and 7 μm are mainly deposited in the alveoli. Very small particles, smaller than about 0.1 μm, have a relatively high alveolar deposition rate, with approximately 50% being deposited. The principles of deposition of particulate matter are outlined elsewhere in this volume. Liquid suspensions may evaporate once inhaled and be absorbed as gas. Gas molecules move to the walls of airways solely by diffusion (see also Chapter 7).[2]

Once inhaled, substances exert their toxic effects in one of several ways (Table 21–1). The agent can be absorbed into the bloodstream and exert systemic toxic effects. The toxin can exert a direct corrosive or irritant effect on the lung, and this stimulates an inflammatory reaction. Simple asphyxia can be caused by an otherwise inert compound that displaces oxygen from the atmosphere. Inhaled toxins can also induce allergic responses and cause cancer, but these topics are dealt with elsewhere in this book.

ASPHYXIATING GASES

Carbon Dioxide

Carbon dioxide is heavier than air and is most commonly encountered in enclosed or poorly ventilated spaces, such as unworked mines, caissons, and tanks. In coal mines it is produced by the oxidation of contaminants of coal on unworked faces and constitutes an important hazard when the face is reopened. Carbon dioxide retention can also be caused by improperly designed or fitted respiratory protective equipment.

Although carbon dioxide is not a particularly toxic gas and is often described as being only a simple asphyxiant at high concentration, it is very far from being without effect at lower levels.[3] Partial pressures of 27 kPa in oxygen have been used to induce surgical anesthesia, and an anesthetic effect can be demonstrated for the gas at arterial levels of 12.5 kPa in healthy people not suffering from respiratory failure.* This represents an inhaled level of between 10% and 11%, although levels of between 7% and 10% have been described as causing a loss of consciousness.[4] A decrement in psychomotor performance can be detected at inspired concentrations of 6.6% but not at inhaled concentrations of 4.5% and 5.5%.[5, 6] The effects seen were a slowing of reasoning without loss of accuracy and an increase in irritability and discomfort.

The major effect of small increases in inhaled carbon dioxide is to stimulate ventilation. At rest, 3% carbon dioxide doubles, 4% triples, and 5% quadruples alveolar ventilation. In a toxic environment, the amount of toxin inhaled will be correspondingly increased. This increase in ventilation above normal is also seen during exercise, although the relative rise is less as the mechanical limits of the lungs and chest are approached.

The symptoms of hyperventilation, headache, and sweating and the signs of bounding pulse and loss of consciousness are familiar to most doctors in a nonindustrial setting. These symptoms and signs are due to the combination of acidosis and catecholamine secretion caused by carbon dioxide retention. Acidosis causes hyperventilation and coma and reduces cardiac output. A rise in circulating catecholamines increases both the force and the rate of cardiac contraction while

---

*kPa = 7.6 mm Hg.

Table 21–1

■

Toxic Gases and Fumes

Agent	Principal Occupations Exposed	Main Mechanism of Injury	Time-weighted Average*	IDLH Level †
Acrolein	Plastic, rubber, textile, resin making	Direct action on mucosa of the eyes and respiratory tract, irritant effects	0.1 ppm	5 ppm
Acrylonitrile	Synthetic fiber, acrylic resin, rubber making	Asphyxiant	2 ppm	4 ppm
Ammonia	Fertilizer, refrigerator, explosive production	Direct action on mucosa of the eyes and respiratory tract, tracheitis and pulmonary edema	25 ppm	500 ppm
Arsine	Smelting, refining	Systemic effects	0.05 ppm	6 ppm
Cadmium oxide fumes	Ore smelting, alloying, welding	Acute tracheobronchitis, pulmonary edema Emphysema, renal effects	0.1 mg/m^3 (40 μg/m^3)	40 mg/m^3
Carbon dioxide	Foundry work, mining	Asphyxiant	10,000 ppm	50,000 ppm
Carbon disulfide	Degreasing, electroplating, sulfur processing	Systemic effects	4 ppm (1 ppm)	500 ppm
Carbon monoxide	Foundry work, petroleum refining, mining	Asphyxiant	35 ppm	1500 ppm
Chlorine	Bleaching, disinfectant and plastic making	Direct action on mucosa of the eyes and respiratory tract, tracheitis and pulmonary edema. Possible chronic effect and airways obstruction	0.5 ppm	25 ppm
Copper fumes	Welding	Systemic effects	0.1 mg/m^3	—
Formaldehyde	Disinfectant, embalming fluid use, paper and photography industry	Direct action on mucosa of the eyes and respiratory tract, dermatitis, and asthma?	1 ppm (0.8 ppm)	100 ppm
Hydrogen chloride	Refining, dye making, organic chemical synthesis	Direct action on mucosa of the eyes and respiratory tract, tracheobronchitis	5 ppm	100 ppm
Hydrogen cyanide	Electroplating, fumigant work, steel industry	Systemic effects	10 ppm	50 ppm
Hydrogen fluoride	Etching, petroleum industry, silk working	Direct action on mucosa of the eyes and respiratory tract, tracheitis	3 ppm	20 ppm
Hydrogen sulfide	Natural gas making, paper pulp, sewage treatment, tannery work, oil well prospecting	Systemic and local effects, pulmonary edema, and asphyxia	10 ppm	300 ppm
Magnesium oxide fumes	Welding, alloy, flare, filament making	Systemic effects	15 mg/m^3	—
Manganese fumes	Foundry work, battery making, permanganate manufacture	Systemic effects, possible predisposition to pneumonia	5 mg/m^3	—
Mercury fumes	Electrolysis	Direct action on mucosa of eyes, gastrointestinal tract, and lung Interstitial pneumonitis, systemic effects	0.1 mg/m^3 (0.05 mg/m^3)	28 mg/m^3
Methyl bromide	Fumigating, dye and refrigerant making	Direct action on mucosa of the eyes and respiratory tract	5 ppm	2000 ppm
Natural gas	Mining, petroleum refining, power plant work	Asphyxiant	—	—
Nitrogen dioxide	Arc welding, dye and fertilizer making, farming	Irritant to respiratory tract, tracheitis, pulmonary edema, and bronchiolitis obliterans	5 ppm (1 ppm)	50 ppm
Osmium tetroxide fumes	Alloy making, platinum hardening	Direct irritation of respiratory tract	0.002 mg/m^3	1 mg/m^3
Ozone	Arc welding, air, sewage and water treatment	Direct irritation of respiratory tract	0.1 ppm	10 ppm
Phosgene	Chemical industry, dye and insecticide making	Direct irritation of respiratory tract, pulmonary edema	0.1 ppm	2 ppm
Platinum, soluble salts (mist)	Alloy, mirror making, electroplating, catalysis, and ceramic work	Asthmatic reactions	0.002 mg/m^3	—
Sulfur dioxide	Bleaching, ore smelting, paper manufacture, refrigeration industry	Direct action on the respiratory tract, bronchitis, exceptional pulmonary edema	2 ppm (0.5 ppm)	100 ppm
Vanadium pentoxide fumes	Glass, ceramic, alloy making, chemical industry (catalysis)	Direct action on respiratory tract, bronchitis, asthma	0.5 mg/m^3 (0.05 mg/m^3)	70 mg/m^3
Zinc chloride fumes	Dry cell making, soldering, textile finishing	Direct action on respiratory tract, irritant	1 mg/m^3	2000 mg/m^3
Zinc oxide fumes	Welding	Systemic effects	5 mg/m^3	—

*Figures in parentheses are National Institute of Occupational Safety and Health (NIOSH) recommendations.
†IDLH, immediately dangerous to life or health.

diverting tissue blood flow to the skin and voluntary musculature. The cardiovascular effects of acidosis are therefore somewhat counteracted in the early stages of carbon dioxide poisoning.[3]

Carbon dioxide may be detected by its ability to extinguish a flame. In mines, a safety lamp is needed, and in other situations, a naked flame is adequate. Once carbon dioxide has been detected, work should not be resumed without breathing apparatus until the gas has been displaced by air.

Inert Gases

All of the inert gases cause simple asphyxia. This is a fairly simple and straightforward concept, and yet asphyxiation from this cause has been an important cause of death in the diving industry for many years (see Chapter 22). Divers breathing compressed air are prone to a battery of ill effects, including narcosis and decompression sickness, some of which are ameliorated by either increasing the concentration of oxygen breathed or changing over to breathing helium and oxygen. Such gas mixtures have to be premixed, and this task is often performed at the diving installation. Death has been caused by switching the diver breathing supply to cylinders, held for gas mixing purposes only, containing inadequate oxygen levels. Such events have led to regulations forbidding the supply of 100% helium and nitrogen to diving installations in the North Sea and to obligatory oxygen analysis of all breathing gas during diving operations. The problem is not unique to diving, and asphyxia due to administration of 100% nitrous oxide to patients, caused by inadvertent switching of the gas supply lines to anesthetic machines, continues to be of concern.

Hydrocarbons

Very high concentrations of short chain length aliphatic hydrocarbons, such as methane and ethane, cause death by simple asphyxia. In addition, alicyclic, aliphatic, and aromatic hydrocarbons may have an anesthetic potency. For aliphatic hydrocarbons, this property is related to chain length, and symptoms of narcosis are accompanied by nausea, headache, and dizziness. Like many volatile anesthetic agents, hydrocarbons may also predispose to cardiac irregularities, including ventricular fibrillation, caused by sensitization of the myocardium to catecholamines.[7] Exposure to aliphatic hydrocarbons by inhalation also causes irritation of the mucous membranes and respiratory tract, and some members of this series of chemicals have individual toxic properties of note. For example, n-hexane causes a polyneuropathy, and 2-nitropropane may cause liver damage and has a carcinogenic potential for this organ.

Carbon Monoxide

Carbon monoxide is a product of incomplete combustion of carbon-containing matter. It is odorless and somewhat lighter than air. It is formed in all fires and is an important cause of death in burning buildings and mines following explosions. While it is familiar as a hazard in garages and kitchens, in industry it may be encountered around blast furnaces and gasworks and in many other situations in which combustion takes place and leaks of exhaust gas can occur. Propane and liquid petroleum gas burners are often used for heating temporary site accommodation and, in the absence of proper ventilation or maintenance, are an important cause of carbon monoxide poisoning. Carbon monoxide poisoning continues to be the commonest cause of death by gassing in industry, and commonly, a number of people are affected in a single incident.

Carbon monoxide acts by combining with hemoglobin to form carboxyhemoglobin in such a way as to reduce the oxygen-carrying power of the blood, its combining power being some 218 times greater than that of oxygen. The plasma half-life of carbon monoxide in someone breathing air is about 5 hours, and this, together with its high affinity for the hemoglobin molecule, makes it accumulate in the body even at low levels of exposure. As the carboxyhemoglobin level increases, the oxygen dissociation curve of the remaining unpoisoned hemoglobin shifts to the left so that less oxygen is available to the tissues.

Severe acute carbon monoxide poisoning causes rapid loss of consciousness with few premonitory symptoms, but headache, dizziness, breathlessness, and nausea may be noted as well as chest pain due to myocardial ischemia. Cyanosis is not a feature; the subject generally looks pallid. The speed of onset of symptoms depends on the concentration of the toxin, and at low levels, a flu-like illness may be simulated which presents with headache, generalized malaise, muscle weakness, nausea, and diarrhea. A history of such problems, perhaps of some months' duration, can often be elicited in the victims of an acute event. Estimation of carboxyhemoglobin in venous blood can be used to confirm the diagnosis. It must be emphasized, however, that the severity of the poisoning does not correlate well with carboxyhemoglobin level, and the physician should be guided by the clinical state of the patient in making therapeutic decisions.

A significant number of survivors, perhaps as high as 10%, go on to develop a posthypoxic cerebral encephalopathy. This may be manifest in a wide range of clinical presentations. After a short recovery period, coma due to cerebral edema may develop. More usually the problem occurs 4 to 6 weeks after the event. Symptoms vary from parkinsonism to those of a neurotic or even psychiatric disorder, and psychosis has been described.[8] Amnesia may be a feature of the condition.[9] The syndrome is without direct treatment, although some 75% recover over a period of several months. A percentage of sufferers, however, will be permanently disabled. Central nervous system imaging may be normal, but degenerative changes in the basal ganglia and elsewhere have been seen in some patients. The cause of this syndrome is unclear, but animal experiments have shown that lipoperoxidation occurs in the brain 90 minutes after removal of the toxin, and this may indicate that tissue free radicals can continue to damage the brain for some time after the initial insult.[10]

Peripheral neuropathy, myositis, and skin blistering have also been described in victims of this toxin, as has pancreatitis. Tissue hypoxia may cause damage to any organ whose circulation was previously impaired by vascular disease, and death or permanent disability may result from acute myocardial or cerebral infarction.[11]

Treatment is by removal of the victim from the toxic area and cardiopulmonary resuscitation if indicated. The mainstay of therapy is the administration of 100% oxygen, and this must be instituted as soon as possible. It should be noted that the standard oxygen administration systems used in hospital do not give more than 60% oxygen, which should be administered with a close-fitting face mask and demand valve system or a suitably modified anesthetic administration circuit. Endotracheal intubation may be required in severe cases, and here oxygen can be administered by positive pressure ventilation. Metabolic acidosis should be treated by the administration of bicarbonate if severe, but treatment of hypoxia usually results in a prompt reversal of this aspect.

Hyperbaric oxygen may be of real value in the treatment of these people. Coma and cardiovascular instability may be rapidly controlled since, while the plasma half-life of carbon monoxide is about 1 hour breathing 100% oxygen at atmospheric pressure, this is reduced to about 20 minutes at three atmospheres absolute, and enough oxygen is dissolved in the plasma at this pressure to reverse tissue hypoxia immediately. If hypoxic brain damage has already occurred, however, coma may persist, although this often reverses spontaneously thereafter. Hyperbaric oxygen is also indicated after significant carbon monoxide poisoning if it can be administered within a reasonable delay, because there is a strong suggestion that the incidence of posthypoxic encephalopathy is reduced by this practice. Preliminary data from an ongoing clinical trial indicate that the incidence of neurological sequelae is lower when hyperbaric oxygen is given within 6 hours of removal from the toxic atmosphere and lipid peroxidation is reversed in the animal model.[12, 13] In any case, it is the authors' practice to treat carbon monoxide–poisoned patients who are unconscious or cardiovascularly unstable with hyperbaric oxygen, if there is reason to assume that they have been unconscious for a period or if there are any residual signs or symptoms of carbon monoxide poisoning. Simple tests of cerebral function are of great use in this context.

The fetus is quite vulnerable to this toxin; pregnant women should receive fetal monitoring, and hyperbaric oxygen is indicated even when the mother is well.[14]

A significant number of patients presenting with carbon monoxide poisoning have inhaled fire smoke, and this produces a number of complications ranging from acute upper airway obstruction due to glottic edema to acute respiratory insufficiency caused by an inhalational pneumonitis. It is important to be sure that the level of care appropriate to the patient can be delivered in the hyperbaric chamber, and, in very ill patients, this may necessitate the presence of intensive care equipment and staff. Smoke inhalation victims, in particular, should not be isolated from such facilities (see also Chapter 19).

Before return to work, it should be clear that the victim has returned to full cerebral function, and a formal neuropsychological assessment may be of use in this respect. Some form of follow-up is required for 2 to 3 months, with a repeat assessment of cerebral function if the patient's condition has deteriorated or if initial testing was abnormal. Victims of even mild poisoning may feel fatigued for some weeks after the event, and headache on wakening in the morning is common during this time.

Detection of carbon monoxide in mines has in the past depended on the use of canaries, which usually respond to the gas by falling off their perches before workers notice any ill effects. While this normally gave ample warning, occasionally in low concentrations of the order of 0.05% carbon monoxide, the bird adapted to the gas, and the worker could collapse while the bird remained well. More accurate methods of measurement are now available from simple detector tubes to highly accurate infrared analyzers, and these should be used in situations in which accumulation of carbon monoxide is possible. Small personal monitors are also available.

Useful information on carbon monoxide poisoning may be obtained from the proceedings of a conference on the subject at the New York Academy of Sciences.[15]

Cyanides

Cyanide may be encountered in industry as sodium or potassium cyanide or as acrylonitrile (vinyl cyanide). Exposure to the inorganic salts may occur in gold extraction, chemical and photographic laboratories, and electroplating, but cases of poisoning are relatively rare. Acrylonitrile is more important as an industrial hazard, since it is used in the production of synthetic rubber. Fumes of this substance may be inhaled or absorbed through the skin by workers loading or unloading tankers or those engaged in the industrial processes.

Hydrogen cyanide is one of the most rapidly acting of poisons. It rises and diffuses rapidly. About 40% of the population cannot smell its sweetish, almond-like odor. Cyanide combines with the ferric iron atom in heme-containing proteins. Its primary action is to act as a poison of cellular respiration, by blocking the enzyme system cytochrome oxidase, and thus preventing the access of oxygen to the tricarboxylic acid cycle. Cyanide reacts very slowly with hemoglobin to form cyanohemoglobin, but the ferric iron in methemoglobin is more effective in competing with cytochrome oxidase for the toxin, although the affinity of cytochrome oxidase for cyanide ion is higher than that for methemoglobin. Cyanide is also metabolized by a mitochondrial enzyme sulfur transferase which used to be called rhodanase. This enzyme catalyzes the reaction of cyanide and thiosulfate to form harmless thiocyanate and sulfite ions. This thiosulfate sulfurtransferase is present in liver, kidney, and other tissues, although little is found in blood. Another sulfur-transferase present in liver, kidney, and blood cells reacts cyanide with β-mercaptopyruvic acid rather than thiosulfate to produce thiocyanate and pyruvic acid. Both enzymes could be involved in the inactivation of cyanide. The enzyme thiocyanate oxidase, however, catalyzes the reverse reaction, and cyanide may be regenerated if thiocyanate excretion is not efficient.

Inorganic cyanides act by ionization in the blood, but acrylonitrile is much less ionized and has a direct toxic action also, perhaps by attacking cellular sulfhydryl groups. It has a direct neurotoxic action and may also be hepatotoxic.

At low doses of cyanide, hyperventilation, dizziness, nausea, trismus, and weakness may occur, and recovery is complete in 15 to 20 minutes after exposure. More severe exposures result in severe nausea, vomiting, dyspnea, coma, and convulsions.

Patients poisoned by cyanide should be removed from the area, and any contaminated skin should be washed. They must receive oxygen by face mask, and the first aid worker should also administer amyl nitrite by inhalation. A blood sample should be taken for cyanide analysis if possible, but in the knowledge that any result will not contribute to the immediate treatment.

Antidotal treatment of cyanide poisoning is based on attempts to compete with cytochrome oxidase for the cyanide and has been reviewed.[16] One of the principles of treatment is to give intravenous or inhaled nitrite, which combines with hemoglobin to produce methemoglobin, followed by thiosulfate. Sodium nitrite, 300 mg, is given over 3 to 20 minutes, and 12.5 g of sodium thiosulfate is then given, which may be repeated in 30 to 60 minutes. Methemoglobinemia may also be produced by 4-dimethylaminophenol. The methemoglobin combines with cyanide to form cyanmethemoglobin, and the thiosulfate provides substrate for the enzyme thiosulfate transulfurase, producing thiocyanate, which is then excreted. A major drawback of this form of treatment has been the loss of oxygen-carrying power of the blood as a result of formation of methemoglobin. Moreover, it is not as effective in acrylonitrile poisoning as in poisoning by more fully ionized cyanide salts. It has been suggested that undue methemoglobin production as a result of this treatment be counteracted by the administration of methylene blue. In reversing methemoglobinemia, however, bound cyanide ions will be released and, in theory, the patient may relapse rather than recover.

Cobalt has the ability to combine with cyanide, and this is now used in therapy. Cobalt ions, however, are toxic in themselves. Chelated cobalt, dicobalt edetate, is less toxic and therefore a more satisfactory therapy which can be given in larger doses. One hundred and fifty milligrams of this substance contains sufficient cobalt to neutralize 40% of an LD50 (50% of lethal dose) of cyanide. A variety of toxic signs and symptoms can be associated with the administration of cobalt edetate, especially if it is administered in the absence of cyanide. The reaction is anaphylactoid in nature, and there are rare reports of collapse and convulsions after administration in the absence of cyanide. Edema of the face is not uncommon, and this may spread to involve the throat, with consequent upper airways obstruction, which may require endotracheal intubation. Other short-term toxic responses include nausea and vomiting, a precipitous drop in blood pressure associated with vasodilation, tachycardia, and angina. Treatment of these reactions is supportive. The circulation and airway must be maintained. Acute hypovolemia should be corrected, and adrenaline and steroids used as indicated for the treatment of cardiovascular collapse and edema of the upper airway. Hydroxycobalamine is less toxic and may be injected intramuscularly or intravenously, but very large volumes are required to neutralize appreciable amounts of cyanide.

When cyanide poisoning is confirmed, and if the condition is sufficiently severe, the patient can be given 600 mg dicobalt edetate. In very severe cases, this should be given over 1 minute; but in less severe instances, the injection should be given over 5 minutes. The injection of each 300 mg should be followed by 50 ml

50% dextrose solution through the same needle since this reduces the toxicity of dicobalt edetate. Cobalt edetate has been shown to reverse cyanide toxicity as long as 6 hours after poisoning, and there is no reason to withhold the treatment simply because of delay. Although inappropriate administration of cobalt edetate is associated with adverse effects, complete recovery from these, with appropriate therapy, is usual. Oxygen should be given, and there is some evidence that high blood levels may speed the detoxification process. Artificial respiration and cardiac massage should be given if necessary until the antidotes work. Hospital admission is required after initial treatment, and victims should be examined to ensure that the hypoxic insult has not resulted in permanent sequelae such as myocardial infarction or brain damage. Latent pulmonary edema can develop owing to the irritant potential of cyanide compounds, and patients may have a significant acidosis after their hypoxic insult. The detailed pharmacology and therapeutic details of the cyanide antidotes and their side effects have been well reviewed.[16a]

Hyperbaric oxygen has been advocated in the treatment of hydrogen cyanide poisoning and should certainly be considered if available and if an adequate standard of care can be maintained in the pressure chamber. It is a logical progression of therapy, especially in the presence of high methemoglobin levels.[17]

Obviously, great care is required in handling cyanides, and workers handling acrylonitrile should be protected by impermeable clothing. If there is any risk of vapor escaping, an independent air supply should be provided. If there is any risk at all of workers being poisoned, there should be cyanide antidote packs and oxygen readily available, and workers should be trained in first aid and in how to deal with an incident.

Hydrogen Sulfide (H$_2$S)

This gas is well known to school children on account of its unpleasant smell, a property which makes it useful as a means of irritating their elders with "stink bombs." It may also occur in coal mines, gas works, tanneries, and rubber works, but poisoning is relatively rare. Accidental industrial exposure in the disposal of chemical wastes may occur,[18] and a number of fatal cases have been reported in the finishing and fishmeal industry.[19] Hydrogen sulfide is also found in natural gas and constitutes a hazard in the oil and gas industry. Several fatalities have been reported in Alberta, in which hydrogen sulfide, or as it is known, "sour gas," has been emitted during drilling for natural gas and oil. It also accumulates occasionally in functioning oil and gas wells and is generated from crude oil by bacterial action.

Beauchamp et al. noted that systemic poisoning occurs only when the amount of hydrogen sulfide absorbed into the blood exceeds that which can be detoxified or eliminated.[20] Low concentrations of gas can be tolerated for long periods without harm; 20 ppm is safe over a 7-hour exposure. The odor is intense and strong but not intolerable at 20 to 30 ppm. The odor threshold for H$_2$S is very low at 0.13 ppm, but olfactory fatigue occurs above 100 ppm, and at lower levels people tend to become accustomed to the smell. After exposure to concentrations above 50 ppm, symptoms are gradually progressive, with painful conjunctivitis, blurred vision, headache, nausea, nasal irritation, rawness of the throat, cough, dizziness, drowsiness, and pulmonary edema. Two hundred to 250 ppm results in severe respiratory irritation, and in addition to this, nausea, vomiting, and dizziness. Death can occur after 4 to 8 hours of exposure at this level. Higher levels cause a more rapid fatal progression. Hydrogen sulfide is an irritant gas, but its major action is to cause chemical asphyxia due to interference with the function of oxidative enzymes, mainly cytochrome oxidase, by binding to iron. Irritancy is caused by the formation of caustic sulfides on contact with moisture.

Treatment of acute hydrogen sulfide poisoning should proceed with the same rapidity as for cyanide intoxication. The victim should be removed to a place of safety and given oxygen to breathe. Nitrites should be given as in cyanide poisoning, but not thiosulfate. Methemoglobin combines and inactivates sulfide as sulfmethemoglobin. Oxygen must be given until oxyhemoglobin levels return to normal, and there is good reason for the use of hyperbaric oxygen in unresponsive cases. Victims should be admitted to a hospital, both because of the severity of this type of toxin and to monitor for the onset of latent pulmonary edema caused by the irritancy of hydrogen sulfide, which may be delayed for up to 72 hours. The patient should also be examined for evidence of myocardial ischemia or infarction and hypoxic brain damage.

Recovery from near fatal poisoning has been observed to result in permanent neurological sequelae, but this is thought to be secondary to brain hypoxia rather than a direct effect of the gas.[21] Hydrogen sulfide at concentrations ranging from 1 to 11 ppm does not affect lung function in exposed workers. In contrast, a 2 ppm exposure for 30 minutes had effects on two asthmatic subjects out of 10 studied. Airway resistance and specific airway conductance changes of greater than 30% were noted, indicating bronchial obstruction.[22]

Phosphine (PH$_3$)

Phosphine is a gaseous agent universally used for the fumigation of bulk quantities of grain, both in storage and during transport. It is colorless and smells of fish or garlic, having an odor threshold of about 2 ppm, which is considerably above the OSHA 8-hour time-weighted average exposure limit of 0.3 ppm. Solid aluminium phosphide is placed on top of the grain, after which the container is sealed. Atmospheric moisture then reacts with phosphide to liberate phosphine gas, which permeates the grain, killing all pests and remaining there until adequate ventilation occurs. The workers most at risk are grain inspectors, and there is a potential for multiple casualties among the crews of freighters.[23, 24] Phosphine poisoning by ingestion of aluminium phosphide tablets is also a well-known cause of death in cases of self-poisoning on the Indian subcontinent.[25, 26]

The mode of action of phosphine in humans is not precisely known, although it has been shown to be a noncompetitive inhibitor of electron transport in mitochondrial cytochrome oxidase in experimental animals.[27] Phosphine is predominantly a systemic toxin, although studies do suggest that it also has a direct irritative effect, and necrosis of the nasal mucosa has been reported.[28] The initial symptoms of poisoning are similar to those of other chemical asphyxiants: headache, nausea or vomiting, shortness of breath, fatigue, and disorientation. Phosphine is also a hepatic and cardiac toxin. Tachycardia with other dysrhythmias is a feature of this agent, and myocarditis leads to cardiac failure and pulmonary edema, which may be delayed in onset. Multiorgan failure is a feature of severe poisoning, which has a very high mortality.

There is no antidote to this toxin, and treatment is directed at respiratory and cardiovascular support as required. Oxygen should be administered and the degree of tissue hypoxia repeatedly assessed by analysis of arterial blood gases and pH. Exposed workers should be observed for at least 48 hours.

There are no reported long-term sequelae of acute poisoning, but this is probably as much a reflection on the lack of appropriate studies as on actual fact, and either neurological or cardiac problems would not be surprising.

IRRITANTS

Airway and pulmonary irritation is caused by the action of the chemical compound involved but can also be caused by inert particles in the respiratory tract. A particle phase, that may be otherwise inert, can also adsorb toxic chemicals which are then deposited in the area of lung affected by that size particle. A good example of this is fire smoke, in which soot particles have a great adsorbency capacity.

The site of action of a particulate irritant depends on its size distribution, as previously discussed. That of a gaseous agent is related to its solubility in water. Highly water-soluble agents are readily absorbed onto mucous membranes and are capable of vigorously attacking the upper respiratory tract. That is not to say, however, that their toxic action is necessarily confined to the upper airway, but that the initial presentation may be as a predominantly upper airway problem. Less soluble agents are not so readily absorbed in the upper airway and may cause damage only by penetration deep into the lung to be taken up predominantly on the terminal bronchioles and alveoli. Again, however, while lower airway signs and symptoms dominate the clinical presentation, they do not rule out the development of upper airway problems, particularly when exposure concentrations are high. Ammonia is an example of the highly water-soluble agents, while phosgene exemplifies the less soluble substances.

An important point to make at this stage is that substances, either particulate or gaseous, that fall out in the airway stimulate airway reflexes (laryngeal spasm, coughing, or bronchoconstriction) that cause the victim to become aware of the toxin and to take avoidance action. Water-insoluble agents and particles that penetrate beyond the second degree bronchi can be inhaled without sensation, and the symptoms and signs of acute or chronic toxicity are the first indication of a problem which may then be irremediable.

Tissue Damage Responses to Irritants

At high concentration, most chemical irritants cause physical disruption of tissues, and this may be sufficient, as in the case of epithelial sloughing with ammonia, to be an immediate threat to life. In survivors of gassing incidents it is more usual, however, for the inflammatory response to the initial tissue damage to be more threatening. The lag time depends on the nature of the toxin involved, but in the case of nitrogen oxides, for example, apparent recovery can be followed by a developing inflammatory process, bronchiolitis obliterans, that can be fatal.

The acute effects of chemical irritants on mucosal surfaces are ulceration, inflammation, and edema with desquamation and hemorrhage into the lumen of the tract involved. The tissue destruction results in white cell invasion, and this may give rise to the adult respiratory distress syndrome which is associated with a high mortality. The acute inflammatory changes may become chronic, and recovery from the initial chemical trauma may be prolonged. Significant destruction of lung connective tissue may lead to bronchiolitis obliterans, chronic obstructive lung disease, and bronchiectasis. It is also becoming increasingly apparent that a single severe exposure or a number of less severe insults may give rise to a reactive airways dysfunction syndrome (RADS).[29]

Clinical Presentation and Treatment of Inhalation Injury

The treatment of inhalational injury may be regarded as standard, whatever the toxin involved. Speedy removal from the toxin is obligatory, and cardiopulmonary resuscitation is performed if required. In view of the potential for the delayed presentation of serious and life-threatening conditions, all those exposed to a potential irritant should be observed, ideally in a hospital, for 24 hours, even if initial symptoms are described as trivial.

Damage to the upper respiratory tract can present as respiratory obstruction in the hours after exposure as inflammation and edema develop in the pharynx, larynx, and upper trachea, with the glottis being the area most commonly affected. The victim has a sore throat and the voice becomes hoarse. Swallowing becomes progressively more difficult and leads to the stage in which oral secretions are drawn into the larynx. As the airway closes, inspiratory stridor develops. In adults this is an extremely grave sign, as it indicates the airway is almost totally occluded. Patients should be managed with the head raised in order to aid venous drainage from the affected area and allowed to breathe fully humidified air which may be oxygen enriched as required. Steroids can be given to reduce edema formation. Patients should be very carefully monitored because the onset of stridor and difficulty in clearing oral secretions are indications for endotracheal intubation. The throat should be examined only by direct visualization at this stage when arrangements are in place for the immediate induction of anesthesia, with muscle relaxation if required and placement of an endotracheal tube either orally or by tracheostomy, since complete respiratory obstruction can be precipitated. Glottic edema usually resolves in a week to 10 days without sequelae.

Pulmonary edema is also an immediate threat to life in severe poisoning. It may present as cyanosis and is manifest by breathlessness and tachypnea. Breathing is painful, and the victim suffers from a cough which may be dry or, more usually, is productive of frothy sputum that is often blood stained. Examination of the chest may reveal the use of accessory muscles of ventilation, indrawing of the intercostal spaces, and a tracheal tug. On auscultation of the chest, there may be generalized crepitations, and partial blockage of airways results in inspiratory and expiratory wheeze. Oxygen should be administered initially in as high a concentration as is practicable and respiration supported if required. Pulmonary edema may be treated by diuretics at this stage. Treatment is monitored by measurement of arterial oxygen saturation by pulse oximetry, analysis of arterial blood gases, and careful observation of the patient with plotting of respiratory rate. A rising respiratory rate is an indicator of impending respiratory failure, as is falling tidal volume. A rising arterial carbon dioxide partial pressure with concurrent hypoxia indicates that respiratory failure has occurred and that ventilatory support is required urgently. This is provided by endotracheal intubation and intermittent positive pressure ventilation, ensuring that the relative humidity of inspired gas is kept at 100%. The aim of therapy is to maintain an optimal level of oxygenation while avoiding concentrations of oxygen much over 60%, which in themselves act as a pulmonary irritant. The introduction of positive end-expiratory pressure helps in the maintenance of arterial oxygen levels by increasing functional residual capacity and preventing airway closure. Increase in mean thoracic pressure, however, can cause pulmonary barotrauma, especially in patients with lung parenchymal injury, and pneumothorax must be treated quickly by chest intubation when it occurs. The leak of fluid from the blood into the lung can cause hypovolemia, which is aggravated by the diuretics which may have been used in the initial treatment of pulmonary edema. Cardiac output is reduced, urine production falls, and there may be a precipitous fall in venous oxygen saturation. Plasma expansion must be carefully managed, since any increase in pulmonary circulatory pressure results in an increase in pulmonary edema formation and reduction of oxygenation. At this stage, since pulmonary vascular resistance is high, central venous pressure may not provide an adequate measure of hypovolemia, and pulmonary artery wedge pressure is used as an estimate of left ventricle filling pressure. This should be kept as low as is compatible with an adequate cardiac output by the judicious administration of plasma expanders and cardiac inotropes. A recent, and as yet experimental, development in the treatment of this phase of pulmonary injury has been the use of nitric oxide by inhalation as a pulmonary capillary vasodilator. If there is extensive damage to the tracheobronchial mucosa, sudden sloughing of necrotic pieces or the dislodgement of casts may result in the obstruction of major airways. The obstruction may be cleared by bronchoscopy but, if the patient's condition permits it, chest physiotherapy can be as effective. The same condition can be caused by sputum retention, and, since sputum production may be profuse, regular tracheal suction and chest physiotherapy are essential if the problem is to be minimized.

Pulmonary edema may develop after inhalation of irritant chemicals, even if initial symptoms are trivial or resolve quickly. The victim becomes breathless, and the clinical picture may develop as described earlier. Pulmonary edema can be confirmed radiologically, but a chest x-ray may be normal in the early stages of interstitial pulmonary edema formation. Although respiratory failure can develop, the situation can usually be managed by the administration of humidified air appropriately enriched with oxygen. Steroid therapy has been advocated in the acute stage of inhalational injury of the lungs. It is not possible, however, to identify a benefit from this therapy, although it is accepted practice to administer steroids in cases of nitrogen dioxide inhalation. Antibiotics should be administered as they are indicated for specific infective problems and not used prophylactically. Respiratory tract infection is the most common complication of inhalational injury, and it is important that treatment does not induce bacterial, fungal, or yeast superinfection with resistant strains of microorganisms.

Long-Term Effects of Inhalational Injury: Reactive Airways Dysfunction Syndrome

Recovery from inhalational injury may be complete with no long-term sequelae. If there has been parenchymal damage, however, or if acute inflammation becomes chronic, long-term pulmonary disease can follow from a single event.

One particular form of chronic lung disease associated with exposure to irritant gases is reactive airways dysfunction syndrome (RADS). This was first described by Brooks et al., who noted the onset of asthma in 10 people, previously without respiratory disease, after a single severe exposure to a respiratory irritant.[29] In all cases, there was persistence of cough, wheezing, and dyspnea of effort after treatment of the initial injury was complete. Methacholine challenge testing demonstrated airways hyperreactivity in all cases, which persisted with symptoms for more than 1 year and often several years after the incident. Bronchial biopsy in two cases showed epithelial cell injury with a chronic nonspecific inflammatory response and without eosinophil infiltration. The authors concluded that the syndrome was not immunologically mediated. Later work has confirmed the observations made by this group, and it seems that the incidence of an asthma-like syndrome after inhalation of irritants may be as high as 10% of those so exposed.[30, 31]

Ammonia

Ammonia is an intensely irritating, highly soluble alkaline gas that is widely used in industry. Important uses include refrigeration, production of fertilizers and explosives, oil refining, and the making of plastics. Exposure to the gas occurs as a result of industrial accidents in which tanks or pipes fracture.

Since ammonia is very water soluble, the brunt of its initial attack is borne by the skin, conjunctivae, and mucous membranes of the mouth and upper respiratory tract. On exposure to the gas, the worker feels intense pain in the eyes, mouth, and throat, and a sense of suffocation. The voice is lost and stridor develops. The patient is cyanotic, with bleeding, ulcerated mouth and nose, and aphonia. There may be corneal opacification. Continued exposure to high concentrations for a minute or less results in death from asphyxiation.

The pathological features of the acute lesion include an acute inflammatory reaction, with edema, ulceration, and desquamation of mucous membranes. Edema of the larynx is the cause of death in very acute cases, supplemented by blockage of airways with desquamated epithelium. Ammonia penetrating into the alveoli causes breakdown of the alveolocapillary membrane, with exudation of blood and edema fluid into alveoli, and this may be apparent radiographically as pulmonary edema.

Follow-up studies of survivors have shown that the initially severe airways obstruction gradually improves, though they may not recover fully for a year or more. There is little evidence that emphysema is an important complication, and it seems likely that in many cases the epithelial surface of the airways is able to regenerate almost completely.[32, 33] That is not to say that the patient does not occasionally suffer prolonged disability from the gassing, and several cases have been reported with persistent chest symptoms due to bronchitis and bronchiectasis following exposure to ammonia,[34–36] although the rate of incidence of this long-term health effect is unknown.

Management of the patient consists of rapid removal from the area by rescuers wearing breathing apparatus, and administration of oxygen. Weakly acidic mouth and eye washes may give some symptomatic relief. In addition to measures directed at ensuring the patient's oxygenation (detailed earlier), chemical burns of the skin should be assessed and an appropriate fluid replacement regimen instituted to avoid cardiovascular shock while ensuring that fluid overload does not complicate any coincident pulmonary edema.

Chlorine

Chlorine is a heavy, irritating gas with a characteristic odor and an odor threshold of 0.06 ppm (although this rises with repeated exposure). It is used widely in industry in the manufacture of alkalis and bleaches and as a disinfectant. It is much less soluble than ammonia and is therefore more likely to affect the whole of the respiratory tract than to cause acute laryngeal edema. Chlorine is commonly stored and transported under pressure, and exposure occurs when tanks or pipes fracture or are damaged.

Slight irritation of the nose can occur at 0.2 ppm, and symptoms include dry throat, cough, and slight breathing difficulty. Shortness of breath is more marked at 1.3 ppm after 30 minutes, and severe headache is usual. Exposure to 14 to 21 ppm results in marked respiratory distress after 30 minutes, with intense coughing, choking, chest pain, and vomiting above 30 ppm. Thirty-five to 50 ppm is lethal in 60 to 90 minutes, and 430 ppm is lethal in 30 minutes. A few breaths at 1000 ppm results in death. Significant exposure results in the production of white or pink sputum.[37] The conjunctivae are sore and reddened. Coarse crackles and often wheezes are heard in the chest. Pulmonary edema is common and may occur almost immediately or be delayed several hours. Hypoxia with a high alveolar-arterial oxygen difference may persist for several days.[38] The radiograph typically shows pulmonary edema (Fig. 21–1).

The pathological changes are of swelling and ulceration of the mucosa, with desquamation into the bronchial lumen, and pulmonary edema with hemorrhage.

Although follow-up studies after single heavy exposures have not shown any long-term effect on survivors,[39] persistent airflow obstruction, reduction in residual volume, and bronchial hyperreactivity have been found in victims 12 years after a single incident.[40] Workers who have experienced multiple chlorine gas exposures have a lower FEV_1:FVC ratio and a lower maximal expiratory flow rate after age and smoking habits are considered.[41]

Oxides of Nitrogen

Nitrogen forms four stable oxides. Nitrous oxide (N_2O) is an anesthetic; nitric oxide (NO) is oxidized in air to nitrogen dioxide, of which there are two forms, NO_2 and N_2O_4. These last two exist in equilibrium as a relatively insoluble, heavy, red-brown gas with an irritating odor. The oxides of nitrogen, and particularly the dangerous dioxide, may be met in several distinct situations in industry, including the handling of fresh silage, arc welding in a confined space, the combustion of nitrogen-containing material, and the production, use, and transport of nitric acid in the chemical industry.

Silo Filling. Ensilage is the agricultural process whereby green crops, particularly grass, alfalfa, and corn, are preserved in a nutritious state after cutting to be fed to livestock in the winter. The crops are packed in a tower or pit at a controlled temperature below 38°C. Oxygen is used up initially, and the carbohydrates in the plant ferment, producing simple organic acids. A side reaction occurs in which nitrates present in the silage, probably largely incorporated from soil treated with nitrogen-rich fertilizer, are oxidized to give off nitrogen dioxide. This process starts

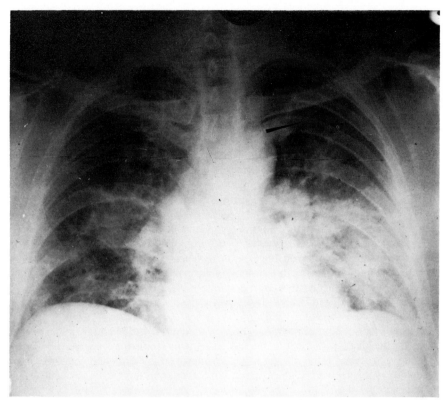

Figure 21-1. Portable chest radiograph of patient exposed to chlorine in an accident at a chemical factory, showing bilateral pulmonary edema. (Courtesy of Dr. F. X. M. Beach.)

a few hours after filling of the silo, reaches a maximum in a few days, and generally ceases within 1 or 2 weeks. However, poisoning has been reported in a man exposed 6 weeks after filling.[42] Farm workers and their families are exposed to this hazard if they enter a silo in the first week after filling, and sometimes even if they approach closely. The disease was known to Ramazzini, who wrote: "... from grain which has been long conserved in a closed chamber, for example in underground places as is the custom of Tuscany, arises an exhalation so dangerous as to be sufficient to cause death to anyone who enters such a place to collect the grain, unless the pernicious air is first allowed to escape for a while."

Arc Welding. The very high temperature of an electric arc causes combination of oxygen and nitrogen from the atmosphere. Many other gases and fumes may be liberated and are normally dispersed by adequate ventilation. If the welder is working in a confined space, such as inside tanks, box girders, or ships' hulls, accumulation of nitrogen dioxide to toxic levels may occur.

Combustion of Nitrogen-Containing Material. Fire smoke from nitrogen-containing materials may contain lethal amounts of nitrogen oxides.[43] A more frequent occurrence is exposure to fumes from burning of dynamite or from shot-firing in coal and metal mines. Usually the ventilation of mines is adequate to remove the fumes rapidly, but injudicious early return to the face after firing may result in dangerous exposures. Very appreciable quantities of nitrogen oxides are also found in the exhaust from internal combustion engines.

Chemical Industry. The most frequent cause of nitrogen dioxide exposure occurs in the chemical industry, in the production, use, and transport of nitric acid. These exposures, as with chlorine and ammonia, usually result from rupture of containers with spillage of the nitric acid, which gives off fumes of nitrogen dioxide when it comes into contact with wood, paper, or other organic material. A risk of exposure may also occur in acid dipping of brass and copper, cleaning of aluminium and copper vats with nitric acid, handling of jet fuel, and nitration of organic compounds.

Clinical Features of Nitrogen Dioxide Inhalation

When inhalation of nitrogen dioxide occurs in the appropriate circumstances, it is called silo filler's disease. The gas is not highly water soluble, and, accordingly, low concentrations are tolerated with only mild upper respiratory tract symptoms. The worker, however, is often aware of the presence of the nitrogen dioxide from its distinctive color as well as from the cough it provokes. The immediate symptoms depend therefore on the concentration of the gas and vary from none to intense choking. Usually, however, they are sufficient to force the worker to leave the site rapidly. With sufficient dose there then follows an episode of coughing, mucoid or frothy sputum production, and increasing dyspnea. Within 1 to 2 hours the patient may be in frank pulmonary edema and cyanosed, with tachypnea, tachycardia, and fine crackles and wheezes throughout the lungs. Alternatively, the patient may simply suffer an increase in dyspnea and cough over several hours, with the symptoms then gradually improving over a 2- to 3-week period. At this stage, when all appears to be well, the disease may relapse rapidly. Fever and chills usher in the relapse, with increasing cyanosis, dyspnea, and generalized lung crackles.[44, 45]

Death from respiratory failure may occur either in the initial or the second stage of the disease. A severe second stage with death may occur even in the absence of a severe initial illness. If the patient survives the second stage, he or she gradually recovers over 2 to 3 weeks. Whether long-term effects occur is not

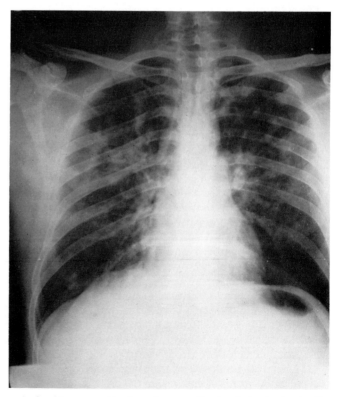

Figure 21–2. Chest radiograph of welder exposed to nitrous fumes working in a fuel tank, showing ill-defined, large nodular opacities throughout both lungs. The patient presented with signs of pulmonary edema and recovered with steroid treatment. (Courtesy of Drs. Glynne Jones and A. C. Douglas.)

certain, though apparently almost complete recovery has occurred in most reported cases.

The radiographic features on the acute initial stage vary from normality to typical pulmonary edema (Fig. 21–2), although most reports mention a nodular component even at the onset. The radiographic picture may then clear, only to show miliary mottling resembling hematogenous tuberculosis as the second stage commences (Fig. 21–3). In severe cases the mottling may become confluent in places.

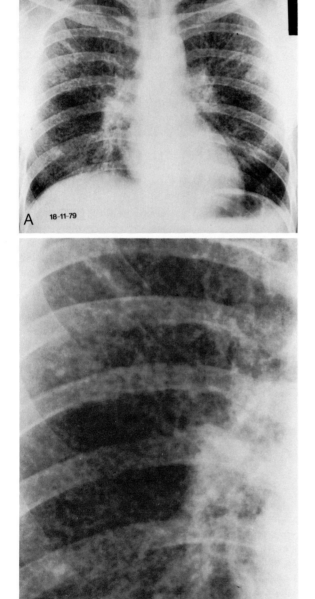

Figure 21–3. A, Chest radiograph of Ontario farmer 10 days after exposure to oxides of nitrogen following opening a silo. Bronchiolitis obliterans is present. The radiographic abnormalities subsequently completely cleared. (Courtesy of Dr. D. Ahmad.) B, Magnified view of A.

Lung function tests in the acute stage show reduction in lung volumes and diffusing capacity, with a low arterial oxygen saturation. Similar findings are recorded in the second stage,[45] though generally they are more marked, and very high alveolar-arterial oxygen gradients may occur.

Follow-up studies have shown varying results. Jones et al. noticed an obstructive lesion with low diffusing capacity in one of their patients,[45] with gradual improvement over 2 months. Moskowitz et al. reported a slow increase in diffusing capacity in one patient over 6 months,[42] whereas Becklake found four of her seven patients to have developed symptoms of dyspnea associated with an obstructive pattern of lung function after recovery from the acute effects of exposure.[46]

Pathological examination of the acute lesion shows extensive mucosal edema and inflammatory cell exudation. The alveolar capillaries are dilated, and edema fluid and blood cells fill the alveoli. The delayed lesion shows the appearance of bronchiolitis obliterans. Small bronchi and bronchioles are packed with an inflammatory exudate which organizes with fibrin, obliterating the whole lumen.[47] Serial lung biopsies in one patient have shown that these lesions may resolve, leaving at 6 months some interstitial collagen and some associated alveolar dilatation.[42]

In addition to a possible long-term effect following acute high-level exposures, it has been suggested that recurrent exposures to relatively low levels of nitrogen dioxide may cause emphysema. In spite of much research, this area remains unclear.[48]

Management

The disease can be prevented through the education of those likely to be exposed. Farm workers should be warned about approaching or entering recently filled silos, notices should be displayed on the silos, and fences should be provided to keep children away. Welders should not be allowed to work in poorly ventilated spaces. In chemical works where the risk obtains, the medical officer should educate workers to seek medical help even if the initial exposure was not very severe, in order to be alert to development of the later sequelae.

Management of the acute attack and of the later episode is as described for inhalational injury with the administration of corticosteroids. Although the disease does not lend itself to the establishment of controlled trials, it is noteworthy that in most reports those subjects given steroids have improved rapidly from the time of administration, while those not so treated have often died.

Those exposed to the nitrogen oxides can also develop a methemoglobinemia, caused by absorption of nitrite into the blood, which can be clinically significant, with levels of up to 44% being reported.[49] Methemoglobinemia should be treated by the intravenous administration of 1 to 2 mg/kg of methylene blue, which may be life-saving.[50]

Ozone

Ozone is present in photochemical smog, in the cockpits of high-flying aircraft (especially of the supersonic type), and in the gas produced by arc welding. In the occupational setting, arc welders using inert gas shielded apparatus are the most likely to be affected by the gas, and their exposure is usually not complicated by the presence of other toxic substances.[51]

Ozone is a respiratory irritant, which also causes headache and drowsiness. Cough, nose and eye irritation, and tightness in the chest are the main symptoms. Severe or fatal cases do not appear to have been reported, though animal studies have shown that high concentrations of gas may induce pulmonary edema. The subject has been comprehensively reviewed by Stokinger.[52] Management depends on recognition of the hazard and its removal by adequate ventilation.

Phosgene (COCl$_2$)

Phosgene is a heavy, colorless gas that liquefies at 8°C. It has a faint odor of new-mown hay, but it is only slightly irritating, so it may be inhaled for prolonged periods without great discomfort. It was responsible for a high proportion of the deaths due to gassing in the First World War. It is now used as a chlorinator in the chemical industry, and it is there that occasional cases of poisoning are reported.[53] Occasionally it may result from use of carbon tetrachloride fire extinguishers.[54]

Phosgene in poisonous doses acts as a powerful oxidant directly on the pulmonary capillary endothelium, producing a large increase in capillary wall permeability and interstitial pulmonary edema which may be massive. An exposed worker usually first develops a cough and after 1 or 2 hours becomes increasingly breathless. Crackles may be heard throughout the lungs, and hypovolemic shock may follow. The mechanism of death is hypoxia due to pulmonary edema. Phosgene is also mildly hydrophilic, and high doses may cause an ulcerative bronchitis and bronchiolitis. In survivors, the pulmonary edema gradually improves over a week, and there is no definite evidence of long-term toxic effects in humans.

Treatment of acute phosgene poisoning should be along the lines detailed earlier for inhalational injury.

Sulfur Dioxide

Sulfur dioxide is a heavy, irritating gas. It occurs chiefly as a general atmospheric pollutant, the result of combustion of coal, oil, and gasoline in towns. Among its important effects are exacerbations of disease in patients with chronic bronchitis and the destruction of the limestone of historic buildings. However, it may also be encountered in industry in the production of paper, in refrigeration plants, in oil refining, in mining, in the manufacture of batteries, and in fruit preserving.

It is a highly water-soluble gas, and the initial effect of exposure to corrosive levels is extreme irritation of the eyes and upper respiratory tract. At low levels (1 to 5 ppm), however, the threshold concentration for eye irritation has been reported as 50% greater than for irritation of the respiratory tract.[55] Exposure to sulfur dioxide levels of more than 10 ppm causes irritation of the eyes, nose, and throat with cough, brochoconstriction, and chest pain. Industrial accidents causing massive exposure have been reported in the mining and paper industries, and the victims of these suffered irritation of the eyes, to the extent of conjunctivitis with ulceration, and upper airway irritation with chest pain, intense dyspnea, and cyanosis.[56–59] Most survivors had a normal chest x-ray, although there were decreased breath sounds with crackles and wheezes on examination of the chest, with hyperemia of the pharyngeal mucosa. The chest x-ray can also show diffuse small opacities and light confluent shadowing. Immediate fatalities were found to have a massive protein-rich pulmonary edema, indicating alveolocapillary membrane damage. The mucosal surface of the airways was intensely inflamed and had sloughed in some instances with bleeding into the bronchial lumen.[57] There was corneal opacification. A case has been reported where the victim recovered sufficiently from the exposure to be sent home only to be taken back to the hospital 10 days later with a dry cough, dyspnea, and profuse mucous secretions. He deteriorated and died of extensive peribronchiolar fibrosis and bronchiolitis obliterans.[56] The survivors of this kind of incident are alleged to develop emphysema with hyperreactivity of the airways.

The immediate treatment of such events is that described for inhalational injury, although sodium bicarbonate solution or aerosol may be helpful in relieving local symptoms. Pain should be relieved by an analgesic of appropriate potency, and there is no real contraindication to opiates, especially if administered with oxygen.

Of more frequent occurrence than acute exposure is prolonged exposure to relatively low levels. There is a considerable body of physiological evidence that sulfur dioxide in low concentrations acts to increase airways resistance, and it is now clear that the combination of exercise and low concentrations of sulfur dioxide (0.5 ppm) may lead to an increase in airways resistance in otherwise asymptomatic asthmatics.[60]

IRRITANT AND TOXIC FUMES

Inhalation Fevers

Exposure to a wide variety of particulate agents may result in a debilitating flu-like illness of short duration which is occasionally associated with the development of chemical pneumonitis and pulmonary edema. Water aerosols contaminated with *Legionella pneumophila* cause Pontiac fever, and aerosols contaminated with a variety of microbacteria cause humidifier fever. Organic dust toxic syndrome (ODTS), or grain fever, is caused by exposure to organic agricultural dusts. Many of these causative agents are also capable of producing other clinical syndromes of greater long-term importance.[61, 62] Although the fume fevers have been described as not causing long-term health effects, such comments are made against a lack of follow-up studies for these conditions. Metal fume fever and polymer fume fever are described here as examples.

Metal Fume Fever

Brass founders' ague, copper fever, brass fever, Monday morning fever, and metal fume fever all are names for a relatively common acute febrile illness. The condition results from the inhalation of minute particles of the oxides of various metals. While zinc, copper, and magnesium are the chief offenders, cadmium, iron, manganese, nickel, selenium, tin, and antimony are in some instances responsible. Metal fume fever occurs as a result of welding operations, and it is particularly common in shipbuilding yards where metal plates are being cut and then welded. The melting of copper and zinc in electric furnaces is also a frequent cause of this condition.[63, 64] Zinc smelting and galvanizing are other common causes of metal fume fever.

The condition can be reproduced in laboratory animals and in human experiments. It has been maintained that fresh fumes are necessary to produce the disease, but most authorities feel that the particle size is the most important factor in the genesis of the condition. There is good evidence to believe that the responsible particles are well below 1.5 μm in size and that most are in the range of 0.02 to 0.25 μm. Their high kinetic energy renders them particularly prone to come into contact with the alveolar walls.

The disease has an acute onset, and although there is no form of chronic metal fume fever, repeated bouts are quite common.[64, 65] It appears likely that resistance to the condition develops after a few days of exposure, but this wears off in a relatively short time, hence the term Monday morning fever. Metal fume fever may occur on the first day a new employee starts work, and there appears to be no latent period for sensitization to occur. The onset of metal fume fever in the absence of prior exposure argues compellingly against an immunological basis for the condition, and suggests that the fever and constitutional symptoms are likely to be caused by chemotaxis of polymorphs, with these cells being responsible for the development of the febrile response.

The symptoms of the disease are the sudden onset of thirst and a metallic taste in the mouth. There is usually a 4- to 8-hour lag before these symptoms occur. Later the subject has rigors, high fever, muscular aches and pains, headaches, and a feeling of generalized weakness. There is profuse sweating, and the condition is often mistaken for influenza. Recurrent attacks have also been mistaken for malaria.

The onset of the muscular pains and rigors may be delayed for 10 to 12 hours following exposure. A leukocytosis is often present. All the symptoms spontaneously subside within 24 to 36 hours.

The diagnosis of metal fume fever is entirely dependent on the history and signs. No specific tests exist for its identification. Most workers are able to recognize it, partly because it is relatively frequent and partly because they have seen their colleagues with repeated attacks and the condition is well known to them. No treatment is known, and the usual folklore remedy of drinking milk is invariably associated with a satisfactory course and few harmful side effects.

Polymer Fume Fever

In 1951, Harris first described polymer fume fever.[66] This condition is characterized by a brief but sharp attack of chest tightness, choking, and a dry cough, and occasionally by rigors. Polymer fume fever is often known as "the shakes." The illness begins several hours after exposure to the heat-degraded polymer, polytetrafluoroethylene (PTFE), also known as Teflon or Fluon. Recovery is rapid, and the condition bears a striking resemblance to metal fume fever. As in the latter condition, repeated attacks are common.[67] PTFE breaks down at a temperature of 250° to 300°C., and when it does, it liberates a collection of aliphatic and cyclic fluorocarbon compounds. Many are powerful irritants which can cause pulmonary edema, and inhalation of high concentrations of polymer fumes causes a direct inhalational injury which can lead to a persistent defect in pulmonary gas transfer. These long-term effects are reviewed by Rose.[61]

The smoking of PTFE-contaminated cigarettes is a factor common to most subjects who develop polymer fume fever. Thus, handlers of PTFE should be advised against smoking while handling the polymer.

Osmium Bronchitis

Osmium is an element which is closely related to platinum and derives its name from the Greek word *osme,* a smell. It is extremely dense, almost three times as heavy as iron, and is found as the ore osmiridium, a natural alloy of osmium and iridium. There are deposits of the ore in Russia, Canada, Colombia, Australia, and the Pacific Northwest in the United States.

The separation of osmium from the other metals with which it is found, such as platinum, is very difficult. Treatment with aqua regia is an essential part of the process. Osmium is used as a catalyst for the synthesis of steroids and ammonia, as an alloy with iridium for the manufacture of nibs and compass needles, in photography, and in electron microscopy.

While the metal itself is innocuous, osmic acid (osmium tetroxide) has very irritant effects similar to those of the halogen gases and is slowly formed when the metal is exposed to air. Osmium tetroxide causes intense conjunctivitis, tracheitis, and bronchitis.[68] Paroxysms of coughing and persistent lacrimation occur after exposure, and blindness following corneal damage can occur. Gastrointestinal disturbances, including nausea and vomiting, occur frequently following prolonged exposure.

Prevention depends on adequate ventilation and on storing osmium tetroxide in sealed containers.

Acid Anhydrides

Acid anhydrides are named after their parent acid and are usually more reactive. Acetic anhydride is the simplest member of the group. Their major application in industry is in the manufacture of alkyl and epoxy resins, which are then used in such products as paints, inks, reinforced plastics, adhesives, and encapsulating and casting compounds. In common with other reactive chemicals such as amines and isocyanates, their major toxic effects are irritation of the skin, eyes, and respiratory tract with induction of pulmonary hypersensitivity. Pulmonary edema due to alveolar injury is also important. Phthalic anhydride, tetrachlorophthalic anhydride, trimellitic anhydride (TMA), hexahydrophthalic anhydride, himic anhydride, maleic anhydride, and pyromellitic dianhydride have been reported to cause asthma. The subject has been reviewed by Venables.[69]

Hemorrhagic pneumonitis following exposure to epoxy resins has been described.[70, 71] The affected subjects had all been exposed to a powder containing a mixture of epoxy resin and TMA in a poorly ventilated workplace. The application of heat or baking to the powder caused liberation of TMA fumes. Those affected complained of cough with repeated hemoptyses. Chest radiography sometimes showed patchy infiltrates, acinous in character and suggesting aspiration of blood. In addition, all subjects developed a hemolytic anemia. Pulmonary function testing revealed a marked hypoxemia and a reduction of the carbon monoxide diffusing capacity (D_LCO), the latter being most prominent when the hemolytic anemia was severe. Earlier, before the anemia became evident, the D_LCO was occasionally increased owing to the soaking up of carbon monoxide by red cells sequestered in the alveoli. Pathologically there was a hemorrhagic pneumonitis with intra-alveolar hemorrhage and alveolar cell hyperplasia (Fig. 21–4). The cessation of exposure usually resulted in the rapid and striking improvement in the condition, with the recurrent hemoptyses disappearing within a few days.

In addition, the inhalation of acid anhydrides leads to a variety of respiratory conditions including rhinitis; TMA flu, a late onset respiratory syndrome with systemic symptoms; asthma; and an irritative bronchitis.[72, 73] The asthma may be of the immediate type with IgE antibodies against TMA protein, or of the delayed type characterized by IgG and IgA antibodies against TMA protein.[74, 75] The subjects with TMA hemorrhagic pneumonitis were noted to have antibodies against TMA human serum albumin and TMA human erythrocytes. The levels of antibody activity resembled those of subjects with a late asthmatic response, in which systemic symptoms were present. IgE-specific antibody for TMA serum albumin was not found in the sera of subjects with hemorrhagic pneumonia, and lung biopsy of such people does not give evidence for an immunological mechanism for this syndrome, which is probably induced by direct chemical injury.[69]

Treatment of acute exposure resulting in pulmonary involvement should be the same as for any inhalational injury. Workers who have become sensitized or who suffer from immunologically mediated disease benefit from transfer to a low-exposure job. Those with late onset asthma or the late respiratory systemic syndrome due to TMA exposure improve both immunologically and clinically. On the other hand, only about 50% of people with IgE-mediated asthma and rhinitis improve after transfer, and this has been ascribed to the degree of worker sensitivity to the agent, very sensitive subjects being affected by windblown TMA.[76]

Vanadium Bronchitis

Vanadium is a metal that is related to niobium and tantalum. It is a rare element and was discovered as a contaminant of iron ore. It occurs naturally as the ore patronite (vanadium sulfate) and also as descloizite (lead zinc vanadate). Deposits of the former are found in Peru and of the latter in South Africa. The metal is isolated by roasting patronite with coal. Vanadium is used in making certain steels, since it removes incorporated oxygen and nitrogen from the steel and also increases its strength. Exposure to vanadium may also occur in the cleaning of boilers that have been used to heat oil, particularly from South America, that is contaminated by the metal.

Mining of the ore has not been noted to lead to harmful effects, and exposure to the metal itself is thought to be innocuous. However, vanadium pentoxide and ammonium metavanadate, both of which are used as catalysts, are definite respiratory hazards and cause occupational asthma.[77, 78] The severity of the respiratory

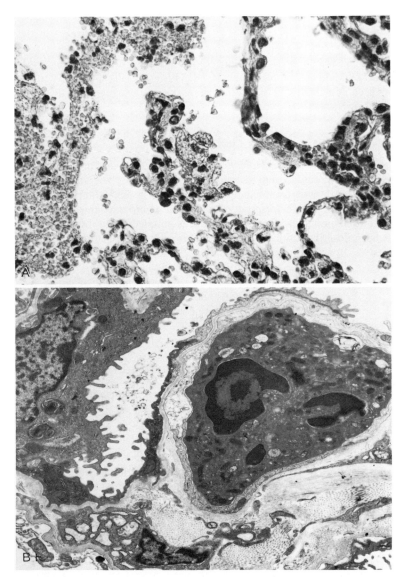

Figure 21–4. Trimellitic anhydride pneumonitis. *A,* Nonspecific alveolar wall injury with intra-alveolar hemorrhage, hemosiderin-laden macrophages, and hypertrophy of the type II pneumocytes. (Courtesy of Drs. A. Herbert and R. Orford.) *B,* Mild focal cytoplasmic edema of pulmonary endothelial cells, suggesting endothelial injury.

effects of vanadium compounds is related to their concentration in the ambient air.[79] Four workers from a vanadium pentoxide refinery were noted to have developed asthma, a green tongue, and upper respiratory tract symptoms. They were not atopic. In one subject the symptoms persisted for 8 weeks in the absence of further exposure.[80] The duration of exposure is also important. Initially there is intense irritation of the eyes with excessive tear production, nasal irritation, sore throat, coughing, and retrosternal discomfort and burning. Bronchitis and a patchy bronchopneumonia may occur. The tongue often becomes greenish. There appear to be no systemic effects from industrial exposure, but the metal is excreted in the urine and feces.

A detailed study of the effects of occupational exposure to vanadium pentoxide has been published.[81] Vanadium exposure increases the number of inflammatory cells in the nasal mucosa, presumably as a result of chemotaxis. Although wheezing occurs more frequently in vanadium pentoxide workers, lung function and chest radiography failed to reveal any evidence of persistent pulmonary disease in the absence of asthma.

Prevention of vanadium bronchitis depends on adequate ventilation, and preferably the process should be completely enclosed. This especially applies when the metal is being used as a catalyst. The wearing of masks and eye goggles is desirable in many circumstances.

Mercury Pneumonitis

Ramazzini, in his treatise *De Morbis Artificium Diatriba,* commented on the association between lung disease and mercury exposure: ''Those who make mirrors become palsied and asthmatic from handling mercury.'' The inhalation of mercury vapor may cause irritation of the respiratory tract with severe tracheitis, bronchitis, bronchiolitis, and pneumonitis. Mercury exposure is an uncommon industrial accident and has been described in extraction of the metal,[82] manufacture of tungsten molybdenum wire,[83] production of thermometers,[84] and cleaning and repairing of tanks and boilers.[85, 86] It has also been described in a domestic setting, in attempts at alchemy, and in the use of mercury-containing paint on boilers.[87, 88] It was formerly used in the manufacture of felt hats and led to tremor and mental deterioration, hence the epithet ''mad as a hatter.'' The common factor has been exposure to mercury vapor in an enclosed space.

The initial symptoms are tightness in the chest and breathlessness starting about an hour after exposure, followed quickly by paroxysmal cough, loss of appetite, fever, restlessness, rigors, and tremor.[86] With severe exposures, the dyspnea may become extreme and death may occur. Otherwise, the symptoms last between a few hours and several days, presumably depending on the dose. With smaller repeated exposures, abdominal pain, diarrhea, and gingivitis may occur. Basal crackles may be heard in the lungs. The chest radiograph may show diffuse patchy changes of pulmonary edema, and lung function tests show a mixed restrictive and obstructive pattern, resolving quite quickly in accord with the patient's clinical improvement.[86] Though mercury may be detected in the serum and urine, initial levels may be surprisingly low, as the mercury is fixed in the tissues. Urinary excretion reaches a peak only 1 to 3 weeks after exposure.[86]

In fatal cases, a diffuse tracheobronchitis and associated acute toxic pneumonitis are found, with alveolar edema and hyaline membranes.[89] Some acute episodes may be followed by a patchy interstitial fibrosis, and in infants pneumothorax and bronchiolitis have been reported as complications. Management of mercury vapor poisoning consists of administration of oxygen and corticosteroids, with general supportive measures if necessary.

Manganese Pneumonitis

Manganese is a silvery-white metal that occurs naturally as pyrolusite. The latter is manganese dioxide and is a black ore found in Russia, India, Morocco, South Africa, and South America. Manganese is used as an alloy to harden steel in the manufacture of such items as rails and mining equipment.

The effects of manganese on the nervous system have been recognized for many years, but some doubt exists as to whether the inhalation of the metal and its salts is harmful to the lungs. Following the construction of a manganese smelting plant in Norway, a tenfold increase in the mortality due to pneumonia was observed in the surrounding area by Riddervold and Halvorsen.[90] While such evidence is circumstantial, Lloyd-Davies described a high incidence of bronchitis and pneumonia in a group of men manufacturing potassium permanganate.[91] Manganese pneumonitis was slow to respond to treatment but apparently left no permanent damage. When mice were exposed to the oxides of manganese, there was a mononuclear interstitial infiltration of the lungs with necrosis and hemorrhage.[91] Further animal studies that tended to confirm the harmful pulmonary effects of manganese were later carried out by Lloyd-Davies and Harding.[92]

Cadmium Lung

Cadmium is a malleable bluish-gray metal which closely resembles zinc. The only naturally occurring cadmium ore is greenockite, but the metal is often present in small quantities in the ores of zinc, copper, and lead. The United States is by far the largest producer of cadmium. The metal is extracted mainly from zinc ores, but some is also obtained from certain lead and copper ores. Cadmium is recovered as a by-product of electrolytic zinc refining and from the fumes of lead and zinc smelting processes. The metal occurs in the form of its oxide, sulfate, or chloride, and subsequently has to be leached, electrolyzed, and precipitated before being cast into bars or anodes for electroplating.

Cadmium resists corrosion and hence is widely used for electroplating. It is also mixed with nickel and silver to form alloys, and is used in nuclear reactors and storage batteries, in the manufacture of jewelry, and in some brazing solders. The ingestion of cadmium salts by mouth leads within 15 minutes to 2 hours to increased salivation, nausea, and vomiting. Later, diarrhea, tenesmus, and shock occur. However, recovery usually starts to take place within 10 hours.

Respiratory and Other Effects

The fumes of cadmium and its compounds are toxic to humans. Exposure occurs mainly from the smelting of ores and from the firing and welding of cadmium-plated metals and alloys. Cadmium fumes are liberated during oxyacetylene cutting of cadmium-coated steel, and the recycling of metallic scrap containing cadmium is hazardous.

ACUTE EXPOSURE

Acute exposure is almost always a consequence of the inhalation of cadmium fumes or dust generated by heating or smelting. Concentrations in the ambient air of between 3 and 100 mg/m³ have been reported.

The effects of acute respiratory exposure develop 3 to 4 hours following exposure and have been well described by Beton et al.[93] These authors reported on five subjects who were severely exposed while dismantling a frame of girders. The fumes were generated by melting cadmium-plated steel bolts with an oxyacetylene torch. Acute exposure is characterized initially by rhinitis, soreness of the throat, cough, a metallic taste in the mouth, and retrosternal discomfort. Later, malaise, rigors, and muscular pains develop in some subjects, along with dyspnea and hemoptysis. The symptoms are similar to those of metal fume fever. Physical signs are relatively nonspecific, but fever and tachypnea are usual. Cyanosis is common, and patchy atelectasis with coarse or medium crackles is often present. The chest film shows either an appearance similar to that seen in pulmonary edema or, alternatively, vague infiltrates in the middle and lower zones.

The necropsy findings in fatal cases are limited mainly to the respiratory tract and kidneys. The trachea and bronchi are inflamed, while the lungs are heavy and filled with edema fluid. Histopathological study of the lungs shows congestion and intra-alveolar hemorrhages. The alveoli are crammed full of large cells showing a deep red cytoplasm when stained with hematoxylin and eosin. These cells are thought to be derived from the alveolar lining cells. Grossly, the kidneys are usually swollen, and there is obvious cortical necrosis that is also microscopically evident. The glomerular vessels are often occluded by thrombi, and the tubules show widespread damage with the presence of proteinaceous and granular casts.

CHRONIC EFFECTS OF THE INHALATION OF CADMIUM

Chronic exposure to cadmium fumes is now known to lead to the development of emphysema. A mortality study of 6995 men exposed to cadmium for more than 1 year between 1942 and 1970 revealed an unexpectedly high incidence of death due to bronchitis which was strongly related to duration and degree of exposure.[94] A later study compared the lung function and chest x-rays of 101 men who had worked for more than 1 year in the manufacture of copper-cadmium alloy with data from a control group matched for age, sex, and employment status.[95] The cadmium workers showed the air flow limitation, lung hyperinflation, and reduced gas transfer typical of emphysema. There was a significant correlation between the degree of pulmonary involvement and the estimated cumulative cadmium exposure.

The symptoms of cadmium emphysema are cough and gradually increasing shortness of breath. The cough is not as productive as that which usually occurs in naturally occurring bronchitis; in fact, bronchitis is reported to be unusual in cadmium emphysema.[96] Physical signs are pertinent to the presence of emphysema, namely, an overdistended and hyperresonant chest with a few scattered wheezes. Anosmia is frequent, as is nasal ulceration. There is often a yellowish band on the incisor and canine teeth; how it originates is not known, but both local and systemic mechanisms have been suggested.

Proteinuria is common and occurs in over 80% of the workers who have been exposed to cadmium for 10 years or more. The protein has a molecular weight of around 20,000 to 30,000. Aminoaciduria has also been reported.[96, 98]

Pulmonary function tests may reveal airways obstruction. The annual decrement in FEV and forced vital capacity is increased in exposed workers.[96] Although chronic cadmium exposure is thought to lead to emphysema, Smith et al. found a restrictive defect in a group of heavily exposed cadmium workers.[99] Five of the 17 showed radiographic evidence of pulmonary fibrosis. Pathological examination of the lungs reveals the presence of marked emphysema in the absence of bronchitis.[100]

Cadmium accumulates primarily in the liver and kidney. In the liver, it stimulates the synthesis of metallothionein, a protein capable of binding to heavy metals, the usual function of which is zinc storage. Cadmium bound to metallothionein then moves in the blood to the kidneys. Damage to renal tubules occurs when the amount of cadmium is too great for the amount of metallothionein synthesized and a toxic amount of free cadmium accumulates. The main effect of cadmium on the kidney is to cause tubular proteinuria, and the changes found in the kidneys in chronic cadmium poisoning vary from no morphological change to severe tubular degeneration. Glomerular filtration has been found to be decreased in cadmium workers, with a positive correlation between markers of glomerular filtration and the estimated cumulative cadmium exposure.[101] Workers who were removed from cadmium exposure because of proteinuria suffered a fall in glomerular filtration rate which was five times faster than that expected owing to aging when followed up over a 5-year period.[102] Liver damage has been reported,[103] and anemia and bone marrow depression may also occur.[104] Finally, no specific treatment is known for either acute or chronic cadmium poisoning, and both British antilewisite (BAL) and ethylenediaminetetraacetic acid (EDTA) are felt to be contraindicated.

OTHER NOXIOUS AGENTS

A variety of other agents may cause an acute rhinitis, tracheitis, and bronchitis when inhaled. Worth special mention as occupational hazards are the hexavalent chromium compounds. These lead to nasal ulceration and perforation, but when inhaled in high concentration may induce a severe tracheobronchitis and pneumonia. The pulmonary effects are usually short-lived, but secondary infection can occur.[105]

Hydrofluoric acid can also induce a severe tracheobronchitis when inhaled. This agent is used as a catalyst in etching and in the refining of metals. Zinc chloride, used in the manufacture of dry cell batteries and in galvanizing iron, has similar effects. Chemical bronchitis and pneumonitis should be treated symptomatically as described previously.

Paraquat

A note should be made of paraquat as an occupational hazard. This highly effective herbicide is used throughout the world in agriculture. It becomes inactive on contact with soil, being adsorbed by clays, and this property is made use of in the management of poisoning by administering fuller's earth. Until recently all reports of poisoning were of accidental or suicidal ingestion of the liquid, but several cases have been reported of lung damage in agricultural workers spraying paraquat.[106, 107] It is probable that the poison is absorbed through the skin rather than through the lungs as an aerosol, and paraquat therefore constitutes a unique occupational lung hazard. There are, however, reports of absorption by aerosol.[108, 109]

The clinical effects of acute oral ingestion are well known, with the lung involved by a progressive fibrosis in fatal cases, although individuals may survive smaller doses with few or no permanent lung sequelae.[110] The chest x-ray findings in paraquat poisoning have been described.[109] Cutaneous absorption from leaking cylinders or from heavy contamination by spray results in skin inflammation and, some days later, pulmonary infiltration, breathlessness, and death from what appears to be pulmonary edema. Smaller doses may be associated with no obvious evidence of disease other than a reduced diffusing capacity, but in such patients biopsies have shown obliterative changes in small pulmonary arteries and interstitial fibrosis.[107] Similar pathological changes have been produced in rats by painting their skin with paraquat.[107] The pulmonary histological appearances of fatal paraquat poisoning are indistinguishable from those seen in animals with acute pulmonary oxygen toxicity,[111] and this agent is thought to disrupt the normal cellular free radical scavenging, leading to unopposed oxidant-induced cell damage by oxygen free radicals and similar molecular species.[112]

Prevention of this disease depends on knowledge of the dangers and the use of protective clothing and boots as well as respirators. Treatment in the event of development of toxicity is supportive and may include the use of corticosteroids.

REFERENCES

1. Health and Safety Commission, Annual Report 1991/2. London, HMSO, 1992.
2. Davies, C.N., Absorption of gases in the respiratory tract. Ann. Occup. Hyg., 29, 13, 1985.
3. Stanford Research Institute. Criteria for a Recommended Standard Occupational Exposure to Carbon Dioxide. Cincinnati, OH, NIOSH, 1976.
4. Prys-Roberts, C., Hypercapnia. *In* Gray, T.C., Nunn, J.F., and Utting, J.E., eds., General Anaesthesia, 3rd ed. London, Butterworths, 1971.
5. Fothergill, D.M., Hedges, D., and Morrison, J.B., Effects of CO_2 and N_2 partial pressures on cognitive and psychomotor performance. Undersea Biomedical Research, 18, 1, 1991.
6. Sayers, J.A., Smith, R.E.A., Holland, R.L., and Keatinge, W.R., Effects of carbon dioxide on mental performance. J. Appl. Physiol., 63, 25, 1987.
7. Zapp, J.A., Jr., The Toxicity of Fire. Medical Division Special Report No. 4. Chemical Centre, MD, Chemical Corps, 1951.
8. Smith, J.S., and Brandon, S., Morbidity from acute carbon monoxide poisoning at three-year follow-up. Br. J. Med., 1, 318, 1973.
9. Min, S.K., A brain syndrome associated with delayerd neuropsychiatric sequelae following acute carbon monoxide intoxication. Acta Psychiatr. Scand., 73, 80, 1986.
10. Thom, S.R., Carbon monoxide-mediated brain lipid peroxidation in the rat. J. Appl. Physiol., 68, 997, 1990.
11. Atkins, E.H., and Baker, E.L., Exacerbation of coronary artery disease by occupational carbon monoxide exposure: a report of two fatalities and a review of the literature. Am. J. Ind. Med., 7, 73, 1985.
12. Thom, S.R., Taber, I., Clark, J.M., and Fisher, A.B., Delayed neuropsychiatric sequelae following CO poisoning and the role of treatment with 100% oxygen or hyperbaric oxygen—a prospective, randomized clinical study. Undersea Biomedical Research, 19(suppl), 47, 1992.

13. Thom, S.R., Antagonism of carbon monoxide-mediated brain lip peroxidation by hyperbaric oxygen. Toxicol. Appl. Pharmacol., 105, 340, 1990.

14. Van Hoesen, K.B., Camporesi, E.M., Moon, R.E., et al., Should hyperbaric oxygen be used to treat the pregnant patient for acute carbon monoxide poisoning? J.A.M.A., 261, 1039, 1989.

15. New York Academy of Sciences, Conference on the Biological Effects of Carbon Monoxide. Ann. N.Y. Acad. Sci., 174, 1, 1970.

16. Shusterman, D.J., Clinical smoke inhalation injury: systemic effects. Occup. Med. State of the Art Reviews, 8, 469, 1993.

16a. Dollery, C., ed., Therapeutic Drugs. Edinburgh, Churchill Livingstone, 1991.

17. Scolnick, B., Hamel, D., and Woolf, A.D., Successful treatment of life-threatening propionitrile exposure with sodium nitrite/sodium thiosulfate followed by hyperbaric oxygen. J. Occup. Med., 35, 577, 1993.

18. Simson, R.E., and Simpson, G.R., Fatal hydrogen sulphide poisoning in association with industrial waste exposure. Med. J. Aust., 1, 331, 1971.

19. Dalgaard, I.B., Decker, F., Fallentin, B., et al., Fatal poisoning and other health hazards connected with industrial fishing. Br. J. Ind. Med., 29, 307, 1972.

20. Beauchamp, P.O., Bus, J.S., Boreiko, C.J., and Andjekovitch, D.A., A critical review of the literature on hydrogen sulphide toxicity. C.R.C. Crit. Rev. Toxicol., 13, 25, 1984.

21. Glass, D.C., A review of the health effects of hydrogen sulphide. Ann. Occup. Hyg., 34, 443, 1990.

22. Jappinen, J., Jones, W., Burjhart, J., and Noonan, G., Exposure to hydrogen sulphide and respiratory function. Br. J. Ind. Med., 47, 824, 1990.

23. Feldstein, A., Heumann, M., and Barnett, M., Fumigant intoxication during transport of grain by railroad. J. Occup. Med., 33, 64, 1991.

24. Wilson, R., Lovejoy, F.H., Rudolph, J., et al., Acute phosphine poisoning aboard a grain freighter. J.A.M.A., 244, 148, 1980.

25. Kabra, S.G., and Narayanan, R., Aluminium phosphide: worse than Bhopal. Lancet, 1, 1333, 1988.

26. Khosla, S.N., Nand, N., and Khosla, P., Aluminium phosphide poisoning. J. Trop. Med. Hyg., 91, 196, 1988.

27. Chefurka. W., Kashi, K.P., and Bond, E.J., The effect of phosphine on electron transport in mitochondria. Pesticide Biochem. Physiol., 6, 65, 1976.

28. Schoonbroodt, D., Guffens, P., Jousten, P., et al., Acute phosphine poisoniong? A case report and review. Acta Clin. Belg., 47, 280, 1992.

29. Brooks, S.M., Weiss, M.A., and Bernstein, I.L., Reactive airways dysfunction syndrome (RADS): persistent asthma syndrome after high level irritant exposure. Chest, 88, 376, 1985.

30. Boulet, L-P., Increases in airway responsiveness following acute exposure to respiratory irritants: reactive airways dysfunction syndrome or occupational asthma? Chest, 94, 476, 1988.

31. Brooks, S.M., Occupational and environmental asthma. In Rom, W.N., ed., Environmental and Occupational Medicine. Boston, Little, Brown and Company, 1992.

32. Levy, D.M., Divertie, M.B., Litzow, T.J., and Henderson, J.W., Ammonia burns of the face and respiratory tract. J.A.M.A., 190, 873, 1964.

33. Walton, M., Industrial ammonia gassing. Br. J. Ind. Med., 30, 78, 1973.

34. Ziskind, M., Ellithorpe, B.D., and Wiles, H., The relationship of lung disease to air pollutants and noxious gases. In Baum, J.L., ed., Textbook of Pulmonary Disease, 2nd ed. Boston, Little, Brown and Co., l974.

35. Leduc, D., Gris, P., Lhereux, P., et al., Acute and long term respiratory damage following inhalation of ammonia. Thorax, 47, 755, 1992.

36. Kass, I., Zamel, N., Dobry, C.A., and Holzer, M., Bronchiectasis following ammonia burns of the respiratory tract. Chest, 62, 282, 1972.

37. Joyner, R.E., and Durel, E.G., Accidental liquid chlorine spill in a rural community. J. Occup. Med., 4, 152, 1962.

38. Beach, F.X.M., Jones, E.S., and Scarrow, G.D., Respiratory effects of chlorine gas. Br. J. Ind. Med., 26, 231, 1969.

39. Jones, R.N., Hughes, J.M., Glindmeycr, H., and Weill, H., Lung function after acute chlorine exposure. Am. Rev. Respir. Dis., 134, 1190, 1986.

40. Schwartz, D.A., Smith, D.D., and Lakshminarayan, S., The pulmonary sequelae associated with accidental inhalational of chlorine gas. Chest, 97, 820, 1990.

41. Salisbury, D.A., Enarson, D.A., Chan-Yeung, M., and Kennedy, S.M., First-aid reports of acute chlorine gassing among pulpmill workers as predictors of lung health consequences. Am. J. Ind. Med., 20, 71, 1991.

42. Moskowitz, R.L., Lyons, H.A., and Cottle, H.R., Silo filler's disease, clinical, physiologic and pathologic study of a patient. Am. J. Med., 36, 457, 1964.

43. Nichols, B.H., The clinical effects of the inhalation of nitrogen dioxide. AJR Am. J. Roentgenol., 23, 516, 1930.

44. Lowry, T., and Schuman, L.M., "Silo filler's disease"—a syndrome caused by nitrogen dioxide. J.A.M.A., 162, 153, 1956

45. Jones, G.R., Proudfoot, A.T., and Hall, J.I., Pulmonary effects of acute exposure to nitrous fumes. Thorax, 28, 61, 1973.

46. Becklake, M.R., Goldman, H.I., Bosman, A.R., and Freed, C.C., The long-term effects of exposure to nitrous fumes. Am. Rev. Tuberc., 76, 398, 1957.
47. McAdams, A.J., Bronchiolitis obliterans. Am. J. Med., 19, 314, 1955.
48. Schlesinger, R.B., Nitrogen dioxide. *In* Rom, W.N., ed., Environmental and Occupational Medicine. Boston, Little, Brown and Company, 1992.
49. Fleetham, J.A., Tunnicliffe, B.W., and Munt, P.W., Methemoglobinaemia and the oxides of nitrogen. N. Engl. J. Med., 298, 1130, 1978.
50. Clutton-Brock, J., Two cases of poisoning by contamination of nitrous oxide with higher oxides of nitrogen during anaesthesia. Br. J. Anaesth., 39, 388, 1967.
51. Challen, P.J.R., Hickish, D.E., and Bedford, J., An investigation of some health hazards in an inert-gas tungsten-arc welding shop. Br. J. Ind. Med., 15, 276, 1958.
52. Stokinger, H.E., Ozone toxicity. A review of research and industrial experience: 1954–1964. Arch. Environ. Health, 10, 719, 1961.
53. Everett, E.D., and Overholt, E.L., Phosgene poisoning. J.A.M.A., 205, 103, 1968
54. Seidelin, R., Inhalation of phosgene in a fire-extinguisher accident. Thorax, 16, 91, 1961.
55. Douglas, R.B., and Coe, J.E., The relative sensitivity of the human eye and lung to irritant gases. Ann. Occup. Hyg., 31, 265, 1987.
56. Galea, M., Fatal sulfur dioxide inhalation. Can. Med. Assoc. J., 91, 345, 1964.
57. Charan, N.B., Myers, C.G., Lakshminarayan, S., and Spencer, T.M., Pulmonary injuries associated with acute sulfur dioxide inhalation. Am. Rev. Respir. Dis., 119, 555, 1979.
58. Härkönen, H., Nordman, H., Korhonen, I., and Winblad, I., Long-term effects of exposure to sulfur dioxide. Am. Rev. Respir. Dis., 128, 890, 1983.
59. Rabinovitch, R., Greyson, N.D., Weiser, W., and Hoffstein, V., Clinical and laboratory features of acute sulfur dioxide inhalation poisoning: two year follow-up. Am. Rev. Respir. Dis., 139, 556, 1989.
60. Sheppard, D., Mechanisms of airway responses to inhaled sulfur dioxide. *In* Loke, J., ed., Lung Bilogy in Health and Disease, Vol. 34. Pathophysiology and Treatment of Inhalation Injuries. New York, Marcel Dekker, 1988.
61. Rose, C.S., Inhalation fevers. *In* Rom, W.N., ed., Environmental and Occupational Medicine. Boston, Little, Brown and Company, 1992.
62. Rask-Andersen, A., and Pratt, D.S., Inhalation fever: a proposed unifying term for febrile reactions to inhalation of noxious substances. Br. J. Occup. Med., 49, 40, 1992.
63. Hamilton, A., and Johnstone, R.T., Industrial Toxicology. New York, Oxford Loose Leaf Medicine, 1945, p. 164.
64. Doig, A.T., and Challen, P.J.R., Respiratory hazards in welding. Ann. Occup. Hyg., 7, 223, 1964.
65. Schiotz, E.H., Welding from the medical point of view. Acta Med. Scand., 121, 557, 1945.
66. Harris, D.K., Polymer-fume fever. Lancet, 2, 1008, 1951.
67. Williams, N., and Smith, F.K., Polymer-fume fever: an elusive diagnosis. J.A.M.A., 219, 1587, 1972.
68. McLaughlin, A.I.G., Milton, R., and Perry, K.M.A., Toxic manifestations of osmium tetroxide. Br. J. Ind. Med., 3, 183, 1946.
69. Venables, K., Low molecular weight chemicals, hypersensitivity, and direct toxicity: the acid anhydrides. Br. J. Ind. Med., 46, 222, 1989.
70. Ahmad, D., Morgan, W.K.C., Patterson, R., et al., Pulmonary haemorrhage and haemolytic anaemia due to trimellitic anhydride. Lancet, 2, 328, 1979.
71. Herbert, F.A., and Orford, R., Pulmonary hemorrhage and edema due to inhalation of resins containing trimellitic anhydride. Chest, 76, 546, 1979.
72. Zeiss, C.R., Patterson, R., Pruzansky, J.H., et al., Trimellitic anhydride induced airways syndromes: clinical and immunologic studies. J. Allergy Clin. Immunol., 60, 96, 1977.
73. Fawcett, I.W., Newman-Taylor, A.J., and Pepys, J., Asthma due to inhaled chemical agents. Clin. Allergy, 7, 1, 1977.
74. Patterson, R., Zeiss, C., Roberts, M., et al., Human anti-hapten antibodies in trimellitic anhydride inhalation reactions. J. Clin. Invest., 62, 971, 1978.
75. Patterson, R., Addington, W., Banner, A.S., et al., Antihapten antibodies in workers exposed to trimellitic anhydride fumes: a potential immunopathogenetic mechanism for the trimellitic anhydride pulmonary disease-anemia syndrome. Am. Rev. Respir. Dis., 120, 1259, 1979.
76. Grammer, L.C., Shaugnessy, M.A., Henderson, J., et al., A clinical and immunological study of workers with trimellitic-anhydride-induced immunologic lung disease after transfer to low exposure jobs. Am. Rev. Respir. Dis., 148, 54, 1993.
77. Symanski, H., Gewerbliche Vanadinschadigungen ihre Enstelung und Symptomatologie. Arch. Gewerbepath., 9, 295, 1939.
78. Williams, N., Vanadium poisoning from cleaning oil fired boilers. Br. J. Ind. Med., 9, 50, 1952.
79. Zenz, C., and Berg, B.A., Human responses to continued vanadium pentoxide exposure. Arch. Environ. Health, 14, 709, 1967.
80. Musk, A.W., and Tees, J.G., Asthma caused by occupational exposure to vanadium compounds. Med. J. Aust., 1, 183, 1982.
81. Kiviluoto, M., Clinical study of occupational exposure to vanadium pentoxide dust. Acta Universitatis Oulensis Series D, Medica No. 72, Medica Publica No. 2. Finland, 1981.
82. Warren, V.A., Toxicology of mercury. Vet. Bureau Med. Bull., 6, 39, 1930.

83. Lewis, L., Mercury poisoning in tungsten-molybdenum wire and rod manufacturing industry. J.A.M.A., 129, 123, 1945.

84. Vroom, F.G., and Greer, M., Mercury vapour intoxication. Brain, 95, 305, 1972.

85. Milne, J., Christophers, A., and De Silva, P., Acute mercurial pneumonitis. Br. J. Ind. Med., 27, 334, 1970.

86. Seaton, A., and Bishop, C.M., Acute mercury pneumonitis. Br. J. Ind. Med., 35, 258, 1978

87. Hallee, T.J., Diffuse lung disease caused by inhalation of mercury vapor. Am. Rev. Respir. Dis., 99, 430, 1969.

88. Natleson, E.A., Blumenthal, B.J., and Fred, H.L., Acute mercury vapour poisoning in the home. Chest, 59, 677, 1971.

89. Matthes, F.T., Kirschner, R., Yow, M.D., and Brennan, J.C., Acute poisoning associated with inhalation of mercury vapour. Pediatrics, 22, 675, 1958.

90. Riddervold, J., and Halvorsen, K., Bacteriological investigations on pneumonia and pneumococcus carriers in Sauda, an isolated industrial community in Norway. Acta Pathol. Microbiol. Scand., 20, 272, 1943.

91. Lloyd-Davies, T.A., and Harding, H.E., Manganese pneumonitis. Br. J. Ind. Med., 3, 111, 1946.

92. Lloyd-Davies, T.A., and Harding, H.E., Manganese pneumonitis, further clinical and experimental observations. Br. J. Ind. Med., 6, 82, 1949.

93. Beton, D.C., Andrews, G.S., Davies, H.J., et al., Acute cadmium fume poisoning—five cases with one death from renal necrosis. Br. J. Ind. Med., 23, 292, 1966.

94. Armstrong, B.G., and Kazantis, G., The mortality of cadmium workers. Lancet, 1, 1424, 1983.

95. Davison, A.G., Fayers, P.M., Newman-Taylor, A.J., et al., Cadmium fume inhalation and emphysema. Lancet, 1, 663, 1988.

96. Bonnell, J.A., Kazantzis, G., and King, E., A follow-up study of men exposed to cadmium oxide fumes. Br. J. Ind. Med., 16, 135, 1959.

97. Lane, R.E., and Campbell, A.C.D., Fatal emphysema in two men making a copper cadmium alloy. Br. J. Ind. Med., 2, 118, 1956.

98. Clarkson, R.W., and Kench, J.E., Urinary excretion of amino acids by men absorbing heavy metals. Biochem. J., 62, 361, 1956.

99. Smith, T.J., Petty, T.L., Reading, J.C., et al., Pulmonary effects of chronic exposure to airborne cadmium. Am. Rev. Respir. Dis., 114, 161, 1976.

100. Smith, J.P., Smith, J.C., and McCall, A.J., Chronic poisoning from cadmium fume. J. Pathol. Bacteriol., 80, 287, 1960.

101. Mason, H.J., Davison, H.G., Wright, A.L., and Guthrie, C.J.G., Relations between cadmium, cumulative exposure, and renal function in cadmium alloy workers. Br. J. Ind. Med., 45, 793, 1988.

102. Roels, H.A., Lauwerys, R.R., Buchet, J.P., et al., Health significance of cadmium induced renal dysfunction: a five year follow-up. Br. J. Ind. Med., 46, 755, 1989.

103. Friberg. L., Chronic cadmium poisoning. Arch. Ind. Hyg., 20, 401, 1959.

104. Berlin, M., and Friberg, L., Bone-marrow activity and erythrocyte destruction in chronic cadmium poisoning. Arch. Environ. Health, 1, 478, 1960.

105. Bidstrup, P.L., Other industrial dusts. In Muir, D.C.F., ed., Clinical Aspects of Inhaled Particles. London, Wm. Heinemann, 1972, p. 162.

106. Jaros, F., Acute percutaneous paraquat poisoning. Lancet, 1, 275, 1978.

107. Levin, P.J., Klaff, L.J., Rose, A.G., and Ferguson, A.D., Pulmonary effects of contact exposure to paraquat: a clinical and experimental study. Thorax, 34, 150, 1979.

108. George, M., and Hedworth-Whitty, R.B., Non-fatal lung disease due to inhalation of nebulized paraquat. Br. Med. J., 280, 902, 1980.

109. Im, J-G., Lee, K.S., Han, M.C., et al., Paraquat poisoning: findings on chest radiography and CT in 42 patients. AJR Am. J. Roentgenol., 157, 697, 1991.

110. Fitzgerald, G.R., Barniville, G., Gibney, R.T.N., and Fitzgerald, M.X., Clinical, radiological and pulmonary functional assessment in thirteen long-term survivors of paraquat poisoning. Thorax, 34, 414, 1979.

111. Rebello, G., and Mason, J.K., Pulmonary histological appearances in fatal paraquat poisoning. Histopathology, 2, 53, 1978.

112. Krall, J., Bagley, A.C., Mullenbach, G.T., and Hallewell, R.A., Superoxide mediates the toxicity of paraquat for cultured mammalian cells. J. Biol. Chem., 263, 1910, 1988.

Barotrauma and Hazards of High Pressure

Stephen J. Watt

■

This chapter covers various physiological and pathological effects associated with work at high pressure or underwater. They affect two groups of workers: caisson workers (who are exposed to a compressed air environment at limited pressure) and divers (who are exposed to various breathing gas mixtures, including air, nitrogen and oxygen, or helium and oxygen at a wide range of pressures).

PHYSICAL PRINCIPLES

Unfortunately, pressure is measured in many units, all of which are in common use in different situations, such as engineering, meteorology, diving, caisson work, and medicine. Some familiarity with these units is necessary for a clear understanding of the effects of work in an environment at increased pressure. At sea level, the pressure exerted by atmospheric air is 1 atmosphere absolute (1 ata); approximately equivalent pressures in other units are as follows:

1 ata
1 bar (1000 millibar)
100 kilo-Pascals (kPa)
14.7 pounds/square inch (psi)
760 mm Hg
10 m of seawater (msw)
33 feet of seawater (fsw)

Only small and clinically insignificant differences exist between these. Beneath sea level, the pressure exerted by water rises linearly with the depth by 1 ata for every 10 msw (33 fsw). Hence, meters or feet of sea water are also used as units of pressure. However, for the calculation of gas effects, the total pressure exerted at depth equals the pressure exerted by water depth plus atmospheric pressure at the surface (i.e., the pressure at 30 msw is equal to 4 ata, that is, 3 ata caused by water depth plus 1 ata caused by environmental pressure at sea level).

The important physical concepts are defined by the gas laws. Boyle's law states that "for a fixed mass of gas at constant temperature the pressure is inversely proportional to the volume," i.e., a balloon containing 1 L of gas at 1 ata pressure (sea level) will contain 500 ml at 2 ata, 250 ml at 4 ata, and so forth. Charles's law states "for a fixed mass of gas at constant pressure, the volume is directly proportional to the temperature (absolute)." Dalton's law states that "in a mixture of gases, the pressure exerted by one of the gases is the same as it would exert if it alone occupied the same volume." This means that the total pressure exerted by a gas mixture is the sum of the partial pressures of all the constituents, e.g., in air at 1 ata, the pressure exerted consists of a partial pressure of approximately 0.79 ata nitrogen and 0.21 ata of oxygen with minor contributions from other gases. Finally, Henry's law states that "at constant temperature, the amount of gas which dissolves in a liquid with which it is in contact is proportional to the partial pressure of that gas." A consequence of these laws is that the amount of nitrogen dissolved in body tissues at sea level relates to both the 0.79-ata partial pressure of nitrogen to which we are exposed and the solubility of nitrogen in the body's tissues. If the pressure changes, in an air environment (79% nitrogen), then the amount of nitrogen absorbed or released when equilibrium has been established will be related to the change in total pressure.

DIVING TECHNIQUES

The technique used depends on the depth and the time required underwater. The simplest form is breath-hold diving, as used in snorkeling. A snorkel tube is used to allow divers to keep their face underwater breathing air from the surface. Brief excursions underwater are made by holding the breath. A face mask which provides an air space in front of the eyes permits improved vision. The air spaces in the lungs, sinuses, and ear cavities and within the face mask are all affected by the pressure change as the diver changes depth.

To remain underwater longer, access to a breathing gas supply is required. The pressure of the breathing gas supply must be almost exactly equal to the diver's ambient pressure at depth. This can be provided by an open "bell," which consists of an upturned bucket or jar into which air is pumped from the surface. Halley's bell (1716) was large enough for two men to sit inside and allowed the divers to make breath-hold dives to and from it. A helmet is really a small bell which gives the diver greater mobility and, when worn combined with a suit, as in standard dress diving suits, also provides greater security. Such systems have been in use since 1837 and remain in use today. These systems require the bell or suit to be flushed with large volumes of breathing gas. On ascent, gas which is dissolved in the body's tissues during the pressure exposure must be released from the body. A slow and staged ascent (decompression) must be required to allow gas to escape without the formation of sufficient bubbles to cause symptoms of decompression illness.

Freedom from direct surface support was made practical by the development of the demand valve; this reduces the air requirement to that of the diver's minute volume and, hence, allows the diver to carry an adequate supply in a reasonably manageable pressure cylinder. Closed-circuit rebreathing systems also permit freedom from the surface but introduce important safety problems in the control of gas concentrations within the circuit and require special training.

In surface-oriented diving, the diver leaves and returns directly to the surface. In deeper dives, a closed (pressurized) bell may be used to transport the diver to the dive site. The diver pressurizes the bell on arrival at the site. This reduces the time spent at pressure and, hence, the duration of the decompression necessary. The bell acts as a safe haven during the dive and finally allows the decompression to take place independent of the bell's position, in effect, on the surface. Such techniques allow divers to work at depths of up to 130 m.

At such depths, the duration of the diver's working time is very limited, and the decompression time is inordinately long. However, once the diver has remained at depth long enough to achieve equilibrium between the environmental gas and the gas in the body tissues (i.e., saturated with gas at that pressure), the required decompression time is thereafter independent of the dive time. In practice, this means that a similar decompression is required for either a 6-hour or a 21-day exposure. More effective use of divers can be achieved by using such "saturation" techniques. Divers are compressed in a living chamber on the surface to a "storage" depth of 10 to 20 m above the working depth. The divers can then transfer from the surface chamber to the work site at depth in a pressurized bell and return to "storage" after the dive. The depth and pressure change in this maneuver is so small that dives of unlimited duration are possible without the requirement for any decompression procedure. The divers may live at pressure at storage depth for several weeks, making excursions to the dive site daily for 8-hour shifts. The decompression may last several days, but the ratio of working time to decompression time is greatly improved. Saturation diving is in widespread use in oil field–related diving throughout the world and is particularly concentrated in the North Sea, off the coast of Great Britain.

CAISSON WORK

A caisson is an enclosed working area constructed so that it can be pressurized with compressed air. Used in civil engineering projects such as tunneling and excavation beneath a water level, the increased air pressure prevents the ingress of water into the caisson and permits work in a dry environment. Major projects, such as the Tyne Tunnel at Newcastle, England, or the Hong Kong Mass Transit Railway, have involved many thousands of compressed-air workers on shift work. Entry to the caisson is through a pressure lock, which also allows controlled decompression at the end of the shift. The pressures involved are generally small when compared with diving (up to 3 ata) and are usually measured in pounds per square inch, but exposures are long. The work load during the shift may be high. Specific decompression procedures have been developed for caisson work. Compression and decompression through large pressure locks is slow and controlled compared with that in surface-oriented diving.

PHYSIOLOGICAL EFFECTS

In most areas of medicine, gas mixtures are described in terms of the percentage of their gas constituents, e.g., 24%, 28%, 40%, or 60% oxygen, and so forth. At stable pressure, this is convenient because the percentage relates directly to the partial pressure responsible for the effect. However, it is essential to convert to the partial pressure when the ambient pressure may alter, since a 0.4-ata partial pressure of oxygen (P_{O_2}) can be achieved by breathing 40% oxygen at an ambient pressure of 1 ata, air at 2 ata, or 4% oxygen at 10 ata. The fact that 2% oxygen is more than adequate to support a diver at a water depth of 200 m provides some insight into the potential for breathing gas–related medical problems during deep diving operations.

A gas's density increases with pressure, and this produces direct effects on ventilation. This may be demonstrated by the measurement of maximum voluntary ventilation, which decreases from approximately 200 L/min at sea level to 85 L/min at 6 ata (50 msw) breathing air.[1] This reduction in ventilatory capacity and the associated increase in the work of breathing necessitate careful control of the work rate by the diver who may be at risk of carbon dioxide retention,[2] a potential cause of loss of consciousness. Indeed, studies have demonstrated that a high proportion of divers have a relatively poor respiratory response to CO_2, possibly as a result of repetitive work in this situation.[3, 4]

Oxygen itself has a variety of toxic effects when breathed at increased partial pressure. At a P_{O_2} of 1.5 ata or more, nervous system effects, which include convulsions and peripheral effects such as muscular twitching, are most important. The risk of nervous system toxicity increases with both P_{O_2} and activity level; e.g., P_{O_2}s of 2.8 ata are widely used in hyperbaric oxygen therapy in a resting patient with minimal risk,[5] but the lower level of 1.5 ata is considered a safe P_{O_2} limit for divers working in the water by the British regulatory authority. Pulmonary oxygen toxicity is dependent on both the P_{O_2} and duration of exposure. It may occur at lower partial pressures and, although it was formerly widely accepted that there were no effects below a Po_2 of 0.5 ata, there is now increasing evidence of subclinical effects, such as increased alveolar permeability, resulting from exposures to as little as 0.35 ata.[6] The risk increases with both the Po_2 and duration of exposure, but brief interruptions to exposure with a normal or reduced Po_2 seem markedly to increase tolerance. The initial symptoms are irritating cough and burning central chest discomfort. Initially, pulmonary function tests are relatively insensitive, but ultimately, with the progression of symptoms and onset of dyspnea, a restrictive ventilatory defect develops. This is reversible, but in severe cases with prolonged exposure and symptoms, there may be progression to pulmonary fibrosis.[7]

Immersion in water induces significant effects on both the cardiovascular and respiratory systems. The differential hydrostatic pressure applied to the body in the water in the upright posture results in a redistribution of blood volume, with an increase in intrathoracic blood volume and an increase in cardiac output.[8] Lung volumes are reduced, with an approximately 5% reduction in vital capacity. The increased pulmonary blood volume also has the effect of decreasing compliance and increasing closing volumes, which tends to increase residual volume and gas trapping. Although immersion contributes to the impairment of ventilatory capacity, there is an associated reduction in alveolar-arterial oxygen tension difference. The net effect is probably not sufficient to induce a significant impairment of exercise capacity.[9, 10]

DISORDERS ASSOCIATED WITH WORK AT PRESSURE

Pulmonary Barotrauma

Barotrauma is tissue damage which results from changes in volume in the gas-containing spaces of the body associated with a pressure change. It may affect any gas space, but particularly, those which are enclosed and unable to communicate with the ambient atmosphere (usually gas at the diver's mouthpiece) are involved. The sites most commonly affected are the middle ear cavity (because of difficulty opening the eustachian tube) and the paranasal sinuses (because of obstruction to the ostia). Rupture of the tympanic membrane or rupture of the paranasal sinus mucosa are the usual results, but more serious effects (such as rupture of the round or oval window, sensorineural deafness, or pneumocephalus) may rarely result. Although reported, barotrauma to the bowel is rare.[11] Gas in dental cavities may result in pain and sometimes explosive ejection of fillings.

The lungs represent the largest gas-containing space within the body, and they are at risk from barotrauma in a variety of situations. Barotrauma may occur during descent (compression) or ascent. Breath-hold (snorkel) divers are at risk of barotrauma if they attempt a deep dive without an adequate inspiration. Remarkably, the depth record for a breath-hold dive stands at 120 m (a pressure of 13 ata).[12] If the dive is commenced with a total lung capacity of 8 L at the surface, the lung gas volume will have been reduced to 615 ml at 120 m, almost certainly well below the residual volume. In most people, this event—lung squeeze—will result in chest pain, dyspnea, and cough with bloody sputum, indicating barotrauma, probably at the alveolar level. Lung squeeze may occur in some other diving situations but is a rare event.

Barotrauma of ascent (burst lung) is both more common and more serious. When the diver breathes compressed gas at depth, e.g., 20 m, if an ascent is made without expiration, the lungs, which might contain 6 L at 20 m, will burst as the gas expands toward 18 L of volume. Any situation which impedes gas flow out of the lungs during an ascent presents a risk for barotrauma. Many of these situations relate to diving practice, and considerable efforts are made during training to ensure both control of breathing and of ascent rates. However, panic associated with the exhaustion of the air supply or a rapid and uncontrolled ascent are frequent precipitants of barotrauma. Theoretically, any pre-existing pulmonary pathological condition which might either lead to obstruction to the exit of the gas or in which there are adjacent areas of lung with differing elasticity may increase the risk of lung rupture as the lung is distended by expanding gas.[13, 14]

When the lung ruptures, gas escaping from the alveoli may move along various routes. Following the path of least resistance within the lung interstitium, the gas tracks to the hilum and, from there, either up into the mediastinum and neck (Fig. 22–1), down into the retroperitoneal space, or by rupturing the parietal

A

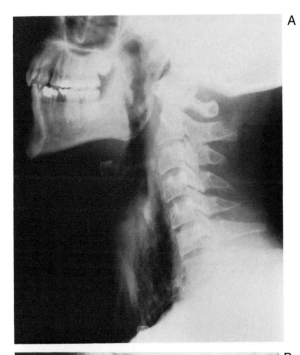

B

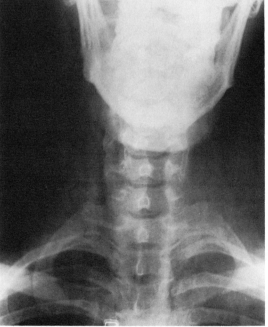

Figure 22–1
Lateral (A) and anteroposterior (B) radiographs of the neck showing gas in the soft tissues after pulmonary barotrauma of ascent.

pleura, into the pleural space.[15–17] Hence, pneumothorax and pneumomediastinum are both common sequelae of pulmonary barotrauma. Gas may also gain access to the pulmonary venous circulation, and in this situation, the expanding volume of gas passes to the left side of the heart and results in cerebral gas embolism. This may occur either with or without other evidence of pulmonary barotrauma.

Pulmonary barotrauma is predominantly a disorder of air diving, and since the volume changes of gas are greatest close to the surface (according to Boyle's law), the symptoms usually present on or soon after arrival at the surface but may be delayed by up to several hours.[18] Cough and hemoptysis may result from alveolar rupture.[19] The symptoms of pneumothorax, pleuritic pain, breathlessness, and cough are typical of the condition in any circumstance. If lung rupture occurs during the ascent some distance from the surface, tension pneumothorax is inevitable at the surface (Fig. 22–2). Likewise, the central chest discomfort, hoarse voice, and breathlessness associated with pneumomediastinum are also typical, although these symptoms may develop after several hours of time lag after surfacing. Only the close temporal relationship with pressure change explains the etiology.

Cerebral air embolism is the most serious pressure-related illness. The presentation is usually a sudden onset of cerebral symptoms, such as hemiplegia, convulsion, or blindness, within the first few minutes after surfacing from a dive. Sudden death may result, possibly from coronary arterial air embolism. Without therapy, the natural history is uncertain; many patients remain permanently disabled, although there is a significant rate of both spontaneous resolution and relapse.[20]

The severity of this illness has resulted in extensive measures to prevent its occurrence. The most vital step involves the training of sport and commercial divers in the necessity for safe practices which prevent rapid or uncontrolled ascent, panic,

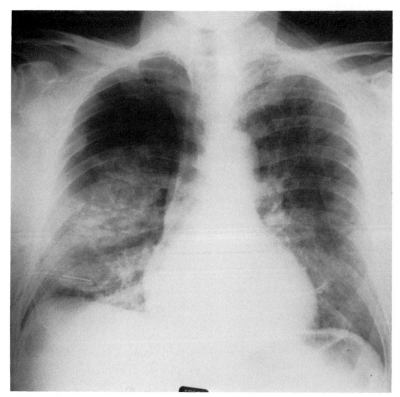

Figure 22–2. Chest radiograph showing right pneumothorax and extensive patchy peripheral shadowing resulting from pulmonary barotrauma of ascent. The diver arrived at the surface with a tension pneumothorax, only partially relieved by intercostal drain at the time of this film.

loss of air supply, or disturbance of normal ventilation during ascent. Considerable efforts are also made during the medical examination of divers to exclude from diving those who have important pulmonary pathological conditions, primarily air-flow obstruction but also focal lung lesions, fibrosis, or other lesions which might affect lung compliance.[21] Despite the theoretical increase in risk associated with such conditions, there is relatively little good evidence that the risk is of significant size. Decreased lung compliance has been found in a group of survivors of pulmonary barotrauma, but it is likely that this abnormality was the consequence rather than the cause of the episode.[22] Numerous anecdotes associate pulmonary pathological conditions with barotrauma. The Diver's Alert Network in the United States has collected reports of many diving accidents. The evidence suggests that the frequency of asthma is over-represented among victims of barotrauma, but this result did not achieve statistical significance. Interpretation is difficult because of the bias against asthmatic divers resulting from normal medical advice to avoid diving.[23]

The treatment of pulmonary barotrauma is dependent on the presentation. Patients with cerebral air embolism should be taken to a recompression chamber for recompression therapy. A delay in receiving therapy greatly reduces the potential benefit, although such therapy may remain valuable even several days after the onset of symptoms. Even moribund patients may make a rapid and complete recovery if recompressed within minutes of presentation; 100% oxygen should be given while the diver awaits recompression therapy (Fig. 22–3).

Pneumothorax and pneumomediastinum should be treated as in any other situation, with analgesia, intercostal drainage, and oxygen as required. Recompression is not normally required unless there are also features of cerebral embolism or a pneumomediastinum has produced potentially life-threatening effects. In this case, recompression will shrink the volume of gas, but therapy is likely to have to be prolonged. When recompression is undertaken for cerebral embolism in association with pneumothorax or mediastinum, the symptoms caused by pneumothorax or pneumomediastinum will be reduced as the gas volume shrinks but will recur on subsequent ascent to the surface. Hence, intercostal drainage of a pneumothorax will usually also be required. Breathing a gas mixture with an elevated P_{O_2} may be valuable in the management of both pneumothorax and pneumomediastinum in a pressure chamber.[24]

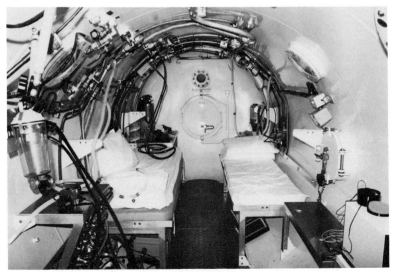

Figure 22–3. Interior of a large medical recompression chamber (Grampian Health Board, Aberdeen, Scotland) showing beds and facilities for medical monitoring, ventilation, and so forth.

Near Drowning

Inhalation of water and loss of the breathing gas supply are common causes for diving fatalities. Entrapment underwater and a loss of the breathing gas supply are obvious precipitants, but poorly fitting or defective demand valves, and training maneuvers such as buddy breathing (where two divers alternately breath from a single demand valve) may lead to water inhalation. Minor degrees of water inhalation occur frequently and may result in other problems, such as the "salt water aspiration syndrome,"[25] respiratory infections, or near drowning. Breathing difficulties underwater commonly result in a rapid ascent to the surface; after this, any neurological symptom, including loss of consciousness, may be diagnosed as cerebral air embolism and considered an indication for urgent recompression therapy. In animal models, inhalation of as little as 1 ml of sea water per kilogram of body weight results in a rapid fall in lung compliance and oxygen saturation.[26, 27] Humans appear not to inhale large volumes of water as they drown,[28] yet substantial acute reductions in dynamic lung volumes have been observed after minor degrees of inhalation injury.[25]

Hence, inhalation of even small amounts of hypertonic seawater may produce almost immediate impairment of lung compliance and ventilation/perfusion imbalance. As a result, the diver has arterial hypoxemia relative to the alveolar PO_2 but with near-normal alveolar partial pressure of carbon dioxide (PCO_2). Both the increased gas density and breathing resistance of equipment may result in some carbon dioxide retention. The increased PO_2 in compressed air breathed at depth may be sufficient to maintain adequate arterial oxygen saturation. However, on ascent to the surface, as the ambient pressure falls, the PO_2 of breathing gas falls to approximately 21 kPa.

Loss of the breathing gas supply at depth produces a situation very similar to a breath-hold dive. Here, alveolar PO_2 falls gradually with an associated increase in alveolar PCO_2 during the dive, but on ascent, both alveolar PO_2 and PCO_2 fall abruptly as atmospheric pressure decreases.[29] The result of this sequence of events may be complete or partial loss of consciousness on or near the surface. The risk of hypoxia inducing a loss of consciousness is enhanced by three factors: the rapid rate of decompression (and hence fall in arterial PO_2) in an emergency ascent, the workload of ascent, and possibly, cerebral vasoconstriction which may occur in response to a transient respiratory alkalosis resulting from the concurrent fall in alveolar PCO_2.[30] Since the circumstances are likely to lead to a rapid ascent rate, the loss of consciousness may be interpreted as air embolism resulting from pulmonary barotrauma. Rapid recovery with the administration of oxygen would be expected, and since an increasing number of diving organizations now carry oxygen for therapy, this situation may be seen more frequently.

Patients with near drowning are inevitably hypoxic, but clinical examination may reveal no other abnormality. The chest radiograph may also be normal or show evidence of pulmonary edema, as in adult respiratory distress syndrome (Fig. 22–4). Pulmonary edema may appear later up to 6 or 12 hours after the incident (secondary drowning) and necessitates admission to the hospital for observation for this period of any near-drowned victim. Management requires administration of oxygen, ventilation, and other supportive measures as necessary and antibiotic treatment of any subsequent infective complication. In most instances, survivors make a complete recovery, but lung function may only recover slowly. Residual damage to small airways function may result.[31] Permanent neurological sequelae are common after incidents involving prolonged loss of consciousness.[32]

Bad Gas

The importance of an accurate analysis of the gas supplied to the diver is clear. There have been a number of fatal and near-fatal accidents when divers were supplied with a hypoxic gas mixture such as 100% helium or nitrogen. In surface-

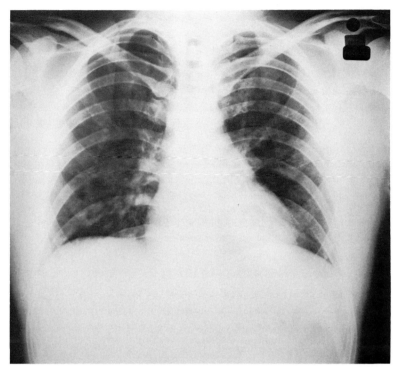

Figure 22–4. Chest radiograph showing extensive peripheral alveolar shadowing in a diver after a near-drowning incident. The diver arrived at the surface unconscious after failure of a demand valve at depth.

supplied diving, continuous on-line analysis of the diver's breathing gas is desirable, with an alternative gas source provided for use in the event of a problem. In sport and scuba diving, the cylinders are usually filled with compressed air, and portable compressors are commonly used to refill cylinders at the dive site. If the air drawn into the compressor becomes contaminated with the exhaust fumes from the compressor engine, the diver may be exposed to small concentrations of carbon monoxide, nitrogen oxides, and other products of combustion. When such gas is breathed at pressure, the effects of small concentrations of toxic gases are magnified, and divers may have symptoms of carbon monoxide poisoning at depth. As in near drowning, the symptoms at depth are partially alleviated by the increased P_{O_2} in the breathing gas at depth, and hence, the symptoms may become more marked as the diver ascends to the surface. This situation may also be confused with other decompression illnesses.

Decompression Sickness

Decompression sickness, known colloquially as ''the bends,'' results from the formation of gas bubbles from gas dissolved within body tissues induced by a reduction in environmental pressure. Bubbles may form in various tissues and result in differing manifestations of the illness. Bubbles that produce their effect locally are likely to be responsible for joint pain and urticarial rash or local skin edema. Neurological symptoms of cerebral or spinal cord origin may result either from bubble emboli or from local bubble formation. It is clear that even symptom-free decompressions are associated with widespread bubble formation, which may be detected by ultrasonic methods, either in the muscles or in the large vessels.[33] Bubbles formed within the venous circulation are subject to the hematological effects induced by the gas-blood interface and are rapidly coated with a protein and platelet complex. Bubble complexes pass through the heart to the pulmonary capillary circulation where most are retained.

There is a significant association between the quantity of bubbles detected by ultrasound and the incidence of symptoms of decompression sickness.[34] It is likely that high bubble loads presented to the pulmonary circulation result in intrapulmonary shunting, with bubbles gaining access to the arterial circulation. Patients with neurological decompression sickness frequently report transient chest discomfort or breathlessness at an early stage of their presentation, which may represent this phase.

Significant pulmonary decompression sickness with acute dyspnea, cough, substernal pain, and cyanosis is uncommon but represents a severe manifestation of decompression sickness, which may precede circulatory collapse. Urgent recompression therapy is required in addition to symptomatic and supportive measures. With therapy, most patients make a good recovery. The outcome in regard to the long-term effects is uncertain. In most patients, the prognosis depends more on the neurological manifestations than on pulmonary effects.

Deep Saturation Diving

Work has become possible at increasingly great depth, and commercial dives to 300 msw are now routine. However, the diving techniques adopted have introduced some additional potential hazards.

This diving practice has many advantages over simple surface-supplied air diving, both in terms of cost effectiveness and diver safety because decompression sickness and barotrauma are rare. However, it has also generated a number of concerns. First, the duration of pressure exposure is considerable, with many divers spending 100 to 150 days a year at pressure. This might be expected to increase any effect associated with breathing dense gas. Second, the exposure to oxygen is considerable. It has become standard practice to use a gas mixture in living chambers at storage depth with a Po_2 between 0.45 and 0.35 ata. Higher partial pressures are used while the diver is working in the water (usually, approximately 0.7 ata) and often during the decompression (0.5 or 0.6 ata) to gain a little time advantage. There is little clinical evidence of respiratory problems resulting from this exposure, but divers who participate in deep experimental dives have been found to experience a small reduction in various lung function parameters, especially the diffusing capacity for carbon monoxide. The values are lower than predive but remain within the normal predicted range and appear to recover slowly after the dive.[35] This effect is attributed to both oxygen exposure and the pulmonary vascular bubble load during the prolonged decompression.

Helium has a remarkably high thermal conductivity. This presents difficulties in maintaining the diver's body heat, and respiratory heat loss becomes of major importance. Heating of the diver's breathing gas is essential at depths below 250 msw, or hypothermia may result from respiratory heat loss alone.

Long-Term Effects on Lung Function

Diving clearly affects lung function. A number of studies have demonstrated that divers have large lung volumes compared with standard prediction equation indices.[36–39] The cause of this appears to be respiratory muscle training which occurs because of the divers' requirement to control their breathing, to breathe dense gas, and to use breathing apparatus with a significant breathing resistance. Even repetitive breath-hold diving can induce an increase in lung volumes, as has been demonstrated in submarine escape tank instructors during a tour of duty.[40] This effect appears to be reversible.

A number of studies have also indicated that divers have lung function indices consistent with a degree of small airways obstruction, particularly decreased expiratory flow rates at low lung volumes.[41–43] The importance of this observation is unclear, and it may be a simple effect of the increase in the total lung capacity associated with training the respiratory muscles. Cross-sectional surveys have also indicated that divers' lung volumes appear to decline at a faster rate than expected, but since the volumes remain above normal, this may only represent a reversible effect and is not evidence for a pathological effect.[44] However, such studies are complicated by the fact that the relationship between lung volumes and age is not linear during the third and fourth decades of life,[45] and this is the age range which includes most active divers. No clinical syndrome of diver's lung has been reported.

More recent studies of saturation divers have again found evidence of reduced air flow at low lung volumes and also suggested that these divers have a small impairment of diffusing capacity, related to their exposure time to saturation diving.[46] However, this population of divers included a substantial number who had undertaken deep experimental dives and may not reflect the pattern in the normal commercial diving population. Deep experimental dives in excess of 300 m have been reported to induce a significant reduction in diffusing capacity which resolved slowly only over a period of months.[35]

A recent study which attempted to separate the effects of the decompression (bubble load) from the effects of oxygen exposure by reproducing the oxygen exposure associated with a 300-m dive at very shallow depth found a small reduction of diffusing capacity, indicating that exposure to elevated Po_2 is at least partially responsible.[47] The small changes in lung function which are observed after deep dives are accompanied by small reductions in aerobic capacity, but the latter is more likely a result of the restrictions on physical activity imposed by life in a pressure chamber during a prolonged decompression.

Breathing dense gases, exposure to elevated Po_2, exposure to the intravascular bubbles associated with decompressions, and the inevitable episodes of minor seawater inhalation may all contribute to a long-term effect on lung function. However, the fact that divers are a selected population with a high level of physical fitness initially, together with the limited duration of a diving career in most cases, may mask the occurrence of a diving-related lung injury, that has not been identified at the present time.

Trauma

With the improvement in diving techniques and the wider application of saturation diving in commercial practice, dysbaric illness has become increasingly rare in commercial diving, and episodes of trauma have become more important. Divers are at considerable risk of mechanical injury from falling debris or equipment and so forth. However, underwater cutting techniques using oxy-arc equipment present a special risk and have been the cause of several explosions underwater. Underwater, a blast may affect the diver directly or after reflection from the sea bed or sea surface. The transmission of the pressure wave through the body may induce substantial injury at gas-tissue interfaces, inducing sinus, ear, and pulmonary barotrauma with pulmonary contusion and pneumothorax. This injury causes considerable pleuritic chest pain impeding ventilation, in addition to the gas-exchange problems associated with the lung injury itself. When this situation has occurred during a saturation dive, there have been considerable problems in the safe decompression of the diver to the surface (Fig. 22–5).

Loss of Consciousness in the Water

Any degree of incapacitation in the water may potentially lead to a fatal incident, usually with drowning as the ultimate cause of death. The diver may lose consciousness for a variety of reasons, most of which involve a failure to control ventilation or the partial pressures of respiratory gases in the tissues. An accurate account of events during the dive is crucial to arrive at the correct diagnosis. A full investigation of such accidents, including an examination of the equipment and an

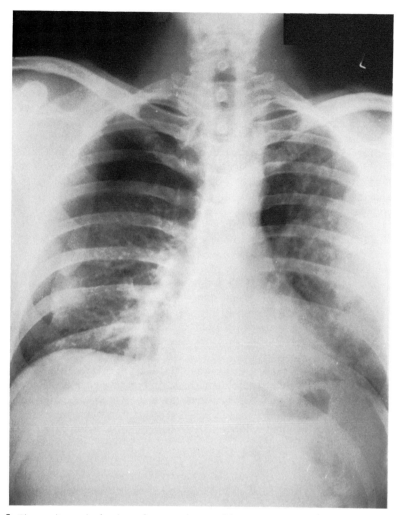

Figure 22-5. Chest radiograph of a diver after an underwater blast injury occurring during a saturation dive showing right pneumothorax and bilateral peripheral shadowing. The latter may represent a pulmonary contusion or the inhalation of sea water. The diver required intercostal drainage during subsequent decompression.

Table 22-1
■
Examples of Causes of Loss of Consciousness During Diving

Diagnosis	Possible Cause	Presentation
Air embolism or pulmonary barotrauma	Failure to exhale on ascent or pulmonary pathological condition	Immediately after surfacing
Decompression illness	Inadequate decompression	After dive
Cerebral oxygen toxicity	High P_{O_2} of breathing gas	During dive or at depth
Hypoxia	Low P_{O_2} of breathing gas	At any phase of dive
Hypercapnia	Hypoventilation caused by gas density	Usually at depth
Nitrogen narcosis	Transient exposure to air during deep helium oxygen dive	At depth
Near drowning	Loss of air supply	At depth or on surfacing
Aspiration of vomit	Secondary to barotrauma or motion sickness	At depth or on surfacing
Hypothermia	Leaking dry suit or poor respiratory gas heating	At any phase of dive
Carbon monoxide toxicity	Contaminated breathing gas	At depth or on surfacing

P_{O_2}, partial pressure of oxygen.

analysis of gas supplies, is also important, both to prevent a recurrence and to explain fully to injured divers the precise cause of the incident. Some of these causes and potential presentations are illustrated in Table 22–1.

REFERENCES

1. Maio, D.A., and Farhi, L.E., Effect of gas density on mechanics of breathing. J. Appl. Physiol., 23, 687, 1967.
2. Wood, L.D.H., and Bryan, A.C., Effect of increased ambient pressure on flow-volume curve of the lung. J. Appl. Physiol., 27, 4, 1969.
3. Song, S.H., Kang, D.H., Kang, B.S., and Hong, S.K., Lung volumes and ventilatory responses to high CO_2 and low O_2 in the ama. J. Appl. Physiol., 18, 466, 1963.
4. Morrison, J.B., Butt, W.S., Florio, J.T., and Mayo, I.C., Effects of increased O_2–N_2 pressure and breathing apparatus on respiratory function. Undersea Biomed. Res., 3, 217, 1976.
5. United States Navy Diving Manual, Oxygen Treatment of Type 2 Decompression Sickness, NAV-SEA 0994-LP-001-9021, revision 2, Vol. 1, 1988.
6. Bruce Davis, W., Rennard, S.I., Bitterman, P.B., and Crystal, R.G., Pulmonary oxygen toxicity—early reversible changes in human alveolar structures induced by hyperoxia. N. Engl. J. Med., 309, 878, 1983.
7. Nash, G., Blennerhasset, J.B., and Pontoppidan, H., Pulmonary lesions associated with oxygen therapy and artificial ventilation. N. Engl. J. Med., 279, 368, 1967.
8. Robertson, C.H., Engle, C.M., and Bradley, M.E., Lung volumes in man immersed to the neck; dilution and plethysmographic techniques. J. Appl. Physiol., 44, 679, 1978.
9. Flynn, E.T., Saltzman, H.A., and Summitt, J.K., Effects of head-out immersion at 19.18 ata on pulmonary gas exchange in man. J. Appl. Physiol., 33, 113, 1972.
10. Prefaut, C., Lupich, E., and Anthonisen, N.R., Human lung mechanics during water immersion. J. Appl. Physiol., 40, 320, 1976.
11. Halpern, P., Sorkine, P., Leykin, Y., and Geller, E., Rupture of stomach in a diving accident with attempted resuscitation. Br. J. Anaesth., 58, 1059, 1986.
12. Bantin, J., Dreams that dollars can buy. Diver, 38, 40, 1993.
13. Maklem, H., Emhjellen, S., and Horgen, O., Pulmonary barotrauma and arterial gas embolism caused by an emphysematous bulla in a scuba diver. Aviat. Space Environ. Med., 61, 559, 1990.
14. Calder, I.M., Autopsy and experimental observations on factors leading to barotrauma in man. Undersea Biomed. Res., 12, 165, 1985.
15. Macklin, M.T., and Macklin, C.C., Malignant interstitial emphysema of the lungs and mediastinum as an important occult complication in many respiratory diseases and other conditions; an interpretation of the clinical literature in the light of laboratory experiment. Medicine, 23, 281, 1944.
16. Schriger, D.L., Rosenberg, G., and Wilder, R.J., Shoulder pain and pneumoperitoneum following a diving accident. Ann. Emerg. Med., 16, 1281, 1987.
17. Rashleigh-Belcher, C., and Ballham, A., Pneumoperitoneum in a sport diver. Br. J. Accident. Surg., 16, 47, 1984.
18. Krzyzak, J., A case of delayed onset pulmonary barotrauma in a scuba diver. Undersea Biomed. Res., 14, 553, 1987.
19. Balk, M., and Goldman, J.M., Alveolar hemorrhage as a manifestation of pulmonary barotrauma after scuba diving. Ann. Emerg. Med., 19, 930, 1990.
20. Leitch, D.R., and Green, R.D., Pulmonary barotrauma in divers and the treatment of cerebral arterial gas embolism. Aviat. Space Environ. Med., 57, 931, 1986.
21. Health and Safety Executive (UK), The medical examination of divers. MA1. London, Medical Division of Health and Safety Executive, 1987, pp. 1–9.
22. Colebatch, H.J.H., Smith, M.M., and Ng, C.K.Y., Increased elastic recoil as a determinant of pulmonary barotrauma in divers. Respir. Physiol., 26, 55, 1976.
23. Corson, K.S., Dovenbarger, J.A., Moon, R.E., Hodder, S., and Bennett, P.B., Risk assessment of asthma for decompression illness. Undersea Biomed. Res. 18(suppl.), 16, 1991.
24. Daugherty, C.G., Inherent unsaturation in the treatment of pneumothorax at depth. Undersea Biomed Res. 17, 171, 1990.
25. Edmonds, C., A salt water aspiration syndrome. Mil. Med., 135, 779, 1970.
26. Modell, J.H., The Pathophysiology and Treatment of Drowning and Near Drowning. Springfield, IL, Charles C Thomas, 1970.
27. Colebatch, H.J.H., and Halmagyi, D.F.J., Lung mechanics and resuscitation after fluid aspiration. J. Appl. Physiol., 16, 684, 1961.
28. Harries, M.G., Drowning in man. Crit. Care Med., 9, 407, 1981.
29. Lanphier, E.H., and Rahn, H., Alveolar gas exchange during breath-hold diving. J. Appl. Physiol., 18, 471, 1963.
30. Ernsting, J., Sharp, G.R., and Harding, R.M., Hypoxia and hyperventilation. In Ernsting, J., and King, P., eds., Aviation Medicine, 2nd ed. London, Butterworths, 1988.
31. Laughlin, J.J., and Eigen, H.E., Pulmonary function abnormalities in survivors of near drowning. J. Paediatr., 100, 26, 1982.

32. Modell, J.H., Graves, S.A., and Kluck, E.J., Near-drowning: correlation of level of consciousness and survival. Can. Anaesth. Soc. J., 27, 211, 1980.
33. Sawatsky, K.D., and Nishi, R.Y., Intravascular Doppler detected bubbles and decompression sickness. Undersea Biomed. Res., 17(suppl.), 34, 1990.
34. Eatock, B.C., Correspondence between intravascular bubbles and symptoms of decompression sickness. Undersea Biomed. Res., 11, 326, 1984.
35. Cotes, J.E., Davey, I.S., Reed, J.W., and Rooks, M., Respiratory effects of a single saturation dive to 300 meters. Br. J. Ind. Med., 44, 76, 1987.
36. Crosbie, W.A., Clarke, M.B., Cox, R.A.F., et al., Physical characteristics and ventilatory function of 404 commercial divers working in the North Sea. Br. J. Ind. Med., 34, 19, 1977.
37. Cimsit, M., and Flook, V., Pulmonary function in divers. *In* Bachrach, A.J., and Matzen, M.M., eds., Proceedings of the Seventh Symposium on Underwater Physiology. Bethesda, MD, Undersea Medical Society, Inc., 1981, pp. 245–255.
38. Clifford, G.M., Smith, D.J., and Searing, C.S.M., A comparison of lung volumes between divers and submariners in the Royal Navy. J. R. Nav. Med. Serv., 70, 143, 1984.
39. Hong, S.K., Rahn, H., Kang, D.H., et al., Diving pattern, lung volumes and alveolar gas of the Korean diving woman (ama). J. Appl. Physiol., 18, 457, 1963.
40. Carey, C.R., Schaefer, K.E., and Alvis, H.J., Effect of skin diving on lung volumes. J. Appl. Physiol., 8, 519, 1956.
41. Crosbie, W.A., Reed, J.W., and Clarke, M.C., Functional characteristics of the large lungs found in divers. J. Appl. Physiol., 46, 639, 1979.
42. Davey, I.S., Cotes, J.E., and Reed, J.W., Does diving exposure induce airflow obstruction? Clin. Sci., 65, 48, 1983.
43. Thorsen, E., Segedal, K., Kambestad, B., and Gulsvik, A., Divers' lung function: small airways disease. Br. J. Ind. Med., 47, 519, 1990.
44. Watt, S.J., Effect of commercial diving on ventilatory function. Br. J. Ind. Med., 42, 59, 1985.
45. Burrows, B., Clive, M.G., Knudson, R.J., et al., A descriptive analysis of the growth and decline of the FVC and FEV_1. Chest, 83, 717, 1983.
46. Thorsen, E., Segedal, K., Myrseth, E., et al., Pulmonary mechanical function and diffusion capacity after deep saturation dives. Br. J. Ind. Med., 47, 242, 1990.
47. Thorsen, E., Segedal, K., Reed, J., et al., Effects of Raised Pressure of Oxygen on Pulmonary Function in Saturation Diving. Report 45-91b. Bergen, Norwegian Underwater Technology Centre, 1992.

Infectious Diseases

Anthony Seaton

■

In general, infection is not an important cause of occupational respiratory disease. There are, however, certain occupations in which the chances of catching such a disease are increased. In some cases, these diseases may be recognized for compensation purposes. Physicians, nurses, veterinary surgeons, medical and bacteriology laboratory workers, farmers, and sewage workers are groups whose contact with an infectious agent or its host may cause disease. In such cases, the connection between occupation and infection is often clear, and preventive measures may normally be taken to avoid the disease.[1]

Less obviously, pneumonia may occur in people as a consequence of workplace exposure. The best known hazard is the *Legionella* species, which by growing in air conditioning and cooling systems has caused outbreaks of often severe pneumonia in a variety of workplaces.[2] It is likely that other organisms can cause similar episodes. The author has investigated one British factory in which four episodes of severe pneumonia, fatal in three cases, occurred in relatively young men over the course of 15 years. All had been exposed to sprayed water from the process, but in no case was the causative organism found. The *Legionella* species was excluded (Fig. 23–1). A similar outbreak, occurring in three men in a steel foundry in Connecticut, was shown to be due to the gram-negative coccobacillus *Acinetobacter calcoaceticus.*[3] Such episodes should remind respiratory physicians that pneumonia is an environmental disease and that the working environment may occasionally be to blame. When a patient of working age presents with pneumonia, an inquiry should be made as to possible exposure to aerosols in the workplace.

Infectious disease may also become an occupational hazard if the job in some way predisposes the workers to the disease either by means of selection, overcrowding, unhygienic conditions, or initiation of another disease that itself predisposes to infection. These mechanisms are exemplified by the increase in mortality rate related to tuberculosis that occurred in Great Britain and other countries during the Industrial Revolution and by the increased susceptibility of silicotic subjects to this disease.

Of all the infectious diseases that are associated with occupation, relatively few can be called strictly pulmonary, although some others, at certain stages, may affect the lung. In the voluntary scheme for reporting occupational lung diseases that has operated in Great Britain since 1989, respiratory physicians had recorded 151 cases of infectious disease up until 1991, although 35 of these were influenza-like illnesses reported in one outbreak. Apart from these, the most common causative organisms were *Coxiella burnetii, Chlamydia psittaci, Legionella pneumophila,* and *Mycobacterium tuberculosis.*

Pulmonary infectious diseases are discussed in detail in standard textbooks of respiratory medicine, and readers are referred to such texts for clinical details.[4] This chapter confines itself to a brief discussion of relevant occupational aspects.

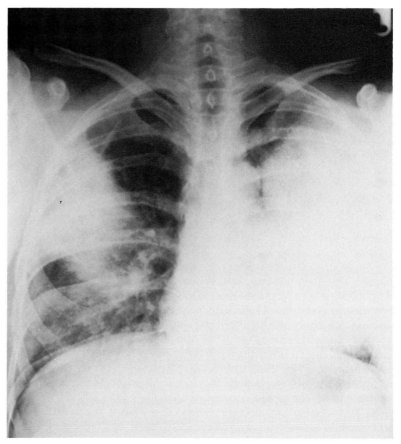

Figure 23–1. Fatal pneumonia in a 40-year-old man after exposure to sprayed water in a factory. Two other workers died from similar disease over a 15-year period.

TUBERCULOSIS

Tuberculosis may occur in three occupational situations. It is a true occupational hazard of physicians and nurses involved in the care of tuberculous patients, of laboratory workers concerned with the identification of the organisms, and of morgue technicians. All such people should be protected by bacille Calmette-Guérin (BCG) inoculation if they were previously tuberculin-negative. Pre-employment and annual radiography is now considered unnecessary in areas with a low incidence of tuberculosis, but such precautions may still be desirable in countries in which the disease is prevalent. The risk of contracting infection with resistant mycobacteria is also somewhat greater among medical personnel, as they have more frequent contact with such organisms. Nevertheless, the treatment is standard, starting with four-drug therapy until the sensitivities are known. It is most unwise to bend the normal rules of therapy to treat a professional colleague.

A second group of workers who contract tuberculosis more frequently than normal are those who work in bars (Fig. 23–2). Alcoholic persons are particularly susceptible to the disease, and it is probable that they play an important part in the spread of this disease in public bars. The presence of crowds with a marked tendency to smoke and cough also probably plays a part. Overcrowding, be it domestic or industrial, is an important factor in the spread of tuberculosis. It was probably the reason why the disease was so prevalent among the makers of boots and shoes in Great Britain in the 1940s.[5]

The third and numerically most important group of occupations in which there

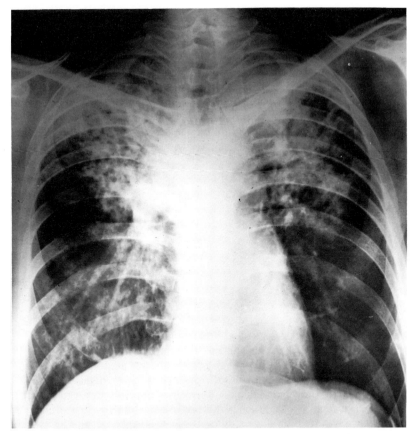

Figure 23–2. Bilateral upper lobe tuberculosis in 45-year-old bartender.

is an increased risk of tuberculosis is that in which silicosis occurs. These diseases occurred together so frequently that until the middle of the 19th century, when the pathological picture of uncomplicated silicosis began to be outlined, a distinction between the diseases was not often made. Aside from any effect the dusty occupations may have had in causing overcrowding, poor living conditions, and so on, silica also acts by potentiating the effect of mycobacterial infection.[6] Even though increasing control of dust in these industries has reduced the prevalence of tuberculosis, the disease remains a fairly common complication. The survey of United States metal miners from 1958 to 1961[7] showed radiographic signs of old or active tuberculosis in 5.3% of silicotic subjects as opposed to 0.6% of nonsilicotic persons. In the same period, British slate workers were shown to have a 0.53% prevalence of bacteriologically active disease.[8] British coal miners, by contrast, were shown to have a lower prevalence of the disease, around 0.14%, although in the 1960s, Enterline showed a raised mortality rate from tuberculosis among United States coal miners.[9] Other studies of slate miners in Britain,[10] metal miners in Sweden,[11] and sandblasters in the United States[12] confirmed that the increased risk still existed among workers exposed to quartz, even in the era of chemotherapy.

The mechanism of the increased risk of tuberculosis in silicotic persons is probably related to the damaging effect of quartz on macrophages. Certainly, *in vitro* sublethal doses of quartz have been shown to allow mycobacteria to grow more rapidly in macrophage cultures.[6] In most cases, the disease process appears to be due to reactivation of an old primary infection rather than to new infection. In previous editions of this book, it was anticipated that the success of antituberculosis campaigns would shortly eliminate the risk of silicotuberculosis in developed countries. The worldwide pandemic of human immunodeficiency virus infection, with its effect on the spread of tuberculosis, has changed this picture, with multidrug-resistant tuberculosis now increasing in the United States.[13] Such optimism was clearly misplaced.

The diagnosis of tuberculosis in patients with silicosis may be difficult because of pre-existing radiologic changes. However, the disease should be suspected in the presence of systemic symptoms (although these may be a feature of accelerated or acute silicosis) and when rapid radiologic change occurs. Features to look for are the rapid appearance of new infiltrates, the development of fluffy consolidation or pleural effusion, and cavitation. However, it may be impossible to differentiate the two diseases radiologically, and the mainstay of diagnosis is demonstration of the bacilli in the patient's sputum.

The treatment of tuberculosis in the presence of pneumoconiosis presents no special problems unless the pneumoconiosis is itself far advanced. The disease appears to respond as well, or almost as well, as uncomplicated tuberculosis to standard chemotherapy.[14–17] Nowadays, the combination of rifampin with isoniazid, pyrazinamide, and ethambutol for 2 months followed by 4 months of rifampin and isoniazid is the treatment of choice. The prevention of tuberculosis in silicotic workers is another matter; there is no consensus. Probably, BCG vaccination in tuberculin-negative silicotic workers is to be avoided because of a risk of enhancing the silicotic process.[18] Moreover, in most developed countries, the risk of infection of tuberculin-negative subjects is still very low. A sensible policy would be to treat tuberculin converters with at least two drugs; many chest physicians, including the author, would use standard chemotherapy in these circumstances.

In epidemic areas, it is likely that tuberculosis promotes the development of progressive massive fibrosis (PMF) in subjects with silicosis and other pneumoconioses. However, it is clear from studies in areas of low tuberculosis prevalence that PMF usually occurs in the absence of tuberculous infection (see Chapters 12 and 15). In the past, treatment of massive fibrosis with antituberculous drugs has been shown to have no effect on the condition,[19] nor has there been any difference in tuberculin skin sensitivity between subjects with and without PMF.[20]

OPPORTUNIST MYCOBACTERIAL INFECTIONS

While the incidence of tuberculosis was declining in the West, there appeared to be a slow but real increase in the number of patients with disease caused by opportunist or atypical mycobacteria.[21–23] It has also been recorded that a high proportion of these patients work in dusty occupations (Fig. 23–3). In one study of 89 subjects with infection with *Mycobacterium avium–intracellulare,* almost one half worked in coal mining or other dusty trades.[22] The same has been found true of subjects with *Mycobacterium kansasii* infection.[24] A British study showed that, of individuals infected with *M. kansasii,* a significantly higher proportion was working in dusty trades at the time of diagnosis than in nondusty trades.[25] In a complementary study comparing patients with *M. kansasii* infection and controls with tuberculosis, the former had a higher frequency of dusty work.[26] It is not clear whether this means that the risk of infection is higher in certain trades or whether the dust load on the lungs impairs the workers' defenses against these organisms.

Further evidence of the importance of opportunist mycobacteria in relation to dust exposure comes from studies of sandblasters in Louisiana and foundry workers in Wisconsin. In the latter, 37% of mycobacterial infections were reported to be due to opportunist organisms, mostly *M. avium–intracellulare.*[27] In Louisiana (where *M. kansasii* is normally the pathogen in around 13% of patients with mycobacterial disease[28]), 41% of silicotic sandblasters with these diseases had *M. kansasii* infection.[12] There are clearly striking geographical differences in the prevalence of these organisms, and much work still needs to be done on their epidemiology and mode of transmission.

An unusual source of infection has recently been described from Australia,

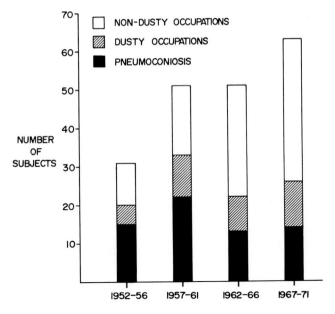

Figure 23–3
Number of patients with pulmonary disease from whom *M. kansasii, M. avium,* and *M. intracellulare* were isolated. Wales 1952–71. (Data from Dr. J. Marks. Tuberculosis Reference Laboratory, Cardiff, Wales.)

where an outbreak of *Mycobacterium bovis* infection caused the death of three seals in a marine park. Subsequently, one of their trainers also fell ill with tuberculosis due to an identical organism.[29] Such infection had not previously been described in seals or been known to be transmitted to humans, and the authors suggested further investigation of its prevalence among such animals. *M. bovis* infection continues to occur in the West, although with a low incidence,[30] and outbreaks still occur in cattle. The clinical picture of infection with opportunist mycobacteria mimics that of tuberculosis (Fig. 23–4). The treatment of *M. kansasii* infection should be rifampin, ethambutol, and another drug to which it is sensitive. It is usually resistant to streptomycin and isoniazid, but it responds well to treatment with appropriate drugs. *M. avium–intracellulare* is resistant to most drugs *in vitro* but nevertheless sometimes responds satisfactorily to standard three- or four-drug regimens given over 2 years.[31] *Mycobacterium malmoense* usually responds to regimens containing rifampin and ethambutol, which may also need to be continued for up to 2 years.[23] In patients in whom the disease pursues a downhill course, surgical treatment may sometimes be necessary.

Although these organisms do not normally spread directly to contacts of the patient, there is some anecdotal evidence of spread between pneumoconiotic workers. In this situation, therefore, contact tracing and radiography should be carried out as for tuberculosis.

Q FEVER

Q fever is an acute febrile illness transmitted by the microorganism *C. burnetii*. The Q stands for "query." When the disease was first described, the organism isolated from the infected abattoir workers had not previously been recognized. The organism causes no clinical illness in animals but is excreted in their milk and products of parturition. Humans may be infected by ingestion or inhalation, and the disease affects predominantly farmers, veterinarians, and slaughterhouse workers. While relatively few cases of occupational cause are currently being reported in Great Britain, serological surveys of farmers have shown a relatively high prevalence of evidence of past infection; 28% of such workers in Northern Ireland had antibodies.[32] In some areas, for example, Australia, the Basque country in Spain, and Nova Scotia in Canada, a high incidence of infection has been reported.[33–35]

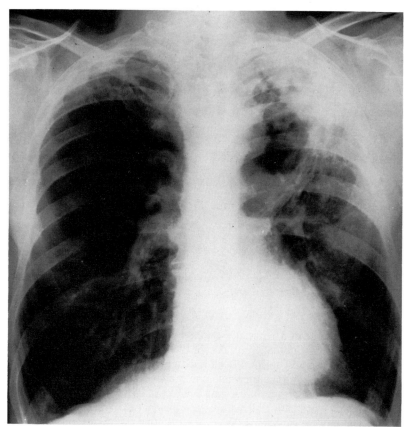

Figure 23–4. *M. kansasii* infection mainly in left upper lobe of a chronic bronchitic worker who had a 30-year history of exposure to dolomite dust in a quarry crushing plant.

However, in most nonagricultural areas, Q fever is responsible for a minority of community-acquired pneumonias, less than 4% in a British survey.[36]

The usual clinical picture is of a disease with a sudden, influenza-like onset, a fever of 38°C to 40°C, and muscular aches. In one half of the patients, a cough develops, and, fairly commonly, areas of consolidation may be seen on the chest radiograph. This consolidation may take up to 1 month to clear and occasionally is associated with a pleural effusion. Rarely, the disease may be complicated by aseptic meningitis, jaundice, or bacterial endocarditis, but it usually runs a benign course.[37, 38]

The differential diagnosis is between influenza and other such respiratory viral diseases; brucellosis; *Mycoplasma,* coxsackievirus, and *Legionella* infections; and infectious mononucleosis. The diagnosis depends on the demonstration of a rising titer of complement-fixing antibodies. The disease is normally self-limiting but responds to tetracyclines.[39, 40]

ANTHRAX

Bacillus anthracis, a large gram-negative rod, is the cause of a virulent disease of livestock that is endemic in the Middle East. The organism contaminates the bones, skin, and hair of dead animals and is liable to infect people who work with these substances. Such workers include those who are employed in making cloth from animal hair, in tanning, in the production of bone-meal fertilizer and glue, and in the importation of animal products. In almost all human cases, the disease takes the form of a primary cutaneous sore associated with extensive edema.[41] The sore starts as a pimple and develops a black central eschar with a ring of purplish vesicles around it. Occasionally, however, in workers exposed to large numbers of anthrax spores dispersed as an aerosol, inhalational anthrax or wool sorters' disease may develop. This is most likely to occur in the sorting and preparation of untreated wool or animal hair imported from the Middle East and India. One important outbreak has been reported in the United States in this century,[42] although the disease used to be more common in Great Britain in the last century. Most outbreaks are sporadic and associated with exposure to spores, the source of which may not be apparent. Thus, the diagnosis is often made post mortem. Relatively recent examples are a man who worked next door to a factory processing Middle Eastern goat hair[43] and a man who had been applying large amounts of bone-meal fertilizer to his garden.[44] Undoubtedly, workers may be exposed to large numbers of spores in the appropriate jobs, and it is surprising that more cases do not occur.[43]

Inhalational anthrax begins insidiously after an incubation period of about 1 week, with slight fever and malaise over a few days. There then develops a severe, short-lived, and usually fatal illness characterized by fever, profuse sweating, dyspnea with cyanosis, and often stridor. Crackles may be heard in the chest, and a pleural effusion may occur. Shock ensues, and the patient usually dies within 24 hours.[42] Pathologically, the disease appears not to be a pneumonia; the evidence indicates that the anthrax spores are engulfed by macrophages and carried to regional lymph nodes, where they germinate and cause a septicemia. The mediastinal nodes show acute inflammation and edema, and this spreads to the other mediastinal structures. Pulmonary edema and pleural effusion may occur.[45]

Anthrax may be controlled by disinfection of imported wool, as occurs in Great Britain, and by vaccination of exposed workers. Ideally, such workers should carry a card warning their physician of the possibility of their contracting anthrax. The disease is diagnosed by an examination of fluid from a skin lesion or by a culture of blood in the generalized disease. If the diagnosis is suspected, it is wise to treat the infection with a combination of penicillin and streptomycin. Severe anthrax septicemia will usually require other measures to combat shock and hypoxemia.

LEGIONNAIRES' DISEASE

Legionnaires' disease is so named because the outbreak that led to the identification of the causative organism occurred at a convention of the American Legion in Philadelphia in 1976. On this occasion, some 180 legionnaires contracted a severe form of the disease, 29 of whom died.[46] The event was sufficiently dramatic to attract national attention, and after the pursuit of several possible causes, the investigators tracked down a previously unknown bacterium, now called *Legionella pneumophila*.[47] The story of this investigation will rank with other classics of epidemiology, such as John Snow's investigation of cholera in London in 1855; coincidentally, both the pump producing infected water in London and the hotel at which the legionnaires were staying in Philadelphia were situated on Broad Streets.[48]

After identification of the organism, with the consequent ability of investigators to detect antibodies and culture *Legionella* from patients, many other outbreaks have been identified, both subsequently and retrospectively. Although sporadic cases occur, it has become clear that unexpected and unpredictable outbreaks, such as that in Philadelphia, are responsible for the bulk of cases. In particular, large hotels and institutions seem to be a frequent site of outbreaks, and investigation has often led to implication of water supplies as the carrier of the organism. In one particularly well-investigated episode, a large number of cases were found among patients, staff, and visitors at a large hospital at a time when a reserve cooling tower was being used for air conditioning. Vapor that contained the organism drifted from the tower into the entry ducts for the cooling system.[49] Work close to outdoor cooling towers is well established as a cause of outbreaks, such as the one that occurred on a power station construction site.[2] Similar studies have pointed to showers as a source of infection, and bacteriological investigation of water in hospitals and hotels has shown *Legionella* to be widely distributed even in places where no recorded cases have occurred.[50] Why outbreaks occur in some circumstances and not in others is not clear, but the dose of the organisms delivered and their virulence may be factors.

The disease itself varies considerably in severity, and judging from serological studies of hotel and hospital staff, subclinical infection may occur. An outbreak in Pontiac, Michigan, diagnosed retrospectively and previously known as Pontiac fever, was relatively mild, and no fatalities occurred.[51] In patients who come to the hospital, the illness is typically severe, with 2 to 10 days of prodromal influenza-like symptoms, confusion, unilateral or bilateral pulmonary consolidation, abnormal liver function, and often hematuria. Almost any pattern of radiographic change, including pleural effusion, may occur. Sputum is usually scanty and nonpurulent, and this, together with the other clinical features and a white cell count not much above normal, often leads to a diagnosis of viral or mycoplasmal pneumonia. The diagnosis may be made by direct immunofluorescent staining of sputum or biopsy material or, after about 1 week, by serology. The treatment may not be successful, but the organism is sensitive to erythromycin and rifampin.

The reason for including this disease among those of occupational origin is that, like allergic alveolitis and humidifier fever, it may be transmitted by water systems in an occupational environment. Outbreaks may therefore be expected to occur among workers in hospitals and large office buildings where a source of warm water is available for bacterial growth and where the water may be circulated as an aerosol throughout the building. Occupational physicians should also be aware of the dangers imposed by work close to cooling towers. These structures are found on most large buildings and within most industrial sites. The plume from the top spreads locally, depending on wind conditions, and may pass unnoticed into adjacent buildings through doors, windows, or air intake ducts. It may pass over outdoor areas where people are at work. If the water in the tower becomes contaminated by the organism, outbreaks, sometimes fatal, may occur.

Conditions that favor the growth of *Legionella* species in water systems are the presence of sludge (which is presumed to supply nutrients), a temperature between 20°C and 45°C, sunlight (which promotes the growth of algae and thus sludge), and recirculation of water by a sump. Legionnaires' disease is now well known to the general public, and both private employers and public corporations have been successfully prosecuted or sued for causing the disease. It is incumbent on employers to take reasonable precautions to prevent outbreaks. These include care at the design and commissioning stage to select systems which reduce the amount of recirculation and aerosolization of water and which are easily accessible for cleaning, steps to prevent drift of contaminated aerosol, regular cleaning and maintenance, and the use of biocides (such as chlorination) if practicable. Particular attention should be paid to the protection of workers engaged in cleaning operations, as these often involve high-pressure jetting, which leads to massive aerosolization of infective material. Employers and owners of buildings should seek advice from the appropriate regulatory authority.

OTHER INFECTIOUS DISEASES

Most of the other occupational infectious diseases are acquired either from contact with animals or in the laboratory.[52] Among these should be mentioned hydatid disease, glanders, brucellosis, psittacosis, and histoplasmosis.

Hydatid disease is relatively common among sheep farmers and their families. It is caused by a cestode organism, *Echinococcus granulosus,* which lives in the

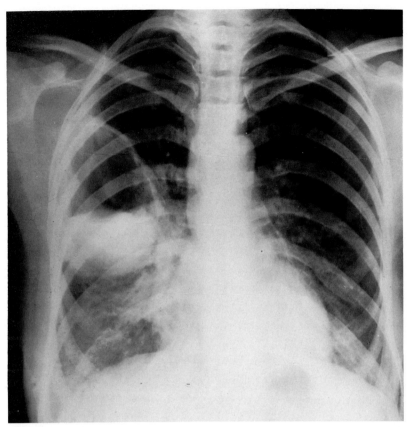

Figure 23–5. Large hydatid cyst in right midzone in a 30-year-old farmer's wife. The patient had coughed up much of the fluid from the cyst, leaving the endocyst visible as a so-called water lily floating on the remaining fluid. Some aspirated fluid accounts for the shadowing in the right lower zone. (Courtesy of Dr. J. Meek.)

gut of dogs. Its ova, liberated in the animal's feces, may be ingested by the secondary host, usually a sheep but occasionally a human. The embryo penetrates the intestinal wall and is trapped in the hepatic or pulmonary capillaries, where it produces the typical hydatid cysts (Fig. 23–5). These present as pulmonary opacities, slowly growing to a large size. Occasionally, the cyst ruptures into the bronchus or pleura. Anaphylactic reactions to the fluid have been described, but more commonly, rupture results in dissemination of the disease through the thoracic cavity.[53] For these reasons, hydatid cysts should be treated. The standard management is surgical,[54] but trials of treatment with drugs have been promising.[55]

Glanders, caused by the organism *Pseudomonas mallei,* is a disease that used to be prevalent among those working with horses. It has now largely been eradicated. In 1947, a small epidemic was described among laboratory workers, to whom it poses an important hazard.[56] The clinical features are of an acute febrile illness with pneumonic consolidation and a tendency to cavitation. A severe disseminated form may occur. The organism in that outbreak was sensitive to sulfonamides.

Allied to glanders is melioidosis, caused by *Pseudomonas pseudomallei.* The disease, which is endemic in Southeast Asia, was significant as a cause of infection of soldiers in South Vietnam. It also can readily be acquired by laboratory workers who handle the organism. It may cause a wide spectrum of illnesses, from an asymptomatic serological reaction to a toxic pneumonitis with formation of multiple pulmonary and systemic abscesses. Melioidosis also responds to sulfonamides, although severe cases in Vietnam required prolonged combination treatment with chloramphenicol, kanamycin, and novobiocin.[57, 58]

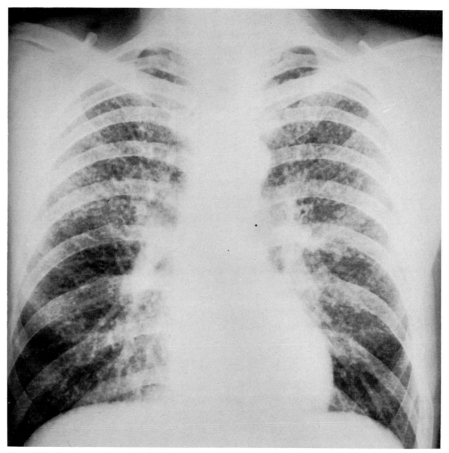

Figure 23–6. Chest radiograph of telephone linesman with acute primary histoplasmosis. The subject had a high fever and myalgia 8 days after installing a telephone conduit in an attic infested by bats.

Brucellosis, a common disease among veterinarians and farmers, is acquired from dealing with the products of abortion in cattle or from drinking infected milk that has not been boiled. It is a generalized disease with multiple clinical manifestations,[59] but cough occurs in approximately one third of those affected. Pneumonia is a rare complication, occurring in severe cases.

Ornithosis, or psittacosis, is endemic in many birds and is an occupational hazard of those who handle them. Poultry farmers, those who deal with poultry carcasses, and veterinarians are at particular risk.[60, 61] The illness varies from a mild influenza-like episode to a serious pneumonia with systemic symptoms. The disease may occasionally be fatal, but normally it responds to tetracycline. Leptospirosis is also occasionally seen as an occupational disease in stevedores, longshoremen, and farm workers.[62] Leptospirosis occasionally presents with a cough and blood-stained sputum. Radiographically, there may be soft exudative parenchymal infiltrates.[63] This disease is contracted either from the usual carriers, i.e., rats, mice, and voles, or from cattle that have themselves been infected.

Histoplasmosis is caused by a fungal intracellular parasite of the reticuloendothelial system, *Histoplasma capsulatum*. It affects a wide range of domestic and wild animals and is endemic in Ontario and in the Mississippi and Ohio Valleys.[64] Farmers in these regions, particularly chicken farmers, are liable to be infected. Occasional outbreaks occur in workers exposed to bats.[65] Normally, infection is either asymptomatic or self-limiting, but single or more often multiple miliary

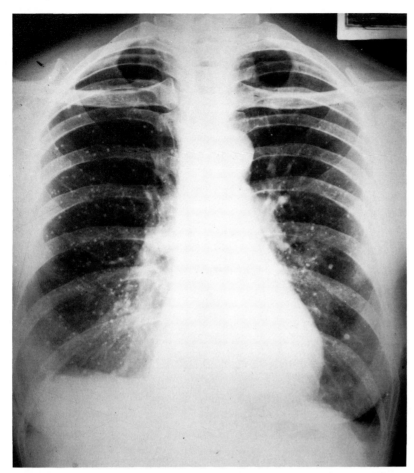

Figure 23–7. Smallpox handler's lung. Chest radiograph taken 10 years after original illness in nurse caring for smallpox patients. Discrete miliary calcification developed 6 years after that initial illness. (From Ross, P. J., Seaton, A., Foreman, H.M., and Morris-Evans, W., Pulmonary calcification following smallpox handler's lung. Thorax, 29, 659, 1974.)

radiographic shadows occur (Fig. 23–6). These have a tendency to calcify. Epidemics of histoplasmosis may occur. They produce an influenza-like illness associated with diffuse pulmonary mottling in those affected. Occasionally, a disseminated infection, requiring treatment with amphotericin B, may occur.[66] Coccidioidomycosis, endemic in semidesert areas of the southwestern United States, Mexico, and South America, may affect people living and working in these areas. Outbreaks have been described in archeologists and laboratory workers.[67, 68] Work with fungi in laboratories has also led to the development of blastomycosis and skin sensitization to *Cryptococcus*.[69, 70]

A historic note might be recorded on smallpox handlers' lung. This was an acute febrile illness occurring in recently immunized subjects who had been in contact with patients with smallpox. An outbreak was described in nurses during the last British epidemic of smallpox. The nurses were shown to have patchy pneumonic consolidation, and it was suggested that the disease was a form of allergic alveolitis.[71] However, follow-up of the patients showed miliary lung calcification (Fig. 23–7), and it now seems likely that the disease was an actual infection, attenuated by vaccination, caused by inhaled smallpox virus, which produced radiographic changes analogous to those of chickenpox.[72]

REFERENCES

1. Sulkin, S.E., and Pike, R.M., Survey of laboratory acquired infections. Am. J. Public Health, 41, 769, 1951.
2. Morton, S., Bartlett, C.L.R., Bibby, L.F., et al., Outbreak of Legionnaires' disease from a cooling water system in a power station. Br. J. Ind. Med., 43, 630, 1986.
3. Cordes, L.G., Brink, E.W., Checko, P.J., et al., A cluster of Acinetobacter pneumonia in foundry workers. Ann. Intern. Med., 95, 688, 1981.
4. Seaton, A., Seaton, D., and Leitch, A.G., Crofton & Douglas's Respiratory Diseases, 4th ed. Oxford, Blackwell Scientific, 1989.
5. Stewart, A.R., and Hughes, J.P.W., Mass radiography in the Northamptonshire boot and shoe industry, 1945–46. B.M.J., 1, 899, 1951.
6. Allison, A.C., and D'Arcy Hart, P., Potentiation by silica of the growth of *Mycobacterium tuberculosis* in macrophage cultures. Br. J. Exp. Pathol., 49, 465, 1968.
7. Public Health Service, Silicosis in the metal mining industry: a re-evaluation, 1958–61. Washington, D.C., Department of Health, Education and Welfare, and Bureau of Mines, 1963.
8. Jarman, T.F., Jones, J.G., Phillips, J.H., and Seingry, H.E., Radiological surveys of working quarrymen and quarrying communities in Caernarvonshire. Br. J. Ind. Med., 14, 95, 1957.
9. Enterline, P.E., Mortality rates among coalminers. Am. J. Public Health, 54, 758, 1964.
10. Glover, J.R., Bevan, C., Cotes, J.E., et al., Effects of exposure to slate dust in North Wales. Br. J. Ind. Med., 37, 152, 1980.
11. Bruce, T., Silicotuberculosis. Scand. J. Respir. Dis., 65(suppl.), 139, 1968.
12. Bailey, W.C., Brown, M., Buechner, H.A., et al., Silico-mycobacterial disease in sandblasters. Am. Rev. Respir. Dis., 110, 115, 1974.
13. Chawla, P.K., Klapper, P.J., Kamholz, S.L., et al., Drug-resistant tuberculosis in an urban population including patients at risk for human immunodeficiency virus infection. Am. Rev. Respir. Dis., 146, 280, 1992.
14. Ramsay, J.H.R., and Pines, A., The late results of chemotherapy in pneumoconiosis complicated by tuberculosis. Tubercle, 44, 476, 1963.
15. MRC/Miners' Chest Diseases Treatment Centre, Chemotherapy of pulmonary tuberculosis with pneumoconiosis. Tubercle, 44, 47, 1963.
16. Jones, F.L., Rifampicin-containing chemotherapy for pulmonary tuberculosis associated with coalworkers' pneumoconiosis. Am. Rev. Respir. Dis., 125, 681, 1982.
17. Dubois, P., Gyselen, A., and Prignot, J., Rifampicin-combined chemotherapy in coalworkers' pneumoconio-tuberculosis. Am. Rev. Respir. Dis., 115, 221, 1977.
18. Snider, R.E., The relationship between tuberculosis and silicosis. Am. Rev. Respir. Dis., 118, 455, 1978.
19. Ball, J.D., Berry, G., Clarke, W.G., et al., A controlled trial of antituberculous chemotherapy in the early complicated pneumoconiosis of coalworkers. Thorax, 24, 399, 1969.
20. Hart, J.T., Cochrane, A.L., and Higgins, I.T.T., Tuberculin sensitivity in coal workers' pneumoconiosis. Tubercle, 44, 141, 1963.
21. Opportunist mycobacteria [editorial]. Lancet, 1, 424, 1981.
22. Schaefer, W.B., Birn, K.J., Jenkins, P.A., and Marks, J., Infection with the Avian-Battey group of mycobacteria in England and Wales. B.M.J., 2, 412, 1969.
23. France, A.J., McLeod, D.T., Calder, M.A., and Seaton, A., *Mycobacterium malmoense* infections in Scotland: an increasing problem. Thorax, 42, 593, 1987.
24. Marks, J., and Jenkins, P.A., The opportunist mycobacteria—a 20-year retrospect. Postgrad. Med. J., 47, 705, 1971.
25. British Thoracic and Tuberculosis Association, Opportunist mycobacterial pulmonary infection and occupational dust exposure: an investigation in England and Wales. Tubercle, 56, 295, 1975.
26. Marks, J., Occupation and kansasii infection in Cardiff residents. Tubercle, 56, 311, 1975.
27. Rosenzweig, D.Y., Silicosis complicated by atypical mycobacterial infection. *In* Transactions of the 26th V.A.-Armed Forces Pulmonary Disease Research Conference. Washington, D.C., U.S. Government Printing Office, 1967, p. 47.
28. Brown, M., Buechner, H.A., Bailey, W.C., and Ziskind, M.M., Atypical mycobacterial pulmonary disease at the New Orleans Veterans' Hospital and Metropolitan New Orleans (Abstract). Am. Rev. Respir. Dis., 103, 885, 1971.
29. Thompson, P.J., Cousins, D.V., Gow, B.L., et al., Seals, seal trainers and mycobacterial infection. Am. Rev. Respir. Dis., 147, 164, 1993.
30. Hardie, R.M., and Watson, J.M., *Mycobacterium bovis* in England and Wales: past, present and future. Epidemiol. Infect., 109, 23, 1992.
31. Hunter, A.P., Campbell, I.A., Jenkins, P.A., and Smith, A.P., Treatment of pulmonary infections caused by mycobacteria of the *Mycobacterium avium-intracellulare* complex. Thorax, 36, 326, 1981.
32. Stanford, C.F., Connolly, J.H., Ellis, W.A., et al., Zoonotic infections in Northern Ireland farmers. Epidemiol. Infect., 105, 565, 1990.
33. Sobradillo, V., Ansola, P., Baranda, F., and Corral, C., Q fever pneumonia: a review of 164 community-acquired cases in the Basque Country. Eur. Respir. J., 2, 263, 1989.
34. Marrie, T.J., Haldane, E.V., Faulkner, R.S., et al., The importance of *Coxiella burnetii* as a cause of pneumonia in Nova Scotia. Can. J. Public Health, 76, 233, 1985.

35. Spelman, D.W., Q fever: a study of 111 consecutive cases. Med. J. Aust., 1, 547, 1982.
36. British Thoracic Society Research Committee, Community acquired pneumonia in adults in British hospitals in 1982–1983. Q. J. Med., 239, 195, 1987.
37. Brown, G.L., Clinical aspects of Q fever. Postgrad. Med. J., 49, 539, 1973.
38. Sawyer, L.A., Fishbein, D., and McDade, J.E., Q fever: current concepts. Rev. Infect. Dis., 9, 935, 1987.
39. Powell, O.W., Kennedy, K.P., McIver, M., and Silverstone, H., Tetracycline in the treatment of Q fever. Australas. Ann. Med., 11, 184, 1962.
40. Sobradillo, V., Zalacain, R., Capelastegui, A., et al., Antibiotic treatment in pneumonia due to Q fever. Thorax, 47, 276, 1992.
41. Christie, A.B., The clinical aspects of anthrax. Postgrad. Med. J., 49, 565, 1973.
42. Plotkin, S.A., Brachman, P.S., Utell, M., et al., An epidemic of inhalation anthrax, the first in the twentieth century. I. Clinical features. Am. J. Med., 29, 992, 1960.
43. La Force, F., Bumford, F.H., Feeley, J.C., et al., Epidemiologic study of a fatal case of inhalation anthrax. Arch. Environ. Health, 18, 798, 1969.
44. Seven, M., A fatal case of pulmonary anthrax. B.M.J., 1, 748, 1976.
45. Albrink, W.S., Brooks, S.M., Biron, R.E., and Kopel, M., Human inhalation anthrax. A report of three fatal cases. Am. J. Pathol., 36, 457, 1960.
46. Frazer, D.W., Tsai, T.R., Orenstein, W., et al., Legionnaires' disease: description of an epidemic of pneumonia. N. Engl. J. Med., 297, 1189, 1977.
47. McDade, J.E., Shepard, C.C., Frazer, D.W., et al., Legionnaires' disease: isolation of a bacterium and demonstration of its role in other respiratory disease. N. Engl. J. Med., 297, 1197, 1977.
48. Weill, H., and Sewell, E.M., In search of the pump handle, 1977. Am. Rev. Respir. Dis., 115, 911, 1977.
49. Dondero, T.J., Rendtorff, R.C., Mallison, G.F., et al., An outbreak of Legionnaires' disease associated with a contaminated air-conditioning cooling tower. N. Engl. J. Med., 302, 365, 1980.
50. Tobin, J. O'H., Swann, R.A., and Bartlett, C.L.R., Isolation of *Legionella pneumophila* from water systems: methods and preliminary results. B.M.J., 282, 515, 1981.
51. Glick, T.H., Gregg, M.B., Berman, B., et al., Pontiac fever. An epidemic of unknown etiology in a health department. I. Clinical and epidemiological aspects. Am. J. Epidemiol., 107, 149, 1978.
52. Occupational hazards for animal workers [editorial]. Lancet, 2, 789, 1981.
53. Xanthakis, D., Ephthimiadis, M., and Papadakis, G., Hydatid disease of the chest: report of 91 patients surgically treated. Thorax, 27, 517, 1972.
54. Lichter, I., Surgery of the pulmonary hydatid cyst—the Barrett technique. Thorax, 27, 529, 1972.
55. Morris, D.L., Dykes, P.W., Dickson, B., et al., Albendazole in hydatid disease. B.M.J., 286, 103, 1983.
56. Howe, C., and Miller, W.R., Human glanders: report of six cases. Ann. Intern. Med., 26, 92, 1947.
57. Patterson, M.C., Darling, C.L., and Blumenthal, J.B., Acute melioidosis in a soldier returning from South Vietnam. JAMA, 200, 447, 1967.
58. Cooper, E.B., Melioidosis. JAMA, 200, 452, 1967.
59. Lula, A.R., Araj, G.F., Khateeb, M.I., et al., Human brucellosis in Kuwait: a prospective study of 400 cases. Q. J. Med., 66, 39, 1988.
60. Psittacosis [editorial]. B.M.J., 1, 1, 1972.
61. Palmer, S.R., Andrews, B.E., and Major, R., A common-source outbreak of ornithosis in veterinary surgeons. Lancet, 2, 798, 1981.
62. Crawford, S.M., and Miles, D.W., *Leptospira hebdomidis* associated with an outbreak of illness in workers on a farm in North Yorkshire. Br. J. Ind. Med., 37, 397, 1980.
63. Poh, S.C., and Soh, C.S., Lung manifestations in leptospirosis. Thorax, 25, 751, 1970.
64. Wheat, L.J., Histoplasmosis. Infect. Dis. Clin. North Am., 2, 841, 1988.
65. Sorley, D.L., Levin, M.L., Warren, J.W., et al., Bat-associated histoplasmosis in Maryland bridge workers. Am. J. Med., 67, 623, 1979.
66. Storch, G., Burford, J.G., George, R.B., et al., Acute histoplasmosis: description of an outbreak in Northern Louisiana. Chest, 77, 38, 1980.
67. Werner, S.B., Pappagianis, D., Heindel, J., and Mickel, A., An epidemic of coccidioidomycosis among archeology students in Northern California. N. Engl. J. Med., 186, 507, 1972.
68. Arupel, N.M., Weiden, M.A., and Galgiani, J.N., Coccidioidomycosis: clinical update. Rev. Infect. Dis., 11, 897, 1989.
69. Baum, G.L., and Lerner, P.I., Primary pulmonary blastomycosis: a laboratory acquired infection. Ann. Intern. Med., 73, 263, 1970.
70. Atkinson, A.J., and Bennett, J.E., Experience with a new skin test antigen prepared from *Cryptococcus neoformans*. Am. Rev. Respir. Dis., 97, 637, 1968.
71. Morris-Evans, W.H., and Foreman, H.M., Smallpox handler's lung. Proc. R. Soc. Med., 56, 274, 1963.
72. Ross, P.J., Seaton, A., Foreman, H.M., and Morris-Evans, W., Pulmonary calcification following smallpox handlers' lung. Thorax, 29, 659, 1974.

24

Occupational Lung Cancer

W. Keith C. Morgan

Robert B. Reger

Percival Pott in 1775 was the first person to attribute the development of cancer to an occupation.[1] He noted that chimney sweeps were particularly prone to scrotal cancer but that the tumor was extremely rare in the general population. Later it became clear that it was the soot that accumulated in the scrotal rugae that was the responsible carcinogen. Subsequently, the development of skin cancer in Lancashire cotton millers, in shale workers in Scotland, and in aniline dye workers in Germany provided a stimulus to the epidemiological investigation of carcinogenesis.

Later, Harting and Hesse observed that there was a vastly increased frequency of lung cancer in metal miners working in the Schneeberg and Jachymov mines of Bohemia, suggesting that there was a carcinogen in the mine environment.[2] It is now realized that it was the radon daughters that are given off by uranium that were responsible for the development of the miners' lung cancer. The uranium mines of Joachimsthal (Jachymov) were found by Madame Curie to contain pitchblende. From this, she isolated radium and polonium. Radium chloride is derived from pitchblende after the extraction of uranium and other minerals. As mentioned previously, it is the radon daughters emitted by the uranium that attach themselves to airborne particles that are subsequently inhaled and lead to the development of lung cancer.

Subsequently, exposures to a number of other substances, including arsenic, asbestos, chromates, nickel, the chloroethers, and other agents were implicated as causes of lung cancer.

In a general context, in the United States, lung cancer mortality accounts for around 22% of deaths in males and 8% of deaths in females. The age-adjusted lung cancer death rates have increased steadily in men from 5 per 100,000 deaths in 1930 to about 180 per 100,000 deaths in 1980.[3, 4] In females, the rate has increased more slowly from 2 to 3 per 100,000 deaths in 1930 to about 34 per 100,000 deaths by the mid-1960s. However, from the mid-1960s to 1986, the female lung cancer mortality rate has increased rapidly to approximately 142 per 100,000 deaths and continues to climb.[3, 4] It has been suggested that the rapid rise in lung cancer among females is a result of the increasing number of women in the work force and because many more women have taken up smoking.[4]

Despite the fact that, over the past two to three decades, a flood of new chemicals has been introduced and marketed commercially, the proportion of cancers induced by occupational exposure remains relatively low, somewhere around 5% to 10% at the most.[5–8] The proportion varies according to the industrial makeup of the country, i.e., whether predominantly industrial or predominantly agricultural. Cigarette smoking is the current cause of 90% to 95% of all lung cancers, and even in those instances where occupational exposure to a known carcinogen has occurred, cigarette smoking usually has acted in the multiplicative or additive manner to increase the risk. Reviews, editorials, and tracts purporting to show that around 30% to 40% of all lung cancer is related to occupation[9] are based on wishful thinking and perhaps a subconscious desire to absolve or excuse the tobacco companies for their reprehensible refusal to accept the fact that tobacco smoking is the single most dangerous environmental killer in the Western world.[4, 10]

CARCINOGENESIS: DEFINITION AND MECHANISMS

The Occupational Safety and Health Administration (OSHA) defines a carcinogen as, "any substance that has validly been shown to produce tumors, either benign or malignant, in animals or which decreases the latent period between exposure and the development of such tumors." This definition places much reliance on animal experiments, and the production of tumors in any species suffices for the substance to be labeled as a carcinogen. Nevertheless, the induction of cancer in experimental animals, with certain recognized exceptions, is uncertain and unpredictable. The likelihood of the successful induction of a tumor depends on the route of administration of the agent being tested, its dose, the duration of exposure, the species of animal, and the age, diet, and sex of the animals used.[11] At the present time, around 175 to 200 substances are recognized as carcinogens by OSHA, but the acceptance of the development of tumors in any one of the vast variety of species in a multitude of differing circumstances, including tumors that may develop spontaneously, increases the number of substances designated as carcinogens by 30 to 40 times.

There is much support for the hypothesis that most cancer originates as a result of alteration in somatic deoxyribonucleic acid (DNA). Furthermore, most carcinogens are also mutagens. Hence, it is often assumed that the carcinogenic potential of a particular agent is related to its ability to damage DNA.[12, 13] There are those, however, who find the enthusiasm of the proponents of the mutagenic hypothesis unconvincing and who suggest that genetic transposition is of more importance.[14]

The layman and the neophyte scientist often pose the question, "What is the cause of cancer?" In doing so, they imply that, first, cancer is a uniform entity of only one type and, second, that it has a single cause. There are those who attribute all cancers to environmental pollution, while others favor viruses or lifestyle. Clearly, both points of view are oversimplification, and a number of considerations need to be borne in mind.

The origin of cancer cannot be explained entirely by the hypothesis that damage to a DNA strand in the chromosome of a somatic cell, given that the damage occurs at a susceptible region, can lead to the development of a clone of cancer cells. This hypothesis has a meretricious veneer of plausibility in that it accommodates the wide range of carcinogens, including radiation and various chemicals. These carcinogens can induce physical damage or react with DNA molecules with a similar result. Such a hypothesis, however, cannot account for the variation in the length of the incubation period of most cancers. When damage occurs at a single position on a DNA strand, why does the affected cell not become an instant nidus for a cancerous clone of cells? Why is it that, as Cairns has observed, chromosomes of cancer cells are most often grossly abnormal in various ways suggesting a gross rearrangement rather than an effect at a single point.[14] While there are plausible explanations to accommodate these observations, the overall likelihood that there is a single cause of cancer is remote.[14]

The observation that persons affected with xeroderma pigmentosum are prone to skin cancer and melanoma is consistent with a simple model since ultraviolet light is known to damage DNA molecules.[14] The inherent defect in this condition involves the biochemical response that is called into play to repair damaged DNA molecules. The question, however, arises as to why persons with this disease are not susceptible to other kinds of cancer caused by carcinogenic agents. It is evident from Cairn's work that human cancer and its cause are not yet understood. The present approach to the problem is best categorized as *hysteron proteron,* i.e., it is difficult to talk about causes when basic mechanisms have still to be elucidated. Until such time as they are understood, it is inappropriate to talk of a single cause, i.e., clinical carcinogens, and to try to postulate that all cancers will respond to a single mode of treatment.

A variety of short-term animal tests are currently used to investigate the mutagenicity of unknown agents. The best known and most widely used is the Ames test, which depends on the ability of the substance in question to influence the mutation rate of a strain of *Salmonella typhimurium* that is nutritionally deficient.[15] The particular strain of *S. typhimurium* used depends on histidine for its growth, but the mutagenic agent will induce reverse mutagens that will permit the bacteria to grow without the presence of histidine. Although the Ames test is widely used and enthusiastically endorsed by many as a powerful tool in the detection of carcinogens, Ames himself has been among the first to warn the test's supporters and enthusiasts that they place too much emphasis on a positive test result. In this connection, it is important to bear in mind that asbestos has only weak mutagenic properties.

Also popular are mammalian cell transformation tests; these depend on the fact that cells in culture are known to affect certain *in vivo* malignancy characteristics. A variety of mammalian cells have been used to separate toxic agents that injure DNA from other agents that do not.[16, 17] A particular type of columnar growth suggests that a substance may be a carcinogen. With such tests, 9 times out of 10, the carcinogen will give positive results, but a significant number of false-positive and false-negative results occur. The cytogenic effects of mutagenic agents in mammalian cells can be determined by cell transformation assays, sister chromatid exchange methods, and other techniques.[16, 17]

The administration of suspected carcinogens to animals that are maintained and killed at intervals to ascertain whether tumors have developed is a more reliable method of detecting carcinogens. As such, animal assays for carcinogens are far more expensive, much more time consuming, and have other drawbacks. Thus, different species often develop different types of tumors when exposed to the same carcinogen. In addition, since animals have a relatively short life span compared with that of humans, it is necessary to administer large doses of the agent to the animals to induce the disease. Carcinogens of low potency may require that the animals have prolonged exposure to the suspected carcinogen. Should the animal be killed prematurely, this may result in false-negative findings. The currently suggested protocol of the National Cancer Institute recommends that the substance being evaluated be administered to two species at two different dose levels and should include 50 male and 50 female animals for each experiment. It is further recommended that the study should continue for the greater part of the animal's normal life span. Comparable controls are mandatory.

INTERNATIONAL AGENCY FOR RESEARCH ON CANCER

The International Agency for Research into Cancer (IARC) has devised a rather elaborate rating system for considering the carcinogenicity of various agents and materials.[18] IARC considers the evidence both in humans and animals in terms of:

1. Sufficient evidence of carcinogenicity.
2. Limited evidence of carcinogenicity.
3. Inadequate evidence of carcinogenicity.
4. Evidence suggesting lack of carcinogenicity.

After a review of all animal and human data relating to the carcinogenicity of an agent, IARC uses an evaluation technique which places the agent into one of five categories:

1. The agent is carcinogenic to humans.
2a. The agent is probably carcinogenic in humans.
2b. The agent is possibly carcinogenic in humans.
3. The agent is not classifiable as to its carcinogenicity to humans.
4. The agent is probably not carcinogenic to humans.

Clearly, groups 2a and 2b are a source of concern and pose difficult problems for exposed workers, industry, and regulatory agencies. For example, an agent may be placed in group 2a (probably carcinogenic to humans) when there exists only limited evidence of carcinogenicity in humans, coupled with sufficient evidence of carcinogenicity in experimental animals. In this instance, limited evidence (humans) means a positive association has been observed between exposure to the agent and cancer for which a causal interpretation is considered to be credible, but chance, bias, or confounding cannot be ruled out with reasonable confidence. Sufficient evidence (animals) relates to an increased incidence of the development of malignant tumors either in (1) multiple species, (2) multiple experiments, or (3) some unusual fashion.

Polychlorinated biphenyls (PCBs), dioxin, silica, and a host of other agents are placed in this category, even though the evidence that, for example, PCBs are carcinogenic in humans is far from compelling and, indeed, is tenuous. Unfortunately, the prevailing philosophy of many governmental agencies is to accept positive animal experimentation results over negative human study findings.

CAUSATION

The assumption of a cause-and-effect relationship between exposure to a certain agent and the development of a disease needs to be considered critically and should not be accepted without adequate validation. Observation may suggest or indicate that certain happenings regularly follow other events or circumstances; from then on, there is often subjective inference that it is essential to confirm. Moreover, causation is seldom related to a single factor or exposure but depends on a series of influences, i.e., a concatenation of events or circumstances. Thus, in lung cancer, for example, there may be multiple exposures, e.g., to asbestos, cigarette smoke, or radon daughters. Other factors, such as heredity and diet, may also be important. Tolstoy realized the distinction between association and cause and effect when he wrote in *War and Peace,* "Whenever I look at my watch and see the hands pointing to ten I hear the bells beginning to ring in the church close by; but I have no right to assume that the movement of the bell is caused by the position of the hands of my watch." When we consider statistical evidence related to a set of data and any inferences drawn from this, it is essential that the evidence be assessed in such a way as to answer the crucial question, "Is there any other explanation for the happenings or facts before us?" To assess whether there is indeed a cause-and-effect relationship, A. Bradford Hill recommended nine criteria that should be used to assess the evidence.[19] These can be shortened to six and include:

1. *Consistency.* The presence of one study purporting to show that a particular agent is harmful is insufficient, and there must be multiple studies with similar results. Thus, almost every study that has been carried out on lung cancer has shown a pre-eminent effect of cigarette smoking in the development of the tumor.
2. *Strength.* Slight increases in the relative risk or the standardized mortality ratio (SMR) in lung cancer or other respiratory diseases for a particular type of work need to be viewed with caution. For example, a SMR that is greater than 100

but less than 200 cannot necessarily be regarded as significant without the most careful exclusion of other factors, which is often difficult or impossible.

3. *Specificity.* Lung cancer is most commonly related to cigarette smoking; however, it is known that the presence of asbestosis in conjunction with cigarette smoking greatly increases the risk. In addition, exposure to radon daughters in the absence of cigarette smoking can cause lung cancer. It is therefore necessary to ascertain whether there has or have been a specific exposure or multiple exposures that may explain the development of the particular type of cancer.

4. *Chronological relationships.* There must be an incubation period from the time of first exposure to the time of the development of a particular disease. It is unreasonable to assume that a 1-year exposure to asbestos, even in a cigarette smoker, will lead to the development of lung cancer within 2, 3, or even 5 years. In general, lung cancer has an incubation period of at least 15 years with the risk for mesothelioma developing for the most part some 25 to 35 years after first exposure.

5. *Dose-response relationship.* There is little doubt that many conditions require a certain cumulative exposure before the disease develops. Thus, there is good evidence to indicate that coal workers' pneumoconiosis will not develop if the dust level is kept below 2 mg/m^3 for a 35-year period.[20] There is similar evidence to indicate that asbestosis and excessive lung cancer will not develop in workers exposed to less than 1 f/cc^3 of asbestos for a working life of 40 years.[21] Although some causal associations may not show an apparent trend with exposure, most of the etiological agents that cause lung cancer, including asbestos, have generally shown an effect that increases with cumulative exposure.

6. *Biological plausibility.* If the disease can also be produced in animals and has similar features to that which occurs in humans, this can be regarded as plausible evidence to support a cause-and-effect relationship. Thus, the development of disease must be in accord with existing biological facts. Clearly, we cannot carry out experiments in humans which might lead to serious disease such as cancer. Nonetheless, Jenner, in his initial experiment to test the efficacy of cowpox vaccination in the control of smallpox, inoculated Billy Phelps. Similarly, John Snow's removal of the Broad Street pump handle to control a cholera epidemic also might be classified as a human experiment.

EPIDEMIOLOGICAL STUDIES

Epidemiological studies in humans might be classified as (1) historical cohort studies, (2) case-control studies, (3) studies of subjects with a particular condition, and (4) record linkage of etiological studies. In general, cohort studies have more power and are more likely to produce valid results. Simple case series, studies of proportional mortality rates, and studies of cancer morbidity are less reliable and are often misleading.

Despite the clear-cut criteria established by A. Bradford Hill,[19] there is little doubt that many studies in man purporting to show an increased risk of cancer, in particular lung cancer, in various occupations, are of dubious validity. This is particularly true of many of the investigations that have attempted to relate exposure to silica, or the fibrosis produced by the dust, to the development of lung cancer. Thus, studies carried out in workers who have been compensated for a particular disease, e.g., silicosis, are much more likely to find symptoms in these patients. It is the symptoms that make these workers seek medical attention and undergo the necessary examinations. In the case of chest disease, the particular symptoms that are a cause of concern are cough, sputum, and shortness of breath, and the most common cause of all three is cigarette smoking. The studies of Ng et al. from Singapore in which a cohort of subjects from the Singapore Silicosis Register were selected is an example in point.[22] The prevalence of smoking in their cohort of silicotic claimants was 91% compared with 60% in the general male population of

Singapore. Thus, the excessive lung cancer SMR in their cohort was derived by comparing silicotic claimants with the general male population of Singapore without taking into account the different smoking habits of the two groups. The overall issue relating to the hypothesized relationship between silica exposure, silicosis, and bronchogenic cancer is covered in Chapter 12.

Large differences in lung cancer rates between occupations exist and are best explained by the prevalence and intensity of smoking habits. The frequency of smoking varies greatly according to the job, religion, and other factors. In an editorial entitled, ''What Proportions of Cancers are Related to Occupation?''[5] the author pointed out the problems associated with comparing the mortality rates from malignant disease by social class in Great Britain. The Registrar General's Decennial Supplement on Occupational Mortality calculates the mortality rates from malignant disease by social class. The 1978 supplement showed a gradient of mortality rates with skilled workers, semiskilled workers, and nonskilled workers having a progressively higher mortality rate from all malignant neoplasms. For example, skilled manual workers had a SMR of 113, and skilled nonmanual workers had a SMR of 91.

The gradient risk is not as steep as we might anticipate, particularly in view of the fact that occupation is only one of the factors that determines social class mortality gradients. Smoking and other habits play a more important role. By determining the risk of lung cancer for various levels of smoking and relating these to social class, it was possible to show that manual laborers had a lung cancer risk of 22% higher than that of administrative and clerical workers. Because lung cancer in Great Britain in men is responsible for just under two fifths of the deaths from all cancers (since that time, i.e., 1978, the incidence of lung cancer in these groups has increased), the effects of smoking and the increased rate of lung cancer would increase the risk in manual workers of all cancers by 9%. Since 1978, there has been a further decline in smoking among all classes, but the decline has been least in blue collar workers. While certain occupations are undoubtedly associated with an increased risk for lung cancer, it is fallacious to assume that it is occupational exposures to carcinogens that are necessarily responsible, and there is little doubt that the most common carcinogen that blue collar workers are exposed to is cigarette smoke. Nonetheless, an increased risk of respiratory cancer exists for several occupations and specific exposures. A description of these follows.

Asbestos

The relationships between asbestos exposure and bronchogenic and other cancers and mesothelioma are discussed in Chapter 14.

Arsenic

Evidence linking arsenic and lung cancer is clear-cut, especially in the mining and smelting industry. Although arsenic was suspected to be a carcinogen in the mid-19th century and was originally thought to be the agent responsible for the deaths of miners in Schneeberg,[2] excessive cases of lung cancer were first observed among workers exposed to sodium arsenic in the manufacture of sheep dip.[23] This industry was investigated in detail in Great Britain by Hill and Fanning[24] who showed that workers involved in the chemical process itself had an increased risk of dying of cancer compared both with other workers in the factory and with the socially comparable male population of the town. The excess of cancers in these men was due to an increase in those tumors that involved the skin and respiratory tract. Investigation of the factory at that time revealed an extremely dusty environment, with chemical evidence of arsenic absorption in the workers.[25] Moreover, virtually all the process workers examined showed clinical evidence of arsenic absorption. The workers examined had increased pigmentation, hyperkeratosis, and warts.

The possible risks of arsenic poisoning and lung cancer have also existed among those involved in the preparation and use of arsenical insecticide sprays.[26, 27] For example, Roth reported that 18 of the 47 German vineyard workers exposed to arsenic who underwent autopsies died of lung cancer.[28] The lung cancer mortality rates of six rural and urban districts of the Moselle and one district of the Ahv[29] indicated that the vineyard districts of the Moselle, in which arsenical insecticides were used, had a higher proportionate mortality rate from lung cancer than did the urban and nonvineyard areas. In addition, the district of Ahv had a lower incidence of lung cancer, which was attributed to the avoidance of arsenical insecticides. All of these substances have now largely been superseded, but arsenic may still be encountered in metal refining and the chemical industry, especially as a contaminant of sulfuric acid. Stringent precautions are necessary to prevent its inhalation or contact with the skin.

Pinto and Bennetter studied active copper smelter workers and pensioners.[30] Although the overall cancer mortality rate was not statistically excessive, the proportionate lung cancer mortality rate in the smelter group was markedly greater than the rate which existed in the state as a whole (8% versus 3%). Milham and Stron examined death certificates from the county where the smelter was located and found 39 deaths caused by lung cancer among county residents who had been employed at the smelter and one lung cancer death in an employee who was not a resident.[31] These 40 lung cancer deaths were clearly excessive given that the expectation was only 18. Lee and Fraumeni[32] studied copper smelter workers exposed to arsenic trioxide between 1938 and 1963 and found that the observed lung cancer deaths were six times higher than expected. A case-control study involving 19 lung cancer cases revealed that 11 lung cancer deaths occurred in men formerly employed at copper smelters; only three deaths occurred among former copper smelter workers in the control group.[33] In addition, in the United States,[34] lung cancer rates that are nearly 10-fold the expected rates have been observed among workers most heavily exposed to arsenic, and convincing dose-response relationships have been obtained relative to cumulative exposure and short-term ceiling levels.[35] Other smelter worker populations have also shown consistent increases in lung cancer rates and modest rate increases for cancers other than those in the lung.[36, 37] Consistent with United States studies, Wall confirmed that the lung cancer risk among Swedish smelter workers was around six to eight times the expected risk.[38]

Chloroethers

Chloroethers are alkylating agents and have been used increasingly in industrial processes as intermediates in organic synthesis, organic solvents, bactericides, fungicides, and cross-linking agents. An alkylating agent with clear carcinogenic potency is bis(chloromethyl) ether (BCME), also known as bischlorodimethyl ether. BCME (and chloromethylmethylether) are unique among causes of human bronchial carcinoma in that their activity was first shown in animal experiments.[39] This led to detailed hygiene and epidemiological studies, which showed a considerably increased risk of oat cell carcinoma in humans.[40, 41]

The carcinogenicity of BCME was first demonstrated in 1968 by skin painting in mice and subcutaneous injection in rats. It was observed that, of 30 mice treated with BCME, papillomata developed in 13; 12 of these progressed to squamous cell carcinomata. These results were confirmed by additional experiments using subcutaneous injections of BCME in newborn mice.[42]

Because industrial exposure to BCME is more likely to be by inhalation rather than cutaneously, several animal inhalation experiments were undertaken. For example, in 1970 and 1971, Laskin et al.[43, 44] reported on rats subjected to inhalation of BCME; carcinoma of the lung was found in five of 19 rats examined by necropsy.

In human studies by Theiss et al.,[45] Figueroa et al.,[40] and Lemen et al.,[41] the incidence of lung cancer was similar: 3% to 5% among manufacturing workers. This was in contrast with the more than 12% found in a study by Sakabe[46] in which five cases of lung cancer occurred among 32 employees exposed to BCME in a dyestuff factory in Japan. Further studies of a chemical manufacturing plant in Philadelphia confirmed the excess of lung cancer and indicated the cause-and-effect relationship of exposure to BCME and the development of lung cancer.[47–49]

The predominance of small cell undifferentiated or oat cell carcinomata noted in these human studies is noteworthy. A similar predominance of this histological type has been noted for bronchogenic cancers associated with radon daughters[50] and nitrogen mustard.[51]

Coke Production

In 1775, Pott[1] provided the initial evidence suggesting that carcinogenic agents are produced during the carbonization or combustion of bituminous coal. Since that time, a great amount of information linking excess cancer at several sites among workers in coal combustion or carbonization occupations has been noted. For example, in the United Kingdom, Doll et al.[52] and Kennaway and Kennaway[53] showed excessive cancer rates for chimney sweeps and several categories of gas works employees. Excess lung cancer rates for gas stokers and coke oven changers were around three times the expected rate.

Workers involved in the destructive distillation of coal (coke production) have been shown by Lloyd[54] to have an increased risk of bronchial carcinoma. Lung cancer mortality rates were twice the expected rate among all coke oven workers, and the rate increased 10-fold among those employed full time for 5 or more years on oven tops. A more recent study of British coke workers[55] also showed an increased risk of death from lung cancer, although of a slightly lower order than that found by Lloyd.[54] Studies in the United States have been greatly extended to evaluate exposure-response relationships for coal tar pitch volatiles and lung cancer.[56, 57] The lung cancer mortality rate among coke oven workers was strongly related to both the duration and intensity of exposure to coke oven fumes. In addition, excessive deaths from prostatic and kidney cancers were also noted, but the excessive mortality rates for these particular cancers did not appear to be dose related.

Chromates

There is no evidence suggesting that trivalent chromium compounds are carcinogenic in humans or animals; however, exposure to certain hexavalent chromium compounds, mainly water-insoluble ones, is related to an increased risk of lung cancer in selected workers. The water-soluble hexavalent chromium compounds, such as chromic acid mist and certain chromate dusts, can also be severe irritants of the nasopharynx, larynx, lungs, and skin.

An early association of lung cancer with exposure to chromium was made by Alwens and Jonas[58] who noted an excessive frequency of lung cancer among workers involved with the heavy metal industry in Germany. Machle and Gregorius[59] reviewed the results from studies in six major United States factories producing chromates. High rates of lung cancer were noted, and the evidence suggested that monochromates (as opposed to dichromates and trivalent chromates) were likely to be responsible for the increased rates. This earlier work was confirmed by Baetjer[60] who studied lung cancer cases and controls at a Baltimore hospital and found a significant link between occupation (as a chromate worker) and bronchogenic cancer. Mancuso and Hueper[61] studied the mortality rates of workers of a chromate plant and found that the proportional mortality rate from lung cancer was 15 times the expected rate in the general population. Evidence was advanced suggesting that the insoluble chromium compounds were causative agents that were responsible for the increases. Later, Enterline[62] reviewed epidemiological evidence regarding the lung cancer mortality rate of workers engaged in chromate ore processing. A lung cancer risk 20 to 30 times greater than that in the general population provided overwhelming evidence related to causation.

The chromium content in the lungs of exposed chromate workers who have died of lung cancer is elevated. For example, the average chromium content in six patients with lung cancer who were chromate workers was 36.7 μg of chromium per gram of lung tissue, whereas a nonexposed lung cancer case would have only around 0.21 μg of chromium per gram of lung tissue.[63] Confirming this work, Kishi et al.[64] evaluated the chromium content of body parts of chromate workers who died of lung cancer. On average, the chromium level in the lungs of chromate-exposed lung cancer cases was 50 times higher than that in controls. Nevertheless, this observation cannot be regarded as a cause-and-effect relationship unless it can be shown that the risk of lung cancer is related to an increasing chromium content.

Without question, excessive exposure to insoluble hexavalent chromium compounds is related to increased lung cancer rates. Workers involved in chromate production and the chromate pigment industry are at highest risk. In addition, it has been suggested that exposure to some soluble hexavalent chromium compounds, including chromium trioxide in electroplating operations, may also increase the risk of bronchogenic cancer.[65, 66]

Nickel

The first human evidence of a relationship between nasal cancer and nickel exposure is contained in a report from the Chief Inspector of Factories in the United Kingdom.[67] Although 10 cases of nasal cancer were initially identified among refinery workers, further follow-up resulted in a total of 52 cases of nasal cancer and 93 cases of lung cancer.[68] Doll et al. later studied workers in the same refinery and reported that deaths from lung cancer were five to 10 times higher than expected among men hired prior to 1925.[69] Deaths from nasal cancers were more than 100 times greater than expected. Nasal cancer excesses have also been reported in nickel refineries worldwide.[70–77]

The study of lung cancer deaths and nickel exposure in the United Kingdom was undertaken by Kreyberg[78] who included in his evaluation the work of others.[73, 79] It was confirmed that nickel refinery workers experienced an excess lung cancer risk compared with appropriate reference populations, and it was also shown that most lung cancers were of the small cell anaplastic and epidermoid cell types. Excess lung cancers were particularly prevalent among cigarette smokers; the role between tobacco smoke and nickel-induced lung cancer remains unclear.

While it has remained a mystery exactly which nickel compounds are human carcinogens, it appears that the cancer risk is associated mostly with the earlier stages of nickel refining.[79] Clearly, the lung and nasal sinuses are the target organs affected. Some evidence does exist, however, that nickel subsulfides and oxides are the most likely carcinogenic agents.[70] On the other hand, no increased cancer risk has been found among aircraft factory workers exposed predominantly to nickel sulfate and chloride.[80]

A recent international committee report on nickel carcinogenesis is enlightening.[81] This review of 10 cohort studies indicated that excess risk has been demonstrated only for sinus and lung cancer. It was also determined that the excess cancer risk was related to workers exposed predominantly to soluble nickel. All forms of nickel were previously considered carcinogenic to humans. However, the international review indicated that workers exposed to pure metallic nickel powder seem not to have an increased risk of lung cancer.[81] Thus, although nickel compounds are considered carcinogenic, metallic nickel is considered only a possible carcinogen in humans. Exposure limits corresponding to the risk of respiratory cancer were set at more than 1 mg/m^3 for soluble nickel and more than 10 mg/m^3 for insoluble nickel. The current threshold limit values offer an order of magnitude safety factor relative to these exposure limit estimates.

Mustard Gas

Mustard gas is an alkylating agent and has effects on cells similar to radiation exposure. Beebe[82] and Case and Lea[83] studied mustard gas exposure during World War I, which provided only hints that the agent might have been responsible for modest increases in lung cancer deaths among veterans. On the other hand, Wada et al. studied mustard gas production workers in Japan and determined that 33 deaths from respiratory tract carcinomata had occurred since 1952.[84] Depending on the reference population used for comparison, respiratory cancer rates were from three- to 40-fold in excess. The confirmed neoplasms were either squamous or undifferentiated and appeared centrally as opposed to peripherally. Also, among British mustard gas workers during World War II, 11 respiratory cancers were identified; only one would have been expected.[85]

Fluorspar

The mineral, calcium fluoride, is used as a flux in steel making and in the production of aluminum and ceramics. It is a source of fluorine for the chemical industry. Although fluorspar is mined worldwide, important deposits have been worked in Newfoundland since the 1930s, and it was here that a detailed investigation of the health of the miners was carried out because of a suspected increased risk in lung cancer.[86] This study showed that fluorspar miners in this region had a death rate from lung cancer 29 times that anticipated from a study of the unexposed population. This difference was not related to cigarette smoking or pneumoconiosis, and environmental investigation showed that the mine air was radioactive to a degree comparable to that found in uranium mines. No radioactive ore was present in the mines, and the activity was shown to emanate from radon daughters dissolved in water that had seeped into the mines. Steps were taken to eliminate the seepage of contaminated water.

Uranium and Radioactive Elements

Uranium occurs as an oxide, as pitchblende, or as a compound oxide with vanadium and potassium known as carnotite. The ore contains amounts of silica varying from 5% to 50%, and uranium mining often therefore entails a risk also of silicosis. It is mined chiefly in Czechoslovakia, the United States, the Congo, Canada, and Australia. Both deep and surface mining are used; the drilling and blasting techniques are similar to those in other forms of hard rock mining.

The crude ore is crushed at the mill, often on the site of the mine, and the uranium is then extracted in the form of a uranite known as yellowcake. This is packed into drums for transport to the user, and dust is liable to be liberated in these two processes. The uranium is then used principally in the production of atomic energy for both peaceful and military purposes but also, to some extent, in the ceramics and chemical industry. Laboratory workers who handle uranium are particularly at risk of toxic effects, which may include lung cancer or fibrosis.

As early as the mid-1500s, fatal lung disease was occurring in miners of uranium-bearing ore in the Erz Mountains of Europe.[87] The excess mortality rate in the Schneeberg metal miners caused by lung carcinoma was likely to be related mainly to the radioactivity of these mines.[88] Harting and Hesse[2] first showed that lung tumors were responsible for three quarters of the deaths of these miners, and it was later confirmed that these tumors were of bronchogenic origin.[88] In 1930, the uranium miners of Joachimsthal were also found to have an increased risk of lung cancer developing.[89] Subsequently, a similar risk was discovered in association with radioactivity in uranium mines in the United States, hard rock miners in the United States, hematite miners in Great Britain,[90] and fluorspar miners in Canada.[86]

The most detailed study of the effects of uranium mining on the lungs was that carried out in the United States between 1950 and 1967.[91] This study demonstrated a mortality rate from lung cancer among the miners than was more than six times of that expected. The mortality rate was related to the calculated cumulative exposure to radiation expressed in working level months. A working level month is defined as an exposure for 170 working hours to a level of radon daughters of 1 L of air resulting in the emission of 1.3×10^5 MeV of potential alpha energy. Even the group of miners with a relatively low exposure to one working level over 10 to 30 years experienced a fourfold increase in the risk of lung cancer. With the higher exposures, the risk was appreciably enhanced to the equivalent of seven or more working levels over 10 or more years.

Further suggestive evidence that radiation is to blame for this excess of lung cancer risk comes from another aspect of the same study.[92] It was shown that small cell undifferentiated cancers became progressively more frequent with greater cumulative radiation exposure. This apparent association of radiation with small cell carcinomata was also found in Joachimsthal and among the fluorspar miners of Newfoundland; a similar association was observed with the radiomimetic agent mustard gas. Studies of uranium miners in Canada also showed an increased proportion of small cell tumors in workers with the highest exposures.[93]

Cigarette-smoking uranium miners in the United States are at greater risk than their nonsmoking coworkers.[94] However, the nonsmoking miners of Joachimsthal still have an increased risk of lung cancer; their tumors take rather longer to develop. Archer et al. showed that the latent period prior to the induction of lung cancer by alpha radiation is shorter the older miners are when they start mining, the more cigarettes they smoke, and the greater the dose of radiation.[95]

Uranium generally represents only 0.5% of the ore, although higher-grade ores may occur, especially close to the surface. Uranium-238 decays to radium-226, and this in turn decays to radon-222. This substance is a gas and emits alpha radiation, as do three of its daughters, polonium-218, -214, and -210. These substances diffuse from the rock into the mine's air, where they become attached to particles of dust or moisture on which they may be inhaled. The alpha particles emitted have a range of sizes in tissue (between 40 to 70 microns), just sufficient for them to damage the nuclei of the basal cells of the bronchial epithelium by ionization. It is assumed that this damage may later lead to malignant change.

The prevention of lung cancer in uranium miners depends on regular measurement of levels of radon daughters, usually by pumping air through a molecular filter and counting the alpha activity in a scintillation counter. Personal radiation badges have also been developed. Where levels are unacceptably high, they should be reduced by ventilation (sealing off unused areas) and by preventing the seepage of water that contains dissolved radon. The individual exposures of miners should be monitored, and the recommendations are that miners should not be exposed to more than 4 working level months in any 1 year or to more than 2 working level months in any 3-month period. Medical supervision should involve excluding subjects with prior chest disease, performing annual or biennial chest radiography, and discouraging smoking. Cytological examination of sputum is not beneficial and has no effect on the prognosis, although it has its advocates.[96] Dust control is of primary importance since the radon daughters are attached to dust particles.

The uranium miner is also at risk for silicosis, although the ventilation necessary to control the radiation hazard is sufficient also to control the silica level. There is limited evidence that chronic irradiation may act in conjunction with silica in producing a modified pulmonary fibrosis in a proportion of the miners.[97]

Workers in a uranium mill may be at risk of malignant disease of the lymphatic and hemopoietic tissues, other than leukemia. One study showed four deaths in a group of 104 workers, compared with the one expected.[98] Clearly, these numbers are very small, and further study is required. Moreover, uranium is toxic to the kidneys. When administered to animals, it causes chronic nephritis. Precautions must therefore be taken to prevent chronic absorption of uranium in the millers by enclosure of the process, rotation of the workers from jobs involving exposure after a short period, and estimation of uranium levels in the urine.

A study of workers at a uranium processing plant involved in nuclear weapons production has so far shown no very convincing evidence of an excess cancer hazard.[99]

Metal Mining

The pneumoconiosis of hematite miners is described in Chapter 16. The novelist A. J. Cronin[100] was one of the first to call attention to the high prevalence of respiratory disease among these miners in the northwest of Great Britain. Subsequent pathological studies[101] suggested that lung cancer was a relatively common cause of death, apparently related to the presence of siderosilicosis. Although it is possible that a combination of iron and silica is carcinogenic to the lungs, an alternative cause was discovered when a survey of radon in British mines revealed high levels in these same hematite mines.[102] A comparison of the mortality rates of hematite miners with those of coal miners and the rest of the population in the same area of Great Britain showed an excess of deaths caused by lung cancer of between 75% and 100%.[90] Death rates among the miners could not be calculated because of unsatisfactory employment figures. This same study demonstrated that up to 40% of these cancers were of the small cell undifferentiated type, a similar proportion to that in uranium miners.[92] The source of radon in these mines is thought to be seepage of water, as in the fluorspar mines. If radiation is the carcinogen, a similar excess cancer mortality risk might not be expected in all hematite mines, but this has not yet been determined. Suggestive evidence, however, comes from a comparison of excess lung cancers in different situations involving exposure to radiation; correction of the cancer mortality rate for the calculated exposure produces closely similar figures.[103]

Underground metal miners in the United States[104] and Sweden[105] have been shown to have an increased lung cancer mortality rate, and this again appears to be associated with irradiation, although the possibility that traces of other carcinogens in the mine's atmosphere might play a part cannot be ruled out. Tin mines are another place where radon daughters might be expected, and raised levels of radiation have been found in British mines. A study of this work force confirmed a small increase in the lung cancer risk for underground miners.[106]

Talc miners and, in fact, all hard rock miners are now considered by some to be at increased risk for bronchogenic cancer.[107, 108] The contaminants of concern in the ore are silica and the nonasbestiform chemical counterparts of amphibole asbestos. Both of these latter issues are covered in Chapters 12, 13, and 14.

Other Agents Suspected of Being a Cause of Respiratory Cancer

In the chemical industry, carcinoma of the nasal sinuses and possibly of the lung appeared to occur unduly frequently in the manufacture of isopropanol.[109] In this industry, propylene gas reacts with arsenic-free sulfuric acid to produce isopropyl sulfates, which are then hydrolyzed to form isopropanol. Isopropyl oil, a volatile substance that is carcinogenic in animals, is given off, and this was suspected to be the offending agent. Measures have been taken to control exposure to this substance, and it is probable that the hazard has been eliminated.

Suspicion has also been raised that printing ink may be a lung cancer hazard; studies in Denmark have shown a sixfold increase in risk in exposed workers,[110] while studies of British newspaper workers have shown a 30% to 40% increase in risk.[111] A slight increase in lung cancer has also been suggested in foundry workers,[112] although the significance of such findings in the absence of information on smoking habits is dubious and there is little hard evidence to support this contention.

It has been suggested that exposures to vinyl chloride monomer might entail an increased risk of lung cancer and liver disease.[113] However, another careful study, taking account of smoking histories, has not shown such an increase in risk.[114] The evidence that vinyl chloride is a respiratory carcinogen is unconvincing, and most studies that show a positive association have not had smoking histories available.[115]

Similarly, there are conflicting reports of an association of lung cancer with beryllium exposure. One showed an inverse relationship to the length of exposure,[116] and others found a small excess risk.[117, 118] The methods used in many of these studies were suspect.[119] The epidemiological evidence that beryllium is a carcinogen was recently reviewed by MacMahon.[120] He reviewed many of the earlier studies and expressed the opinion that they were poorly designed and overinterpreted. Small excesses of lung cancer were incorrectly attributed to beryllium when smoking, almost certainly, was responsible. Likewise, excess lung cancer rates have been reported in the aluminum industry, especially in the former Soviet Union.[121, 122] In none of these situations is there convincing proof of human lung carcinogenesis.[123]

It should be noted that adenocarcinoma of the nasal cavity and sinuses, a rare tumor, has been shown to be associated with woodworking, principally in the furniture industry, and with leather in boot and shoe manufacturing.[124]

Acrylonitrile is used in the manufacture of plastics, synthetic rubber, and fibers. An association between lung cancer and exposure to acrylonitrile was noted by O'Berg.[125] Subsequent studies purport to confirm this association but were based on small numbers of subjects and lack information on smoking.[126, 127] At the present time, there is no definite evidence that acrylonitrile is indeed a carcinogen.

Formaldehyde is used widely for making adhesives for plywood and manufacturing rubber, leather, explosives, and dyes. It is also used by morticians and in the fixing of tissues for pathological examinations. It is found in cigarette smoke and car exhausts. The evidence that formaldehyde is a carcinogen is weak. In a large study of 26,561 subjects, Blair et al. could find no increased risk.[128] Sterling and Weinkam reanalyzed data from the same cohort with what appears to have been a preconceived desire to show that increased cumulative exposure to formaldehyde was associated with an increased risk of lung cancer.[129] In doing so, they did not apparently realize that increasing exposure to formaldehyde was likely to be confounded by an increased exposure to cigarette smoke.

A number of other agents have been suggested as possible carcinogens. These include acetaldehyde; however, the data for this agent are inconclusive and indeed inadequate to make a judgment.[130] In addition, synthetic fibers made of glass, rock wool, slag wool, and ceramic fibers have the physical characteristics that suggest that, under such circumstances, they could be carcinogens. Thus, they occur as long thin fibers, some of which may persist for some considerable time in the lungs when inhaled. Several epidemiological investigations of workers exposed to glass fibers, rock wool, and slag wool have been conducted in the United States and Europe. The results do not provide sufficient evidence to establish them as a cause of lung cancer (see also Chapter 13).[131]

The possible relationship between silica exposure, silicosis, and lung cancer is currently a source of contention. Although this has been discussed in Chapter 12, we disagree with most of the conclusions stated there. Neither are we impressed with the IARC pronouncement in relation to silica as a carcinogen. Although the literature is replete with studies purporting to show an association between exposure to silica and lung cancer, the results have been inconsistent. Many of the studies have been seriously flawed, both as far as design and analysis have been concerned. Seldom have so many positive studies failed so frequently to fulfill A. Bradford Hill's criteria, to which reference was made earlier in this chapter.[19] Thus, although some studies have shown an association between silicosis and lung cancer, others have shown an association between silica exposure and lung cancer in the absence of silicosis. In many investigations, no obvious dose-response relationship was present. Other studies have shown a relationship between silicosis of the lymph nodes and lung cancer[132] but no such association between parenchymal disease, i.e., silicosis and lung cancer. Many studies relied on subjects who were listed on a

Silicosis Register or who had been awarded workers' compensation. As such, a greater proportion of these subjects were smokers compared with the controls.[22] Compensation was and is frequently awarded on the basis of respiratory impairment whether or not the x-ray finding is positive. Should the radiograph show simple pneumoconiosis and should the subject have airways obstruction, it is frequently assumed that there is a cause-and-effect relationship. This we know to be fallacious, and almost invariably, the cause of the patient's chronic airflow limitation is cigarette smoking. In other instances, there have been exposures to other known carcinogens. These include radon daughters, polycyclic hydrocarbons, chromium, asbestos, and nickel. There has been a regrettable tendency to endorse silica as a carcinogen, a view that holds favor with many lawyers who envision the carcinogenic consequences of silica exposure as another lucrative source of litigation. The acceptance of the association between silica and lung cancer by many physicians and health workers is a classic example of the Gold effect.[133] Suffice it to say that we are not convinced that there is such a relationship[134] and neither is McDonald.[135]

PREVENTION

The prevention of respiratory cancer among workers exposed to carcinogens encountered in the workplace can be effected in several ways. These include the elimination or reduction of exposures to the appropriate carcinogen by cutting down on the number of cigarettes smoked and, possibly, by chemoprevention. The concept of screening for early disease and the prevention of lung cancer has been tried and, for the most part, found wanting.[136]

Changes in industrial methods or processing have eliminated or reduced exposures to chloromethyl ethers and greatly reduced the risk of lung and nasal cancer related to nickel exposure. The combination of decreasing exposure to asbestos fibers and a reduction in cigarette smoking has likewise had a great effect on reducing asbestos-induced lung cancer.

Occupational exposure plays an important role in the development of lung cancer in a selected minority of workers, somewhere around 5% to 8%. However, cigarette smoking is of paramount importance and is the single most important preventable cause of this condition and of cancer in general. As more and more work sites forbid smoking on the job, then the death rate will decline even further. The screening of workers at high risk of lung cancer by means of serial chest films and sputum cytological examination offers a meretricious veneer of plausibility but has proved ineffective.[136]

Both epidemiological and experimental evidence indicates that dietary factors may modify the risks of lung cancer. For the most part, attention has been concentrated on vitamin A and carotenoids.[137] Additional studies are in progress. These are random trials designed to determine if the administration of beta-carotene or carotenoids reduces the risk of lung cancer. At the present juncture, it is impossible to give a definite answer.

CODA

The general acceptance of a number of agents as "probable" and "possible" carcinogens, e.g., PCBs, Agent Orange, silica, and so forth, is often a result of what has been termed the "Gold effect." This is named after Professor T. Gold who first described the phenomenon.[133] In most instances, when one or two persons have a preconceived notion that a particular agent is harmful and likely to be a carcinogen, they pass on this information to a physician or the media. This calls attention to the hypothesis and stimulates investigations. Some of these are poorly designed, and most yield equivocal or contradictory results but suffice to suggest a possible relationship between exposure to the agent concerned and the development of cancer.

Armed with the inconclusive and the indefinite, a few medical or scientific adherents of the hypothesis organize a meeting or symposium. Many of those who attend have a morbid desire to prove that everything is a carcinogen and represent the radical rump of those environmentalists who subscribe to the notion that all cancer is caused by occupational or environmental exposures. Unfortunately, the objective and disinterested eschew the meeting. Subsequently, the proceedings of the meeting are published with great fanfare, with prominence being given to those with the most tendentious views.

A clique or sect is then established to publicize the concept that a particular agent is a carcinogen. As a result, a host of gullible and usually young investigators who believe almost all they read are stimulated to carry out investigations of their own. In doing so, some, if not most, adopt and mimic the same flawed methods used by early workers and come to the same predictable but erroneous conclusions.

As more articles are published, the consensus undergoes transmogrification into an overwhelming majority. Meta-analyses are published purporting to show a conclusive association, but the authors forget that negative findings seldom appear in journals. The process is furthered by the failure of many physicians and scientists to voice their doubts publicly. Moreover, once the idea or concept has become accepted by "reputable" journals, it becomes almost impossible to eradicate. Orthodox conformity is the criterion by which most articles are accepted for publication, and few dare to oppose the tyranny of the majority. Moreover, what journal is interested in publishing negative results?

Now that the hypothesis has received the blessing of so-called informed opinion, the sect thereafter resorts to *ex cathedra* pronouncements. What began as a barely conceivable hypothesis in short order becomes generally accepted, rapidly progresses to established fact, and finally becomes an incontrovertible self-evident reality. Those with the courage to differ from the accepted norm are designated as "industry's eccentric reactionaries." Crass exaggeration, but very little removed from reality!

Finally, it must be borne in mind that, although great harm can be done by failing to diagnose a disease, equally great harm can be done by diagnosing disease when none exists. The same principle operates in the designation of carcinogens. Patients who have been told they have been exposed to a carcinogen and are likely to have cancer develop when this is not the case have been done a tremendous disservice. In this context, Thomas Huxley's apothegm reigns supreme, "Blind faith is the one unpardonable sin, skepticism the supreme virtue."

REFERENCES

1. Pott, P., Chirurgical Observations Relative to the Cataract, the Polypus of the Nose, the Cancer of the Scrotum, the Different Kind of Ruptures and the Mortification of the Toes and Feet. London, 1775.
2. Harting, E.F., and Hesse, W., Der Lungenkrebs, die Bergkrankheit in der Schneeburger Gruben. Vjschr. Gericht. Med., 31, 102, 1879.
3. Surgeon General, Reducing the Health Consequences of Smoking. Office of Smoking and Health, Rockville, MD, Department of Health and Human Services, 1989.
4. Shopland, D.R., Eyre, H.J., Pechacek, T.F., Smoking attributable cancer mortality in 1991. J. Natl. Cancer Inst., 83, 1142, 1991.
5. Editorial, What proportion of lung cancers are due to occupation? Lancet, 2, 1238, 1978.
6. Abelson, P.H., Cancer opportunism and opportunity. Science, 11, 206, 1979.
7. Morgan, W.K.C., Industrial carcinogens: the extent of the risk. Thorax, 34, 431, 1979.
8. Higgins, J., and Muir, C.S., Carcinogenesis: misconceptions and limitations to cancer control. J. Natl. Cancer Inst., 63, 1291, 1979.
9. Bridbord, K., Decoufle, P., Fraumeni, J., et al., Estimates of the fraction of cancer in the United States related to occupational factors. Report prepared by National Cancer Institute, National Institute of Environmental Health Sciences, National Institute for Occupational Safety and Health, Washington, D.C., Dept. Health, Education and Welfare, 1978.
10. Doll, R., and Peto, R., The causes of cancer. J. Natl. Cancer Inst., 66, 1197, 1981.

11. McLean, A.E.M., Diet and the chemical environment as modifiers of carcinogenesis. *In* Doll, R., and Vodopila, I., eds., Host Environmental Interactions in the Etiology of Cancer in Man. Lyon, International Agency for Research on Cancer, 1973, pp. 223–232.

12. Paterson, M.C., Environmental carcinogenesis and imperfect repair of DNA in *Homo sapiens. In* Griffin, A.C., and Shaw, C.R., eds., Carcinogenesis: Identification and Mechanisms of Action. New York, Raven Press, 1979, pp. 251–286.

13. Meselson, M., and Russell, K., Screening for carcinogens. *In* Hiatt, H.H., Watson, J.D., and Winston, J.A., eds., Origins of Human Cancer. New York, Cold Spring Harbor Laboratory, 1977, pp. 1473–1481.

14. Cairns, J., The origin of human cancers. Nature, 289, 353, 1981.

15. Ames, B.M., and Cooper, K., Does carcinogenic potency correlate with mutagenic potency in the Ames assay? Nature, 274, 19, 1978.

16. Bridges, J.W., and Fry, J.R., Mammalian short term tests for carcinogens. *In* Dayan, A.D., and Brimblecombe, R.W., eds., Carcinogenicity Testing, Principles, and Problems. Lancaster, UK, MTP Press, 1978, pp. 29–52.

17. Lambert, B., and Erikkson, G., Effects of chemotherapeutic agents on testicular DNA synthesis in the rat. Evaluation of a short term test for studies of chemicals and drugs in vivo. Mutat. Res., 68, 275, 1979.

18. Saracci, R., The IARC monograph program on the evaluation of the carcinogenic risk of chemicals to humans as a contributor to the identification of occupational carcinogens. *In* Peto, R., and Schneiderman, M., eds., Banbury Report 9. Quantification of Occupational Cancer. New York, Cold Spring Harbor Laboratory, 1981.

19. Hill, A.B., A Short Textbook of Medical Statistics. Sevenoaks, U.K., Hodder and Stoughton, 1977, pp. 285–296.

20. Reisner, M.T.R., Results of epidemiologic studies on the progression of coal workers' pneumoconiosis. Chest, 78(suppl.), 406, 1980.

21. Neuberger, H., and Kundi, M.I., Individual asbestos exposure, smoking, and mortality: a cohort study in the asbestos cement industry. Br. J. Ind. Med., 47, 615, 1990.

22. Ng, T.P., Chan, S.L., and Lee, J., Mortality of a cohort of men in a silicosis register: further evidence of an association with lung cancer. Am. J. Ind. Med., 17, 163, 1990.

23. Henry, S.A., Industrial Maladies. London, Legge, 1934.

24. Hill, A.B., and Fanning, E.L., Studies of the incidence of cancer in a factory handling inorganic compounds of arsenic. I. Mortality experience in the factor. Br. J. Ind. Med., 5, 1, 1948.

25. Perry, K., Bowler, R.G., Buckell, H.M., et al., Studies of the incidence of cancer in a factory handling inorganic compounds of arsenic. II. Clinical and environmental investigations. Br. J. Ind. Med., 5, 6, 1948.

26. Mabuchi, K., Lilienfeld, A.M., and Snell, L.M., Cancer and occupational exposure to arsenic: a study of pesticide workers. Prev. Med., 9, 51, 1980.

27. Oh, M.G., Holder, B.B., and Gordeon, H.L., Respiratory cancer and occupational exposure to arsenic. Arch. Environ. Health, 29, 250, 1974.

28. Roth, F., Late consequences of chronic arsenicism in Moselle vine dressers. Dtsch. Med. Wochenschr., 82, 211, 1957.

29. Roth, F., Arsenic liver tumors (haemangioendothelioma). Z. Krebsforsch, 61, 468, 1975.

30. Pinto, S.S., and Bennetter, B.M., Effect of arsenic trioxide exposure on mortality. Arch. Environ. Health, 7, 583, 1963.

31. Milham, S., Jr., and Stron, T., Human arsenic exposure in relation to a copper smelter. Environ. Res., 7, 172, 1974.

32. Lee, A.M., and Fraumeni, J.H., Jr., Arsenic and respiratory cancer in man: an occupational study. J. Natl. Cancer Inst., 42, 1045, 1969.

33. Kuratsune, M., Tokundime, S., Shirakusa, T., et al., Occupational lung cancer among copper smelters. Int. J. Cancer, 13, 552, 1974.

34. Lee-Feldstein, A., Cumulative exposure to arsenic and its relationship to respiratory cancer among copper smelter employees. J. Occup. Med., 28, 296, 1986.

35. Welch, K., Higgins, I., Oh, M., and Burchfield, C., Arsenic exposure, smoking, and respiratory cancer in copper smelter workers. Arch. Environ. Health, 37, 325, 1982.

36. Enterline, P.E., and Marsh, G.M., Mortality studies of smelter workers. Am. J. Ind. Med., 1, 251, 1980.

37. Enterline, P.E., and Marsh, G.M., Cancer among workers exposed to arsenic and other substances in a copper smelter. Am. J. Epidemiol., 116, 895, 1982.

38. Wall, S., Survival and mortality patterns among Swedish smelter workers. Int. J. Epidemiol., 9, 73, 1980.

39. Nelson, N., Carcinogenicity of halo ethers. N. Engl. J. Med., 288, 1123, 1973.

40. Figueroa, W.G., Razzkowski, R., and Weiss, W., Lung cancer in chloromethyl ether workers. N. Engl. J. Med., 288, 1096, 1973.

41. Lemen, R.A., Johnson, W.M., Wagoner, J.K., et al., Cytologic observations and cancer incidence following exposure to BCME. Ann. N. Y. Acad. Sci., 271, 71, 1976.

42. Gafafar, W.M., Reese, W.H., and Rutter, H.A., Induction of lung adenomas in newborn mice by bis (chloromethyl) ether. Toxic Appl. Pharmacol., 15, 92, 1969.

43. Laskin, S., Drew, R.T., Cappielo, V.P., et al., Inhalation carcinogeneicity of alpha halo-ethers. *In*

British Occupational Hygiene Society, Walton, W.H., ed., Inhaled Particles III. Old Woking, Surrey, U.K., Unwin Bros. Ltd., 1971.

44. Laskin, S., Kuschner, J., Drew, R.T., et al., Tumors of the respiratory tract induced by inhalation of bis (chloromethyl) ether. Arch. Environ. Health, 23, 135, 1971.

45. Theiss, A.M., Hay, W., and Zeller, H., Zur Toxikologie von Dischlorodimethylather-Verdacht, auf kanzerogene Wirking auch bein Menschen. Zentralbl. Arbeitsmed., 23, 97, 1973.

46. Sakabe, H., Lung cancer due to exposure to bis (chloromethyl) ether. Ind. Health, 11, 145, 1973.

47. Weiss, W., Moser, R.L., and Auerbach, O., Lung cancer in chloromethyl ether workers. Am. Rev. Respir. Dis., 120, 1031, 1979.

48. Weiss, W., Epidemic curve of respiratory cancer due to chloromethyl ethers. J. Natl. Cancer Inst., 69, 1265, 1982.

49. Weiss, W., Lung cancer due to chloromethyl ethers: bias in cohort definitions. J. Occup. Med., 31, 102, 1989.

50. Saccamano, G., Archer, V.E., Auerbach, O., et al., Histologic types of lung cancer among uranium miners. Cancer, 275, 15, 1971.

51. Yamanda, A., On late injuries following occupational inhalation of mustard gas with special reference to carcinoma of the respiratory tract. Acta Pathol. Jpn., 13, 131, 1963.

52. Doll, R., Vessey, M.P., Beasley, R.W.R., et al., Mortality of gas workers—final report of a prospective study. Br. J. Ind. Med., 29, 394, 1972.

53. Kennaway, E.L., and Kennaway, N.M., A further study of the incidence of cancer of the lung and larynx. Br. J. Cancer, 1, 260, 1947.

54. Lloyd, J.W., Long term mortality of steelworkers. Respiratory cancer in coke plant workers in Britain. Am. J. Ind. Med., 4, 691, 1983.

55. Hurley, J.F., Archibald, R.M., Collings, P.L., et al., The mortality of coke workers in Britain. Am. J. Ind. Med., 4, 691, 1983.

56. Redmond, C.K., Cancer mortality among coke oven workers. Environ. Health Perspect., 52, 67, 1983.

57. Rockette, H.E., and Redmond, C.K., Selection, follow-up, and analysis in the coke oven study. Natl. Cancer Inst. Monograph, 67, 89, 1985.

58. Alwens, W., and Jonas, W., Chromat-Lungen Krebs. Acta Unio Internationalis Contra Cancrum, 3, 103, 1938.

59. Machle, W., and Gregorius, F., Cancer of the respiratory system in the United States chromate producing industry. Public Health Rep., 63, 1114, 1948.

60. Baetjer, A.M., Pulmonary carcinoma in chromate workers. I. A review of the literature and report of cases. Arch. Ind. Hyg. Occup. Med., 2, 485, 1950.

61. Mancuso, T.F., and Hueper, W.C., Occupational cancer and other health hazards in a chromate plant: a medical appraisal. I. Lung cancers in chromate workers. Ind. Med. Surg., 20, 358, 1951.

62. Enterline, P.E., Respiratory cancer among chromate workers. J. Occup. Med., 16, 523, 1974.

63. Tsuneta, Y., Ohsaki, Y., Kimura, K., et al., Chromium content of lungs of chromate workers with lung cancer. Thorax, 35, 294, 1980.

64. Kishi, R., Tamuri, T., Uchino, E., et al., Chromium content of organs of chromate workers with lung cancer. Am. J. Ind. Med., 11, 67, 1987.

65. Sorahan, T., Burges, D.C.L., and Waterhouse, J.A.H., A mortality study of nickel chromium workers. Br. J. Ind. Med., 44, 803, 1987.

66. Coultas, D.B., and Samet, J.M., Occupational lung cancer. Clin. Chest Dis., 13, 341, 1992.

67. Chief Inspector of Factories, Annual Report of the Chief Inspector of Factories for the Year 1932. London, H.M. Stationery Office, 1933, p. 103.

68. Chief Inspector of Factories, Annual Report of the Chief Inspector of Factories for the Year 1950. London, H.M. Stationery Office, 1952, p. 145.

69. Doll, R., Morgan, L.G., and Speizer, F.E., Cancers of the lung and nasal sinuses in nickel workers. Br. J. Cancer, 24, 623, 1970.

70. Committee of Medical and Biologic Effects of Environmental Pollutants (CMBEFEP), Nickel. Washington, D.C., National Academy of Sciences, 1975.

71. Mastromatteo, E., Nickel: a review of its occupational health aspects. J. Occup. Med., 9, 127, 1967.

72. Virtue, J.A., The relationship between the refining of nickel and cancer of the nasal cavity. Can. J. Otolaryngol., 1, 37, 1972.

73. Pederson, L.E., Hogetveit, A.C., and Anderson, A., Cancer of respiratory organs among workers at a nickel refinery in Norway. Int. J. Cancer, 12, 32, 1973.

74. Konetzke, G.W., Berufiche Krebserkrankungen durch Arsen and Nickel sowei deren Verbindugen. Dtsch. Ges. Wesen., 29, 1334, 1974.

75. Sakyn, A.V., and Shabynina, N.K., Epidemiology of malignant neoplasms at nickel smelters. Gig. Tr. Prof. Zabol., 17, 25, 1973.

76. Tatarskaya, A.A., Cancer of the respiratory tract in people engaged in the nickel industry. Vopr. Onkol., 123, 58, 1967.

77. Tatarskaya, A.A., Occupational cancer of upper respiratory passages in the nickel industry. Gig. Tr. Prof. Zabol., 9, 22, 1965.

78. Kreyberg, L., Lung cancer in workers in a nickel refinery. Br. J. Ind. Med., 35, 109, 1978.

79. Loken, A.C., Lung cancer in nickel workers. Tidsskr. Nor. Laegeforen., 70, 376, 1950.

80. Bernacki, E.J., Parsons, G.E., and Sunderman, F.W., Jr., Investigation of exposure to nickel and

lung cancer mortality. Case control study at aircraft engine factory. Am. J. Clin. Lab. Sci., 8, 190, 1978.

81. Report of the International Committee on Nickel Carcinogenesis in Man. Scand. J. Work Environ. Health, 6, 1, 1990.

82. Beebe, G.W., Lung cancer in World War I veterans: possible relation to mustard gas injury and 1918 influenza epidemic. J. Natl. Cancer Inst., 25, 1231, 1960.

83. Case, R.A.M., and Lea, A.J., Mustard gas poisoning, chronic bronchitis, and lung cancer. Br. J. Prev. Soc. Med., 9, 62, 1955.

84. Wada, S., Miyanishi, M., Nishimoto, Y., et al., Mustard gas as a cause of respiratory neoplasia in man. Lancet, 1, 1161, 1968.

85. Manning, K.P., Skegg, D.C.G., Stell, P.M., and Doll, R., Cancer of the larynx and other occupational hazards of mustard gas workers. Clin. Otolaryngol., 6, 165, 1981.

86. deVillicrs, A.J., and Windish, J.P., Lung cancer in a fluorspar mining community. I. Radiation, dust, and mortality experience. Br. J. Ind. Med., 21, 94, 1964.

87. Agricola, A.C., De Re Metallica. 1557. Translated by Hoover, H.C., and Hoover, L.C. New York, Dover Publications, 1950.

88. Arnstein, A., Sozialhygienische Untersuchungen uber die Bengleute in den Schneeberger Kobalt-Gruben, insbesodere uber des Borkommen des sogenannten "Schneeberger Lungenkrebses" Osterreich Sanitatswesen Wien Arbeit., a.d. Geb. I. Soz. Med. Beihefte, 5, 64, 1913.

89. Pichan, A., and Sill, H., Cancer of the lung in the miners of Jachymov. Am. J. Cancer, 16, 681, 1932.

90. Boyd, J.T., Doll, R., Faulds, J.S., et al., Cancer of the lung in iron ore (haematite) workers. Br. J. Ind. Med., 27, 97, 1970.

91. Lundin, F.E., Lloyd, J.W., Smith, E.M., et al., Mortality of uranium miners in relation to radiation exposure, hard rock mining, and cigarette smoking—1950 through September 1967. Health Phys., 16, 571, 1969.

92. Saccomanno, G., Archer, V.E., Auerbach, O., et al., Histologic types of lung cancer among uranium miners. Cancer, 27, 515, 1971.

93. Chovil, A., The epidemiology of primary lung cancer in uranium miners in Ontario. J. Occup. Med., 23, 417, 1981.

94. Archer, V.E., Wagoner, J.K., and Lundin, F.E., Uranium mining and cigarette smoking effects on man. J. Occup. Med., 15, 204, 1973.

95. Archer, V.E., Health concerns in uranium mining and milling. J. Occup. Med., 23, 502, 1981.

96. Saccomanno, G., Saunders, R.P., Archer, V.E., et al., Cancer of the lung: the cytology of sputum prior to the development of carcinoma. Acta Cytol., 9, 413, 1965.

97. Trapp, E., Renzetti, A.D., Kobayashi, T., et al., Cardiopulmonary function in uranium miners. Am. Rev. Respir. Dis., 101, 27, 1970.

98. Archer, V.E., Wagoner, J.K., and Lundin, F.E., Cancer mortality among uranium mill workers. J. Occup. Med., 15, 11, 1973.

99. Polednak, A.P., and Frome, E.L., Mortality among men employed between 1943 and 1947 at an uranium processing plant. J. Occup. Med., 23, 169, 1981.

100. Cronin, A.J., Dust inhalation by haematite miners. J. Ind. Hyg., 8, 291, 1926.

101. Faulds, J.S., and Stewart, M.J., Carcinoma of the lung in hematite miners. J. Pathol. Bacteriol., 72, 353, 1956.

102. Duggan, M.J., Soilleux, P.J., Strong, J.C., and Howell, D.M., The exposure of United Kingdom miners to radon. Br. J. Ind. Med., 27, 106, 1970.

103. Archer, V.E., Lung cancer among populations having lung irradiation. Lancet, 2, 1261, 1971.

104. Wagoner, J.K., Miller, R.W., Lundin, F.E., et al., Unusual cancer mortality amongst a group of underground metal miners. N. Engl. J. Med., 269, 706, 1963.

105. Axelson, O., and Rehn, M., Lung cancer in miners. Lancet, 2, 706, 1971.

106. Fox, A.J., Goldblatt, P., and Kinlen, L.J., A study of the mortality of Cornish tin miners. Br. J. Ind. Med., 38, 378, 1981.

107. Reger, R.B., and Morgan, W.K.C., On talc, tremolite, and tergiversation. Br. J. Ind. Med., 47, 505, 1990.

108. International Agency for Research on Cancer, IARC Monograph of the Evaluation of the Carcinogenic Risk of Chemicals to Humans, Vol. 42. Lyon, International Agency for Research on Cancer, 1987.

109. Weil, C.S., Smyth, H.F., and Nale, T.W., Quest for suspected industrial carcinogen. Arch. Ind. Hyg., 5, 535, 1952.

110. Ask-Upmark, E., Bronchial carcinoma in printing workers. Dis. Chest, 27, 427, 1955.

111. Moss, E., Scott, T.S., and Atherley, G.R.C., Mortality of newspaper workers from lung cancer and bronchitis 1952–66. Br. J. Ind. Med., 29, 1, 1972.

112. Egan-Braum, E., Miller, B.A., and Waxweiler, R.J., Lung cancer and other mortality patterns among foundrymen. Scand. J. Work Environ. Health, 7(suppl.), 147, 1981.

113. Buffler, P.A., Wood, S., Eifler, C., et al., Mortality experience of workers in a vinyl chloride monomer production plant. J. Occup. Med., 21, 195, 1979.

114. Theriault, G., and Allard, P., Cancer mortality of a group of Canadian workers exposed to vinyl chloride monomer. J. Occup. Med., 23, 671, 1981.

115. Heldacs, S.S., Langard, S.L., and Andersen, A., Incidence of cancer among vinyl chloride and polyvinyl chloride workers. Br. J. Ind. Med., 41, 25, 1984.

116. Mancuso, T.F., Relation of duration of employment and prior respiratory illness to respiratory cancer among beryllium workers. Environ. Res., 3, 251, 1970.
117. Mancuso, T.F., Mortality study of beryllium industry workers' occupational lung cancer. Environ. Res., 21, 48, 1980.
118. Infante, P.F., Wagoner, J.K., and Sprince, N.L., Mortality patterns from lung cancer and nonneoplastic respiratory disease among white males in the Beryllium Case Registry. Environ. Res., 21, 25, 1980.
119. Round the World Column. The beryllium dispute. Lancet, 1, 202, 1978.
120. MacMahon, B., The epidemiological evidence on the carcinogenicity of beryllium in humans. J. Occup. Med., 36, 15, 1994.
121. Konstantinov, F.G., and Kuzminykh, A.I., Tarry substances and 3,4-benzopyrene in the air of electrolytic shops of aluminum works and their carcinogenic significance. Hyg. Sanit., 36, 368, 1971.
122. Litvinov, N.W., Goldberg, M.S., and Kimina, S.N., Morbidity and mortality in man caused by pulmonary cancer and its relation to the pollution of the atmosphere in the areas of aluminum plants. Acta Unionis Internationalis Contra Cancrum, 19, 742, 1963.
123. Gibbs, G.W., Mortality Experience in Eastern Canada. I. In Hughes, J.P., ed., Health Protection in Aluminium Production, Vol. 2. London, International Primary Aluminium Institute, Haymarket, 1981.
124. Acheson, E.C., Cowdell, R.H., and Rang, E., Adenocarcinoma of the nasal cavity and sinuses in England and Wales. Br. J. Ind. Med., 29, 1, 1972.
125. O'Berg, M.T., Epidemiologic study of workers exposed to acrylonitrile. J. Occup. Med., 22, 245, 1980.
126. O'Berg, M.T., Chen, J.L., Burke, C.A., et al., Epidemiologic study of workers exposed to acrylonitrile. An update. J. Occup. Med., 27, 835, 1985.
127. Werner, J.B., and Carter, J.T., Mortality of United Kingdom acrylonitrile polymerisation workers. Br. J. Ind. Med., 38, 247, 1981.
128. Blair, A., Stewart, P., and O'Berg, M., Morbidity among industrial workers exposed to formaldehyde. J. Natl. Cancer Inst., 76, 1071, 1986.
129. Sterling, J.B., and Weinkam, J.J., Reanalysis of lung cancer mortality in a National Cancer Institute study on mortality among industrial workers exposed to formaldehyde. J. Occup. Med., 30, 895, 1988.
130. International Agency for Research on Cancer, IARC Monograph on the Evaluation of the Carcinogenic Risk of Chemicals to Humans. Allyl Compounds, Aldehydes, Epoxides, and Peroxides, Vol. 36. Lyon, International Agency for Research on Cancer, 1985.
131. International Agency for Research on Cancer, IARC Monograph on the Evaluation of Carcinogenic Risk in Humans. Manmade Mineral Fibers and Radon, Vol. 3. Lyon, International Agency for Research on Cancer, 1988.
132. Hnizdo, E., and Sluis-Cremer, G.K., Silica exposure, silicosis, and lung cancer: a mortality study of South African gold miners. Br. J. Ind. Med., 48, 53, 1991.
133. Lyttleton, R.A., The Gold effect. In Duncan, R., Weston-Smith, M., eds., Lying Truths: A Critical Scrutiny of Current Beliefs and Conventions. Oxford, Pergamon Press, 1979, pp. 182–198.
134. Reger, R.B., and Morgan, W.K.C., Silica: is it a carcinogen? J. Occup. Health Safety Aust. N. Z., 6, 481, 1990.
135. McDonald, J.C., Silica, silicosis, and lung cancer. Br. J. Ind. Med., 46, 289, 1989.
136. U.S. Preventive Services Task Force Screen for Lung Cancer and Guide to Clinical Preventive Services, An Assessment of the Effectiveness of 169 Interventions. Baltimore, Williams and Wilkins, 1989, p. 67.
137. Zegler, R.G., A review of epidemiologic evidence that carotenoids reduce the risk of cancer. J. Nutr., 119, 116, 1989.

Index

Note: Page numbers in *italics* refer to illustrations; page numbers followed by t refer to tables.

A

(A-a)O₂ (alveoloarterial oxygen gradient), 54, 54t
  measurement of, for assessment of disability, 74–75, *75*
  use of, in epidemiological studies, 96
Abietic acid, chemical formula of, *477*
Abrasive(s), aluminum-containing, effects of, 416
Absolute risk, assessment of, 87
Acceptable risk, assessment of, 87
Accident(s), during diving, 607–608, *608*, 608t
Accuracy, of epidemiological studies, 89, *90*
ACGIH (American Conference of Governmental Industrial Hygienists), respirable fraction curve of, *161*
  standard on inhalability of aerosols of, 159
Acid anhydride(s), chemical formula of, *476*
  toxicity of, 587–588, *589*
Acid-base balance, 59–61
Acrolein, toxicity of, 570t
Acrylonitrile, exposure to, and lung cancer, 636
  toxicity of, 570t, 573–575
Acute nonbyssinotic respiratory disease, 498–499
Adenopathy, hilar, with chronic berylliosis, *423*
Adhesion molecule(s), in alveolocapillary unit, 207–208
Aerodynamic diameter (d$_{ae}$), of particles, 159, *159*
Aerosol(s), alveolar, measurement of, criteria for, 160–161, *161*
  coarse, measurement of, *166–169*, 166–170
    criteria for, 158–159, *159*
  definition of, 112
  fibrous, measurement of, criteria for, 161
  fine, measurement of, criteria for, 160–161, *160–161*
  in humidifiers, 560
  inhalability fraction of, 158–159, *159*, 162–163
    measurement of, with static sampler, 167, *167*
  measurement of, 158–180
    critique of, 162
    for multiple fractions, 174, *174–175*
    instruments for, commercial availability of, 180, 180t
      direct reading, 178–179
    sampling probes for, accuracy of, 164–165, *165*
    sampling system components for, 176–178
    scientific aspects of, 164–166, *165*
    spectrometers for, 174–176, *176–177*
    standards for, 162–163
    strategies for, 163–164
  respirable fraction of, 160–161, *161*, 163
    measurement of, 170–173, *170–173*
  thoracic, measurement of, 173
    criteria for, 160, *160*, 163
  tracheobronchial, measurement of, criteria for, 160–161, *160–161*
Age, and alveoloarterial oxygen gradient, *75*

Age *(Continued)*
  and degree of impairment, 71
  and maximal oxygen consumption, *67*
  and reference values from pulmonary function testing, 97–99, *98*
  and risk of allergic alveolitis, 528
Agricola, 2, 222
Agricultural worker(s), inhalation disease in, 559t
Air, asbestos in, measurement of, 314–315
Air embolism, cerebral, with pulmonary barotrauma, 602
Air flow, laminar, 40
  resistance to, with use of respirator, 186–187
  turbulent, 40
  type of, and dust deposition, 113
Air leak(s), in respirators, prevention of, 184
Air-purifying respirator(s), 182–183
Airway(s), anatomical differences in, and deposition of dust, 114
  pathological reactions to dust in, 127t
Airway(s) obstruction, dust exposure and, 507–509, *510*
  forced expiratory volume in, 39, *39*
  from hard metal disease, 442–443, 447
  residual volume/total lung capacity percentage in, *37*, 37–38
  reversibility of, pulmonary function testing for, 99–100
  vital capacity in, *37*
Airway(s) resistance (Raw), 40–41, *41*
Allergic alveolitis, 123–124, 133, 525–548
  bacterial, 526t
  caused by animals, 526t, 554–557
  caused by birds, 526t, 554–556, *555*
  centrilobular distribution of, 535, *536*
  challenge testing for, 544–545, *546–547*
  chemical, 526t, 557–558
  clinical features of, 526–528, *527*
  diagnosis of, 543
  epidemiology of, 525–526, 526t
  examination for, 544
  extrinsic, 123–124
    from dust exposure, 133
  from hard metal disease, 442–443
  from Pauli's reagent, before challenge testing, 545, *546*
  fungal, 526t, 548–554
  history in, 543
  immunological findings in, 544
  isocyanide, 526t, 557
  lung biopsy for, 545
  pathogenesis of, 538, 541–543
  pathological findings in, 535, *536–537*, 538, *539–542*
  pulmonary function in, 533, 535, 535t
    testing of, 544
  radiographic features of, 528, *529–534*, 533, 544

643

ISBN 0-7216-4671-9

90038

9 780721 646718